CARDIOLOGY
1997

James T. Willerson, MD

William C. Roberts, MD

Charles E. Rackley, MD

Thomas P. Graham, Jr., MD

Dean T. Mason, MD

William W. Parmley, MD

Copyright © 1997
Futura Publishing Company, Inc.

Published by
Futura Publishing Company, Inc.
135 Bedford Road
Armonk, New York 10504

ISBN #: 0-87993-677-0
ISSN #: 0275-0066

Printed in the United States of America.

ⓧ Printed on acid-free paper.

Cardiology
1997

JAMES T. WILLERSON, MD
Edward Randall III Professor and Chairman
Department of Internal Medicine
The University of Texas—Houston Medical School
Chief of Medical Service
Hermann Hospital
Medical Director, Chief of Cardiology,
and Director of Cardiology Research
Texas Heart Institute
Houston, Texas
Editor in Chief, Circulation

William C. Roberts, MD
Executive Director
Baylor Cardiovascular Institute
Dean, A. Webb Roberts Center
for Continuing Education
Baylor University Medical Center
Dallas, Texas
Editor in Chief, The American Journal
of Cardiology
Editor in Chief, The Baylor University
Medical Center Proceedings

Charles E. Rackley, MD
Professor of Medicine
Division of Cardiology
Department of Medicine
Georgetown University Medical Center
Washington, D.C.

Thomas P. Graham, Jr., MD
Professor of Pediatrics
Director of Pediatric Cardiology
Vanderbilt University Medical Center
Nashville, Tennessee

Dean T. Mason, MD
Physician in Chief, Western Heart Institute
Chairman, Department of
Cardiovascular Medicine
St. Mary's Medical Center
at Golden Gate Park, San Francisco
San Francisco, California

William W. Parmley, MD
Professor of Medicine
University of California
San Francisco, School of Medicine
San Francisco, California
Editor in Chief, Journal of the
American College of Cardiology

**Futura Publishing
Company, Inc.**
Armonk, NY

Preface

Cardiology 1997, the 17th volume to be published in this series, is a compilation of more than 700 summaries highlighting the major emphases in the cardiologic literature of 1996. This book is intended to serve as an overview of the current trends in basic and clinical research and in clinical applications both for adult and pediatric cardiology.

Research in the area of atherosclerosis continues to focus on the mechanisms involved in atherogenesis, with emphasis in recent years on the role of platelets, platelet products, and growth factors. More insights have also been gained regarding the characteristics of unstable plaque. In addition to plaque erosion, which leads to platelet aggregation, thrombosis, and vasoconstriction, vulnerable plaques have been found to have temperature heterogeneity. To detect this heterogeneity, researchers have developed a method of infrared imaging. If vulnerable areas of plaque can be identified at the time of arteriography, it may become possible to aim treatment at these specific sites, thus preventing the cascade of events leading to myocardial infarction or stroke.

The role of lipids in atherogenesis and the effects of lipid-lowering agents in many patient subgroups are also being refined. In a 5-year study in which pravastatin lowered the rate of coronary events, the investigators concluded that the benefits of cholesterol-lowering therapy extend to many patients with coronary disease who have more average serum cholesterol and low-density lipoprotein (LDL) values. In addition, combination therapy has been effective in several clinical trials, including the Regression Statin Study Trial (REGRESS) wherein calcium channel blockers plus pravastatin may have acted additionally to retard the progression of established coronary atherosclerosis.

Promising treatment has also been shown for patients with unstable angina. Several studies have tested the effects of platelet inhibitors of platelet glycoprotein IIb/IIIa receptors. In a Canadian trial that evaluated the effect of lamifiban, a nonpeptide platelet glycoprotein IIb/IIIa antagonist, the incidence of death and acute myocardial infarction at 1 month was reduced in patients with unstable angina. These patients were also protected from severe ischemic events during the infusion period (3 to 5 days). In a randomized multicenter trial, integrelin was shown to reduce the number and duration of Holter ischemic events in patients with unstable angina.

Platelet glycoprotein IIb/IIIa receptor blockade has also been effective in improving outcomes in patients undergoing direct and rescue percutaneous transluminal coronary angioplasty (PTCA). In the Evaluation of c7E3 for Prevention of Ischemic Complications (EPIC) trial, chimeric 7E3 Fab (c7E3) therapy resulted in a decreased incidence of acute ischemic events and possibly of clinical restenosis after PTCA.

Coronary stenting also has the potential to improve results after PTCA by reducing the rate of restenosis to 12% to 25%; however, data on the long-term outcomes of stent implantation are not yet available. Newer heparin-coated stents, used in conjunction with antiplatelet drugs, appear to have eliminated the need for anticoagulant therapy. This concept of stent management was tested in the BENESTENT-II Pilot Study. No thrombosis occurred during any of the study's 4 phases, and the overall clinical success rate at discharge was 99%. The restenosis rate overall was 13%, and a favorable event-free survival was shown after 6 months.

Many pharmacological agents have been tested in efforts to combat congestive heart failure (CHF). The one most emphasized in clinical trials in the past year was carvedilol, a third-generation β-blocking agent with vasodilator properties. At therapeutic doses, carvedilol blocks all 3 adrenergic receptors that mediate a positive inotropic response in human cardiac myocytes. Investigators in the PRECISE trial examined carvedilol's effect on 2 groups of patients: those with mild symptoms and those with moderate-to-severe heart failure. When carvedilol was used with standard therapy including an angiotensin-converting enzyme (ACE) inhibitor, there was a reduction in clinical progression of CHF in patients who were mildly symptomatic. Carvedilol also produced important clinical benefits, including better survival, in those patients with moderate-to-severe CHF who were treated with digoxin, diuretics, and an ACE inhibitor. In a multicenter, placebo-controlled trial, carvedilol was the first β-blocking agent to show a significant decreased mortality in patients with CHF. When 3 groups in the study were combined, the all-cause mortality risk was lowered by 73% in the carvedilol-treated subjects.

Pharmacological trials are ongoing to test the efficacy of various drug therapies for other types of chronic conditions affecting the heart. In the treatment of pulmonary hypertension, for example, short-term infusion of prostacyclin resulted in better prognoses in patients who had a decrease in total pulmonary vascular resistance of more than 50%. In another study, patients with severe pulmonary hypertension who were given epoprostenol, a form of prostacyclin, also showed symptomatic and hemodynamic improvement and had improved survival rates when compared with patients who did not take epoprostenol.

In the subspecialty of pediatric cardiology, surgical techniques for correcting congenital heart defects continue to be refined, offering hope for survival and good quality of life to many young patients. In children, cardiomyopathy, for which there is little surgical treatment, remains a leading cardiac cause of death. One group of researchers described differential diagnoses for genetic conditions. They classified these conditions as inborn errors of metabolism, malformation syndromes, neuromuscular disorders, and familial isolated cardiomyopathy disorders. This type of approach should hasten the day when genetic testing and treatment for some rare cardiomyopathic conditions will be possible.

The preceding are only a few of the many recent developments in cardiology that are described in this text. Because we could only summarize these developments, we have included references citing the full-length articles at the end of each chapter. This series is intended to keep anyone involved in the treatment of patients with cardiovascular disease aware of continuing developments is this rapidly changing field of medicine. We hope you will find this book useful.

Acknowledgments

The contributors of *Cardiology 1997* spent many hours gleaning the most recent developments from the literature to create this volume of current, important trends in the field of cardiology. Dr. Robert's articles were chosen from *The American Journal of Cardiology;* Dr. Rackley's were from *Arteriosclerosis, Thrombosis, and Vascular Biology;* and Dr. Parmley's were from the *Journal of the American College of Cardiology.* Dr. Graham's selections for the pediatric section were taken from a variety of medical journals. My summaries were from *Circulation* and several general medical journals, including *The New England Journal of Medicine, The Lancet,* and the *Annals of Internal Medicine.*

In addition to the painstaking task of selection, several individuals also assisted in preparing these summaries for publication. We are grateful to Rebecca Teaff and Suzy Lanier for editorial assistance and to Leslie Flatt, Marie Young, Linda B. Maddox, Joy Phillips, Barbara Capps, and Angie Esquivel for typing the summaries in this volume. We also are grateful to Ann Kerr of Futura Publishing Company for editorial coordination of this project.

We owe many thanks to Dr. William C. Roberts for serving as editor of this volume for the past 16 years. I am particularly grateful for his encouragement and direction in this transition of editorship. Finally, I would like to thank Futura Publishing Company for continuing their tradition of excellence in bringing this book to the medical community.

James T. Willerson, MD

Contents

Cardiology
1997

Conversion of Units

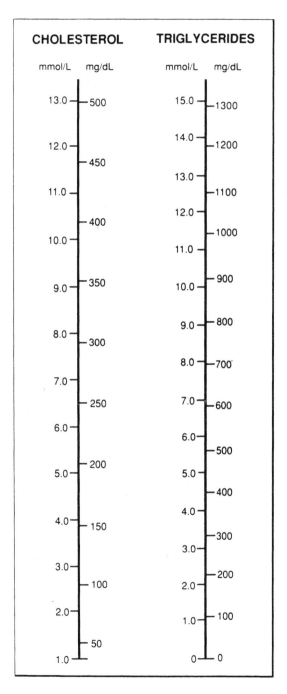

Cholesterol mg/dL = mmol/L x 38.6
Triglyceride mg/dL = mmol/L x 88.5

1

Atherosclerosis

Biology of Atherosclerotic Plaques

Lesion Morphology

Increasing evidence suggests that complement activation might represent an important mechanism in early atherogenesis. Thus, complement components, in particular the membrane attack complex, have been isolated from human atherosclerotic lesions. Furthermore, complement activation is known to occur in atherosclerotic lesions induced in experimental animals, and the severity of cholesterol-induced plaques is markedly reduced in complement-deficient animals. During atherogenesis, monocytes are recruited into the arterial wall, and a potent chemoattractant for monocytes, monocyte chemotactic protein-1, is expressed by vascular smooth muscle cells. Torzewski and coworkers[1] in Cambridge, United Kingdom, hypothesized that the generation of membrane attack complexes on smooth muscle cells during the activation of complement might lead to the release of monocyte chemotactic protein-1 and hence to monocyte recruitment. In this study, membrane attack complexes were generated on human smooth muscle cells *in vitro* by sequential addition of the purified complement components C5b6, C7, C8, and C9. The supernatant of the culture was chemotactic for freshly isolated peripheral blood monocytes in a modified Boyden chamber. The chemotactic activity of the supernatant was abolished by antimonocytes chemotactic protein-1 blocking antibodies, but not by an isotype-matched antibody against an irrelevant antigen. The release of chemotactic activity was dependent on the dose of membrane attack complexes formed on smooth muscle cells and was demonstrated within 10 minutes of exposure of the cells. The data supported the hypothesis that complement-mediated release of monocyte chemotactic protein-1 from smooth muscle cells might be important in the recruitment of monocytes into the developing atherosclerotic lesion and could be an important initiating event in atherogenesis.

Chemotaxis/Inflammatory Atherogenesis

Interleukin-8 is a chemotactic peptide produced by macrophages that may be involved in the recruitment of inflammatory cells into atherosclerotic plaque. Apostolopoulos and coinvestigators[2] in Victoria, Australia, studied *in vitro* interleukin-8 production by macrophages isolated from carotid plaques and noncarotid plaques from the same patients. Interleukin-8 produced by atherosclerotic macrophages was demonstrated to be biologically active in a neutrophil chemotaxis assay. Interleukin-8 messenger RNA (mRNA) was detectable in plaque macrophages and blood monocytes from these patients, but blood monocytes from normal donors did not exhibit detectable interleukin-8 mRNA. Interleukin-8 mRNA was localized in macrophage-rich areas of atherosclerotic plaques by *in situ* hybridization. These studies demonstrated that macrophages from atherosclerotic plaques showed an enhanced capacity to produce interleukin-8 compared with normal and patient blood monocytes, and that macrophages are a major site of interleukin-8 mRNA production in atherosclerotic plaque. These results provided further evidence for a pro-inflammatory role for macrophages in atherosclerosis.

Wang and coinvestigators[3] in Wilmington, Delaware, investigated the gene expression and enzyme kinetics of acyl coenzyme A:cholesterol acyltransferase in human monocytes, macrophages, and foam cells. Northern blot analysis, in which a coding region of human acyl cholesterol transferase cDNA was used as the probe, showed that each of the cell types exhibited 4 mRNA transcripts. The levels of the 4.2 and 3.7 kb acyl cholesterol transferase transcripts were 3- and 6-fold higher, respectively, in macrophages than in monocytes. These transcripts were expressed at the same high levels after conversion of macrophages to foam cells. In contrast, the 6.3 and 4.4 kb transcripts for the acyl cholesterol transferase were expressed at a relatively constant level in all 3 cell types. The expression of mRNA for glyceraldehyde phosphate dehydrogenase, the control gene in this study, was also expressed at a constant level in each of the cell types. The increase in acyl cholesterol transferase mRNA was accompanied by changes in the kinetic properties of the enzyme. Although not definitive, the concomitant changes in mRNA and the $\dot{V}_{max}$ strongly suggested that the amount of acyl cholesterol transferase protein increased on conversion of monocytes to macrophages. These data showed that acyl coenzyme A:cholesterol acyl transferase in monocytes can be regulated by both substrate and gene expression.

LDL-Mediated Monocyte Chemotaxis

Monocyte migration into the vessel wall is an early step in atherogenesis. Even though a number of chemotactic factors have been identified, the regulation of the chemotactic response is not clearly understood. As a release of arachidonic acid has been implicated in monocyte chemotaxis, Kreuzer and coworkers[4] in Heidelberg, Germany, studied the influence of low-density lipoprotein (LDL), which can supply this fatty acid to cells, on the chemotactic mobility of monocytes. Migration of human monocytes U937 cells was abolished by a 30-hour incubation in medium containing lipoprotein-depleted 10% fetal calf serum. Thereafter, human very low-density lipoprotein (VLDL), LDL, acetyl LDL, methyl LDL, high-density lipoprotein (HDL), free cholesterol, linoleic acid, oleic acid, or arachidonic acid was added. At the end of varying incubation periods (0.5–8 hours), chemotaxis, viability, and cellular cholesterol content were measured. In the same experimental setting, the investigators also studied the effects of the pharmacological agents chloroquine, indomethacin, and acetyl salicylic acid on LDL-mediated chemotaxis. Chemotaxis was restored by LDL in a dose- and time-dependent manner, beginning at concentrations as low as 5 μg/mL and in incubations as brief as 30 minutes. The other lipoproteins tested (VLDL, HDL, acetyl LDL, and methyl LDL, as well as free cholesterol) had no comparable effect on chemotaxis. Viability and total cholesterol content did not differ among the groups. Simultaneous incubation of cells with chloroquine, indomethacin, and acetyl salicylic acid reduced restitution of chemotaxis by LDL by 71%, 82%, and 68%, respectively. In contrast, the agents had only slight inhibitory effects on the chemotactic mobility of serum-controlled cells. Incubation with linoleic acid showed a 60% restoration of chemotaxis, whereas arachidonic acid stimulated chemotaxis by 140% compared with the positive control. Preincubation of LDL with a monoclonal antibody MB47 directed against LDL resulted in a significantly reduced migratory response. The data suggested a novel cyclooxygenase-dependent regulatory mechanism of chemotaxis by LDL.

Platelet-Derived Growth Factor in Hypercholesterolemic Patients

Platelet-derived growth factor is implicated in the accumulation of smooth muscle cells in atherosclerotic lesions after monocyte migration through the vascular endothelium. Billett and coworkers[5] in Nottingham, United Kingdom, showed a 15- to 20-fold increase in expression of platelet-derived growth factor A and B genes (as measured by a quantitative reverse transcription-polymerase chain reaction assay of mRNA concentration) in circulating monocytes of hypercholesterolemic and hyperlipidemic patients compared with normocholesterolemic individuals. Strong positive correlations between platelet-derived growth factor A and B mRNA concentrations indicated that the 2 genes were coordinately regulated in mononuclear cells in both normal and hypercholesterolemic individuals. Platelet-derived growth factor gene expression in patients correlated with concentrations of plasma total cholesterol and of LDL cholesterol, a proven risk factor for atherosclerosis (Figure 1-1). Activation of monocyte plasma platelet-derived growth factor expression may be an important component of the atherosclerotic risk associated with raised cholesterol levels and may represent an essential step in the early stages of atherogenesis. However, the marked increases in platelet-derived growth factor mRNA levels in patients with modest hypercholesterolemia compared with normal subjects suggested that other factors were involved. The relationship of monocyte platelet-derived growth factor expression to other atherosclerotic risk factors and to the different stages of atherosclerosis needs to be carefully evaluated.

Heparin-Binding Epidermal Growth Factor-Like Growth Factor in Atherosclerosis

Nakata and colleagues[6] in Osaka, Japan, have shown *in vitro* that heparin-binding epidermal growth factor-like growth factor (HB-EGF) is a mitogen

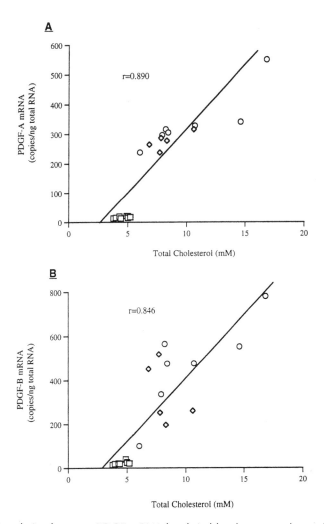

FIGURE 1-1. Correlation between PDGF mRNA levels in blood mononuclear cells and plasma total cholesterol concentrations. Lines were drawn using a least-squares algorithm. A, PDGF-A mRNA: r = .890, p<.001. B, PDGF-B mRNA: r = .846, p<.001. □ represents normocholesterolemic individuals; ◇, HL individuals; and ○, FH individuals. Reproduced with permission from Billett et al.[5]

and chemoattractant for vascular smooth muscle cells, suggesting a role for HB-EGF in the pathogenesis of atherosclerosis. They investigated the localization of HB-EGF in both normal and atherosclerotic human coronary arteries in an effort to elucidate the possible role of this growth factor in the formation of atherosclerotic lesions. The immunohistochemical localization of HB-EGF, smooth muscle cells, macrophages, and epidermal growth factor receptors was examined in human coronary arteries obtained at autopsy. The medial smooth muscle cells of coronary arteries in neonates, infants, and children consistently synthesize HB-EGF protein. In normal adults, however, the relative number of HB-EGF positive medial smooth muscle cells decline gradually with age after approximately 30 years of age. In nonatherosclerotic coronary arteries with diffuse intimal thickening, smooth muscle cells of the intima, especially those located in the area of the medial side of the intima, were strongly positive for HB-EGF. In atherosclerotic plaques of coronary arteries with eccentric intimal thickening, both smooth muscle cells and macrophages in and around the core lesions, in addition to the intimal and medial smooth muscle cells located adjacent to the plaque, produced HB-EGF protein (Figure 1-2). A strong immunostaining of epidermal growth factor receptors was observed in these smooth muscle cells, suggesting an association of the HB-EGF and epidermal growth factor receptor expression. Thus, these data suggest that the HB-EGF

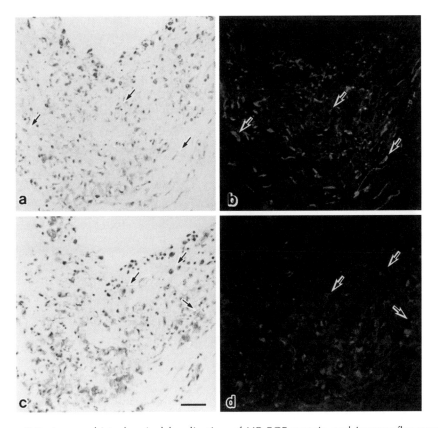

FIGURE 1-2. Immunohistochemical localization of HB-EGF protein and immunofluorescent localization of smooth muscle cells or macrophages by double immunohistostaining in sections from the left anterior descending coronary artery with atherosclerotic plaque (53-year-old woman, case 16). a, Immunohistochemical localization of HG-EGF in the atherosclerotic plaque (antibody H-6). b, Localization of smooth muscle cells detected by anti-α-smooth muscle cells actin monoclonal antibodies in the same section. c, Immunohistochemical localization of HB-EGF in the atherosclerotic plaque (antibody H-1). d, Detection of macrophages in the plaque by HAM56 in the same section as in c (a, b, c, and d, x140; bar = 70μm). Many HB-EGF-positive cells were observed in the intima of this atherosclerotic plaque (a, c). Relatively large cells with a granular staining pattern of the cytoplasm were identified as macrophages; small and round or spindle-shaped cells were identified as smooth muscle cells (b, d). Cells indicated by arrows in a and b are the same smooth muscle cells; cells indicated by arrows in c and d are the same macrophages. Reproduced with permission from Nakata et al.[6]

may play a role in the migration of smooth muscle cells from media to intima, the proliferation of smooth muscle cells, and the interaction between smooth muscle cells and macrophages in the process of coronary atherogenesis.

Interleukin-1β in Ischemic Heart Disease

Interleukin-1β is known to have a number of effects on the different cell types present within coronary arteries. Galea and coinvestigators[7] in Sheffield, United Kingdom, identified the location and phenotype of cells containing interleukin-1β in human coronary specimens from patients suffering from either coronary atherosclerosis or cardiomyopathy, and they correlated the presence of interleukin-1β with disease severity. Luminal endothelial cells, adventitial vessel wall cells, and macrophages were double labeled immunohistochemically for interleukin-1β protein in a cell type-specific monoclonal antibody for either endothelial cells or macrophages. *In situ* hybridization was performed to locate the presence of interleukin-1β mRNA within the coronary artery wall. In this study, interleukin-1β protein was found to be increased in the advent tissue wall vessels of atherosclerotic coronary arteries compared with coronary arteries from nonischemic cardiomyopathic hearts. This increase was directly proportional to the severity of coronary atherosclerosis. Interleukin-1β protein was also detected in luminal endothelium and macrophages of atherosclerotic coronary arteries and coronary arteries from nonischemic cardiomyopathic hearts. Interleukin-1β mRNA was found in luminal endothelial cells, adventitial vessel endothelial cells, and macrophages. The investigators concluded that interleukin-1β is produced by endothelial cells and macrophages in coronary arteries from ischemic hearts and, to a lesser extent, from nonischemic cardiomyopathic hearts.

C-Type Natriuretic Peptide in Atherogenesis

Naruko and colleagues[8] in Kyoto, Japan, studied 33 coronary artery segments harvested at autopsy: 10 were normal with diffuse intimal thickening, and 23 had atherosclerotic lesions. Samples were snap-frozen and processed for immunohistochemical staining. For the identification of C-type natriuretic peptide (CNP), a mouse monoclonal antibody was used. Antibodies to other cellular constituents were also used to stain smooth muscle cells, macrophages, and endothelial cells. CNP was present in several cell types, including CNP-positive endothelial cells and normal arterial segments. Hypercellular atherosclerotic lesions showed distinct CNP positivity of smooth muscle cells and macrophages, but a decrease in positivity of endothelial cells. Advanced atherosclerotic lesions contained CNP-positive macrophages, but the smooth muscle cells within the fibrous cap and the endothelial cells were virtually CNP-negative. These data suggest that CNP may have functional significance in atherogenesis.

Angiotensin-Converting Enzyme Levels in Atherosclerosis

Diet and colleagues[9] in Stanford, California, studied tissue angiotensin-converting enzyme (ACE) levels in human coronary artery disease to identify potential mechanisms of ACE inhibitors. They examined ACE expression immunohistochemically in nonatherosclerotic and diseased human coronary arteries. In nonatherosclerotic arteries, ACE immunoreactivity was found in luminal and adventitial vasa vasorum endothelium. In early- and intermediate-stage atherosclerotic lesions, ACE was detected in regions of fat-laden macrophages and in association with T lymphocytes. In advanced lesions, ACE immunoreactivity was localized to the endothelium of the microvasculature throughout the plaques. Immunoreactive angiotensin II was also detected in these areas. ACE expression in macrophages was further examined by *in vitro* experiments with a monocytoid cell line. ACE activity was induced 3-fold after differentiation of the cells into macrophages and was further increased after stimulation with acetylated LDL. Thus, these observations demonstrate that significant sources of tissue ACE in human atherosclerotic plaques are regions of inflammatory cells, especially those clustered macrophages, as well as microvessel endothelial cells. ACE accumulation within the plaque may contribute to an increased production of local angiotensin that may participate in the pathobiology of coronary artery disease (CAD).

Ultrastructural Studies of Restenotic Tissue

In animal studies, smooth muscle cell phenotype conversion has been suggested to be an essential prerequisite for subsequent migratory and proliferative events leading to (neo)intima formation. To determine ultrastructural characteristics of individual smooth muscle cells and to relate them to specific lesion types and intimal cell density, Bauriedel and associates[10] from Tübingen, Federal Republic of Germany, used transmission electron microscopy and histology to compare atherectomy samples from 17 restenotic and 32 primary coronary and peripheral lesions. Ultrastructural analysis of cell-rich tissue, predominantly of restenotic origin, revealed smooth muscle cells full of synthetic organelles. Moreover, these cells were frequently found to be surrounded by loose extracellular matrix and partially fragmented basement membrane components. In contrast, plaques exhibiting low cell density, as exclusively seen with primary lesions, displayed an extensive build-up of extracellular matrix containing sparse numbers of microfilament-rich smooth muscle cells. The central finding of the study is a morphometrically quantitated, 2-fold greater volume fraction of synthetic organelles (V_S) within smooth muscle cells in restenotic versus primary plaques, indicating a more dedifferentiated cellular phenotype as a typical feature of restenotic lesions. Equally enhanced V_S values were seen for restenotic coronary and peripheral plaques. No V_S decrease was observed during time after angiography (2 to 30 months) regardless of previous revascularization procedures (balloon angioplasty or atherectomy). Despite intra- and interlesional variability, V_S and intimal cell density were strongly correlated. This correlation was observed more often with clinical restenoses and, importantly, in a portion (10% to 15%) of primary lesions. Data from restenotic lesions indicate that a dedifferentiated smooth muscle cell phenotype, pericellular matrix disintegration, and intimal hypercellularity are long-lasting biological responses to previous smooth muscle cell injury. Similar tissue characteristics expressed in several primary lesions suggest that comparable pathogenic mechanisms are related to the progression and/or acuity of chronic lesions.

Mast Cells in Rupture-Prone Areas of Atheromas Produce TNF-α

Kaartinen and colleagues[11] in Helsinki, Finland, have shown that mast cells are present in coronary atheromas and localize to the erosion or rupture site of atheromas in patients with AMI. In this report, they identified the presence of tissue necrosis factor (TNF)-α, a proinflammatory cytokine, in mast cells of human coronary atheromas. From samples of 37 coronary arteries from subjects autopsied, sections of the bifurcation areas of the LAD were stained immunohistochemically for mast cells and TNF-α. In addition, macrophages, T lymphocytes, smooth muscle cells, and endothelial cells were evaluated for their content of TNF-α. In normal intimas and fatty streaks, none of the cell types studied were TNF-α-positive. In 14 of 24 atheromas found, TNF-α-positive cells were present. Among the total number of mast cells, 23% stained for TNF-α. Among the macrophages, 1% stained for TNF-α, and of the smooth muscle cells, 0.4% stained for TNF-α. The majority (55%) of TNF-α-positive mast cells in the atheromas were located in the shoulder region, 35% were in the cap, and 10% were in the core regions. Immunoelectron microscopy showed that TNF-α in mast cells resided within their cytoplasmic secretory granules. Thus, these data demonstrate the presence of mast cells with TNF-α-containing secretory granules, especially in the shoulder region of human coronary atheroma. By releasing their TNF-α, mast cells may play an active role in the inflammatory lesions of these rupture-prone areas of atheromas.

Active Tissue Factor in Coronary Atheroma

Marmur and colleagues[12] obtained directional coronary atherectomy specimens from 63 lesions in human coronary atheroma and analyzed them with the use of a quantitative tissue factor-specific activity assay. The median content of tissue factor was 10 ng/g per plaque. After homogenization of the specimens, tissue factor activity was detected in 28 of 31 lesions (90%) (Figure 1-3). With a polyclonal antihuman tissue factor antibody, the use of immunohistochemistry detected tissue factor antigen in 43 of 50 lesions (86%). Tissue factor antigen was expressed in cellular and acellular areas of the plaque. Histologically defined thrombus was present in 19 of the 43 lesions with detectable tissue factor antigen and in none of the 7 lesions without detectable tissue factor antigen. Tissue factor antigen was undetectable with immunohisto-

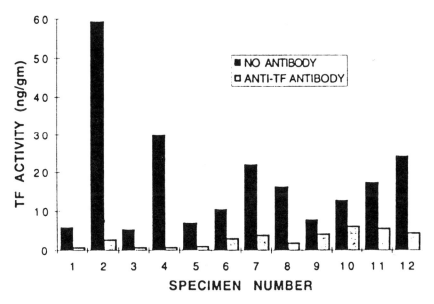

FIGURE 1-3. Tissue factor (TF) activity measurements in homogenized coronary atherectomy specimens preincubated *in vitro,* with or without an antihuman TF antibody. Each set of specimens (n = 12) is derived from a single lesion. Procoagulant activity is markedly diminished in the portion of the specimen pretreated with anti-TF antibody. Reproduced with permission from Marmur et al.[12]

chemistry in 4 of 13 restenotic lesions and in 3 of 37 *de novo* lesions. Thus, these data suggest that tissue factor may contribute to the procoagulant activity of many atherosclerotic lesions treated with directional coronary atherectomy.

Coronary Plaque Erosion as a Cause of Coronary Thrombosis

Farb and colleagues[13] in Washington, D.C., compared the incidence and morphological characteristics of coronary thrombosis associated with plaque rupture versus thrombosis in eroded plaques without rupture in 50 consecutive cases of sudden death due to coronary artery thrombosis. Plaque rupture of a fibrous cap with communication of the thrombus with a lipid pool was found in 28 cases. Thrombi without rupture were present in 22 cases, all of which had superficial erosion of a proteoglycan plaque. The mean age at death was 53 years in plaque rupture versus 44 years in eroded plaques without rupture. In the plaque-rupture group, 5 of 28 (18%) were women versus 11 of 22 (50%) men with eroded plaques. The mean percent luminal area of stenosis was 78% in plaque rupture and 70% in superficial erosion. Plaque calcification was present in 69% of ruptures versus 23% of erosions. In plaque ruptures, the fibrous cap was infiltrated by macrophages in every instance, and T cells in 75% of cases, compared with 50% by T cells and 32% by macrophages in superficial erosions. Clusters of smooth-muscle cells adjacent to the thrombi were present in 95% of erosions versus 33% of ruptures. Thus, erosion of proteoglycan-rich and smooth muscle cell-rich plaques lacking a superficial lipid core or plaque rupture is a frequent finding in sudden death due to coronary thrombosis, comprising 44% of cases in the present study. These lesions are more often seen in younger individuals and women, they have less luminal narrowing and less calcification, and less often have foci of macrophages and T cells compared with those site of plaque rupture.

Thermal Detection of Cellular Infiltrates in Atherosclerotic Plaques

Casscells and colleagues[14] in Houston, Texas, tested the hypothesis that vascular thrombotic events may be predicted by heat released by activated macrophages either on the plaque surface or under a thin cap. They measured the intimal surface temperatures at 20 sites in each of 50 samples of carotid artery plaque taken at endarterectomy from 48 patients. The living samples were probed with a thermistor, which included a 24-gauge needle-tip with an accuracy of 0.1°C and a time contrast of 0.15 seconds. The tissues were then fixed and stained. The atherosclerotic plaques showed several regions in which the surface temperatures varied reproducibly by 0.2° to 0.3°C, but 37% of plaques had substantially warmer regions (0.4–2.2°C). Points with substantially different temperatures could not be distinguished from one another by the naked eye, and such points were sometimes very close to one another (<1 mm apart). Temperature correlated positively with cell density (r = 0.68, p = .0001) and inversely with the distance of the cell clusters from the luminal surface. Most cells were macrophages. Infrared thermographic images also revealed heterogeneity in temperature among the plaques. Thus, living atherosclerotic plaques show thermal heterogeneity, which raises the possibility that an infrared catheter, or other techniques that can localize heat or metabolic activity, might be able to identify plaques at high risk of rupture or thrombosis.

Oxidation of Lipids/Antioxidants

Oxidized LDL and Growth of Human Monocyte-Derived Macrophages

The growth of murine peritoneal macrophages is induced by oxidized LDL, and lysophosphatidylcholine plays an important role in its mitogenic activity. Sakai and coinvestigators[15] in Kumamoto, Japan, examined oxidized LDL-induced macrophage growth with human monocyte-derived macrophages. The cell growth of human macrophages was significantly induced by oxidized LDL, but not by acetylated LDL. The treatment of acetyl-LDL with phospholipase A_2, however, led to a marked increased in the mitogenic activity, with a concomitant conversion of 75% of its phospholipids to lysophosphatidylcholine. The growth-simulating activity became positive only when both acetyl-LDL and lysophosphatidylcholine were co-incubated, although neither of them exhibited cell growth-promoting activity. These results suggested that oxidized LDL could stimulate the growth of human monocyte-derived macrophages, and lysophosphatidylcholine might play an essential role in the mitogenic activity of oxidized LDL.

New Functional Domain in Binding of Oxidized LDL

Uptake of oxidized LDL by macrophages is 1 of the key events implicated in the initiation and perpetuation of atherosclerotic lesions. One of the major scavenging receptors that binds modified LDL on macrophages is CD36. The domain on CD36 implicated in the binding of oxidized LDL remains to be elucidated. In a study by Navazo and coinvestigators[16] in Paris, France, COS cells transfected with human CD36 cDNA bound fluorescein isothiocyanate (FITC)-oxidized human LDL in a dose-dependent saturable manner. This binding was inhibited by an excess of oxidized LDL, but not by native LDL. Anti-CD36 monoclonal antibodies completely inhibited oxidized LDL binding to human CD36-transfected COS cells. Cells transfected with a chimeric human CD36 construct, resulting from the swapping of human domain 155-183 with its murine counterpart, resulted in low binding of oxidized LDL. In contrast, cells transfected with a chimeric CD36 construct resulting from the swapping of murine domain 155-183 with its human counterpart resulted in high binding of oxidized human LDL. Binding of oxidized LDL to cells transfected by chimeric construct mhm 155-183 were only partially blocked by anti-CD36 monoclonal antibodies. In the present study, the investigators have demonstrated for the first time an important functional domain (encompassing amino acids 155-183) on CD36 involved in the binding of oxidized LDL. In addition, the binding site for human LDL on murine CD36 seems to be different from its human counterpart.

Human Monocytes/Macrophages Release TNF-α in Response to Oxidized LDL

The uptake of oxidatively modified LDL by intimal macrophages is believed to play a key role in the development of atherogenesis. A study by Jovinge and coinvestigators[17] in Stockholm, Sweden, demonstrated that oxidized LDL in low concentrations activates monocyte/macrophage release of factors that stimulate smooth muscle cell growth, whereas higher concentrations are inhibitory. Exposure of monocytes/macrophages to oxidized LDL increased expression of TNF-α mRNA, but had no effect on interleukin-1β platelet-derived growth factor B or heparin-binding epidermal growth factor-like mitogen mRNA levels. Oxidized LDL also stimulated monocyte/macrophage release of TNF-α in a dose-response manner with maximal effect at an LDL concentration of 8 μg/mL. Addition of TNF-α-blocking antibodies to condition medium from monocytes/macrophages already exposed to oxidized LDL reduced mitogenic activity by 45%. Stimulation of TNF-α release by oxidized LDL was associated with activation of transcription factor AP-1, whereas the activity of transcription factor nuclear factor-kB remained unchanged. These findings suggested that enhanced secretion of TNF-α by macrophages exposed to oxidized LDL may be involved in the formation of atherosclerotic lesions.

In Vivo *Oxidized LDL: Contribution to LDL Oxidation and Dense LDL Subpopulations*

Sevanian and colleagues[18] in Los Angeles, California, studied the oxidative modification of LDL, which is thought to be a radical-mediated process involving lipid peroxides. The small dense LDL subpopulations are particularly susceptible to oxidation, and individuals with high proportions of dense LDL are at a greater risk for atherosclerosis. An oxidatively modified plasma LDL, referred to as LDL$^-$, is found largely among the dense LDL fractions. LDL$^-$ and dense LDL particles also contain much greater amounts of lipid peroxides compared with total LDL or the more buoyant LDL fractions. The content of LDL$^-$ in dense LDL particles appears to be related to copper- or heme-induced oxidative susceptibility, which may be attributable to peroxide levels. The rate of lipid peroxidation during the antioxidant-protective phase (lag period) and the length of the antioxidant-protective phase (lag time) are correlated with the LDL$^-$ content of total LDL. Once LDL oxidation enters the propagation phase, there is no relationship to the initial LDL$^-$ content or total LDL lipid peroxide or vitamin E levels. Beyond a threshold LDL$^-$ content of around 2%, there is a significant increase in the oxidative susceptibility of the nLDL particles, and this susceptibility becomes more pronounced as the LDL$^-$ content

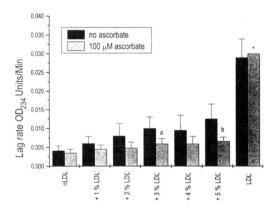

FIGURE 1-4. Bar graph shows effect of ascorbic acid on LDL oxidation rate during lag phase (lag rates). Rates of Cu^{2+}-induced oxidation are presented on the basis of the change in conjugated diene absorbance (OD$_{234}$) per minute while monitoring the samples at 25°C. Oxidation rates are shown for mixtures of nLDL and LDL$^-$ and pure nLDL and pure LDL$^-$ alone. Results are mean ± SE from three independent experiments except for LDL$^-$ treated in the presence of ascorbate (indicated by asterisk), which is mean ± SE of two determinations. aP<.05 nLDL + 3% LDL$^-$ absence vs presence of ascorbate; bP<.01 nLDL + 5% LDL$^-$ absence vs presence of ascorbate (all by paired Student's *t* test). Reproduced with permission from Sevarian et al.[18]

increases. Unmodified normal LDL is resistant to copper- or heme-induced oxidation. The oxidative susceptibility is not influenced by vitamin E content in LDL, but is strongly inhibited by ascorbic acid in the medium (Figure 1-4). Involvement of LDL$^-$-associated peroxides during the stimulated oxidation of LDL is suggested by the inhibition of unmodified LDL oxidation when LDL$^-$ is treated with ebselen prior to its addition to unmodified LDL. Populations of LDL enriched with LDL$^-$ appear to contain peroxides at levels approaching the threshold required for progressive radical propagation reactions. The investigators postulated that elevated LDL$^-$ may constitute a pro-oxidant state that facilitates oxidative reactions in the vascular components.

Antioxidants Alone and Combined with Monounsaturated Fatty-Acid Enriched Diets

Previous studies have demonstrated that compared with more buoyant LDL, dense LDL is more susceptible to oxidation and less readily protected from oxidation by antioxidant enrichment. However, diets enriched in monounsaturated fatty acids appear particularly effective in protecting dense LDL from oxidation. Therefore, Reaven and associates[19] in LaJolla, California, evaluated in 12 noninsulin-dependent diabetes mellitus subjects the effects of supplementation with α-tocopherol (1600 U/day) and probucol (1 gm/day) alone and in combination with a monounsaturated fatty acid-enriched diet on LDL and LDL subfraction susceptibility to oxidation and monocyte release of superoxide anion. Subjects received either α-tocopherol or probucol for 4 months, and during the 4th month, both groups also received a monounsaturated fatty acid-enriched diet. α-Tocopherol levels were significantly increased in LDL and LDL subfractions after 3 months of supplementation. Monounsaturated fatty acid-enriched diets led to further increases in α-tocopherol in LDL fractions in the α-tocopherol group, as well as in those receiving probucol. In the α-tocopherol-supplemented group, lag times were increased significantly for all LDL fractions, although the absolute increase was least for dense LDL. Although probucol supplementation increased lag times of LDL and LDL subfractions 3- to 4-fold, dense LDL was still more readily oxidized. In both the α-tocopherol- and probucol-supplemented groups, the benefit of adding monounsaturated fatty acid-enriched diets was greatest for the dense LDL with further increase in lag time of 26% and 18%, respectively. Neither antioxidant supplementations nor the addition of a monounsaturated fatty acid-enriched diet reduced unstimulated or phorbol ester-stimulated monocytes superoxide anion production. These data demonstrated the markedly different effects that antioxidants and diet may have on different LDL subfractions, which may be particularly important in individuals with noninsulin-dependent diabetes mellitus who frequently have increased amounts of dense LDL.

Coenzyme Q and Oxidation

There is considerable interest in the ability of antioxidant supplementation, in particular with vitamin E, to attenuate LDL oxidation, a process implicated in atherogenesis. Because vitamin E can also promote LDL lipid peroxidation, Thomas and coworkers[20] in Sydney, Australia, investigated the effects of supplementation with vitamin E alone or in combination with coenzyme Q on the early stages of the oxidation of isolated LDL. Isolated LDL was obtained from healthy subjects before and after *in vitro* enrichment with vitamin E or dietary supplementation with vitamin E and/or coenzyme Q. LDL oxidation initiation was assessed by measurement of the consumption of vitamin E and cholesteryl esters containing polyunsaturated fatty acids and by the accumulation of cholesteryl ester hydroperoxides during incubation of the LDL in the transition of metal-containing Ham's F-10 medium in the absence and presence of human monocyte-derived macrophages. Native LDL contained 8.5 molecules of vitamin E and 0.5 to 0.8 molecules of ubiquinol-10 per lipoprotein particle. Incubation of this LDL and Ham's F-10 medium resulted in a time-dependent loss of vitamin E with concomitant stoichiometric conversion of the major cholesteryl esters to their respective hydroperoxides. Monocyte-derived macrophages enhanced this process. LDL lipid peroxidation occurred via a radical chain reaction in the presence of vitamin E, and the rate of this oxidation decreased on vitamin E depletion. *In vitro* enrichment of LDL with vitamin E resulted in an LDL particle containing 6-fold to 7-fold more vitamin E, and such enriched LDL was more readily oxidized in the absence and presence of monocyte-derived macrophages compared with native LDL. *In vitro* vitamin E-deficient LDL, isolated from a patient with familial isolated vitamin E deficiency, was highly resistant to Ham's F-10-initiated oxidation, whereas dietary supplementation with vitamin E restored the oxidizability of the patient's LDL. Oral supplementation of healthy individuals for 5 days, with either vitamin E or coenzyme Q, increased the LDL levels of vitamin E and ubiquinol-10 by 2 to 3 or 3 to 4 times, respectively. Vitamin E-supplemented LDL was significantly more prone to oxidation, whereas ubiquinol-10 enriched LDL was more resistant to oxidation initiation by Ham's F-10 medium than native LDL. Co-supplementation with both vitamin E and coenzyme Q resulted in LDL with increased levels of vitamin E and ubiquinol-10, and such LDL was markedly more resistant to initiation of oxidation than native or vitamin E-enriched LDL. These results demonstrated that oral supplementation with vitamin E alone resulted in LDL that is more prone to oxidation initiation, whereas co-supplementation with coenzyme Q not only prevented this prooxidant activity of vitamin E, but also provided the lipoprotein with increased resistance to oxidation.

Effect of Dietary Fat on LDL Oxidation

Mata and coinvestigators[21] in Madrid, Spain, subjected 42 healthy men and women to 4 consecutive dietary periods differing in the fat content of saturated fatty acids, monounsaturated fatty acids, and polyunsaturated fatty acids. Plasma lipids, vitamin E, and *in vitro* LDL oxidation were examined during each period. Adhesion of human monocytes to cultured human endothelial cells was used as a functional test to identify differences in the biological properties of LDL from each dietary period. Consumption of a saturated fat-rich diet resulted in higher LDL cholesterol than did consumption of monoun-saturated fatty acids or polyunsaturated fatty acid-rich diets. HDL cholesterol was lower during both polyunsaturated fatty acid-rich diets than during the saturated fatty acid diets and the monounsaturated fatty acid-rich diets. LDL resistance to copper-induced oxidation, expressed as lag time, was highest during the monounsaturated fatty acid-rich diets and lowest during the polyunsaturated fatty acid and saturated fatty acid-rich diets. LDL induction of monocyte adhesion to endothelial cells was lower during the monounsaturated fatty acid-rich diet than during the other periods. The highest monocyte adhesion was obtained during the polyunsaturated fatty acid and the saturated fatty acid dietary periods. In conclusion, a monounsaturated fatty acid-rich diet benefits plasma lipid levels more than a saturated fatty acid-rich diet. Furthermore, this diet resulted in an increased resistance of LDL to oxidation and a lower rate of monocyte adhesion to endothelial cells than the other dietary fats examined.

α-Tocopherol in Reducing Risk of AMI

Stephens and colleagues[22] in the United Kingdom tested the hypothesis that treatment with a high dose of α-tocopherol reduces subsequent risk of AMI and cardiovascular death in patients with CAD. They used a double-blind, placebo-controlled study with stratified randomization of 2002 patients with angiographically proven CAD. The patients were followed up for a median of 510 days, with a range of 3 to 981 days. One thousand thirty-five patients were assigned to receive α-tocopherol capsules containing 800 IU daily for the first 546 patients and 400 IU daily for the remainder; 967 received identical placebo capsules. The primary end points were a combination of cardiovascular death and nonfatal AMI, as well as nonfatal MI alone. Plasma α-tocopherol concentrations measured in subsets of patients rose in the actively treated group from a baseline mean value of 34.2 μmol/L to 51 μmol/L with 400 IU daily and 64.5 μmol/L with 800 IU daily, but did not change in the placebo group. α-Tocopherol treatment significantly reduced the risk of the primary trial end point of cardiovascular death and nonfatal AMI (41 vs. 64 events; relative risk 0.53). The beneficial effects on this composite endpoint were due to a significant reduction in the risk of nonfatal AMI (14 vs. 41,023, p = .005). However, there was a nonsignificant excess of cardiovascular deaths in the α-tocopherol group (27 vs. 23). All cause mortality was 36 of 1035 α-tocopherol-treated patients and 27 of 967 placebo-treated patients. These data suggest that in patients with angiographically proven symptomatic CAD, α-tocopherol treatment substantially reduces the risk of nonfatal AMI with beneficial effects apparent after 1 year of treatment.

Supplementary Antioxidant Vitamin Intake: Effect on Arterial Wall Thickness

Azen and colleagues[23] in Los Angeles, California, explored the association of self-selected supplementary antioxidant vitamin intake on the rate of pro-

TABLE 1-1
On-Trial Annualized Rate of Intima-Media Thickness Change (mm/y) Between High and
Low Vitamin E and Vitamin C Intake Groups

| | High* | | Low* | | |
Vitamin Intake	No.	Mean ± SD	No.	Mean ± SD	P†
Supplemenatry vitamin E					
Drug group	11	−0.017 ± 0.019	62	−0.025 ± 0.033	.46
		(−0.020 ± 0.033)		(−0.024 ± 0.032)	.71
Placebo group	11	0.008 ± 0.023	62	0.023 ± 0.020	.02
		(0.008 ± 0.021)		(0.023 ± 0.020)	.03
All subjects	22	−0.005 ± 0.025	124	−0.001 ± 0.036	.52
		(−0.004 ± 0.036)		(−0.001 ± 0.035)	.70
Supplementary vitamin C					
Drug group	18	−0.017 ± 0.027	55	−0.026 ± 0.032	.29
		(−0.019 ± 0.032)		(−0.025 ± 0.032)	.50
Placebo group	11	0.017 ± 0.018	62	0.022 ± 0.022	.52
		(0.019 ± 0.021)		(0.021 ± 0.021)	.71
All subjects	29	−0.004 ± 0.029	117	−0.001 ± 0.036	.64
		(−0.005 ± 0.036)		(−0.001 ± 0.035)	.61

* High and low groups defined at 100 IU per day for vitamin E and 250 mg per day for vitamin C, respectively.

† Probability value obtained from two-sample t test (first entry) and from ANCOVA adjusted for total cholesterol, LDL cholesterol, and diastolic blood pressure at baseline (second entry). Reproduced with permission from Azen et al.[23]

gression of early atherosclerosis. They used data from the Cholesterol Lowering Atherosclerosis Study (CLAS), an arterial imaging trial in which nonsmoking men, aged 40 to 59 years, with previous coronary artery bypass surgery were randomly assigned to either colestipol/niacin and diet or placebo and diet. The rate of progression of early atherosclerosis was determined in 146 individuals by use of high-resolution B-mode ultrasound quantification of the distal common carotid artery far wall intima-media thickness. From the nutritional supplement database, 22 subjects had on-trial average supplementary vitamin intake of 100 IU or more per day (high users), and 29 subjects had average on-trial supplementary vitamin C intake of 250 mg per day or more (high users). Within the placebo group, less carotid intimal-medial thickness progression was found for high supplementary vitamin E users than for the low vitamin E users (Table 1-1). No effect of vitamin E within the drug group itself was found, and no effect of vitamin C within the drug or placebo group was found. Thus, these data suggest that supplementary vitamin E intake may be effective in reducing the progression of atherosclerosis in individuals not treated with lipid-lowering drugs while the atherosclerotic process is still confined to the arterial wall.

Autoantibody Titers to Oxidized LDL in Coronary Artery Disease

Oxidation of LDL is considered the initial step in the atherosclerotic process. Autoantibodies to oxidized LDL have been detected in human serum. Bui and investigators[24] from Washington, D.C., used an enzyme-linked immunosorbent assay technique to measure autoantibody titers in 63 normal individuals and patients with CAD. Thirty-five patients underwent coronary angiography for suspected CAD. Patients were divided into the following categories: group 1, 20 healthy young volunteers; group 2, 8 patients age-matched to the catheterization patients; group 3, 10 patients with normal coronary angiograms; and group 4, 25 patients with angiographic CAD. Autoantibody titers to oxidized LDL were group 1, 0.142 ± 0.023; group 2, 0.197 ± 0.039; group 3, 0.183 ± 0.038; and group 4, 0.340 ± 0.026. There was no statistical difference between groups 1, 2, and 3, but the difference between these groups and group 4 was highly significant. This study demonstrates that 1) autoantibodies to oxidized LDL can be detected in normal individuals and in patients with abnormal coronary angiograms and 2) significantly higher titers of autoantibodies to oxidized LDL were seen in patients with angiographic evidence of CAD.

Human Antioxidized LDL Autoantibodies

Autoantibodies to oxidized LDL have been reported in normal subjects and in patients with arteriosclerosis, but their possible pathogenic role is not yet well defined. One important problem is the existence of contradictory data reported by different groups concerning the associations between antioxidized LDL antibodies and the presence or progression of arteriosclerotic lesions. Such contradictions led Mironova and coinvestigators[25] in Charleston, South Carolina, to conduct further investigations to isolate and characterize antioxidized LDL antibodies by affinity chromatography with the use of oxidized LDL cross-linked to Sepharose. Antioxidized LDL antibodies were isolated from selected serum samples obtained from 8 subjects. Seven of them (6 patients and 1 control subject) had high levels of antioxidized LDL antibodies during screening. The other subject, a healthy volunteer, had a low level of antibody. All purified antibodies contained immunoglobulin G (IgG) (subclasses 1 and 3) as the predominant isotype and were primarily specific for oxidized LDL, but showed some cross-reactivity with malondialdehyde-modified LDL and native LDL. Two other purified antibodies cross-reacted with cardiolipin. The investigators determined average dissociation constants for the antioxidized LDL antibodies purified from 5 individuals, which varied between 2.4×10^{-7} and 7.5×10^{-7} mol/L, whereas the average dissociation constant of rabbit hyperimmune anti-LDL antibody was determined to be 2.7×10^{-8} mol/L. In conclusion, the investigators purified human autoantibodies reactive with oxidized LDL that appeared to be predominantly of moderate-to-low affinity and of variable cross-reactivity. The predominance of IgG1 and IgG3 antibodies is significant from the standpoint of potential pathogenicity because these 2 subclasses activate the classic complement pathway system and have the highest binding affinities for Fc gamma receptors on phagocytic cells.

Human Endothelial Cells and Oxidized LDL

Oxidized LDL, a causal factor in atherosclerosis, is cytotoxic and triggers the expression of various heat-shock proteins, among which is heat-shock protein 70, in cultured animal and human cells. Heat-shock proteins constitutively act as molecular chaperones and, in situations of stress, protect other cellular proteins from potential denaturation caused by cytotoxic stimuli. Zhu and coinvestigators[26] in Milano, Italy, examined the sensitivity of endothelial cells to oxidized LDL toxicity and, accordingly, the level of heat-shock protein 70 expression, which depended on cell density. Whereas confluent cells were relatively resistant to oxidized LDL toxicity and were not induced to express heat-shock protein 70 when challenged with the lipoprotein, sparse cells exhibited a concentration- and time-dependent expression of inducible heat shock protein 70, which increased up to 5- to 6-fold in unchallenged cells. Neither the activity of the receptors recognizing oxidized LDL nor potentially protective cell products affected the stress response. Rather, the investigators demonstrated that cell proliferation, which is high for sparse cultures and wound healing, is responsible for these observations. The investigators also demonstrated that the lipid moiety of oxidized LDL essentially accounts for the heat-shock protein-inducing effect of the lipoprotein. Oxidized LDL has been detected in atherosclerotic lesions, which also show an increase of immunoreactive heat-shock protein 72/73. The investigators speculated that *in vivo* rapidly growing cells, such as those of lesion-prone areas, are more sensitive to the toxicity of oxidized LDL than are acquiescent cells and that an increased expression of heat-shock protein 70 may allow proliferating cells an increased chance of survival.

Endothelial Function, Vasodilation, Vascular Remodeling, and Inflammation

Coronary Constrictor Effects of Endothelin

Pernow and colleagues[27] in Stockholm, Sweden, compared the effects of endothelin-1 and big (precursor) endothelin-1 on coronary blood flow in relationship with plasma endothelin-1 and big endothelin-1 levels in healthy subjects. The peptides were infused intravenously at rates of 0.2, 1, and 8 pmol/kg per minute. Each dose was administered for 20 minutes, except for the highest dose of endothelin-1, which was administered for 10 minutes. Endothelin-1 and big endothelin-1 evoked dose-related increases in mean arterial blood pressure from 93 to 107 mm Hg and from 89 to 122 mm Hg, respectively, at the highest dose. Endothelin-1 and big endothelin-1 reduced coronary sinus blood flow measured by thermodilution by a maximum of 25% and 28%, and they increased coronary vascular resistance by 50% and 107%, respectively. Coronary sinus, but not arterial, oxygen saturation was reduced in association with a reduction in coronary sinus blood flow. The effects of endothelin-1 and big endothelin-1 were similar at corresponding time points. During infusion of endothelin-1, a 19% extraction of endothelin-1 was observed over the coronary bed. Administration of big endothelin-1 elevated arterial plasma endothelin-1 levels by 2-fold and, after correction for local extraction of endothelin-1, a myocardial production of endothelin-1 was observed. Thus, endothelin-1 and big endothelin-1 induce comparable increases in blood pressure and coronary vasoconstriction in humans *in vivo*. The data also suggest removal of circulating endothelin-1 and big endothelin-1 and a local conversion of big endothelin-1 into endothelin-1 within the coronary vascular bed.

Vascular Cell Adhesion Molecules

O'Brien and colleagues[28] in Seattle, Washington, studied the arterial distribution of the leukocyte adhesion molecules E-selectin, intercellular adhesion molecule-1 (ICAM-1), and vascular cell adhesion molecule-1 (VCAM-1) in human atherosclerosis in 99 coronary artery segments (65 with atherosclerotic plaque and 34 controls) using immunohistochemistry to identify E-selectin, ICAM-1, VCAM-1, macrophages, smooth muscle cells, and T lymphocytes. For each segment, the presence or absence of adhesion molecules was determined at the arterial lumen, on intimal neovasculature, and on intimal neoendothelial cells. Each segment was scored for intimal macrophage and T-lymphocyte densities on a semiquantitative scale of 0 to 3. In atherosclerotic plaques, the prevalence of E-selectin, ICAM-1, and VCAM-1 on plaque neovasculature was 2-fold higher than their prevalences on arterial luminal endothelium. E-selectin was the only adhesion molecule for which expression on arterial luminal endothelial cells was more prevalent in plaques than in control segments. Increased plaque intimal macrophage density was associated with expression of VCAM-1 on neovasculature and on neoendothelial cells. Increased plaque intimal T-lymphocyte density was associated with the presence of both ICAM-1 and VCAM-1 on neovasculature and on neoendothelial cells. Thus, in atherosclerotic plaques, the expression of all 3 leukocyte adhesion molecules was more prevalent on intimal neovasculature than on arterial luminal endothelium. Furthermore, the presence on neovasculature and nonendothelial cells of VCAM-1 and ICAM-1 was strongly associated with increased intimal leukocyte accumulation. These data suggest that leukocyte recruitment through and/or activation of intimal neovasculature may play important roles in the pathogenesis of human atherosclerosis.

Intercellular Adhesion Molecule-1 and L-Selectin and Chronic Inflammation

Atherosclerosis is increasingly thought to be a chronic inflammatory disease. Inflammation requires transmigration of leukocytes from the circulation to the tissues. Adhesion of leukocytes to endothelial cells is the initial event in an inflammatory response, and it is mediated by expression of several adhesion molecules. In this study, Haught and associates[29] from Gainesville, Florida, and Ridgefield, Connecticut, characterize the contribution of circulating ICAM-1 and L-selectin in patients with different CAD diseases. Serum concentrations of circulating ICAM-1 and L-selectin were measured by enzyme-linked immunosorbent assay in 31 patients with stable angina, 30 patients with unstable angina, 18 patients with AMI, and 20 healthy individuals as a control group. All patients underwent coronary angiography. Mean circulating ICAM-1 levels were higher in patients with stable angina (249 ± 16 ng/mL), unstable angina (260 ± 16 ng/mL), or AMI (261 ± 24 ng/mL) compared with those in individuals in the control group (171 ± 11 ng/mL). In contrast, levels of L-selectin were lower in patients with stable angina (1.2 ± 0.1 μg/mL), unstable angina (1.1 ± 0.6 μg/mL), or AMI (1.1 ± 0.1 μg/mL) compared with those in individuals in the control group (1.8 ± 0.1 μg/mL). No difference was found in circulating ICAM-1 or L-selectin levels among patients with stable angina, unstable angina, or AMI. No correlation was seen between circulating ICAM-1 or L-selectin levels and extent (or severity) of CAD or leukocyte count. L-selectin expression was observed to be depressed in patients with severe angina compared with that in members of the control group. To examine the mechanism of reduction in L-selectin levels and L-selectin expression on leukocytes, leukocytes from the control group were stimulated *in vitro*. Stimulation of leukocytes resulted in a rapid down-regulation of surface L-selectin expression, measured by flow cytometry, similar to the suppressed expression of L-selectin found on leukocytes from patients with CAD. In conclusion, altered circulating ICAM-1 and L-selectin levels in patients with CAD reflect the presence of a chronic inflammatory process. This inflammatory process results in down-regulation of leukocyte expression of L-selectin and, thus, lower circulating L-selectin levels.

Cell Adhesion Molecules in Dyslipidemia

Hackman and colleagues[30] in Houston, Texas determined whether dyslipidemia is associated with increased expression of cell adhesion molecules by examining the levels of soluble ICAMs, including soluble intercellular adhesion molecule-1 (sICAM-1), soluble vascular cell adhesion molecule-1 (sVCAM-1), and soluble E-selectin in patients with either hypercholesterolemia or hypertriglyceridemia and in control subjects matched for age and sex. Patients with hypertriglyceridemia had significantly higher levels of sVCAM-1 compared with patients with hypercholesterolemia and control subjects. Levels of sICAM-1 were increased in both the hypercholesterolemic and hypertriglyceridemic groups compared with the control individuals. Levels of sE-selectin were higher in the hypercholesterolemic patients than in the control subjects. Ten hypercholesterolemic patients were treated aggressively with atorvastatin alone or a combination of colestipol and either atorvastatin or simvastatin for a mean of 42 weeks and had an average LDL cholesterol reduction of 51%. Comparison with soluble cell adhesion molecules (CAMs) before and after treatment showed a significant reduction only in sE-selectin, not for sVCAM-1 or sICAM-1. The authors concluded that although severe hyperlipidemia is associated with increased levels of soluble cell adhesion molecules, aggressive lipid-lowering treatment had limited effect on their levels, and the soluble cellular adhe-

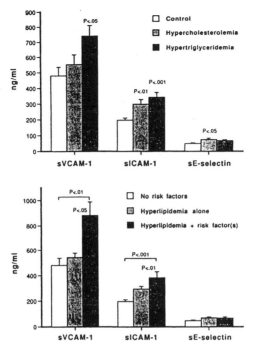

Figure 1-5. Top, Mean values and standard errors of sVCAM-1, sICAM-1, and sE-selectin in the 3 subject groups. Open bars represent control subjects (n = 13), light shaded bars indicate subjects with hypercholesterolemia (n = 14), and dark shaded bars indicate subjects with hypertriglyceridemia (n = 13). Significant differences between the groups with hyperlipidemia and the control group are shown with respective p values. Bottom, Comparison of levels of sVCAM-1, sICAM-1, and sE-selectin when additional risk factors such as hypertension, diabetes mellitus, tobacco use, or history of vascular disease are taken into consideration. Open bars represent control subjects with normal lipids and no risk factors (n = 13), light shaded bars represent patients with hyperlipidemia alone (elevated LDL-C or elevated triglyceride level) (n = 19), and the dark shaded bars indicate patients with hyperlipidemia and at least 1 other risk factor such as hypertension, diabetes mellitus, tobacco use, or history of vascular disease (n = 8). Significant differences between the group with hyperlipidemia with risk factor(s) and the control group are shown with respective p values above the bracket. Significant differences between the group with hyperlipidemia with risk factor(s) and hyperlipidemia alone are shown with respective P values below the bracket. Reproduced with permission from Hackman et al.[30]

sion molecules in patients with hyperlipidemia may be a marker for atherosclerosis (Figure 1-5).

Effect of Flavonoids on Endothelial Cell Expression of Adhesion Molecules

Wolle and coworkers[31] in Ann Arbor, Michigan, examined the effect of flavonoids on the endothelial cell expression of adhesion molecules, an early step in inflammation and atherogenesis. Addition of TNF-α to human aortic endothelial cells led to the induction of VCAM-1 expression and enhancement in expression of ICAM-1. A flavonoid (PD098063) markedly inhibited TNF-induced VCAM-1 cell surface expression in a concentration-dependent fashion with half maximal inhibition at 19 μmol/L, but it had no effect on ICAM-1 expression. Another structurally distinct flavonoid similarly selectively decreased VCAM-1 expression. The inhibition in cell-surface expression of VCAM-1 by PD098063 correlated with decreases in steady state mRNA levels, but there was no effect on ICAM-1 mRNA levels. The decrease in VCAM-1 mRNA level was not due to changes in mRNA stability, but rather resulted from a reduction in the rate of transcription of the gene. However, electrophoretic mobility shift assays, using nuclear extracts from TNF-induced human aortic endothelial cells treated with PD098063, failed to show a decrease in the activation of NF-kB, indicating that inhibition of activation of this transcription factor may not be its mode of action. Similarly, PD098063 did not affect chloramphenicol acetyltransferase reporter gene activity in TNF-inducible minimal VCAM-1 promoter constructs containing 2 NF-kB sites. This suggests that the compound did not affect the transactivation driven by these sites. The investigators concluded that this compound selectively blocked agonist-induced VCAM-1 protein and gene expression in human aortic endothelial cells by NF-kB-independent mechanisms.

Down-regulation of Nitric Oxide Synthase in Endothelial Cells

Because endothelium-dependent vasodilation is altered in atherosclerosis, and enhanced monocyte/endothelial interactions are implicated in early atherosclerosis, Marczin and coinvestigators[32] in Augusta, Georgia, evaluated the effect of monocytes on the endothelial nitric oxide pathway by estimating release of biologically active nitric oxide from cultured endothelial cells and levels of constitutive nitric oxide synthase. Nitric oxide release was estimated in a short-term bioassay using endothelial cell-induced cyclic guanosine monophosphate (cGMP) accumulation in vascular smooth muscle cells. Exposure of smooth muscle cells to porcine aortic endothelial cells and human aortic endothelial cells produces large increases in the content of cGMP in smooth muscle cells; this increase was prevented by N^G-nitro-L-arginine methyl ester, the inhibitor of endothelial nitric oxide synthase. Confluent monolayers of porcine aortic endothelial cells and human aortic endothelial cells co-cultured with monocytes also stimulated smooth muscle cGMP formation; however, nitric oxide release from these cultures was attenuated in a cocultured time (2–48 hours)- and monocyte concentration-dependent manner. This effect of monocyte adhesion appeared to be selective for nitric oxide release because other biochemical pathways, such as atriopeptin- and isoproterenol-induced cyclic nucleotide accumulation within the endothelial cells, were not altered by monocytes. The effects of adherent monocytes or nitric oxide release were mimicked by monocyte-derived cytokines TNF and interleukin-1α. Furthermore, the conditioned medium of monocytes contained significant quantities of these cytokines. Conditioned medium, as well as monocytes physically separated from the endothelial cells, attenuated nitric oxide release, suggesting that soluble factors may mediate the effects of monocytes. An interleukin-1β neutralizing antibody fully prevented the nitric oxide dysfunction in response to directly adherent monocytes. Superoxide dismutase catalase, 4, 5-dihydroxy-1,3-benzene disulfonic acid, and exogenous L-arginine failed to improve nitric oxide relief. This suggests that oxidant stress-induced inactivation of nitric oxide or limited substrate availability were not primarily responsible for the inhibiting effects of monocytes. Western blot analysis revealed reduced quantities of constitutive nitric oxide synthase in monocyte/endothelium cocultures, as well as in human aortic endothelial cells treated with monocyte condition serum or TNF-α. Thus, adhesion of monocytes to endothelial cells and monocyte-derived secretory products down-regulate steady-state levels of constitutive nitric oxide synthase, an event associated with attenuated release of biologically active nitric oxide. This mechanism may potentially contribute to diminished endothelium-dependent and nitric oxide-mediated vasodilation in early atherosclerosis.

Nitric Oxide in Pulmonary Vascular Resistance

Cooper and colleagues[33] in Boston, Massachusetts, tested the hypothesis that in conscious adults the endothelium, through nitric oxide production, is important in maintaining basal pulmonary vascular resistance, and it can increase nitric oxide production further in response to receptor-mediated stimulation, leading to further pulmonary artery vasodilation. In this study, pulmonary arterial resistance vessel function was studied within the distribution of a segmental lower lobe pulmonary artery in 8 conscious adults, 37 to 76 years old, undergoing cardiac catheterization. Segmental blood flow was determined with the use of a Doppler-tip guidewire and quantitative angiography. Drugs were administered locally within the segmental artery through an infusion catheter. The N^G-monomethyl-L-arginine (L-NMMA) was used as a specific inhibitor of nitric oxide production, whereas acetylcholine was used to test receptor-mediated vasodilation. To demonstrate that vasodilation to acetylcholine was nitric oxide-dependent, acetylcholine response was tested alone, in the presence of L-NMMA, and in the presence of a control constrictor, phenylephrine. Basal pulmonary vascular resistance was nitric oxide-dependent because L-NMMA infusion resulted in a dose-dependent decrease in local flow velocity, with flow decreasing 33% at the highest dose of L-NMMA (Figure 1-6). Acetylcholine infusion resulted in a dose-dependent increase in flow velocity. The acetylcholine response was at least in part nitric oxide-dependent because it was diminished by the presence of L-NMMA. The effect of L-NMMA on the acetylcholine response was not due to nonspecific preconstriction because L-NMMA diminished the acetylcholine response significantly more than did the endothelium-independent constrictor, phenylephrine, despite comparable preconstrictions. Thus, these data demonstrate that in healthy conscious adults, normal basal pulmonary resistance is maintained in part by continuous local production of

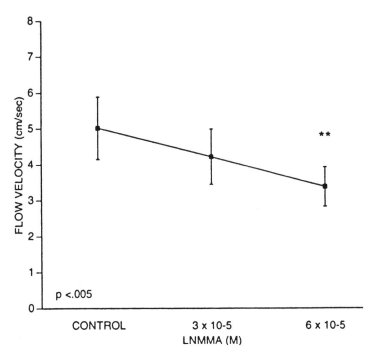

FIGURE 1-6. Dose-response curve of pulmonary segmental arterial Doppler flow velocity during L-NMMA infusion. Values are mean ± SEM. p<.005 by repeated-measures ANOVA, n=6. **p<.01 vs control. Reproduced with permission from Cooper et al.[33]

nitric oxide, and the local nitric oxide production is responsive to receptor-mediated stimulation, which leads to further vasodilation.

Nitric Oxide Production in Hypercholesterolemia

N^G-monomethyl-L-arginine, a specific inhibitor of nitric oxide synthesis, was used to investigate the effects of inhibition of nitric oxide synthesis on the coronary conductance and resistance vessels in hypercholesterolemic patients by Shiode and associates[34] from Hiroshima, Japan. Acetylcholine (3 and 30 μg/min) was administered to 10 hypercholesterolemic and 10 control patients before and after N^G-monomethyl-L-arginine (25 μmol/min) infusion. Epicardial coronary diameter was measured by quantitative angiography, and coronary blood flow was derived from Doppler flow-velocity and coronary diameter measurements. In hypercholesterolemic patients, acetylcholine-induced dilation of epicardial arteries was attenuated, and the percentage increase in coronary blood flow caused by acetylcholine was smaller than that in control patients. N^G-monomethyl-L-arginine attenuated acetylcholine-induced dilation of epicardial arteries in control patients. It had no effect on coronary blood flow responses to acetylcholine in both patient groups, but it significantly decreased the baseline coronary diameter and coronary blood flow in both groups. These results indicated that hypercholesterolemia impaired the acetylcholine-induced dilation of the conductance and resistance coronary vessels. This impairment in the conductance vessels was dependent on nitric oxide production; that of resistance vessels was not. The basal release of nitric oxide in conductance and resistance vessels was preserved in hypercholesterolemic patients.

L-Arginine Supplementation and Endothelium-Dependent Coronary Vasodilation

Egashira and colleagues[35] from Fukuoka, Japan, examined whether supplementation with L-arginine, a precursor of endothelium-derived nitric oxide, improves endothelium-dependent coronary vasodilation in patients with angina and normal coronary arteriograms. The effects of intracoronary infusion of L-arginine (50 mg/min) on acetylcholine-induced coronary vasomotion were studied in 8 patients and 8 control subjects. The responses of the large epicardial coronary artery diameter and coronary blood flow were measured with coronary arteriography and an intracoronary Doppler catheter, respectively. Acetylcholine increased coronary blood flow with modest vasoconstriction of the large coronary artery without altering arterial pressure and heart rate. The acetylcholine-induced increase in coronary blood flow was less in patients than in normal control subjects. L-Arginine significantly augmented the coronary blood flow responses to acetylcholine in the patients, but not in control subjects (Figure 1-7). L-Arginine did not alter responses of the large coronary artery in either group. Thus, these data indicate that L-arginine improves endothelium-dependent vasodilation of coronary microcirculation in patients with microvascular angina.

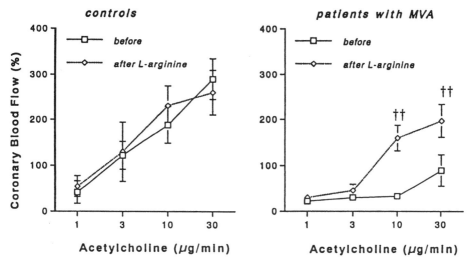

FIGURE 1-7. Effect of intracoronary infusion of L-arginine on acetylcholine-induced coronary vasodilation in control subjects (left) and patients with angina pectoris and normal coronary arteriograms (right). MVA indicates microvascular angina. [++]p<.01 vs. before L-arginine by 2-way ANOVA and multiple comparison tests. Reproduced with permission from Egashira et al.[35]

Aging-Associated Endothelin Dysfunction Reversed by L-Arginine

An impaired response to acetylcholine with aging has been demonstrated in humans. However, the mechanisms underlying this impaired response of the coronary microvasculature remain to be determined. Chauhan and colleagues[36] from Cambridge and London, United Kingdom, evaluated whether this selective impairment of endothelium-dependent function may be reversible by administration of L-arginine. They infused the endothelium-independent vasodilators papaverine and nitroglycerin and the endothelium-dependent vasodilator acetylcholine into the left coronary artery of 34 patients aged 27 to 73 years (with typical chest pain, negative exercise test results, completely normal findings on coronary angiography, and no coronary risk factors). Coronary blood flow was measured with an intracoronary Doppler catheter. The papaverine and acetylcholine infusions were repeated in 14 patients after an intracoronary infusion of L-arginine (160 μmol/min for 20 minutes). There was a significant negative correlation between aging and the peak coronary blood flow response evoked by acetylcholine. However, there was no correlation between aging and the peak coronary blood flow response to papaverine. The peak coronary blood flow response evoked by acetylcholine was normalized after L-arginine infusion. These authors concluded that aging selectively impairs endothelium-dependent coronary microvascular function and that the impairment could be restored by administration of L-arginine, a precursor of nitric oxide.

Antioxidant Therapy in Endothelial Dysfunction

Levine and colleagues[37] in Boston, Massachusetts, hypothesized that an antioxidant, ascorbic acid, would improve endothelium-dependent arterial dilation in patients with CAD. Brachial artery endothelium-dependent dilation in response to hyperemia was assessed by high-resolution vascular ultrasound before and 2 hours after oral administration of either 2 g of ascorbic acid or placebo in 46 patients with documented CAD (Figure 1-8). Plasma ascorbic acid concentration increased 2.5-fold 2 hours after treatment. In the prospectively identified patients with an abnormal baseline response, ascorbic acid produced marked improvement in dilation, whereas placebo had no effect. Ascorbic acid had no effect on hyperemic flow or arterial dilation to sublingual nitroglycerin. These data suggest that ascorbic acid reverses endothelial vasomotor dysfunction in the brachial circulation of patients with CAD. They suggest that increased oxidative stress contributes to endothelial dysfunction in patients with atherosclerosis and that endothelial dysfunction may respond to antioxidant therapy.

Oxidative Stress as a Determinant of Coronary Endothelial Dysfunction

Anderson and colleagues[38] in Alberta, Canada, evaluated endothelium-dependent coronary vasomotion in response to acetylcholine (10^{-8}–10^{-6}

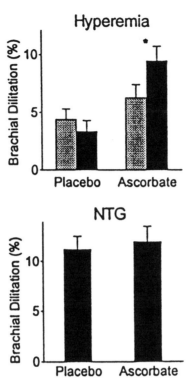

FIGURE 1-8. Brachial artery dilation in response to hyperemia or nitroglycerin (NTG). Patients referred for cardiac catheterization underwent brachial ultrasound imaging according to the protocol described in "Methods." The dilation response to hyperemia (top) was measured before (shaded bars) and after (solid bars) placebo (n = 20) or ascorbic acid (n = 26) administration. The response to NTG (bottom) was determined after placebo or ascorbic acid as described in "Methods." Data are presented as mean ± SEM. *Significant effect of ascorbate treatment compared with placebo, p = .0007 by ANOVA. Reproduced with permission from Levine et al.[37]

mol/L) in 23 hypercholesterolemic patients (mean age 56 years) after 1 year of therapy with the American Heart Association Step I Diet (7 patients), lovastatin plus cholestyramine (7 patients), or lovastatin plus the antioxidant probucol (9 patients). The susceptibility of LDL to oxidation was determined by measuring the lag phase of conjugated diene formation induced by copper. Patients treated with lovastatin plus probucol had prolongation of the lag phase (to 263 minutes) compared with diet alone (91 minutes) or lovastatin plus cholestyramine (118 minutes) (Figure 1-9). By multivariate analysis, the lag phase was a significant predictor of acetylcholine vasomotor response, independent of the effect of cholesterol-lowering treatment. Thus, in patients treated with lipid-lowering agents, the vasodilator response to acetycholine is related to the susceptibility of LDL to oxidation. These findings indicate that oxidative stress is an important determinant of the coronary endothelial dysfunction observed in patients with atherosclerosis and hypercholesterolemia.

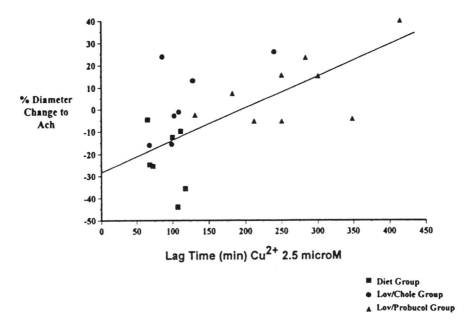

FIGURE 1-9. Relation between endothelium-dependent coronary vasomotion and the lag time to conjugated diene formation after 1 year of therapy. Increased lag time indicates decreased susceptibility to oxidation. Ach indicates acetylcholine. r = .62, p = .002. Reproduced with permission from Anderson et al.[38]

Brachial Artery Vasoactivity: Correlation with Cholesterol Levels

Current National Cholesterol Education Program guidelines consider desirable total and LDL cholesterol levels to be less than 200 and less than 160 mg/dL, respectively, for healthy individuals without multiple coronary risk factors. To determine the extent to which these levels affect vascular function, Vogel and associates[39] from Baltimore, Maryland, assessed flow-mediated (endothelium-dependent) brachial artery vasoactivity noninvasively before, during, and after cholesterol lowering using simvastatin (10 mg/day) in 7 healthy middle-aged men with cholesterol levels meeting current recommendations. Flow-mediated brachial artery vasoactivity was measured using 7.5 MHz ultrasound and expressed as percent diameter change from baseline to hyperemic conditions (1 minute after 5 minutes of blood pressure cuff arterial occlusion). After 2, 4, and 12 weeks of cholesterol-lowering therapy, flow-mediated vasoactivity rose from 5.0% ± 3.6% at baseline to 10.5% ± 5.6%, 13.3% ± 4.3%, and 15.7% ± 4.9%, respectively, as cholesterol fell from 200 ± 12 to 161 ± 18, 169 ± 16, and 153 ± 11 mg/dL (Figure 1-10). Vasoactivity and cholesterol returned to baseline levels 12 weeks after simvastatin discontinuation. Overall, vasoactivity was found to correlate inversely with cholesterol levels. These data suggest that flow-mediated brachial artery vasoactivity responds rapidly to changes in cholesterol levels and that endothelial function improves by lowering cholesterol levels below recommendations of current guidelines.

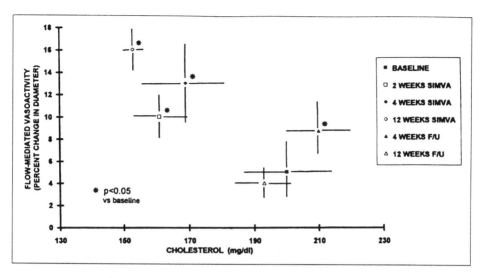

FIGURE 1-10. Mean brachial artery vasoactivity and corresponding total cholesterol levels are plotted for measurements obtained at baseline, during simvastatin (SIMVA) treatment, and during follow-up (F/U). Reproduced with permission from Vogel et al.[39]

Quinapril Improves Endothelial Vasomotor Dysfunction

Mancini and colleagues[40] for the Trial on Reversing ENdothelial Dysfunction Study Investigators (TREND Trial) determined whether the ACE inhibitor quinapril might improve endothelial dysfunction in normotensive patients with CAD and no congestive heart failure (CHF) or major lipid abnormalities. Using a double-blind, randomized, placebo-controlled design, investigators measured the effects of quinapril (40 mg daily) on coronary artery diameter responses to acetylcholine using quantitative coronary angiography. The primary response variable was the net change in the acetylcholine-provoked constriction of target segments between the baseline and 6-month follow-up angiograms. The constrictive responses to acetylcholine were comparable in the placebo (n = 54) and quinapril (n = 51) groups at baseline. After 6 months, only the quinapril group showed significant net improvements in response to acetylcholine (Figure 1-11). Thus, in this study, ACE inhibition with quinapril improved endothelial dysfunction in patients who were normotensive and who did not have severe hyperlipidemia or evidence of CHF. These protective effects may be due to attenuation of the superoxide-generating effects of angiotensin II and/or enhancement of endothelial cell release of nitric oxide as a result of diminished breakdown of bradykinin.

Impaired Endothelial Function in Hypertension

The objective of this investigation was to evaluate the role of hypertension in endothelial function, changes in which are known to be an early event of

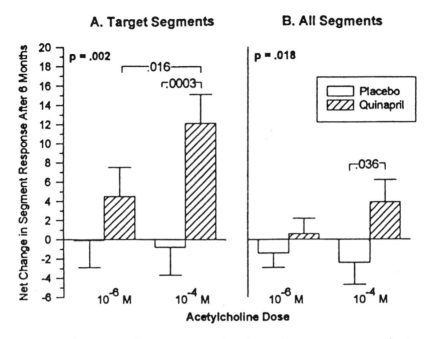

FIGURE 1-11. A, The primary efficacy parameter (net change in segment response after 6 months in the target segment, expressed as a percent ± SE, plotted on y axis) for 2 concentrations of acetylcholine (x axis). B, Analysis of all segments. Overall differences in response between the placebo and quinapril groups were significant for the target segment analysis (P = .002) and for all segments (P = .018). At the 10^{-4} mol/L dose, the difference between the placebo and quinapril groups was significant for both the target vessel analysis (P < .0003) and for all groups (P = .036). Reproduced with permission from Mancini et al.[40]

atherosclerosis. Iiyama and associates[41] from Suita, Japan, assessed endothelial function in 13 individuals with normal blood pressure (BP) and 13 individuals with essential hypertension who had never been treated for hypertension or hyperlipidemia and who had no history of smoking or coronary or cerebrovascular disease. B-mode ultrasonography was used to measure the diameter of the brachial artery. Endothelium-dependent dilatation was assessed as the change in diameter of the artery during reactive hyperemia. Endothelium-independent dilatation was evoked as a control by sublingual administration of isosorbide dinitrate. Despite similar ages and lipid and glucose levels in the study groups, endothelium-dependent dilatation was less in patients with hypertension (13% ± 1.6%) than in individuals with BP (19% ± 1.9%), whereas isosorbide dinitrate-induced changes were similar. Systolic and diastolic BP we're significantly correlated with endothelium-dependent vasodilatation, but not with the change by isosorbide dinitrate. These results suggest that endothelial dysfunction exists in patients with hypertension and precedes overt atherosclerotic disease.

Endothelial Vasoconstriction in Cocaine Use

Cocaine use has been associated with AMI, stroke, and intestinal infarction. Previously demonstrated effects of the drug, including increased heart rate and blood pressure and increased vascular tone may not fully explain the sporadic nature of these vascular events where the occurrence of ischemia is remote from acute administration. Havranek and colleagues[42] from Denver, Colorado, Los Angeles, California, and Dallas, Texas, evaluated endothelium-dependent vasorelaxation in long-term users of cocaine as a potential mechanism for such events remote from acute drug use. Using plethysmography, they evaluated the change in forearm blood flow in response to intra-arterial acetylcholine and nitroprusside in 10 long-term cocaine users and 13 control subjects of similar age who had not used cocaine. Mean forearm blood flow during acetylcholine infusion was significantly lower in cocaine users than in control subjects. During nitroprusside infusion, there was no difference between cocaine users and control subjects. Cigarette smoking did not explain the differences between cocaine users and control subjects. Acetylcholine elicited coronary vasoconstriction in 8 of 10 subjects who were long-term cocaine users. These authors concluded that endothelium-dependent vasorelaxation is impaired in long-term users of cocaine, and that this endothelial dysfunction is a potential mechanism for vasoconstrictive events remote from acute drug use.

Arterial Remodeling in the Superficial Femoral Artery

Pasterkamp and colleagues[43] in Utrecht, The Netherlands, assessed local arterial remodeling by analyzing 45 artery segments at 0.5-cm intervals over a length of 10 to 15 cm in 20 patients studied by 30-MHz intravascular ultrasound before balloon angioplasty of the superficial femoral artery (370 cross sections) and 25 femoral artery segments postmortem (551 cross sections). In each cross-section, the area surrounded by the internal elastic lamina and the plaque area were measured. The internal elastic lamina area was larger in the cross-section with the largest plaque area than in the cross section with the smallest plaque area. A significant positive correlation was found between plaque area and internal elastic lamina area for the pooled data (Figure 1-12). In 12 of 20 and 16 of 25 individual arterial segments, there was no significant correlation between plaque area and internal elastic lamina for either intravascular ultrasound or histology, respectively. There was a large variation in the correlation of the regression of plaque to internal elastic lamina area and slope (Figure 1-13). Thus, this study demonstrates that in the majority of atherosclerotic femoral arteries, significant compensatory enlargement could not be demonstrated. The data suggest that arterial remodeling in response to plaque formation may vary among individuals.

Atherogenesis/Thrombosis

Hemostasis, Thrombin Markers, and Other Risk Factors for Coronary Artery Disease

Studies suggest that thrombosis is important in the progression of athero-sclerotic lesions. Biochemical markers prothrombin fragment 1-2 and fibrino-

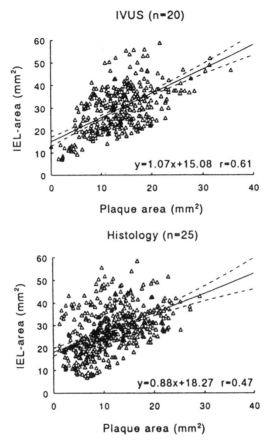

FIGURE 1-12. Relation between the plaque area and the area encompassed by the internal elastic lamina (IEL-area) for the pooled cross sections obtained with intravascular ultrasound (IVUS; left) and history (right). (IVUS: 370 cross sections, y = 1.07x + 15.08, r = .61, p<.01; histology: 551 cross sections, y = 0.88x + 18.27, r = .47, p<.01). Note that the slope of the regression line is close to 1.0. Reproduced with permission from Pasterkamp et al.[43]

peptide A reflect *in vivo* thrombin generation and activity, respectively. As such, they are markers that might be associated with cardiovascular risks. From the Cardiovascular Health Study, a cohort study of 5201 persons over 65 years of age, Cushman and colleagues[44] in Colchester, Vermont, selected 399 persons free of clinical cardiovascular disease at the baseline examination for study of specialized markers of hemostasis. The investigators reported the cross-sectional relationship of the thrombin markers to cardiovascular disease, risk factors, and measures of subclinical cardiovascular disease. The range of fragment 1-2 was 0.12 to 0.85 nmol/L. The range of fibrinopeptide A was 0.9 to 44.1 μg/L. High levels of fragment 1-2 and fibrinopeptide A were associated with age, with levels higher in women than in men. Fragment 1-2 was associated with smoking; high levels of triglyceride, creatinine, and C-reactive protein; and low levels of glucose. Fibrinopeptide A was associated with C-reactive protein and the apolipoprotein(a) and lower ankle-brachial index. There were no significant associations of the thrombin markers with race, fibrinogen, alco-

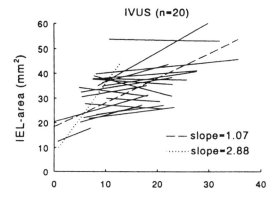

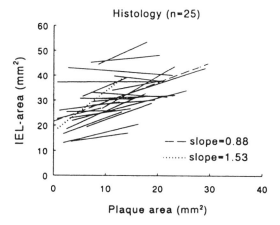

FIGURE 1-13. Linear regressions of the individual arterial segments, the pooled data, and the cross sections that contained the least amount of plaque (reference site, dotted lines) obtained with intravascular ultrasound (IVUS; top) and histology (bottom). In the case of the reference cross sections, the steep slopes (2.88 and 1.53) of the regression line are compatible with variations in original vessel size rather than with overcompensatory enlargement. The length of the regression lines represents the ranges in plaque area. IEL-area indicates area encompassed by the internal elastic lamina. Reproduced with permission from Pasterkamp et al.[43]

hol consumption, diabetes, or most measures of subclinical cardiovascular disease. The study findings support the hypothesis that physiological interrelationships exist between cardiac risk factors, hemostatis, inflammation, and the progression of atherosclerosis.

Factor VII Coagulant Activity and Cardiovascular Risk Factors

Factor VII coagulant activity has been found to be related to cardiovascular risk factors and may be an independent predictor of CAD. Whether these associations are due to changes in factor VII activation rather than factor VII concentration remain unclear. Therefore, Scarabin and coinvestigators[45] in Paris,

France, investigated the relation between activated factor VII and CAD risk factors in healthy subjects (336 men and 348 women) aged 25 to 64 years. In addition to direct quantitation of activated factor VII, by use of a recombinant, truncated tissue factor, factor VII activity and factor VII antigen levels were measured by standard procedures. There were highly significant correlations between the 3 techniques of factor VII assay. Plasma factor VII coagulant activity and activated factor VII levels increased with age in both sexes, but the increase was significantly greater in women than in men. At younger ages, mean values of factor VII coagulant activity and activated factor VII were significantly lower in women than in men, whereas at older ages, the reverse was observed. After adjustment for age, postmenopausal women had significantly higher mean levels of factor VII coagulant activity and activated factor VII than did premenopausal women. Hormone replacement therapy significantly reversed the rise in factor VII coagulant activity in postmenopausal women, and a similar trend in activated factor VII was also observed. Age, sex, and menopause-related changes in factor VII coagulant activity were partly explained by a higher proportion of fully active factor VII molecules, as indicated by significant differences in activated factor VII activity to factor VII antigen ratio. Oral contraceptive use was associated with high factor VII coagulant activity level, and this effect was mainly due to an increase in factor VII antigen. Levels of activated factor VII were positively correlated with serum cholesterol concentrations in both sexes. There were no strong associations between activated factor VII levels and other CAD risk factors, including smoking habits, alcohol consumption, blood pressure, obesity, glucose, triglycerides, and serum lipoprotein(a) concentration. Multiple regression analysis showed independent effects of age and cholesterol levels on activated factor VII in men, whereas age and menopausal status were the main predictors of activated factor VII in women. These results show that factor VII activation is associated with CAD risk factors. These findings are consistent with a possible role of factor VII in the pathogenesis of CAD. Furthermore, the investigators' data suggested that the dramatic rise in CAD incidence in postmenopausal women, as well as the cardioprotective effect of estrogen, may be mediated through factor VII and blood coagulation.

Visceral Fat and Plasma Hemostatic Factors

The associations between abdominal visceral fat and the plasma hemostatic system were examined in 38-year-old healthy men (n = 52) by Targher and Associates[46] in Verona, Italy, with a wide range of fatness and fat distribution. Plasma hemostatic factors and metabolic parameters, including glucose tolerance, were measured; body fatness and adipose tissue distribution were assessed by using computed tomography. The men with more visceral fat had a less favorable metabolic profile than did the men with less visceral fat. They also had significantly higher plasma fibrinogen, factor VIII clotting activity, tissue-type plasminogen activator antigen and plasminogen activator inhibitor-1 activity, and lower basal tissue-type plasminogen activator activity. After adjustment for plasma insulin, the men with larger abdominal visceral fat area still had significantly higher plasminogen activator inhibitor-1 activity, but no difference was found in any of the other hemostatic factors. In multiple linear regression analysis, abdominal visceral fat area was a positive predictor of plasminogen activator inhibitor-1 activity, but it failed to show any significant association with other hemostatic factors after controlling for plasma insulin. These results suggest the presence of relations between abdominal visceral fat and several hemostatic factors that are largely mediated by concomitant alterations in plasma insulin concentration. In addition, these results suggested that abdominal accumulation of visceral fat is an independent predictor of plasminogen activator inhibitor-1 activity.

The Association Between Antithrombin and Atherosclerosis

Antithrombin is a potent inhibitor of thrombotic tendency. Whether atherosclerotic disease is associated with high or low antithrombin is unclear. Studies of the relation between antithrombin and the presence of arterial disease have shown contrasting results. van der Bom and coinvestigators[47] in Rotterdam, The Netherlands, evaluated a single-center, population-based cohort study of 7983 subjects aged 55 years and older for the association between atherosclerosis and antithrombin. The ratio of ankle-to-arm blood pressure is a graded marker for atherosclerosis and provides the opportunity to investigate nonlinear associations. In the first 1427 participants of the Rotterdam Study who did not use anticoagulants, both antithrombin and the ratio of ankle-to-arm blood pressure were measured. In men, the association between the 2 was quadratic: antithrombin activity was increased in men with moderate peripheral arterial atherosclerosis compared with those without; in men with more severe atherosclerosis, it was decreased. (Figure 1-14). In women, the association was linear: a decreased ratio of ankle-to-arm pressure was associated with increased antithrombin activity. These associations were independent of smoking, body mass index, serum lipids, fibrinogen, and factor VIIc. The investigators proposed that antithrombin activity rises in response to increased risk of cardiovascular disease and also in response to the presence of atherosclerosis, whereas antithrombin may decrease with increasing severity of the atherosclerotic process in men. This may explain the contrasting results found in previous studies. Changes in antithrombin over time might be useful in predicting the risk of cardiovascular disease and progression.

Vitamin E Inhibits Platelet Aggregation and Adhesion

Freedman and colleagues[48] in Boston, Massachusetts, evaluated mechanisms by which vitamin E inhibits platelet aggregation and adhesion. This inhibition of platelet aggregation and adhesion may contribute to the protective effect that vitamin E (α-tocopherol) exerts in patients with CAD. Using gel-filtered platelets derived from platelet-rich plasma treated with α-tocopherol (500 μmol/L) or vehicle (0.5% ethanol), the authors found that inhibition of platelet aggregation by α-tocopherol was closely linked to its incorporation into

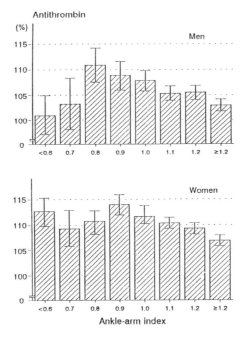

FIGURE 1-14. Antithrombin activity by ankle-arm index for men and women. Values are mean and SE, adjusted for age. Reproduced with permission from van der Bom et al.[47]

platelets. Platelet incorporation of α-tocopherol was associated with significant reduction in platelet sensitivity to aggregation by adenosine 5′-diphosphate, arachidonic acid, and phorbol ester by approximately 0.15-, 2-, and 100-fold, respectively. Platelets treated similarly with a butylated hydroxytoluene, another potent lipid-soluble antioxidant, did not demonstrate any change in sensitivity to these agents. Platelet incorporation of α-tocopherol inhibited phorbol ester-induced stimulation of platelet protein kinase C in 15 normal subjects; oral supplementation with α-tocopherol (400 to 1200 IU per day) resulted in an increase in platelet α-tocopherol that correlated with marked inhibition of phorbol ester-mediated platelet aggregation. Platelets derived from these subjects after supplementation demonstrated apparent complete inhibition of protein kinase C stimulation by phorbol ester. These data suggest that platelet incorporation of α-tocopherol at levels attained with oral supplementation is associated with inhibition of platelet aggregation through a protein kinase C-dependent mechanism. These data may help explain 1 possible mechanism for the observed beneficial effect of α-tocopherol in preventing the development of progressive CAD in patients.

Implications of Silent, Multiple Lacunar Stroke

Silent lacunar stroke, often found in the elderly, has been proposed as a predisposing condition for clinically overt stroke. However, the risk factors related to this condition have not been thoroughly studied. Kario and coinvestigators[49] in Hyogo, Japan, conducted brain MRI and measured the levels of fibrinogen, molecular markers of coagulation activation and endothelial cell damage, and lipid profiles, including lipoprotein(a), in 178 asymptomatic, high-risk Japanese subjects (aged 44–93 years). The investigators also studied 32 symptomatic patients with lacunar stroke. The prevalence of silent lacunar stroke increased with age up to 85 years, but decreased with age in those 85 years old and older. Of the 160 elderly subjects, 84 (53%) had one or more lacunar infarcts, and the remaining 76 were considered as the nonlacunar group. Fibrinogen and F1 + 2 levels in the silent lacunar group were significantly higher than those in the nonlacunar group. Mean lipoprotein(a) levels and the prevalence of subjects with a lipoprotein(a) level greater than 30 mg/dL were significantly higher in the symptomatic lacunar group than in the nonlacunar group, whereas these levels in the silent lacunar group were intermediate to those in the other 2 groups. When the investigators further classified the silent lacunar group into these 3 subgroups based on the number of lacunes, levels of lipoprotein(a) and markers of coagulation activation and thrombomodulin were significantly higher, and lipoprotein(a) levels greater than 30 mg/dL were more common in the numerous-lacune than in the few-lacune subgroups. The investigators concluded that silent lacunar stroke was often found in asymptomatic, high-risk, elderly Japanese patients and that silent multiple lacunar stroke was associated with hypercoagulability, endothelial cell damage, and high levels of lipoprotein(a).

Thrombotic Risk with Antiphospholipid Antibodies

Antiphospholipid antibodies are associated with thrombosis, but the mechanisms of this thrombotic tendency are unknown. Reverter and coinvestigators[50] in Barcelona, Spain, investigated the ability of antiphospholipid antibodies to induce tissue factor expression on human monocytes in 56 patients: 12 with systemic lupus erythematosus and antiphospholipid antibodies and previous thrombosis, 12 with systemic lupus and antiphospholipid antibodies but no thrombosis, 15 with lupus without antiphospholipid antibodies or thrombosis, 11 with primary antiphospholipid syndrome with thrombosis, and 6 asymptomatic subjects with antiphospholipid antibodies. A double direct immunofluorescence technique was used, and procoagulant activity in viable and disrupted cells was measured after plasma incubation for 6 hours to 37°C with normal mononuclear cells. Hemostasis regulatory proteins, prothrombin fragment 1 + 2, and prothrombin-antithrombin III complex levels were determined. Increased tissue-factor expression and procoagulant activity were observed using plasma samples from lupus patients with antiphospholipid antibodies and thrombosis and from primary antiphospholipid syndrome patients, but not in the patients with lupus and antiphospholipid antibodies but no thrombosis, patients with lupus without antiphospholipid antibodies, or asymptomatic patients with antiphospholipid antibodies. Purified antiphospholipid immunoglobulins from 1 primary antiphospholipid syndrome and 2 lupus patients added to normal plasma showed a significant increase in both

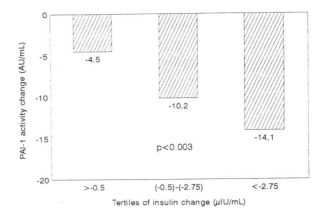

FIGURE 1-15. Bar graph shows median PAI-1 activity decrease from NCEP to MUFA diets, according to tertiles of insulin decrease from NCEP to MUFA diets. Reproduced with permission from Lopez-Segura et al.[51]

tissue-factor expression and procoagulant activity compared with purified anti-phospholipid antibodies from 2 lupus patients without thrombosis. The addition of nonspecific IgG from 3 lupus patients without antiphospholipid antibodies and from 3 control subjects did not increase tissue factor expression. Low free-protein S was seen in 8 patients. Increased tissue factor expression and low free-protein S correlated with thrombosis and with higher prothrombin fragment 1 + 2 and thrombin-antithrombin III values. These observations may contribute to a further understanding of the thrombotic risk in antiphospholipid antibody patients.

Effects of Diet on Coagulation and Hemostasis

An increase in levels of plasma plasminogen activator inhibitor type 1 is one of the hemostatic alterations in patients with CAD. Despite growing interests in the fibrinolytic system, few studies have been undertaken to determine the effect exerted on it by the different dietary fatty acids. Lopez-Segura and colleagues[51] in Cordoba, Spain, investigated the effect of a monounsaturated fat-rich diet in comparison with a low-fat diet (National Cholesterol Education Program Step I Diet), on factors involved in blood coagulation and fibrinolysis. The investigators also determined the effect of dietary cholesterol on these blood parameters. Twenty-one young, male, healthy volunteers followed 2 low-fat/high-carbohydrate diets for 24 days each with 115 or 281 mg of cholesterol per 1000 KCAL per day and 2 oleic acid-enriched diets with the same dietary cholesterol as the low-fat/high-carbohydrate diets. Plasma levels of fibrinogen, thrombin-antithrombin complexes, prothrombin fragments 1 + 2, plasminogen, α_2 antiplasmin, and tPA were not significantly different among the experimental diets used in this study. Consumption of the diet rich in monounsaturated fat resulted in a significant decrease in both plasminogen activator inhibitor-1 plasma activity and antigenic plasminogen activator inhibitor-1 compared with the carbohydrate rich diet. (Figure 1-15). The addition of dietary cholesterol to each of these diets did not result in any significant additional effect. Changes in insulin level and plasminogen activator inhibitor-1 activity were possibly correlated. In conclusion, consumption of diets rich in monounsaturated fatty acids decreases plasminogen activator inhibitor-1 plasma activity, which is accompanied by a parallel decrease in plasma insulin levels.

Effects of Diet and Exercise in Overweight, Postmenopausal Women

Svendsen and coworkers[52] in Kolding, Denmark, assessed the short- and long-term effects of an energy-restrictive diet, with or without exercise, on plasminogen activator inhibitor-1 antigen and plasminogen activator inhibitor-1 activity, tissue-type plasminogen activator antigen, and fibrinogen serum levels. Healthy, overweight postmenopausal women were randomly assigned to 1 of 3 groups: control, 4200 kJ/d diet, or 4200 kJ/d diet with combined aerobic and anaerobic exercise. Plasminogen activator inhibitor-1 activity and plasminogen activator inhibitor-1 antigen, tissue-type plasminogen activator antigen, and fibrinogen levels were measured at baseline, after a 12-week intervention, and after a further 6-month follow-up. Plasminogen activator inhibitor-1 antigen and activity and tissue-type plasminogen activator antigen were positively correlated with serum triglyceride levels, the abdominal-to-total-body fat ratio, fasting blood glucose, and systolic blood pressure, and they were negatively correlated with HDL cholesterol and sex-hormone binding globulin. The diet led to profound decreases and normalization of plasminogen activator inhibitor-1 activity, plasminogen activator inhibitor-1 antigen, and tissue-type plasminogen activator antigen, but exercise conferred no additional effect. Fibrinogen did not change. In follow-up, no significant changes were seen. In conclusion, plasminogen activator inhibitor-1 antigen and activity, as well as tissue-type plasminogen activator antigen, appear to be part of the metabolic syndrome X. The diet appeared to make the blood less thrombogenic in the short term, but exercise added no effect.

Aspirin as an Antithrombin Inhibitor in Hypercholesterolemia

Recent evidence indicates that aspirin inhibits thrombin generation in clotting blood. Szczeklik and coinvestigators[53] in Kracow, Poland, noticed that this effect was less pronounced in patients with hypercholesterolemia. The aim of their study was to prove this observation. The effects of aspirin on thrombin generation were evaluated in (1) 46 healthy volunteers, 2 hours after ingestion of a single 500-mg dose and (2) 28 survivors of myocardial infarction who took 300 mg aspirin per day for 2 weeks. In both populations, 2 well-matched subgroups were distinguished, by using a serum cholesterol level of 6.2 mmol/L (240 mg/dL) and LDL cholesterol of 4.0 mmol/L (155 mg/dL) as borderline. Thrombin generation was monitored *ex vivo* in blood emerging from a skin microvascular injury and additionally in a single-dose study *in vitro* in re-calcified plasma. Aspirin depressed thrombin generation in the group of sub-jects with serum cholesterol less than 6.2 mmol/L and LDL cholesterol less than 4.0 mmol/L, but not in the group with high blood cholesterol levels. Inhibi-tory effects of aspirin were more pronounced after the 2-week treatment than after a single dose. There was a significant correlation between total serum cholesterol or LDL cholesterol and total amount of thrombin generated after aspirin treatment. In subjects with high blood cholesterol levels, thrombin gen-eration was not affected by aspirin. Blunting of aspirin action in hypercholes-terolemia might be explained by (1) alterations in platelet lipid protein matrix that render their membrane protein less accessible for acetylation by aspirin, and (2) changes in composition and structure of plasmin lipoproteins that diminish the chance of aspirin to interact with thrombin.

Fibrinogen Concentrations and Lipid Profiles

Hyperfibrinogenemia and dyslipoproteinemia characterized by reduced HDL_2 cholesterol and elevated levels of small dense LDL particles are risk factors for CAD. However, the relation between fibrinogen and lipoproteins, in particular LDL subfractions, is uncertain. Halle and coworkers[54] in Freiburg, Germany, therefore measured serum fibrinogen levels and serum concentra-tions of cholesterol and apolipoproteins of VLDL, IDL, 6 LDL, and 2 HDL subfractions by using the technique of density gradient ultracentrifugation in 132 nonsmoking men without evidence of CAD or AMI. When the individuals were divided into quartiles according to their fibrinogen values, men within the highest fibrinogen quartile had significantly higher concentrations of small dense LDL, apolipoprotein B, and lower concentrations of HDL_2 than did men in the lower fibrinogen quartiles. Multivariant regression analysis revealed that the association between fibrinogen in small, dense LDL particles was indepen-dent of serum triglycerides, cholesterol, body mass index, and age. In contrast, the relation between fibrinogen and HDL_2 cholesterol was primary influenced by triglyceride and cholesterol and not independently influenced by fibrinogen. There were no significant differences between the quartiles in terms of insulin, glucose, insulin resistance, free fatty acids, lipoprotein(a) and blood pressure. This study showed that fibrinogen is associated with expression of a more atherogenic LDL subfraction phenotype independent of body mass index, age, other serum lipids, and insulin resistance in a healthy male nonsmoking popu-lation. The reason for this association is uncertain. These findings reinforce the evidence that fibrinogen should be determined when assessing coronary risk.

Coagulation and Dyslipidemia

Tissue-factor pathway inhibitor, a Kunitz-type inhibitor of the extrinsic coagulation pathway; factor VII coagulant; and the fibrinolytic factors plasmin-ogen activator inhibitor-1 and tPA have been studied in various hyperlipidemias. In this study by Zitoun and associates,[55] when compared with a normal lipidemic group, mean tissue-factor inhibitor activity was 70% higher in type IIa hyperlipidemia, 36% higher in type IIb hyperlipidemia, and lower by 13% in type IV hyperlipidemia. Tissue-factor inhibitor was correlated with LDL cholesterol, total cholesterol, apolipoproteins AI and B and lipoprotein(a). Tissue-factor inhibitor was negatively correlated with the triglyceride levels: correlation was dependent on LDL cholesterol and HDL cholesterol levels, which were decreased in type IV hyperlipidemia. Factor VII coagulant activity was increased by 30% in both type IV and type IIb hyperlipidemia and was correlated with triglyceride levels. Factor VIIa was not significantly increased in any group when compared with the control group. Factor VIIc was correlated with triglyceride level, whereas factor VIIa was not. Interestingly, factor VIIa was correlated with factor VIIc in the control group, as well as in the hyperlipidemic group. These results favor the hypothesis that higher factor VIIc concentrations in hyperlipidemic patients are likely due to enhancement or synthesis of factor VII and that a part of this factor VII circulates in an activated chemical form. Compared with the control group, plasminogen activator inhibitor activity was 2-fold higher in type IIa hyperlipidemia, 3-fold higher in type IIb hyperlipidemia, and 4-fold higher in type IV hyperlipidemia. Plasminogen activator inhibitor-1 activity correlated with triglyceride levels, apoprotein B levels, and total cholesterol levels. These correlations were dependent on apolipoprotein B and probably reflect the correlation between plasminogen activated inhibitor-1 and VLDL. In contrast, tPA level was normal in the different hyperlipidemias. No correlation was found between tissue-factor inhibitor, factor VIIc, and plasminogen activator inhibitor-1. Variation of tissue-factor inhibitor activity appears to be related to the variations of its main lipoprotein carriers: LDL, HDL, and lipoprotein (a). The association in hypertriglyceridemic patients of hypercoagulability and hyperfibrinolysis may explain thrombosis predisposition of some of these patients. The investigators suggest it would be interesting to study the increased levels of endothelium-derived tissue factor pathway inhibitor in plasma induced by the injection of heparin.

Triglyceride-Rich Lipoproteins and the Coagulation Pathway

In vitro studies in purified plasma systems have suggested that triglyceride-rich proteins such as chylomicrons, VLDL, and their remnants promote activation of factor VII through activated factor XII and the intrinsic coagulation pathway. Silveira and coworkers[56] in Stockholm, Sweden, specifically examined the roles of factors XII, XI, and IX in activation of factor VII during alimentary lipemia *in vivo* in humans and addressed the issue of whether generation of activated factor VII is accompanied by increased thrombin production. For this purpose factor XIIa, factor VIII activation peptide, VIIa prothrombin fragment 1 + 2, and thrombin-antithrombin complex were determined in plasma samples taken before, and 3, 6, and 9 hours after an intake of a mixed meal type of oral fat-load in 24 healthy men. The VIIa response to fat intake was also determined in 7 patients with single coagulation-factor deficiency, of whom 2 were deficient in factor XII, 2 in factor XI, and 3 in factor VIII. Post-prandial activation of factors VIII and VII occurred in the healthy individuals, whereas the plasmin levels of factor XIIa did not change in response to the test meal. Factor VIIa increased in the postprandial period in the 2 factor XII-deficient patients who underwent the oral fat-tolerance test, but appeared to remain unchanged in the factor XI- and factor VIII-deficient patients. There-fore, the current concept that the activation of factor XII plays a pivotal role in initiating the sequences of events linking postprandial lipemia to activation factor VII is contradicted by the present study. Whether activation of factor XI by triglyceride-rich lipoproteins initiates these reactions needs to be demon-strated in future studies.

Coagulation Pathway Inhibitors

Tissue-factor pathway inhibitor, a protease with 3 tandem Kunitz-type domains, inhibits the initial reaction of the tissue-factor-mediated coagulation pathway. Tissue-factor pathway inhibitor occurs in a free and a lipoprotein-associated form in plasma as well as an endothelial cell-associated form on vascular walls. In a previous study, Kokawa and associates[57] in Osaka, Japan, had demonstrated that free-form tissue-factor pathway inhibitor activity was lower in hyperlipidemic patients. In the present study, the investigators estab-lished a new enzyme immunoassay method for measuring free-form tissue-factor pathway inhibitor antigen; this new method used a monoclonal antibody that recognized the K3 domain of free-form tissue-factor pathway inhibitor, but not lipoprotein-associated tissue-factor pathway inhibitor. Free-form tis-sue-factor pathway inhibitor antigen was significantly lower in hyperlipidemic patients compared with those in normolipidemic individuals. The investigators applied this new method to measure the amount of endothelial cell-associated tissue-factor pathway inhibitor, which can be released by heparin injection, as "free-form tissue-factor pathway inhibitor." The investigators found that free-form tissue-factor pathway inhibitor antigen in plasma was positively corre-lated with the endothelial cell-associated form. These results indicated that both of these forms of tissue-factor pathway inhibitor were in equilibrium *in vivo* and that the new method could be used for assessing changes in the levels of endothelial cell-associated tissue-factor pathway inhibitor antigen and, hence, for assessing thrombotic tendencies in various disease states.

Gemfibrozil—Treatment of Combined Hyperlipoproteinemia

Hypertriglyceridemia is linked to impaired fibrinolytic function, and lipid-lowering treatment with fibric acid derivatives could hypothetically improve fibrinolysis in this condition. Bröijersen and coworkers[58] in Stockholm, Swe-den, conducted a double-blind, placebo-controlled, crossover study of gemfi-brozil treatment on fibrinolytic function in 21 men with combined hyperlipo-proteinemia. Measurements were performed at rest and during mental stress, and after venous occlusion. The patients had clearly disturbed fibrinolytic function, with elevated plasminogen activator inhibitor-1 activity at rest. Gemfibrozil reduced plasma total and VLDL cholesterol, as well as all triglyceride fractions, whereas HDL cholesterol increased. Total triglyceride levels were reduced by 57%. Fasting serum insulin levels were not altered by gemfibrozil treatment. Plasma levels of plasminogen activator inhibitor-1 activity and tissue-type plasminogen activator activity or antigen were unaffected by gemfibrozil treatment both at rest and during the provocations. The levels of D-dimer, plasmin/antiplasmin complex, and fibrinogen were also unaffected by gemfibrozil treatment. Mental stress elevated tissue-type plasminogen activator activity and lowered plasminogen activator inhibitor-1, but treatment effects did not differ by analysis on change in values. Venous occlusion reduced plasminogen activator inhibitor-1 activity, whereas tissue-type plasminogen activator activity and plasmin/antiplasmin complex increased during both treatments. Thus, gemfibrozil treatment did not improve fibrinolysis or lower fibrinogen levels in men with combined hyperlipoproteinemia despite marked reduction of plasma triglyceride levels. It seemed unlikely that improved fibrinolysis explained the primary preventive effect of gemfibrozil.

Lipid Metabolism and Genetics

Cellular Markers in Hypercholesterolemia

Mononuclear phagocytes play a major role in the development of vascular lesions in atherogenesis. The goal of a study by Rothe and associates[59] in Regensburg, Germany, was to characterize circulating blood monocyte subpopulations as potential cellular markers of systemic immunologic abnormalities in hypercholesterolemia. In normal subjects, 3-parameter immunophenotyping of whole blood revealed that 61% of monocytes showed "bright" expression of the lipopolysaccharide receptor and Fc gamma receptor without expression of Fc gamma-RIII. Other monocyte subsets were characterized by the simultaneous expression of both Fc gamma-R, isolated expression of Fc gamma-RIII, or high expression of CD33 with only dim expression of CD14, respectively. The smallest subset of monocytes differed from the predominant population of CD14 Bright CD64+ CD16−− monocytes by additional expression of neural cell adhesion molecule. In a group of hypercholesterolemic patients, HDL cholesterol levels were negatively correlated to the population size of CD64− CD16+− monocytes. In both healthy subjects and hypercholesterolemic patients, the rare apolipoprotein E3E4 and E4E4 phenotypes were associated with a tendency toward a larger population CD64−− and CD16+ monocytes. Expression of the varied activation antigen CD45 RA by peripheral blood mononuclear phagocyte showed a positive correlation to plasma levels of the atherogenic lipoprotein LDL and lipoprotein(a). These data suggested that systemic abnormalities in mononuclear phagocyte subpopulations may play a role in the pathogenesis of atherosclerosis.

Cholesterol Biosynthesis

The objective of a study by Jones and coworkers[60] in Quebec, Canada, was to measure the response of cholesterol biosynthesis in subjects to 3 different amounts of dietary cholesterol: 50 (low), 350 (medium), and 650 (high) mg cholesterol per 2800 kcal. Individuals with low (n = 7), normal (n = 12), and elevated (n = 11) plasma cholesterol concentrations consumed, in random order, solid food test diets (15%, 55%, and 30% of energy as protein, carbohydrate, and fat respectively) at each dietary cholesterol level. The 3 diets were consumed for 4 weeks each, and each dietary phase was separated by a 4-week washout. During the final week of each diet, 0.7 g D_2O was given per kilogram of body water, and deuterium incorporation into the high-cholesterol pool was measured for 24 hours. Urinary mevalonate levels were also determined in samples obtained during 2 consecutive 24-hour periods. Both techniques provided measurements of whole-body cholesterol biosynthesis. In all subjects, the cholesterol synthesis rate as measured by deuterium incorporation was significantly lower after the transition from low-to-medium and low-to-high cholesterol diets. Urinary malvalonate excretion decreased after the change from medium-to-high and low-to-high cholesterol diets. Although correspondence between the 2 methods was poor, they both indicated some suppression of cholesterol synthase by dietary cholesterol. The response of cholesterogenesis to different amounts of dietary cholesterol was related to the rate of synthesis under depressed conditions of the low cholesterol diet. These findings indicate modest down-regulation of synthesis in response to dietary cholesterol in humans, independent of plasma cholesterol levels.

Lipid-Lowering in Cholesterol-Induced LDL

One form of hypercholesterolemia is characterized by high levels of LDL cholesterol and normal levels of LDL-apolipoprotein(B). The reason for hypercholesterolemia, therefore, is enrichment of LDL particles with cholesterol. Vega and Grundy,[61] in Dallas, Texas, have previously reported that about one-third of patients with primary moderate hypercholesterolemia have this lipoprotein pattern and have no apparent abnormality in LDL-apolipoprotein(B) metabolism. These investigators conducted a study designed to determine whether the combination of the Step I Diet (30% of total calories as fat, <10% saturated fatty acids, and <300 mg per day per cholesterol), with or without cholestyramine therapy, would correct the hypercholesterolemia in patients of this type. Ten hypercholesterolemic men of this type were identified and recruited into the study. Their LDL cholesterol levels were greater than 160 mg/dL, and LDL-apolipoprotein(B) levels were less than 120 mg/dL. For patient selection, the subjects were challenged with a high-fat diet (40% of total calories as fat, 18% saturated fatty acids, and 400 mg/day cholesterol) for 6 weeks to confirm persistence of a high LDL cholesterol/apolipoprotein(B) ratio. Thereafter, the subjects were started on a Step I Diet, and lipoprotein analyses were repeated. Finally, cholestyramine (16 g per day) was added to the Step I Diet.

TABLE 1-2
Lipoprotein Cholesterol and Cholesterol Ratios

	High Fat Diet	Step I Diet	Cholestyramine Therapy
Non-HDL cholesterol, mg/dL	218 ± 19	201 ± 33*	177 ± 33‡
Total plasma apo B, mg/dL	129 ± 14	131 ± 21*	116 ± 22‡
Non-HDL cholesterol/total apo B ratio	1.69 ± 0.12	1.53 ± 0.11†	1.54 ± 0.09†
VLDL + IDL cholesterol, mg/dL	38 ± 7	34 ± 10*	37 ± 12*
VLDL + IDL apo B, mg/dL	26 ± 5	24 ± 8*	23 ± 8*
VLDL + IDL cholesterol/apo B ratio	1.46 ± 0.25	1.42 ± 0.17*	1.61 ± 0.29*

* Not significantly different compared with high-fat diet.
† Significantly lower than high-fat diet ($P<.01$).
‡ Significantly lower than Step I Diet ($P<.01$).
Reproduced with permission from Vega and Grundy.[61]

The Step I Diet alone significantly reduced the LDL cholesterol-apolipoprotein(B) ratios and produced a trend toward lowering LDL cholesterol levels. Cholestyramine therapy further reduced LDL cholesterol levels and maintained a normal LDL cholesterol-apolipoprotein(B) ratio (Table 1-2). Thus, the investigation confirmed the existence of a form of moderate hypercholesterolemia that arose from a defect in LDL composition. In addition, the study demonstrated that the combination of the Step I Diet and cholestyramine therapy corrected the defect and normalized LDL levels and LDL composition.

LDL-Receptor Binding and LDL Subclass

Campos and coworkers[62] in San Francisco, California, examined differences in LDL receptor-binding affinity among LDL particles of different size in competitive binding assays in human skin fibroblast and LDL from subjects with a predominance of large, medium, and small LDL. Among 57 normolipidemic subjects with LDL cholesterol levels less than 160 mg/dL, binding affinity was reduced by 16% in those with predominantly large LDL and by 14% in those with small LDL compared with most subjects who had a predominance of medium-size LDL. Affinity was also reduced in all LDL-size subgroups of 66 subjects with LDL cholesterol greater than 160 mg/dL. Differences in LDL receptor-binding affinity were further investigated by using LDL density subfractions from 3 subjects with predominantly large and small particles. The binding affinity of LDL-II was similar for patterns A and B and 30% lower in the LDL-III from both groups. The binding affinity of LDL-I in pattern A was lower than that in LDL-II and LDL-I from pattern B. After incubation with a monoclonal antibody that specifically blocked the LDL receptor-binding of apolipoprotein E, LDL-I from 2 pattern B subjects showed substantially lower binding affinity than in pattern A, a result consistent with the finding of a higher apolipoprotein E content in pattern B LDL-I. Thus, factors associated with variations in particle size and apolipoprotein E content in LDL subclasses in normolipidemic subjects contributed to the differences in LDL receptor binding that may result in differing metabolic behavior *in vivo*.

LDL Subfraction in Human Plasma

By using fast protein lipid chromatography, Demuth and coinvestigators[63] in Paris, France, isolated from human plasma a minor electronegative LDL subfraction designated LDL-. After immunoaffinity chromatography against apolipoprotein(a) and apolipoprotein A-I, LDL- represented 8% of total LDL. Compared with the major LDL subfraction, designated LDL +, LDL- contained similar amounts of thiobarbituric acid-reactive substances, conjugated dienes, and vitamin E, and had a similar lipid/protein ratio and mean density. Moreover, the apolipoprotein B of LDL- was not aggregated, and its LDL receptor-binding activity was slightly increased. These results were consistent with the nonoxidized nature of LDL-. LDL- showed increased levels of sialic acid, apolipoprotein C-III, and apolipoprotein E (Table 1-3). Compared with LDL +, LDL- displayed enhanced cytotoxic effects on cultured human umbilical vein endothelial cells, as shown by lactate dehydrogenase assay, neutral red uptake, and morphological studies. The investigators also studied the relationship of LDL- to age and plasma lipid levels in 133 subjects. The percentage of contribution of LDL- to total plasma LDL correlated with age, total cholesterol, and LDL cholesterol. In conclusion, this study showed that LDL-, a circulating human plasma LDL, is an electronegative native LDL subfraction with cytotoxic effects on endothelial cells. This subfraction, which correlated positively with common atherosclerotic risk factors, might induce atherosclerosis by actively contributing to alteration of the vascular endothelium.

TABLE 1-3
Chemical Composition of LDL(+) and LDL(−) Subfractions

	Chromatographic Subfractions	
	LDL(+)	LDL(−)
Lipid and protein composition, wt/wt %*		
Triglycerides	7.3 ± 0.7	6.9 ± 1.3
Cholesteryl esters	38.7 ± 1.1	36.9 ± 2.5
Free cholesterol	9.6 ± 0.7	10.2 ± 0.5
Phospholipids	20.1 ± 1.2	21.4 ± 1.4
Proteins	24.3 ± 1.2	24.6 ± 1.2
Lipid/protein ratio	3.1 ± 0.2	3.1 ± 0.2
Apolipoprotein content, protein %		
Apo C-III	0.14 ± 0.04	1.43 ± 0.21†
Apo E	0.10 ± 0.05	1.64 ± 0.26‡
Sialic acid content, nmol/mg protein	28.9 ± 3.3	38.1 ± 5.2†
Lipoperoxidation product content, nmoL/mg protein		
T-BARS	1.2 ± 0.6	1.6 ± 0.8
Conjugated dienes	36.0 ± 14.0	38.0 ± 16.0
Vitamin E content, nmol/mg protein	18.3 ± 2.0	17.3 ± 1.8

Values are mean ± SD of triplicate determinations on seven separate LDL preparations.

* The percentage of each component within each subfraction was calculated by taking the sum of the masses of the individual components (triglycerides, cholesteryl esters, free cholesterol, phospholipids, and protein) in each subfraction as 100%. Cholesteryl ester content was calculated as 1.68 × (total cholesterol-free cholesterol).

† $P < .01$, ‡ $P < .0005$, Student's paired t test, for LDL(−) vs LDL(+).

Reproduced with permission from Demuth et al.[63]

Fish-Eye Disease

A 53-year-old man with a severely reduced HDL cholesterol level, dense corneal opacities, normal renal function, and premature CAD was investigated by Kuivenhoven and colleagues[64] in Amsterdam, The Netherlands, together with 16 members of his family. The proband was diagnosed with fish-eye disease. As in previously reported patients with fish-eye disease, the endogenous plasma cholesterol esterification rate was near normal, yet lecithin:cholesterol acyltransferase activity was almost absent when measured with exogenous HDL analogues used as substrates. Direct sequencing of the transferase gene revealed 2 novel missense mutations in exon 1 and exon 4, resulting in the substitution of PRO[10] with Gln(P10Q) and Arg[135] with Gln(R135Q), respectively. The missense mutations were located on different alleles. Genetic analysis by polymerase chain reaction revealed 4 carriers of the P10Q and 3 carriers of the R135Q defect. Functional assessment of both missense mutations revealed that when exogenous HDL analogues were used as substrates, the specific activity of the acyltransferase was 18% of wild type; however, when LDL was used as a substrate, the activity was 146% of wild type. By contrast, acyltransferase was inactive against both substrates. Thus, the investigators concluded that the acyltransferase mutation was causative for complete acyltransferase deficiency, and the clinical phenotype of fish-eye disease seen in the patient was due to the PRO[10] mutation. The presence of premature CAD in the absence of other risk factors in this new case of fish-eye disease raises questions regarding the risk of atherosclerosis, which has previously been reported to be nonexistent.

Premature Atherosclerosis in Patients with Chylomicronemia

Benlian and colleagues[65] at the University of British Columbia prospectively evaluated patients with lipoprotein lipase deficiency for atherosclerosis. Patients with lipoprotein lipase deficiency usually present with chylomicronemia in childhood. This syndrome has been considered nonatherogenic, primarily because of the low levels of LDL cholesterol. Evidence of carotid, peripheral, and coronary atherosclerosis was sought in 4 patients, including 2 men and 2 women with the phenotype of familial chylomicronemia by clinical examination over a period of 14 to 30 years and by Doppler ultrasonography and exercise tolerance testing after the age of 40. Angiography was performed when indicated. Lipoprotein lipase deficiency was assessed *in vivo* and *in vitro* by functional assays and DNA-sequence analysis. All 4 patients had a profound functional deficiency of lipoprotein lipase with a reduced enzymatic mass due to missense mutations on both alleles of the lipoprotein lipase gene. In all 4 patients, peripheral or coronary atherosclerosis, or both, was observed before the age of 55 years. Despite following a low-fat diet in which fat comprised 10% to 15% of the daily caloric intake, the patients had hypertriglyceridemia with a mean serum triglyceride level of 2621 mg/dL, low plasma levels of HDL cholesterol (17 mg/dL), and very low levels of LDL cholesterol (28 mg/dL).

Three patients had 1 risk factor for atherosclerosis, whereas in 1 male patient, heavy smoking and diabetes were associated with an accelerated course of the disease. Thus, premature atherosclerosis can occur in patients with familial chylomicronemia as a result of mutations in the lipoprotein lipase gene. Defective lipolysis may increase susceptibility to atherosclerosis in humans.

Fenofibrate-Induced Modulation of Atherogenic Dense LDL Profile in Combined Hyperlipidemia

Guérin and colleagues[66] in Paris, France, investigated the effect of fenofibrate on plasma cholesteryl ester transfer protein activity in relation to the quantitative and qualitative features of apolipoprotein B- and apolipoprotein A-I-containing lipoprotein subspecies in 9 patients presenting with combined hyperlipidemia. Fenofibrate (200 mg/day for 8 weeks) induced significant reductions in plasma cholesterol (-16%), triglyceride (-44%), VLDL cholesterol (-52%), LDL cholesterol (-14%), and apolipoprotein B (minus 15%) levels and increased HDL cholesterol (15%) and apolipoprotein A-1 (12%) levels. An exogenous cholesteryl ester transfer assay revealed a marked decrease of 26% in total plasma, cholesteryl ester transfer protein-dependent cholesteryl ester transfer activity after fenofibrate treatment. Concomitant with the pronounced reduction in VLDL levels, the rate of cholesteryl ester transfer from HDL to VLDL was significantly reduced by 38%, whereas no modification in the rate of cholesteryl ester exchange between HDL and LDL occurred after fenofibrate therapy. Combined hyperlipidemia is characterized by an asymmetrical LDL profile in which small dense LDL subspecies predominate. Fenofibrate quantitatively normalized the atherogenic LDL profile by reducing levels of dense LDL subspecies by 21% and inducing an elevation of 26% in LDL's subspecies of intermediate density, which possessed optimal binding affinity for the cellular LDL receptor. However, no marked qualitative modifications in the chemical composition or size of LDL particles were observed after drug treatment. Interestingly, the HDL cholesterol concentration was increased by fenofibrate therapy, whereas no significant change was detected in total plasma HDL mass. In contrast, the HDL subspecies pattern was modified as the result of an increase in the total mass, at the expense of reductions in the total mass of HDL_{2b} and HDL_{3c}. Such changes are consistent with a drug-induced reduction in cholesteryl ester transfer protein activity. In conclusion, the overall mechanism involved in the fenofibrate-induced modulation of the atherogenic-dense LDL profile in combined hyperlipidemia primarily involved reduction in cholesteryl ester transfer from HDL to VLDL together with normalization of the intravascular transformation of VLDL precursors to the receptor-active LDLs of intermediate density.

Effect of Cholesteryl Ester Transfer Protein on Lipid Metabolism

To evaluate the independent effect of cholesteryl ester transfer protein on HDL concentrations in humans, Foger and coinvestigators[67] in Innsbruck,

Austria, measured lipids, lipoproteins, postprandial lipemia after an oral fat load, cholesteryl ester transfer protein mass, and the activities of cholesteryl transfer protein, lipoprotein lipase, and hepatic lipase. The study group comprised 16 healthy, normotriglyceridemic men and 23 men with moderate, primary hypertriglyceridemia who were on an American Heart Association Step I diet. Fasting triglycerides and postprandial lipemia were increased and HDL cholesterol was decreased in hypertriglyceridemic men compared with control subjects. In the normotriglyceridemic group, cholesteryl ester transfer protein mass and activity were directly related to lipoprotein lipase activity. After statistical adjustment for this close association, no significant relationship of cholesteryl ester transfer protein to HDL cholesterol independent of lipoprotein lipase activity could be demonstrated in the normotriglyceridemic subjects. In contrast, cholesteryl ester transfer protein was unrelated to lipoprotein lipase activity in the hypertriglyceridemic subjects, but cholesteryl ester transfer protein concentration showed a close inverse relationship to HDL cholesterol. Structural equation modeling of the association structures between HDL fasting and postprandial triglycerides, endothelial lipases and cholesteryl ester transfer protein in both groups indicated that the overall regression models for the 2 groups differed. Specifically, the associations between cholesteryl ester transfer protein mass and activity and HDL cholesterol differed between both routes. Investigators concluded that high-normal cholesteryl ester transfer protein levels lower HDL cholesterol in nonsmoking, nonobese men with moderate, primary hypertriglyceridemia on a hypolipidemic diet, but do not lower HDL cholesterol in healthy, normal triglyceridemic men on an unrestricted diet. Thus, variation in cholesteryl ester transfer protein plasma concentration may contribute to the high triglyceride, low HDL phenotype.

Effects of Fenofibrate on Triglyceride-Rich Lipid Metabolism

The 2 major subclasses of HDL contain apolipoprotein A-I only or both apolipoprotein A-I and apolipoprotein A-II. McPherson and coworkers[68] in Ottawa, Canada, studied 13 hypertriglyceridemic subjects before and after fenofibrate therapy. Fenofibrate treatment resulted in a decrease in total cholesterol of 19%, triglycerides of 48%, and VLDL cholesterol of 70%, and a 28% increase in HDL cholesterol with no significant change in the proportion of lipoprotein A-I and lipoprotein A-I/A-II particles. The abundance of cholesteryl ester transfer protein mRNA in peripheral adipose tissue decreased with treatment in 4 of 5 patients studied; however, no change occurred in plasma cholesteryl ester transfer protein mass. Using an isotopic transfer assay, the investigators demonstrated that both lipoprotein A-I and lipoprotein A-I/A-II participated in the cholesteryl ester transfer reaction with no change after fenofibrate therapy. This finding suggested that the marked increase in HDL cholesterol during fenofibrate therapy is due to normalization of plasma triglycerides and, hence, decreased opportunity for mass transfer of lipids between HDL and triglyceride-rich protein *in vivo*. In this population of hypertriglyceridemic subjects, cholesteryl ester transfer protein was distributed in both lipoprotein A-I and lipoprotein A-I/A-II subfractions of HDL, with preferential association with the smaller lipoprotein A-I pool. Nonetheless, the lipoprotein A-I/A-II fraction of HDL contributed significantly to the total cholesteryl mass transfer in normolipemic plasma. Lipoprotein A-I/A-II is an efficient donor for cholesteryl ester transfer to triglyceride rich protein, and its lower affinity for cholesteryl ester transfer protein may, in fact, facilitate neutral lipid transfer either by a shuttle mechanism or by formation of a ternary complex.

Lipid Metabolism/HDL

Hepatic lipase has demonstrated a dual role in plasma lipid transport in that it participates in the removal of remnants of triglyceride-rich lipoproteins from the circulation and in the metabolism of plasma HDL. Mowri and colleagues[69] in Houston, Texas, investigated the substrate properties for hepatic lipase of HDL differing in density and apolipoprotein composition. Rates of fatty acid liberation were 2-fold higher in HDL_2, compared with the respective HDL_3 subspecies. Within each density class, enzyme-catalyzed fatty acid release was nearly 2-fold higher from HDL containing apolipoprotein A-II than from HDL devoid of apolipoprotein A-II. When native HDL_3 devoid of apolipoprotein A-II was reconstituted with dimeric apolipoprotein A-II *in vitro*, rates of fatty-acid liberation in reconstituted particles were similar to those in native HDL_3 containing apolipoprotein A-II. HDL containing apolipoprotein A-II competed more effectively with small VLDL for binding of hepatic lipase than did HDL devoid of apolipoprotein A-II. HDL_3, particularly apolipoprotein A-II-containing HDL_3, reduced lipolysis of triglyceride and total fatty-acid liberation in small VLDL. The investigators concluded that the substrate properties of HDLs for hepatic lipase were influenced by both their size and apolipoprotein A-II content. Moreover, size, as well as apolipoprotein A-II content, may indirectly affect remnant clearance.

Clinical Metabolism Study of Apolipoprotein A-I HDL

Apolipoprotein A-I is the principal protein component of plasma HDL. Tissue culture studies have suggested that lipid-free apolipoprotein A-I may, by recruiting phospholipids and unesterified cholesterol from cell membranes, initiate reverse cholesterol transport and provide a nidus for the formation, via lipid poor, pre-β-migrating HDLs, of spheroidal α-migrating HDLs. Apolipoprotein A-I has also been shown to inhibit hepatic lipase and lipoprotein lipase *in vivo*. To further study its functions and fate *in vivo*, Nanjee and coinvestigators[70] in London, United Kingdom, gave lipid-free apolipoprotein A-I intravenously on a total of 32 occasions to 6 men with low HDL cholesterol (30–38 mg/dL) by bolus injection (25 mg/kg) and/or by infusion over 5 hours. The procedure was well tolerated; there were no clinical, biochemical, or hematologic changes, and there was no evidence of allergic, immunologic, and acute phase responses. The 5-hour infusions increased plasma total apolipoprotein A-I concentration in a dose-related manner by 10 to 50 mg/dL after which it

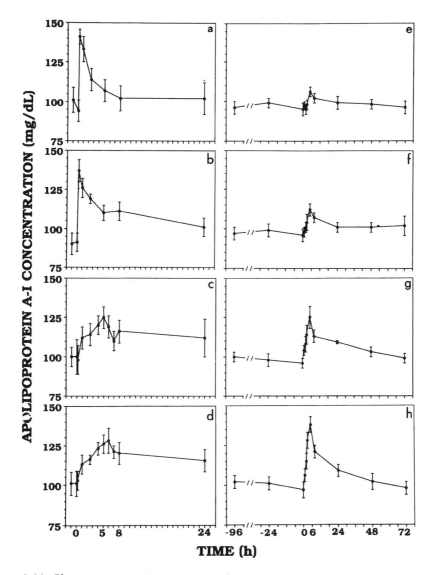

FIGURE 1-16. Plasma concentration-time curves for total apolipoprotein A-I. Left panels (series I) show results obtained after administration of 25 mg apolipoprotein A-I per kilogram of body weight IV by (a) bolus injection, (b) bolus injection with intralipid coinfusion, (c) 5-hour infusion, and (d) 5-hour infusion with intralipid coinfusion. Right panels (series II) show results obtained with 5-hour infusions (all without intralipid) at rates of (e) 1.25 mg·kg^{-1}·h^{-1}, (f) 2.5 mg·kg^{-1}·h^{-1}, (g) 5.0 mg·kg^{-1}·h^{-1}, and (h) 10 mg·kg^{-1}·h^{-1}. Results are means ± SEM of 4 subjects. Note that left and right panels have similar scales on the y axes (concentration) but different x axes (time). Reproduced with permission from Nanjee et al.[70]

decreased, with a half-life of 15 to 54 hours (Figure 1-16). Coinfusion of intralipid reduced the clearance rate. The parent volume of distribution exceeded the known extracellular space in humans, suggesting extensive first-pass clearance by 1 or more organs. No apolipoprotein A-I appeared in the urine. Increases in apolipoprotein A-I mass were confined to the pre-β region on cross immunoelectrophoresis of plasma and to HDL size particles on size exclusion chromatography. Increases were recorded in HDL phospholipids, but not in HDL unesterified or esterified cholesterol. Increases also occurred in LDL phospholipids and in VLDL cholesterol, triglycerides, and phospholipids, but not in plasma total apolipoprotein B concentration. These results can all be explained by combined inhibition of hepatic lipase and lipoprotein lipase activities. Because of the effects that this would have had on HDL metabolism, no conclusions can be drawn from these data about the role of lipid-free apolipoprotein A-I in the removal of phospholipids and cholesterol from peripheral tissues in humans. The kinetic data suggested to the investigators that the fractional catabolic rate of lipid-free apolipoprotein A-I exceeds that of spheroidal HDLs and is reduced in the presence of phospholipids.

Clinical Metabolism Study of Thyroid-Hormone Triiodothyronine and Apolipoprotein A-I

Apolipoprotein A-I is the principal protein component of HDL cholesterol. The thyroid hormone triiodothyronine is known to be a potent mediator of expression of apolipoprotein A-I structural gene. Using complex segregation analysis, Blangero and associates[71] in San Antonio, Texas, detected a major gene influencing plasma concentration of apolipoprotein A-I and examined its interaction with triiodothyronine serum level in Mexican Americans participating in the San Antonio Family Heart Study. Strong evidence for a major locus with two alleles (A and *a*) determining apolipoprotein A-I level was obtained when interaction with triiodothyronine was allowed. The major gene appeared not to be linked to the apolipoprotein A-I structural gene structural locus. Genotypes differed significantly in their relation to triiodothyronine level. The 2 alleles' genotypes showed a positive relationship with triiodothyronine level, whereas the rarer allele homozygote showed a strong positive relationship with triiodothyronine. The relative variance in apolipoprotein A-I concentration to this major gene varied from 56% to 18% depending on triiodothyronine levels. On average, a major gene accounts for 30% of apolipoprotein A-I variation, and shared household effects account for an additional 11%. These findings suggested that thyroid hormone has an important role in the genetic control of lipoprotein metabolism.

Paraoxonase and Lipid Metabolism

Paraoxonase, an enzyme associated with the HDL particle, hydrolyzes paraoxon, the active metabolite of the insecticide parathion. Several studies have shown that paraoxonase levels in humans have a distribution characteristic of 2 alleles, 1 with low activity and the other with high activity. Paraoxonase also has arylesterase activity, which does not exhibit activity polymorphism and can therefore serve as an estimate of enzyme protein. Although the ability of paraoxon to irreversibly inhibit lipoprotein lipase has been exploited experimentally for many years, the role of plasma paraoxonase and lipoprotein metabolism is unknown. Nevin and colleagues,[72] in Seattle, Washington, examined 72 normal individuals for paraoxonase genotypes, plasma paraoxonase and arylesterase activities, post-heparin lipoprotein lipase and hepatic lipase activities, and lipoprotein levels to determine whether (1) paraoxonase activity or genotype determines lipoprotein levels via an effect on lipoprotein lipase or hepatic lipase activities or (2) variation in lipoprotein lipase and hepatic lipase activities determines HDL levels and indirectly affects paraoxonase activity and protein levels in plasma. In the entire group, paraoxonase activity was related to arylesterase activity and genotype. Whereas arylesterase activity was correlated with HDL cholesterol and apolipoprotein A-I levels, neither arylesterase nor paraoxonase was correlated with lipoprotein lipase or hepatic lipase activity. Furthermore, lipoprotein lipase activity was possibly correlated and hepatic lipase inversely correlated with HDL cholesterol and apolipoprotein A-I levels, whereas lipoprotein lipase was inversely correlated with triglyceride levels. The paraoxonase genotypes of a study group were 30 individuals homozygous for the low activity allele, 38 heterozytes, and 4 individuals homozygous for the high activity allele (Figure 1-17). Paraoxonase genotype accounted for ≈.75 of the variation in paraoxonase activity. Paraoxonase activity was linearly related to arylesterase activity within each subgroup. No difference in either lipoprotein lipase or hepatic lipase was seen as a function of paraoxonase genotype nor were differences seen in the plasma triglyceride or HDL cholesterol

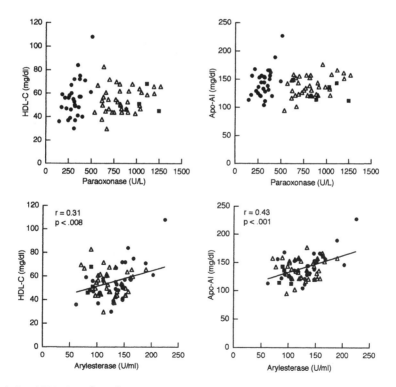

FIGURE 1-17. HDL-C and apolipoprotein A-I versus paraoxonase activity (upper panels) and arylesterase activity (lower panels) for homozygous-low (●), heterozygous (△), and homozygous-high (■) individuals. Reproduced with permission from Nevin et al.[72]

by genotype. The relation between lipoprotein lipase and hepatic lipase in components of HDL in the paraoxonase genotype subgroups in general reflected the association seen in the group as a whole. Multivarianalysis showed that lipoprotein lipase, hepatic lipase, and arylesterase, a measure of paraoxonase mass, were independent predictors of HDL cholesterol, while paraoxonase genotype or activity was not. Thus, variation in lipoprotein lipase and hepatic lipase appears to be significantly related to HDL cholesterol and apolipoprotein A-I levels. The levels of HDL are a major correlate of paraoxonase protein level, whereas paraoxonase genotype is a major predictor of plasma paraoxonase activity.

Effects of Fish Oil on Oxidation Resistance of VLDL and LDL

In hypertriglyceridemic patients, the addition of fish oil to the diet causes a marked reduction in the concentration of triglyceride-rich lipoprotein in the serum. Hau and coworkers[73] in Leiden, The Netherlands, investigated the effects of fish oil on the oxidation resistance of VLDL and LDL in hypertriglyceridemic patients. Nine male patients received 1 gm per day of fish oil (containing 56% n-3 polyunsaturated fatty acids and 1 U α-tocopherol per gram) for 6 weeks followed by 5 gm per day for an additional 6-week period. Copper-in-

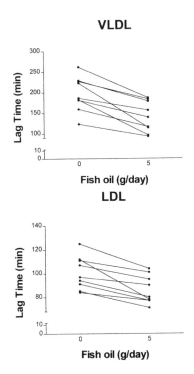

FIGURE 1-18. Lag times of VLDL (top) and LDL (bottom) oxidation *in vitro* at baseline and after 6 weeks of 5 g/d fish oil. $P = .001$ for both by paired Student's t test. Reproduced with permission from Hau et al.[73]

duced oxidation of VLDL and LDL was measured by continuous monitoring conjugated dieners. Supplementation with 1 gm per day of fish oil causes hardly any changes in the n-3 polyunsaturated fatty acid content of lipoprotein or lipoprotein concentrations in the serum. However, supplementation with 5 gm/day resulted in a significant increase of n-3 polyunsaturated fatty acid content in VLDL and LDL: decreases in serum triglycerides, VLDL triglycerides, and VLDL cholesterol concentrations, respectively; and an increase in LDL cholesterol. The lag times of VLDL and LDL oxidation decreased from 197 to 140 minutes, respectively (Figure 1-18). At the end of the 5 gm per day supplementation, the lag times of VLDL and LDL oxidation were correlated with the respective n-3 polyunsaturated fatty acid content. Before and at the end of supplementation with 5 gm per day, the lag times and propagation rates of VLDL oxidation also correlated with the total number of double bonds in all polyunsaturated fatty acids of VLDL. The investigators concluded that fish oil supplementation strongly reduced serum concentrations of total triglycerides, VLDL triglycerides, and VLDL cholesterol. However, in hypertriglyceridemic patients, fish oil supplementation increased the serum LDL cholesterol concentration and the susceptibility of VLDL and LDL to oxidation.

Lipids—Prognosis

Variation at Apolipoprotein(a) Gene Locus as a Determinant of Coronary Artery Disease Risk

A high plasma concentration of lipoprotein(a) has been suggested as a risk factor for CAD, but some recent prospective studies have questioned the significance of lipoprotein(a). Lipoprotein(a) concentrations are determined to a large extent by the hypervariable apolipoprotein(a) gene locus on chromosome 6q2.7, which contains a variable number of identical, tandemly arranged, transcribed kringle IV type 2 repeats. The number of these repeats correlates inversely with plasma lipoprotein(a) concentration. Lingenhel and colleagues[74] in Innsbruck, Austria, analyzed whether apolipoprotein(a) gene variation is associated with CAD. Apolipoprotein(a) genotypes were determined by pulsed-field gel electrophoresis/genomic blotting in CAD patients who had undergone angiography and control subjects matched for age, sex, and ethnicity and were related in lipoprotein(a) concentration, apolipoprotein(a) isoform and plasma, and disease status. Apolipoprotein(a) alleles with low kringle IV copy number and high lipoprotein(a) concentration were significantly more frequent in the CAD group, whereas large, nonexpressed alleles were more frequent in control subjects. The odds ratio for CAD increased continuously with a decreasing number of kringle IV repeats and ranged from 0.3 in individuals with greater than 25 kringle IV repeats on both alleles to 4.6 in those with less than 20 repeats on at least 1 allele. This investigation provided direct genetic evidence that variation at the apolipoprotein(a) gene locus, which determines lipoprotein(a) levels, is also a determinant of CAD risk.

Lipoprotein(a) Levels in Atherosclerotic Vascular Disease in Familial Hypercholesterolemia

There is considerable variation in the severity of cardiovascular disease among patients with familial hypercholesterolemia. Some reports have suggested that plasma lipoprotein(a) may explain such variation and that familial hypercholesterolemic patients deficient in LDL receptors, especially those with CAD, tend to have elevated lipoprotein(a) levels. Carmena and associates[75] in Montreal, Canada, investigated the possible role of the LDL receptor in determining plasma lipoprotein(a) in a genetically homogeneous familial hypercholesterolemic population and the contribution of lipoprotein(a) to cardiovascular risk. A total of 98 familial hypercholesterolemic subjects in 66 healthy first- and second-degree relatives from 30 families with familial hypercholesterolemia (based on the French-Canadian greater than 10-kb deletion of the LDL receptor gene) were studied. A reference group of 392 normolipidemic French-Canadian participants in a Heart Health Survey was used for comparison. Familial hypercholesterolemic subjects were subdivided into subsets of 63 individuals free from atherosclerotic vascular disease and 35 individuals with atherosclerotic vascular disease. A complete cardiovascular evaluation was performed, and plasma lipid, lipoprotein, and lipoprotein(a) were measured in all subjects in the absence of medication. Apoprotein(a) phenotype was determined in 112 of familial hypercholesterolemic and nonfamilial hypercholesterolemic subjects. The log-transformed values for plasma lipoprotein(a) were not significantly different among the 3 groups. The distribution of the lipoprotein(a) phenotypes did not differ between the familial hypercholesterolemic and nonfamilial hypercholesterolemic groups. Comparison of 2 age- and sex-matched subgroups of familial hypercholesterolemic subjects with and without atherosclerotic vascular disease failed to show any differences in lipoprotein(a) level. However, mean lipoprotein(a) log values in the reference group were significantly lower than values obtained for the total familial hypercholesterolemic group but were not different from those of the unaffected family members. Thus, in this sample, the LDL receptor appeared not to influence plasma lipoprotein(a) levels; rather, these levels reflect shared apolipoprotein(a) genes. The cardiovascular risk in this group of patients with familial hypercholesterolemia was related to age, male sex, and total LDL cholesterol and higher apolipoprotein B, but not lipoprotein(a) levels.

Hypertriglyceridemia and Elevated Lipoprotein(a) as Risk Factors for Coronary Events

Assmann and associates[76] from Münster, Germany, analyzed cardiovascular risk factors in 4849 male participants, aged 40–65 years, in an 8-year follow-up of the Prospective Cardiovascular Münster (PROCAM) study. One hundred eighty-one definite nonfatal AMIs, 49 fatal AMIs, and 28 sudden cardiac deaths were observed. Multiple logistic function analysis confirmed that age, LDL cholesterol, HDL cholesterol, systolic blood pressure, cigarette smoking, diabe-

Relation Between Values of Age-Standardized Risk and Development of Major Coronary Events Over Eight Years

| | Major Coronary Events | | |
| | Absent (n = 4.381) | Present (n = 258) | p Value |
Variable			
Cholesterol (mg/dL)	224 (41)	252 (52)	<0.001
HDL cholesterol (mg/dL)	46 (12)	40 (10)	<0.001
LDL cholesterol (mg/dL)*	148 (36)	175 (41)	<0.001
LDL cholesterol/HDL cholesterol ratio*	3.4 (1.2)	4.6 (1.6)	<0.001
Triglycerides (mg/dL)†	133	175	<0.001
Systolic blood pressure (mm Hg)	133 (19)	140 (22)	<0.001
Diastolic blood pressure (mm Hg)	87 (11)	89 (13)	<0.001
Body mass index (kg/m²)	26.3 (3.0)	26.7 (2.9)	<0.05
Fasting blood glucose (mg/dL)	102 (20)	109 (37)	<0.01
Uric acid (mg/dL)	5.7 (1.1)	5.8 (1.1)	NS
Lp(a) (g/L)†‡	0.05	0.09	<0.05

* Major coronary events: absent, n = 4,255; major coronary events: present, n = 246.
† Geometric mean.
‡ Major coronary events: absent, n = 828; major coronary events: present, n = 33.
Values are mean [SD] unless otherwise indicated.
HDL = high-density lipoprotein; LDL = low-density lipoprotein; Lp(a) = lipoprotein(a).
Reproduced with permission from Assman et al.[76]

tes mellitus, angina pectoris, and family history of AMI were important cardiovascular risk factors. This analysis revealed a significant and independent association between serum levels of triglycerides and the incidence of major coronary events. The relation between lipoprotein(a) levels and the occurrence of major coronary events was analyzed in a subgroup of 878 men. Thirty-three probands with major coronary events had significantly higher geometric mean levels of lipoprotein(a) than did 828 men who did not experience major coronary events (0.09 vs. 0.05 g/L). Thus, in addition to established risk factors, serum levels of triglycerides and lipoprotein(a) are sensitive indicators of increased risk for major coronary events (See Table 1-4 and Figure 1-19).

Lipoprotein(a) is not a Predictor of Myocardial Infarction

Lipoprotein(a) is considered a risk factor for the development of CAD. There is conflicting evidence regarding the risk of AMI from lipoprotein(a). Kinlay and colleagues[77] from Newcastle, New South Wales, Australia, did a population-based case–control of 893 men and women to evaluate whether lipoprotein(a) concentrations were risk factors for a first acute and recurrent AMI. Compared with control subjects without a previous AMI, median lipoprotein(a) concentrations increased from case patients with a first AMI (15 mg/L higher) to control patients with a previous AMI (159 mg/L higher) and case patients with a previous AMI (60 mg/L higher). Women had significantly higher lipoprotein(a) concentrations than did men (median 71 mg/L higher). The highest quintile of lipoprotein(a) was a significant risk factor for a first AMI (odds

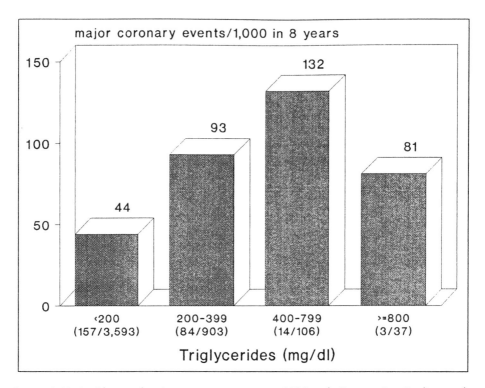

Figure 1-19. Incidence of major coronary events per 1000 male Prospective Cardiovascular Münster Study participants aged 40 to 65 years over an 8-year period according to triglyceride levels. There were 258 events among 4/639 men. Reproduced with permission from Assmann et al.[76]

ratio = 1.77, CI = 1.03 to 3.03). In those with a previous AMI, however, the highest quintile was not associated with recurrent AMI (odds ratio = 0.84, CI = 0.30 to 2.37). These authors concluded that high lipoprotein(a) concentrations may be a marker of vascular or tissue injury or may be associated with other genetic or environmental factors that cause acute myocardial infarction. However, levels of lipoprotein(a) are not predictive of AMI.

Elevated Lipoprotein(a) Does Not Increase Risk of Coronary Atherosclerosis in Older Women

Sunayama and colleagues[78] in Tokyo, Japan, determined serum lipoprotein(a) concentrations in 354 women and 706 men with or without angiographically defined CAD. The age-specific impact of elevated lipoprotein(a) of 30 mg/dL or greater on CAD was examined in each sex. In the younger age group (<55 years of age), elevated lipoprotein(a) was independently associated with CAD in both sexes. The age-specific adjusted odds ratio declined with age, and elevated lipoprotein(a) no longer conferred an increased CAD risk in either elderly men or women 65 years of age or older. In the age group of 55 to 64

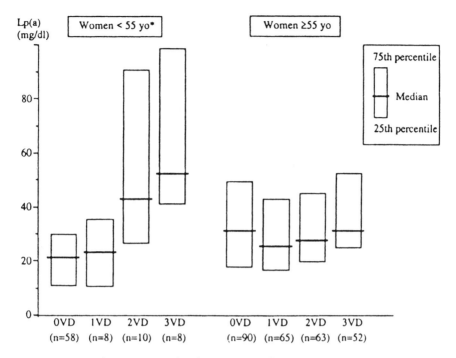

Figure 1-20. Serum lipoprotein(a) distributions according to angiographic diagnostic groups in women younger than 55 years and those 55 years of age or older. Lipoprotein(a), lipoprotein(a); 0VD, patients without significant stenosis; 1VD, those with 1-vessel disease; 2VD, those with 2-vessel disease; and 3VD, those with 3-vessel disease. *p<.01, testing for equality of distributions among 4 diagnostic groups (Kruskal-Wallis test). Reproduced with permission from Sunayama et al.[78]

years, elevated lipoprotein(a) was positively associated with CAD for men, but not for women (Figure 1-20). These data suggest that for both sexes, elevated lipoprotein(a) appears to be an independent risk factor for premature CAD and the importance of lipoprotein(a) appears to decrease with age. However, in women, the risk estimate lipoprotein(a) began to decline at an age approximately 10 years younger than for men.

Carotid Artery Wall Thickness and Lipoprotein(a): Predictors by Sex and Race

The association of lipoprotein(a) with preclinical atherosclerotic disease is not well established in any racial group, particularly African Americans. Schreiner and colleagues[79] in Minneapolis, Minnesota, examined the relationship of lipoprotein(a) with preclinical extracranial carotid atherosclerosis in middle-aged black and white participants in the Atherosclerosis Risk in Communities study. Study participants (15124 black and white men and women) who were 45 to 64 years old at baseline were examined from 1987 through 1989. Carotid intima-media far-wall thickness was determined by B-mode ultrasonography and expressed as the overall wall-thickness mean at 6 sites to approximate atherosclerosis in the carotid system. Lipoprotein(a) was measured as its total protein component, lipoprotein(a) protein, by a double-antibody technique for apolipoprotein(a) detection. Lipoprotein(a) protein levels were higher in blacks than in whites. Mean carotid wall thickness (in millimeters) varied by race and gender. Multivariable-adjusted lipoprotein(a) protein was independently associated with wall thickness in white men and black men; among women, however, this association appeared to be stronger when smoking and diabetes were present. Among white women who smoked, the difference in wall thickness was 0.051 mm compared with 0.032 mm for former/never smokers and 0.21 mm in black female diabetics compared with 0.031 mm in black female nondiabetics. The results suggested that lipoprotein(a) is associated with preclinical carotid atherosclerosis in both blacks and whites, but that this association may be affected by the presence of other cardiovascular risk factors, particularly in women.

Lipid Regression Trials and Prognosis

Long-Term Effects of Lipoprotein(a) in Plasma Samples: Epidemiological Studies

Prospective case-control studies investigating lipoprotein(a) as a risk factor for atherosclerosis have measured lipoprotein(a) in frozen samples stored for up to nearly 20 years. Kronenberg and associates[80] in Innsbruck, Austria, therefore prospectively examined the influence of long-term plasma sample storage on measured values, depending on the molecular weight of apolipoprotein(a) isoforms. Apolipoprotein(a) phenotyping was performed on 310 plasma samples, and lipoprotein(a) was measured after 3 years and 28 months of storage at $-80°C$. The value of both measurements correlated significantly for both low- and high-molecular weight apolipoprotein(a) phenotypes. Nevertheless, the investigators detected, on average, a small decrease of 5%, which was statistically significant. The absolute and relative lipoprotein(a) decrease over time became larger with a decreasing number of kringle IV repeats of apolipoprotein(a), and lipoprotein(a) decreased markedly more in subjects with a low molecular weight compared with those with high molecular weight apolipoprotein isoforms. More than 70% of the absolute lipoprotein(a) decrease in the total sample was caused by samples with low molecular weight apolipoprotein(a) isoforms which represented only 27% of the sample. Low molecular weight apolipoprotein(a) isoforms are reported more frequently in patients with atherothrombotic disease compared with control subjects. Measurements of lipoprotein(a) in several-year-old frozen samples is therefore likely to result in a preferential decrease and false lower lipoprotein(a) concentrations in patient groups compared with control groups. The negative results of some prospective studies with retrospective measurements of lipoprotein(a) may be caused by such an artifact.

Apolipoprotein E and LDL Size in a Biethnic Population

Polymorphisms in the apolipoprotein E phenotype (especially E_4) are associated with increased cardiovascular risk and, particularly, with increased concentrations of LDL cholesterol. Little is known, however, about whether alterations in LDL size are associated with apolipoprotein E_4. Haffner and coinvestigators[81] in San Antonio, Texas, determined LDL size by gradient gel electrophoresis, and apolipoprotein E phenotype was determined by isoelectric focus in 337 nondiabetic subjects from the San Antonio Heart Study, a population-based study of diabetes and cardiovascular risk factors in Mexican American and non-Hispanic whites. Apolipoprotein E_4 was associated not only with increases in LDL cholesterol concentrations, but also with decreased LDL size. After adjustment for age, sex, body mass index, waist-to-hip ratio, triglycerides, HDL cholesterol, fasting insulin, and diabetic status, the apolipoprotein E phenotype remained significantly related to LDL size in both men and women. Variations in apolipoprotein E phenotype are associated not only with changes in absolute concentration of LDL cholesterol, but also with changes in composition. These changes are only partly explained by associations of apolipoprotein E with insulin, triglycerides, and HDL cholesterol.

Apolipoprotein E as a Predictor of Coronary Artery Disease

Wilson and coworkers[82] in Framingham, Massachusetts, undertook a meta-analysis to assess the impact of apolipoprotein E alleles ($\epsilon2$, $\epsilon3$, $\epsilon4$) on coronary disease in 14 published observational studies (9 clinical coronary disease and 5 coronary angiography). In comparison with $\epsilon3$, the $\epsilon4$ allele was associated with greater odds for CAD, and summary estimates of the odd ratios and for both sexes combined were odds ratio = 0.98 for $\epsilon2$ and odds ratio = 1.26 for $\epsilon4$. Separate analyses for men and women showed similar associations. In angiographic studies, the relative odds for significant CAD among both sexes combined was odds ratio 0.76 for $\epsilon2$ and odds ratio 1.1 for $\epsilon4$. The overall impression is that $\epsilon4$ is associated with clinical and coronary disease and the results are similar in men and women.

Apolipoprotein E Lipid Profile in American Indians

Apolipoprotein E is an important genetic factor in the development of cardiovascular disease, which is the leading cause of death among American Indians. Kataoka and colleagues[83] in Washington, D.C., investigated the occurrence of the apolipoprotein E alleles and the relation between apolipoprotein E polymorphism and blood lipoproteins and apolipoprotein protein in members of 13 American Indian communities in 3 geographic areas. The frequencies of the $\epsilon2$ alleles in American Indians are significantly lower than those in white Americans with the lowest frequencies of $\epsilon2$ in American Indians who reside in Arizona. Levels of LDL cholesterol and apolipoprotein B were highest in those with $\epsilon 4$ and lowest in those with $\epsilon 2$. Concentrations of HDL cholesterol and apolipoprotein A-I, however, tended to be lowest in $\epsilon 4$ and highest in $\epsilon 2$. Concentrations of total and VLDL triglycerides were lowest in the small $\epsilon 3$ group and higher in groups $\epsilon 2$ and $\epsilon 4$. Differences in concentrations of LDL cholesterol, HDL cholesterol, apolipoprotein B and apolipoprotein A-I with apolipoprotein E polymorphism were greater in woman than in men and differences in total and VLDL concentration by apolipoprotein E phenotype were greater in men. Relations of total and VLDL triglycerides with apolipoprotein E phenotype were stronger in women after menopause. In addition, differences in nearly all lipid and lipoprotein concentrations between post-menopausal women and premenopausal women were greater if they had $\epsilon 2$. Relations between apolipoprotein E phenotype and lipoproteins were seen in individuals with diabetes mellitus, as well as in nondiabetics. Apolipoprotein E was significantly related to glucose control in diabetic women: those with $\epsilon 3$ had higher glucose and hemoglobin A1C concentrations. These findings showed that (1) American Indians have low frequencies of apolipoprotein $\epsilon 2$; (2) apolipoprotein E phenotype can influence levels of VLDL, LDL, HDL, apolipoprotein B, and apolipoprotein A-I; (3) the associations of apolipoprotein E polymorphisms with lipid parameters differ between men and women; and (4) the associations in women of apolipoprotein E polymorphisms with lipid parameters are modified by menopausal status.

Poland and the United States Collaborative Study of Cardiovascular Epidemiology

HDL cholesterol levels are inversely related to CAD risk, and HDL cholesterol distributions vary among countries. Poland is one of the few developed countries in which CAD rates are increasing at the same time that United States rates have been falling, but whether these differences are explained by differences in risk factors such as HDL cholesterol has not been determined. To examine this possibility, levels of HDL cholesterol and its subfractions were compared by Broda and coworkers[84] in Warsaw, Poland, and compared in United States and Polish urban and rural men and women aged 45 to 64 years. Age-adjusted HDL cholesterol means were 0.20 mmol/L higher in urban Polish men and 0.37 mmol/L higher in rural Polish men than in their United States counterparts; means in urban Polish women were 0.06 mmol/L higher than in their United States counterparts and in rural Polish women 0.09 mmol/L higher than in their United States counterparts. Adjustment for age, education, alcohol intake, smoking, body mass index, heart rate, and menopause status in women had little effect on differences. Means of HDL_2 and HDL_3 levels showed similar between-country differences, although differences were minimal for HDL_2 in urban men and women, and HDL_3 means did not differ between rural women. Body mass index was inversely related to HDL cholesterol and both subfractions in all gender or country-site strata, and alcohol was directly related to HDL cholesterol in all strata, except Polish women. Cigarette smoking was negatively related to HDL cholesterol in both subfractions in all United States samples, except HDL_2 in urban men, whereas in Polish samples, significant associations were found only in urban women for HDL cholesterol and in rural and urban women for HDL_3. Age, heart rate, and education showed inconsistent or no association with HDL cholesterol and its subfractions in either country. This profile of HDL cholesterol and its subfractions in Polish samples contrasts sharply with the opposite trend in CAD morality rates, which suggests either that other risk factors may account for the trends or that the relation between HDL cholesterol and CAD may differ between the 2 countries.

LDL-Apheresis Plus Simvastatin Versus Simvastatin Alone

Kroon and colleagues[85] in Nijmegen, The Netherlands, assessed the effect of aggressive lipid lowering with LDL-apheresis in a randomized study in 42 men with hypercholesterolemia and severe coronary atherosclerosis. For 2 years, 42 men were treated with either biweekly LDL-apheresis and medication or medication alone. In both groups, a dose of simvastatin of 40 mg/day was administered. Baseline LDL cholesterol was 7.8 $mmol/L^{-1}$ and 7.9 $mmol/L^{-1}$ in the apheresis and medication groups. The mean reduction in LDL cholesterol was 63% in the apheresis and 47% in the medication group. Primary quantitative coronary angiographic endpoints were changes in average mean segment diameter and minimal obstruction diameter. No differences between the apheresis and medication groups were found in mean segment diameter or in minimal obstruction diameter expressed as means per patient. On the basis of coronary segment, mean percent stenosis of all lesions showed a tendency to decrease. However, only in the apheresis group did more minor lesions disappear. With bicycle exercise testing, the time to 0.1 mV ST-segment depression increased significantly by 39%, and the maximal level of ST depression decreased significantly by 0.07 mV in the apheresis group versus no change in the medication group. Thus, these data demonstrate that 2 years of lipid lowering with medication alone or LDL apheresis with medication showed angiographic arrest of the progression of CAD (Tables 1-5 and 1-6).

Angiographic Changes in Patients on a Low-Fat Diet and Exercise Program

Niebauer and associates[86] from Leipzig, Germany, randomly assigned 113 patients with serum LDL cholesterol (<210 mg/dL) and CAD to an intervention group (n = 56) or a control group (n = 57). The intervention program consisted of daily exercise and a low-fat diet according to the American Heart Association's recommendation phase III; patients in the control group received "usual care" rendered by their private physician. After 1 year, complete data were available for all 92 patients (intervention: n = 40; control: n = 52) who underwent repeat coronary angiography. During the study course, patients in the intervention group showed an increase in apolipoprotein A-I (123 ± 18 vs. 129 ± 20 mg/dL) and apolipoprotein A-I/B (1.3 ± 0.4 vs. 1.5 ± 0.4) and a decrease in apolipoprotein B (99 ± 20 vs. 89 ± 18 mg/dL), while apolipoprotein A-II

TABLE 1-5
Changes in Lipids and Lipoproteins: Baseline and Treatment Levels

| | Apheresis (n=21) | | | | | Medication Only (n=21) | | | Difference |
	Basal	Before	After	Interval Mean	% Change	Basal	Mean	% Change	p
Total cholesterol, mmol·L^{-1}	9.72 ± 1.84	5.60 ± 1.26	2.06 ± 0.46	4.63 ± 1.18	−52.9 ± 6.6	9.85 ± 2.17	5.95 ± 1.60	−39.5 ± 7.7	.005
Triglycerides, mmol·L^{-1}	2.32 ± 1.03	1.83 ± 0.76	0.48 ± 0.28	1.83 ± 0.76	−17.4 ± 24.4	2.64 ± 1.33	1.84 ± 0.89	−26.5 ± 20.3	.38
LDL cholesterol, mmol·L^{-1}	7.78 ± 1.86	3.72 ± 1.26	0.82 ± 0.41	2.95 ± 1.13	−62.9 ± 8.3	7.85 ± 2.34	4.13 ± 1.58	−47.4 ± 8.1	.01
HDL cholesterol, mmol·L^{-1}	0.93 ± 0.18	1.09 ± 0.20	1.08 ± 0.20	1.09 ± 0.20	+17.7 ± 13.6	0.92 ± 0.19	1.05 ± 0.22	+13.7 ± 10.9	.23
Lipoprotein(a), mg·dL^{-1}	57.0 ± 63.9	59.1 ± 68.8	13.8 ± 15.3	44.5 ± 54.3	−18.6 ± 18.0	38.4 ± 39.7	44.5 ± 45.7	+14.9 ± 16.3	.02
Apolipoprotein A1, g·L^{-1}	1.43 ± 0.29	1.34 ± 0.17	1.08 ± 0.13	1.34 ± 0.17	−5.3 ± 13.0	1.46 ± 0.38	1.33 ± 0.21	−5.4 ± 16.8	.89
Apolipoprotein B, g·L^{-1}	2.59 ± 0.47	1.65 ± 0.43	0.45 ± 0.16	1.32 ± 0.35	−49.0 ± 7.6	2.60 ± 0.61	1.74 ± 0.47	−31.0 ± 17.0	.003

Data are mean ± SD. Apheresis group: 52 measurements per patient. Medication group: 26 measurements per patient. Before indicates pretreatment levels (C$_{MAX}$); after, posttreatment levels (C$_{MIN}$); interval mean, time-averaged levels (C$_{AVG}$), calculated as follows: C$_{AVG}$ = C$_{MIN}$ + 0.73 (C$_{MAX}$ − C$_{MIN}$) (see text); % change, difference between basal and mean levels; p, probability values of differences between interval mean in the apheresis group and mean levels in the medication group (t test or Mann-Whitney U test where appropriate). To convert values for total cholesterol to mg/dL, multiply by 38.67; to convert values for triglycerides to mg/dL, multiply by 88.57. Reproduced with permission from Kroon et al.[85]

remained unchanged (38 ± 6 vs. 38 ± 6 mg/dL). In the control group, there were no significant changes (apolipoprotein A-I, 124 ± 17 vs. 128 ± 13 mg/dL; apolipoprotein A-II, 38 ± 6 vs. 39 ± 6 mg/dL; apolipoprotein B, 100 ± 21 vs. 99 ± 16 mg/dL; apolipoprotein A-I/B, 1.3 ± 0.3 vs. 1.4 ± 0.5). As previously reported, there was a significant retardation of progression in patients in the intervention group (progression 23%, no change 45%, regression 32%) compared with the control group (progression 48%, no change 35%, regression 17%). Although retardation of progression was significantly associated with

TABLE 1-6
Results of Quantitative Computer Analysis of the Coronary Angiographies: Baseline and at the End of the Study

| | Apheresis | | | | Medication Only | | | | Difference |
	No.	Baseline	Follow-up	Change	No.	Baseline	Follow-up	Change	p
Per-patient analysis	20				20				
Mean segment diameter, mm		2.65 ± 0.49	2.63 ± 0.41	−0.01 ± 0.16		2.58 ± 0.51	2.60 ± 0.48	0.03 ± 0.16	.46
Minimal obstruction diameter, mm		1.93 ± 0.43	1.92 ± 0.40	−0.01 ± 0.13		1.89 ± 0.50	1.90 ± 0.46	0.01 ± 0.11	.54
Percent stenosis									
20%–50%		31.3 ± 5.5	31.9 ± 5.8	0.6 ± 2.3		33.2 ± 5.4	33.9 ± 4.4	0.7 ± 3.5	.65
>50%		...	...	...		...	...	...	...
Per-segment analysis	173				178				
Mean segment diameter, mm		2.59 ± 0.96	2.59 ± 0.95	0.00 ± 0.24		2.56 ± 1.00	2.59 ± 0.97	0.02 ± 0.24	.29
Minimal obstruction diameter, mm		1.93 ± 0.93	1.92 ± 0.92	−0.01 ± 0.26		1.89 ± 0.98	1.90 ± 0.94	0.01 ± 0.26	.48
Percent stenosis									
20%–50%	177	30.1 ± 7.6	29.6 ± 11.4	−0.6 ± 8.4	161	32.8 ± 8.6	32.0 ± 11.5	−0.8 ± 9.1	.82
>50%	18	56.0 ± 7.6	52.5 ± 12.4	−3.5 ± 9.5	25	57.0 ± 6.6	52.6 ± 11.8	−4.5 ± 12.3	.78

Data are mean ± SD. Change indicates difference of follow-up minus baseline; p, probability value of treatment effect comparing changes in the apheresis group with the changes in the medication group (t test). In the per-patient analysis, mean percent stenoses >50% were not present. Reproduced with permission from Kroon et al.[85]

an increase in apolipoprotein A-I/B and a decrease in apolipoprotein B, these gave way in multivariate analysis to changes in total cholesterol/HDL cholesterol, absolute levels of LDL cholesterol, and, in a subgroup of patients, to leisure-time physical activity. These data demonstrate that an intervention based on a low-fat diet and intensive physical exercise is capable of improving apolipoprotein levels, associated with retardation of progression of CAD. However, total cholesterol/HDL cholesterol and LDL cholesterol appear superior to apolipoproteins as metabolic markers for effective treatment in patients with CAD.

Triglyceride-Rich Lipoproteins and Coronary Artery Disease

Accumulating evidence suggests that triglyceride-rich lipoproteins contribute to CAD. Using data from the Monitored Atherosclerosis Regression Study, an angiographic trial of middle-aged men and women randomized to lovastatin or placebo, Mack and colleagues[87] in Los Angeles, California, investigated relations between lipoprotein subclasses and progression of coronary artery atherosclerosis. Coronary artery lesion progression was detected by quantitative coronary angiography in low-grade (<50% diameter stenosis), high-grade (≥50% diameter stenosis), and all coronary artery lesions in 220 baseline/2-year angiogram pairs. Analytical ultracentrifugation was used to measure lipoprotein masses that were statistically evaluated for treatment group differences and relationships to progression of coronary artery atherosclerosis. All LDL, intermediate density lipoprotein, and VLDL masses were significantly lowered and all HDL masses were significantly raised with lovastatin therapy. The mass of smallest LDL, all VLDL subclasses, and peak LDL flotation rate were significantly related to the progression of coronary artery lesions, specifically low-grade lesions. Greater baseline levels of HDL_3 were related to a lower likelihood of coronary artery lesion progression. In multivariate analyses, small VLDL and HDL_3 mass were the most important correlates of coronary artery lesion progression (Table 1-7). These results provided further evidence for the importance of triglyceride-rich lipoproteins in the progression of CAD. In addition, these results present new evidence for the possible protective role of HDL_3 in the progression of coronary artery lesions. More specific information on coronary artery lesion progression may be obtained through the study of specific apolipoprotein B-containing lipoproteins.

Atherosclerotic Lesion Progression with Lovastatin in Smokers

Waters and colleagues[88] in Hartford, Connecticut, assessed the effects of smoking on the evolution of coronary atherosclerosis by serial angiography. Ninety smokers with coronary atherosclerosis with fasting serum cholesterol levels between 220 and 300 mg/dL were enrolled in a randomized, double-blind, placebo-controlled trial of cholesterol-lowering therapy, along with 241 nonsmokers and exsmokers. Lovastatin at a mean dose of 36 mg/day lowered

TABLE 1-7
Multivariate Models of Coronary Artery Lesion Progression

Lipoprotein Subclass	Placebo		Lovastatin		Combined	
	<50%S (n=105)	All Lesions (n=106)	<50%S (n=112)	All Lesions (n=114)	<50%S (n=217)	All Lesions (n=220)
Baseline						
HDL$_3$ per 30 mg/dL	...	...	...	0.7 (0.5–1.0)	...	0.7 (0.6–1.0)
On-trial						
IDL per 20 mg/dL	...	2.7 (1.1–6.3)	...	...	...	...
Small VLDL per 30 mg/dL	2.4 (1.2–4.8)	...	...	...	2.1 (1.3–3.4)	1.7 (1.1–2.8)
Intermediate VLVL per 30 mg/dL	...	2.2 (0.9–5.1)	...	...	...	...
Peak LDL flotation rate	...	...	0.5 (0.2–1.0)	...	...	...

Numbers are OR (95% CI). For placebo and drug groups, baseline levels of significant on-trial lipoprotein subclasses were forced into the model. For the combined group, treatment group and baseline levels of significant on-trial lipoprotein subclasses were forced into the model. Reproduced with permission from Mack et al.[87]

total and LDL cholesterol by 21% and 29%, respectively, but these levels changed by less than 2% in placebo-treated patients. Coronary arteriography was repeated after 2 years in 72 smokers, and their 557 lesions were measured blindly with an automated quantitative system, along with 1752 lesions in 227 nonsmokers. Coronary change score, the per-patient mean of the minimal luminal diameter changes for all qualifying lesions, worsened by 0.16 mm in smokers and by 0.07 mm in nonsmokers in the placebo group. Lovastatin-treated smokers had less worsening than placebo-treated smokers. One or more coronary lesions progressed in 16 of 34 lovastatin-treated smokers and in 28 of 38 placebo-treated smokers (47% vs. 74%) (Table 1-8). In the placebo group, new coronary lesions developed in 21 of 38 smokers and in 28 of 115 nonsmokers (55% vs. 24%). Fewer lovastatin-treated smokers developed new lesions (Table 1-9). Thus, smoking accelerates coronary progression and new lesion formation as assessed by serial quantitative coronary arteriography. Lovastatin attenuates the progression of coronary atherosclerosis and delays or prevents the development of new lesions in smokers.

TABLE 1-8
Quantitative Coronary Arteriographic Measurements

	Lovastatin Smokers	Placebo Smokers	Lovastatin Nonsmokers	Placebo Nonsmokers	Lovastatin All Patients	Placebo All Patients
Patients	34	38	112	115	146	153
Lesions	256	301	839	913	1095	1214
MLD pre	1.54 ± 0.21	1.55 ± 0.30	1.54 ± 0.27	1.48 ± 0.31	1.54 ± 0.25	1.49 ± 0.31
MLD post	1.47 ± 0.23	1.39 ± 0.25	1.50 ± 0.29	1.40 ± 0.32	1.49 ± 0.27	1.40 ± 0.30
MLD change	−0.07 ± 0.15*	−0.16 ± 0.16*	−0.04 ± 0.13	−0.07 ± 0.15	−0.05 ± 0.13†	−0.09 ± 0.16†

MLD indicates minimal lumen diameter in millimeters.

* $p=.024$; † $p=.010$.
Reproduced with permission from Waters et al.[88]

TABLE 1-9
Results for Categorical End Points for Smokers and Nonsmokers

End Point	Lovastatin Smokers (n = 34)	Placebo Smokers (n = 38)	p*	Lovastatin Nonsmokers (n = 112)	Placebo Nonsmokers (n = 115)	p*	p: All Smokers vs. Nonsmokers†
Progression only	15	26	.058	33	50	.038	.002
Any progression	16	28	.029	46	58	.183	.026
Regression only	7	2	.075	7	8	1.000	.105
Any regression	8	4	.206	20	16	.470	.850
New lesions	5	21	<.001	18	28	.139	.007
New occlusions	4	6	.740	11	13	.830	.448
Recanalizations	0	0	1.000	7	2	.099	.090

Progression only and regression only categories exclude patients with mixed changes, is, progression of one lesion and regression of another. Any progression and any regression include patients with mixed changes.

* Fisher's exact test; † Mantel-Haenszel test. Reproduced with permission from Waters et al.[88]

Nonimaging Lipid-Lowering Trials

Colestipol/Niacin Plus Diet or Placebo Plus Diet on Cholesterol Lowering

Azen and colleagues[89] in Los Angeles, California, used data from CLAS and randomly assigned 162 nonsmoking, 40- to 59-year-old men with previous coronary artery bypass grafting (CABG) to colestipol/niacin plus diet or placebo plus diet. Atherosclerosis change on 2-year coronary arteriograms was evaluated by a consensus panel and by quantitative coronary angiography. Using quantitative coronary angiography, the average per-subject change in percent diameter stenosis and minimal lumen diameter was identified. The benefits of colestipol/niacin therapy on coronary atherosclerosis were determined with annual follow-up for an average of 7 years for all patients completing the 2-year angiographic study. Clinical coronary events, including the need for revascularization, nonfatal AMI, and coronary death were documented. The risk of clinical coronary events was related to coronary lesion progression. New lesion formation in bypass grafts and progression of mild/moderate lesions were predictive of clinical coronary events. Changes in minimal luminal diameter contributed significantly to their prediction of clinical coronary events (Table 1-10). The data obtained in this study demonstrate that in this population of nonsmoking men with previous CABG, both the consensus panel and quantitative coronary angiography-based end points of CAD progression predict clinical coronary events of the need for future revascularization, nonfatal AMI, and coronary death. Subjects who demonstrate greater coronary artery lesion progression have an increased risk of future clinical coronary events.

Effect of Pravastatin on Coronary Events After Myocardial Infarction

Sacks and his colleagues[90] for the Cholesterol and Recurrent Events trial investigators (CARE Study) determined whether lowering serum cholesterol

TABLE 1-10
Adjusted RRs of Any Coronary Event and Nonfatal MI/Coronary Death per 10%S Increase
in %S and per 0.3-mm Decrease in MLD by QCA Stratified
by Lesion Location and Lesion Severity

	Measure	RR (95% CI)*	p†
Any coronary event‡			
All lesions	%S	2.2 (1.4, 3.5)	<.001
	MLD	2.1 (1.5, 2.9)	<.001
Lesion severity			
Mild/moderate (<50%S)	%S	2.1 (1.4, 3.0)	<.001
	MLD	1.8 (1.4, 2.4)	<.001
Severe (≥50%S)	%S	0.8 (0.5, 1.2)	.30
	MLD	0.8 (0.5, 1.2)	.24
Lesion location			
Native arteries	%S	1.5 (1.1, 2.2)	.05
	MLD	1.5 (1.0, 2.0)	.04
Proximal to grafts	%S	1.2 (0.9, 1.6)	.27
	MLD	1.3 (0.9, 1.7)	.11
Distal/unrelated to grafts	%S	1.2 (0.9, 1.7)	.26
	MLD	1.3 (0.9, 1.9)	.15
Bypass grafts	%S	1.6 (1.2, 2.1)	<.01
	MLD	1.5 (1.2, 1.7)	<.001
Nonfatal MI/coronary death			
All lesions	%S	2.0 (1.1, 3.7)	.03
	MLD	1.8 (1.2, 2.3)	<.01
Lesion severity			
Mild/moderate (<50%S)	%S	1.9 (1.2, 3.1)	<.01
	MLD	1.7 (1.2, 2.3)	<.01
Severe (≥50%S)	%S	0.6 (0.3, 1.2)	.12
	MLD	0.6 (0.4, 1.2)	.13
Lesion location			
Native arteries	%S	1.8 (1.2, 2.9)	<.01
	MLD	1.6 (1.1, 2.5)	.03
Proximal to grafts	%S	1.5 (0.9, 2.2)	.08
	MLD	1.5 (1.0, 2.1)	.05
Distal/unrelated to grafts	%S	1.4 (0.9, 2.2)	.10
	MLD	1.4 (0.8, 2.2)	.22
Bypass grafts	%S	1.5 (1.1, 2.0)	.04
	MLD	1.3 (1.1, 1.5)	<.01

* Calculated for native arteries and bypass grafts. RRs adjusted for treatment group and CLAS-II continuation status and calculated per 10%S change in %S and per 0.3-mm change in MLD. The cutoff points of 10%S and 0.3 mm are twice the measurement error for %S and MLD on short-term repeat angiograms, respectively.
† Likelihood ratio test for RR = 1 after adjustment for treatment assignment and CLAS II continuation status.
‡ Any coronary event: CABG, PTCA, nonfatal MI, or coronary death. Reproduced with permission from Azen et al.[89]

values in patients with "average" serum cholesterol levels has a benefit on survival and morbidity in patients with coronary heart disease. In a double-blind trial lasting 5 years, they administered either 40 mg of pravastatin per day or placebo to 4159 patients (3583 men and 576 women) with myocardial infarction who had plasma total cholesterol levels of less than 240 mg/dL (mean 209 mg/dL) and LDL cholesterol values of 115 to 174 mg/dL (mean 139 mg/dL)

(Table 1-11). The primary end point in this study was a fatal coronary event or a nonfatal myocardial infarction.

The primary end point was reached in 10% of the pravastatin-treated patients and in 13% of those treated with placebo, an absolute difference of 3 percentage points and a 24% reduction in risk (p = 0.003) (Figure 1-21). Coronary bypass surgery was required in 7.5% of patients treated with pravastatin and 10% of those in the placebo group, a 26% reduction (P = 0.005) (Figure 1-21). Coronary angioplasty was required in 8% of the pravastatin group and 11% of the placebo group (p = 0.01). The frequency of cerebrovascular accidents was reduced by 31% by pravastatin therapy (p = 0.03). There were no significant differences in overall mortality or mortality from noncardiovascular causes. Pravastatin lowered the rate of coronary events more among women than among men. The reduction in coronary events was also greater in patients with higher pretreatment levels of LDL cholesterol.

The authors conclude from this study that the benefit of cholesterol-lowering therapy extends to many patients with coronary disease who have average serum cholesterol and LDL values.

Simvastatin in the Reduction of Serum Cholesterol

To evaluate the effects of short-term cholesterol lowering treatment on myocardial effort ischemia, de Divitiis and associates[91] from Naples, Italy, randomly allocated 22 patients with stable effort ischemia and mild-to-moderate hypercholesterolemia (LDL cholesterol 160 to 220 mg/dL) at baseline in 2 groups. Group A comprised 12 patients treated with simvastatin (10 mg twice daily); group B comprised 10 patients treated with placebo. All patients underwent a treadmill electrocardiography test; total cholesterol, HDL and LDL cholesterol, triglycerides, plasma, and blood viscosity were measured. All tests were repeated after 4 and 12 weeks. For 18 of the same patients (11 taking simvastatin, 7 receiving placebo), forearm strain-gauge plethysmography was performed at baseline and after 4 weeks, both at rest and during reactive hyperemia. At 4 and 12 weeks, group A showed a significant reduction in total cholesterol and LDL, with unchanged HDL, triglycerides, blood, and plasma viscosity. Effort was unmodified; ST-segment depression at peak effort and ischemic threshold were significantly improved after 4 and 12 weeks with unchanged heart rate times systolic blood pressure product. A significant increase in the excess flow response to reactive hyperemia was detected in group A; group B showed no changes in hematochemical and ergometric parameters. These data suggest that cholesterol-lowering treatment is associated with an improvement in myocardial effort ischemia; this might be explained by a more pronounced increase of coronary blood flow and capacity of vasodilation in response to effort.

Lovastatin in African Americans

A paucity of substantive data from clinical drug trials is available, specifically evaluating the effects of therapy for hypercholesterolemia in African

TABLE 1-11
Baseline Characteristics of Patients in the Placebo and Pravastatin Groups*

Characteristic	Placebo (n = 2078)	Pravastatin (n = 2001)
General		
Age (yr)	59 ± 9	59 ± 9
Sex (%)		
Female	14	14
Male	86	86
Race (%)		
White	92	93
Other	8	7
Country of residence (%)		
United States	66	66
Canada	34	34
Hypertension (%)	43	42
Current smoker (%)	21	21
Diabetes (%)	15	14
Body-mass index†	28 ± 4	28 ± 4
Blood pressure (mm Hg)		
Systolic	129 ± 18	129 ± 12
Diastolic	79 ± 10	79 ± 10
Cardiovascular status		
Months from myocardial infarction to randomization	10 ± 5	10 ± 5
Type of myocardial infarction (%)		
Q wave	61	61
Other	38	38
Angina (%)	20	21
Congestive heart failure (%)	4	4
CABG (%)	28	26
PTCA (%)	32	34
CABG or PTCA (%)	54	54
Thrombolysis (%)	40	42
Ejection fraction (%)	53 ± 12	53 ± 12
Medication use		
Aspirin (%)	83	83
β-blocker (%)	39	41
Nitrate (%)	33	32
Calcium-channel blocker (%)	38	40
ACE inhibitor (%)	14	15
Diuretic agent (%)	11	11
Insulin (%)	2.6	2.4
Oral hypoglycemic agent (%)	7	5‡
Estrogen (% of women)	10.3	8.4
Plasma lipids§		
Cholesterol (mg/dl)		
Total	209 ± 17	209 ± 17
VLDL	27 ± 16	27 ± 16
LDL	139 ± 15	139 ± 15
HDL	39 ± 9	39 ± 9
Triglycerides (mg/dL)	155 ± 61	156 ± 61

* Plus-minus values are means ± SD. Except for the use of oral hyperglycemic agents, differences between the groups were not significant. CABG denotes coronary artery bypass grafting, PTCA percutaneous transluminal coronary angioplasty, ACE angiotensin converting enzyme, VLDL very low-density lipoprotein, LDL low-density lipoprotein, and HDL, high-density lipoprotein.

† The body mass index is the weight in kilograms divided by the square of the height in meters.

‡ <0.05 for the comparison with the placebo group.

§ To convert values for cholesterol to millimoles per liter, multiply by 0.02586. To convert values for triglycerides to millimoles per liter, multiply by 0.01129.

Reproduced with permission from Sacks et al.[90]

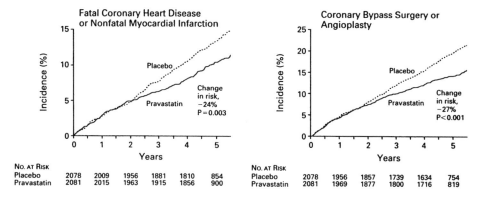

FIGURE 1-21. Kaplan-Meier estimates of the incidence of coronary events in the pravastatin and placebo groups. The left-hand panel shows data for the primary end point—fatal coronary heart disease or nonfatal myocardial infarction. The right-hand panel shows data for coronary bypass surgery or angioplasty. Changes in risk are those attributable to pravastatin. p values and changes in risk are based on Cox proportional-hazards analysis. Reproduced with permission from Sacks et al.[90]

Americans, even though a substantial number are candidates for medical advice and intervention for high blood cholesterol. The efficacy and safety of lovastatin in 459 African Americans with hypercholesterolemia were studied by Prisant and associates[92] from multiple United States medical centers in the Expanded Clinical Evaluation of Lovastatin study, a multicenter, double-blind, diet- and placebo-controlled trial. This trial involved 8245 patients who were randomly assigned, regardless of race, to receive placebo or lovastatin at doses of 20 mg once daily, 40 mg once daily, 20 mg twice daily, or 40 mg twice daily for 48 weeks. Among African Americans, lovastatin produced sustained, dose-related decreases in LDL cholesterol (20% to 38%), total cholesterol (14% to 28%), and triglycerides (8% to 15%) (Table 1-12). From 75% to 96% of African Americans treated with lovastatin achieved the National Cholesterol Education Program goal of LDL cholesterol less than 160 mg/dL, and from 33% to 71%

TABLE 1-12
Mean Percent Change from Baseline in Plasma Lipid/Lipoprotein Levels

		Treatment Group			
		Lovastatin (mg)			
Lipid/Lipoprotein	Placebo	20 qpm	40 qpm	20 bid	40 bid
LDL cholesterol*	−1 (12)	−20 (13)	−26 (15)	−30 (16)	−38 (14)
HDL cholesterol	2 (13)	5 (12)	5 (14)	6 (12)	5 (14)
Total cholesterol*	0 (8)	−14 (10)	−19 (11)	−22 (12)	−28 (11)
Triglycerides†	6	−8	−13	−11	−15

* All pairwise comparisons of lovastatin with placebo were significant ($p < .001$) using t test.

† Median triglyceride values are presented. The differences between placebo and all lovastatin groups were significant ($p < .001$) using the Wilcoxon rank-sum test.

Values are expressed as percent changes from baseline (SD).

Reproduced with permission from Prisant et al.[92]

achieved the goal less than 130 mg/dL. The safety profile of lovastatin in African Americans was generally favorable. A relatively high incidence of creatine kinase levels greater than the upper limit was observed in African-Americans during the study, ie, 63% in the placebo group and similar levels in lovastatin treatment groups. Lovastatin is highly effective and generally well tolerated as therapy for primary hypercholesterolemia in African Americans.

Lipids: Clinical Guidelines and Cost Effectiveness

Abnormal Lipoprotein Levels in a Biracial Population

Gidding and associates[93] from Chicago, Illinois, examined the prevalence of abnormal LDL and HDL cholesterol levels in young adults to determine the ability of National Cholesterol Education Program Adult Treatment Panel (ATP) guidelines to identify persons with elevated LDL cholesterol; to compare other algorithms with those of the ATP; and to determine the contributions of race, gender, and other CAD risk factors for identifying patients with elevated LDL and low HDL cholesterol. The cohort was population-based, aged 23 to 35 years, and included relatively equal numbers of blacks and whites, and men and women. The prevalence of LDL cholesterol of 160 mg/dL or greater (>4.1 mmol/L) was 5% in black women, 4% in white women, 10% in black men, and 9% in white men. ATP identified most participants with elevated LDL cholesterol (range: 58.8% of white men to 70.7% of black women). Lipoprotein panels would have been required in 6% to 7% of women and in 15% to 18% of men. Algorithms that used nonlipid risk factors required more lipoprotein panels and identified fewer additional participants at risk. The prevalence of HDL cholesterol of less than 35 mg/dL (0.9 mmol/L) was 3% in women, 7% in black men, and 13% in white men. Algorithms that used nonlipid risk factors before measuring HDL cholesterol would require HDL cholesterol measurements in 35% of whites and 56% of blacks, but reduced sensitivity for identifying low HDL cholesterol (range: 58% in white men to 93% in black women). In young adults, algorithms based on nonlipid risk factors and family history have lower sensitivity, and increase rather than decrease the number of fasting lipoprotein panels required when compared with ATP levels.

Cost-Effectiveness of Pravastatin

Ashraf and associates[94] from several United States medical centers analyzed the cost-effectiveness in pravastatin in secondary prevention of CAD. The projected risk model in 445 male patients with established CAD and moderately elevated serum LDL cholesterol used results data from 2 placebo-controlled plaque regression trials: Pravastatin Limitation of Atherosclerosis in the Coronary Arteries, and Pravastatin, Lipids, and Atherosclerosis in the Carotids. Framingham Heart Study data were used to project the risk of mortality 10 years after AMI for incremental male patients in the placebo group who had AMI.

TABLE 1-13
Hospitalization and Post-Event Follow-up Incremental Costs

Time Period	MI	Angina Pectoris	Stroke*	Congestive Heart Failure
Initial hospitalization	$18,614	$17,140	$7,366	$12,949
Year 1 follow-up	$2,142	$3,140	$5,434	$2,881
Year 2 follow-up	$898	$1,896	$892	$1,637
Year 3 follow-up	$898	$1,896	$892	$1,637
Year 4 follow-up	$812	$1,724	$806	$1,465
Year ≥5 follow-up†	$812	$1,724	$806	$1,465

* Follow-up cost for stroke does not include possible nursing home or home health care costs.
† Only MI has >5 years of follow-up.
MI = myocardial infarction.
Reproduced with permission from Ashraf et al.[94]

A Markov process was used to estimate life-years saved, and decision analysis was used to estimate cost. Depending on the patient-risk profile, the midrange estimated cost per life-year saved with pravastatin in secondary prevention of CAD varied from $7,124 to $12,665, which is favorable compared with other widely accepted medical interventions (Table 1-13 and Figure 1-22).

Insulin Research/Diabetes Mellitus

Insulin Resistance Syndrome: Related Gene Effects

Insulin resistance is part of a metabolic syndrome that includes noninsulin-dependent diabetes mellitus, dyslipidemia, obesity, and hypertension. It has

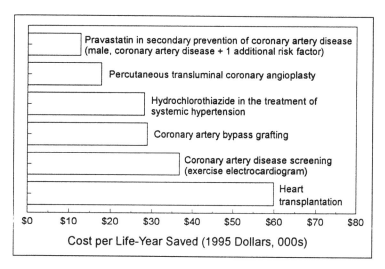

FIGURE 1-22. Estimates (adjusted to 1995 dollars) of other medical interventions for cardiovascular disease. Reproduced with permission from Ashraf et al.[94]

been hypothesized that insulin resistance represents the primary physiological defect underlying the syndrome. Because insulin resistance is at least partially genetically determined, Mitchell and coworkers[95] in San Antonio, Texas, hypothesized that genes influencing insulin resistance would have pleiotropic effects on a number of other traits, including triglyceride and HDL cholesterol levels, body mass index and body fat distribution, and blood pressure levels. To investigate this hypothesis, the investigators analyzed data obtained from individuals in 41 families enrolled in the San Antonio Family Heart Study. Statistical methods that take advantage of the relatedness among individuals were used to differentiate between genetic and nongenetic contributions to phenotypic variation between traits. Serum levels of fasting and 2-hour insulin were used as a measure of insulin resistance. The genetic correlations were high between insulin levels and each of the following: body mass index, HDL level, waist-to-hip ratio, and subscapular-to-triceps ratio, indicating that the same gene, or set of genes, influenced each pair of traits. In contrast, the genetic correlations of insulin levels with systolic and diastolic blood pressures were low. The investigators had previously shown that a single diallelic locus accounts for 31% of the phenotypic variation in 2-hour insulin levels in this population. The investigators conducted a bivariate segregation analysis to see if the common genetic effects on insulin and the other traits could be attributable to the single locus. The results indicated a significant effect of the 2-hour insulin locus on fasting insulin levels with the high insulin allele associated with higher levels of fasting insulin, but lower levels of body mass index. There were no detectable effects of the locus on HDL level, triglyceride level, subscapular-to-triceps ratio, or blood pressure. Overall, the results suggested that a common set of genes influencing insulin levels also influenced other insulin resistance syndrome-related traits although, for the most part, the pleiotropy was not attributable to the 2-hour insulin level major locus.

Insulin Sensitivity and Atherosclerosis

Howard and colleagues[96] in Winston-Salem, North Carolina, evaluated insulin sensitivity by the frequently sampled intravenous glucose tolerance test and compared insulin sensitivity with intimal-medial thickness of the carotid artery as an index of atherosclerosis using noninvasive B-mode ultrasonography. The relations between insulin sensitivity and atherosclerosis were evaluated in 398 black, 457 Hispanic, and 542 non-Hispanic white individuals. There was a significant negative association between insulin sensitivity and the intima-medial thickness of the carotid artery both in Hispanics and in non-Hispanic whites. This effect was reduced, but not totally explained by adjustment for traditional cardiovascular risk factors, glucose tolerance, measures of adiposity, and fasting insulin levels. There was no association between insulin sensitivity and intimal-medial thickness of the carotid artery in blacks. The association between insulin sensitivity and intimal-medial thickness was stronger for the internal carotid artery than for the common carotid artery in all ethnic groups. Thus, these data suggest that higher levels of insulin sensitivity are associated with less atherosclerosis in Hispanics and non-Hispanic whites, but not in blacks.

Insulin Resistance and Nicotine Gum

Eliasson and colleagues[97] in Göteborg, Sweden, examined insulin sensitivity and cardiovascular risk profile in 20 healthy, nonobese, middle-aged men who were long-term users of nicotine-containing chewing gum and in 20 matched control subjects who did not use nicotine. Long-term use of nicotine-containing chewing gum was associated with insulin resistance and hyperinsulinemia (Figure 1-23). The degree of insulin sensitivity correlated negatively to the extent of nicotine use measured as plasma cotinine levels. These data suggest that nicotine is a major constituent in cigarette smoke that leads to insulin resistance, metabolic abnormalities associated with the insulin resistance syndrome, and possibly increased cardiovascular morbidity. Thus, the authors suggest that the use of nicotine replacement therapy during smoking cessation should be for only a limited period of time.

Endothelial Function and Insulin Resistance

Mäkimattila and colleagues[98] in Helsinki, Finland, determined whether chronic hyperglycemia is associated with defects in endothelium-dependent vasodilation *in vivo* and whether defects in the hemodynamic effects of insulin

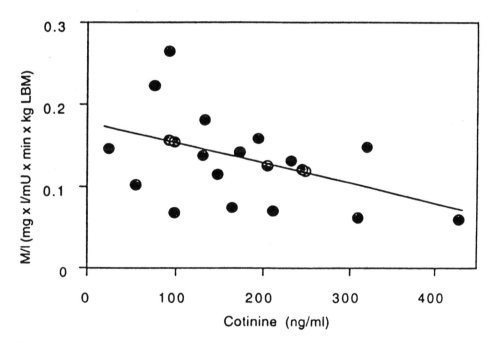

Figure 1-23. A, C-peptide levels (μg/L) (mean ± SEM) in the fasting state and during clamp steady state in NGCs and nonsmokers. Degree of suppression: nonsmokers 0.7 ± 0.1; NGCs, 0.2 ± 0.1 (p = .0013). **p<.01; ***p<.001. Be, Insulin levels (mU/L) (mean ± SEM) in the fasting state and during clamp steady state in NGCs and nonsmokers. *p<.05; ***p<.001. Reproduced with permission from Eliasson et al.[97]

explain insulin resistance. Vasodilator responses to brachial artery infusions of acetylcholine, sodium nitroprusside, and N^G-monomethyl-L-arginine and, on another occasion, *in vivo* insulin sensitivity measured by a euglycemic insulin clamp combined with the forearm catheterization technique, were determined in 18 patients with insulin-dependent diabetes mellitus and 9 normal subjects. At identical glucose and insulin levels, insulin stimulation of whole-body and forearm glucose uptake was 57% reduced in the insulin-dependent diabetic patients compared with normal subjects (p<0.001). The defect in forearm glucose uptake was attributable to a defect in glucose extraction, not blood flow. With the group of insulin-dependent diabetes mellitus patients, hemoglobin A_{1c} was inversely correlated with forearm blood flow during administration of acetylcholine, but not sodium nitroprusside. The ratio of endothelium-dependent to endothelium-independent blood flow was approximately 40% lower in patients with poor glycemic control than in normal subjects or patients with good or moderate glycemic control (Figure 1-24). The data suggest that chronic hyperglycemia is associated with an impaired endothelium-dependent vasodilation *in vivo* and with a glucose extraction defect during insulin stimulation. Thus, chronic hyperglycemia appears to impair vascular endothelial function and insulin action by distinct mechanisms.

Endothelium-Dependent and Endothelium-Independent Vasodilation in Insulin-Dependent Diabetes Mellitus

Vascular complications in diabetes mellitus are associated with endothelial dysfunction. Whether endothelium-dependent vasodilation is impaired in normo-albuminuric patients with insulin-dependent diabetes mellitus is controversial. Using a noninvasive echo-Doppler method, Lambert and colleagues[99] in Amsterdam, The Netherlands, investigated endothelium-dependent and endothelium-independent vasodilation in the brachial artery of patients with insulin-dependent diabetes mellitus. The study comprised 52 normo-albuminuric and normotensive patients with insulin-dependent diabetes mellitus (average age, 32 years; duration of diabetes, 15 years) and 52 healthy control subjects (comparable for age and sex). Brachial artery diameter was measured at baseline, during postocclusion reactive hyperemia, and after 400 μg of glyceryl trinitrate given sublingually. Vasodilation was expressed as the percentage change relative to the baseline diameter. Baseline flow and blood pressure were similar for insulin-dependent diabetes mellitus patients and control subjects. Baseline vessel diameter was slightly larger in insulin-dependent diabetes mellitus patients compared with control subjects. The endothelium-dependent dilation in insulin-dependent diabetes mellitus patients was decreased (12% vs. 16%), as was glyceryl trinitrate-induced vasodilation 15% vs. 18%). After correction for the difference in baseline diameter, endothelium-dependent dilation and trinitrate-induced dilation were not different between the groups. Glyceryl trinitrate-induced vasodilation decreased slightly with an increase in diabetes duration. There was no relation between the vasodilatory responses and hemoglobin A1c. In normo-albuminuric insulin-dependent diabetes mellitus patients, endothelium-dependent, as well as

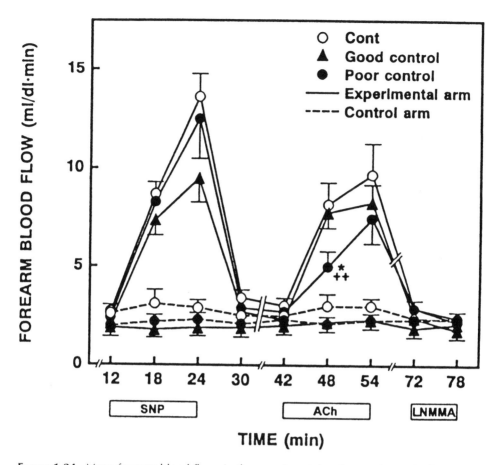

FIGURE 1-24. Mean forearm blood flows in the experimental and control arms in the normal subjects (Cont, n=9), and in the IDDM patients in good control (Good control, n=9) and poor control (Poor control, n=9). Glycemic control was defined according to the HbA_{1c} concentration. *p<.05 for IDDM patients in Good vs. Poor control; ‡p<.02 for IDDM patients in Poor glycemic control vs. Cont. Reproduced with permission from Mäkimattila et al.[98]

endothelium-independent vasodilation is normal when the difference in baseline diameter is taken into account.

Vascular Reactivity in Insulin-Dependent Diabetes Mellitus

Endothelial dysfunction is assumed to be an early event in the development of atherosclerosis. Like other risk factors, diabetes is assumed to produce its adverse effects in part by effects on endothelial dysfunction. Clarkson and colleagues[100] from London, England, and Camperdown, New South Wales, Australia, evaluated whether endothelial function was impaired in the large vessels of asymptomatic young adults with insulin-dependent diabetes and whether endothelial dysfunction was related to the duration or control of diabetes, small vessel disease, or other vascular risk factors. These authors compared 80 young adults with insulin-dependent diabetes (age 15 to 40 years) with a mean diabetes duration of 13 ± 8 years, with 80 matched nondiabetic control subjects. Using high-resolution vascular ultrasound, they measured brachial artery responses to reactive hyperemia (with increased flow causing endothelium-dependent dilation) and sublingual nitrate (causing endothelium-independent dilation). Flow-mediated dilation was significantly impaired in diabetic subjects (5.0% vs. 9.3% in control subjects). The ratio of flow-mediated dilation to nitrate-induced dilation was significantly lower in diabetic subjects, indicating that impaired dilation to increased flow was out of proportion to the impairment of the nitrate response in these subjects (15.6% vs. 19.7% in control subjects). On multivariate analysis, flow-mediated dilation was inversely related to both the duration of diabetes and LDL cholesterol levels. These authors concluded that vascular reactivity is impaired in the systemic arteries of asymptomatic young adults with insulin-dependent diabetes and may represent early large-vessel disease. The degree of impairment was related to the duration of diabetes, and these patients appeared particularly vulnerable to damage from LDL cholesterol, even at levels considered acceptable in nondiabetic subjects. These data provide additional information that the common final pathway of all risk factors for CAD may be through endothelial dysfunction and its accompanying adverse effects.

Risk Factors in Insulin-Dependent Diabetes Mellitus

Insulin-dependent diabetes mellitus increases the risk of developing CAD compared with that seen in the general population, whereas the sex differential in rates of CAD is considerably reduced in insulin-dependent diabetes mellitus populations. To further the understanding of these observations, Lloyd and coworkers[101] in Pittsburgh, Pennsylvania, examined the effects of gender on baseline risk factors for CAD incidence. Participants in the Pittsburgh Epidemiology of Diabetes Complications Study were recruited from the Children's Hospital of Pittsburgh Insulin Dependent Diabetes Mellitus Registry and had been diagnosed between 1950 and 1980. Subjects completed a series of questionnaires and were given a full clinical examination at baseline (1986–1988) and every subsequent 2 years. The report was based on the first 4 years of follow-up. Similar incidence rates of new CAD events were observed in men and women. In neither sex was glycemic control a predictor of later CAD. Sex-specific Cox proportional hazards models showed that for men, duration of insulin-dependent diabetes mellitus, HDL cholesterol, fibrinogen, hypertension, and smoking were all significantly associated with the onset of CAD. Hypertension, fibrinogen, and smoking were all replaced by nephropathy when this latter variable was added to the model. For women, duration, hypertension, waist-to-hip ratio, physical activity, and depressive symptomatology were all significant independent predictors of CAD. Nephropathy status did not enter the model for women. Whereas 4-year incidence of CAD in IDDM varies little by sex in this population, the predicted risk factors varied considerably. In particular, the effect of renal disease was stronger in men, whereas the cluster of physical activity, waist-to-hip ratio, and depressive symptomatology were more important in women. These results may help explain the relatively greater impact of insulin-dependent diabetes mellitus on CAD risk for women and suggest new potential preventive approaches.

Vasodilation in Noninsulin-Dependent Diabetes Mellitus

Previous studies have suggested that patients with insulin-dependent diabetes mellitus demonstrate impaired endothelial-dependent vasodilation. Williams and colleagues[102] from Boston, Massachusetts, sought to determine whether nitric oxide-mediated vasodilation is abnormal in patients with noninsulin-dependent diabetes mellitus. Vascular reactivity was measured in the forearm resistance vessels of 21 patients with noninsulin-dependent diabetes mellitus and in 23 matched healthy controls. Each subject was pretreated with aspirin to inhibit endogenous production of vasoactive prostanoids. Forearm blood flow responses to methacholine chloride and nitroprusside were significantly attenuated in diabetic compared with nondiabetic subjects. By contrast, the response to verapamil was not different between the 2 groups. These authors concluded that nitric oxide-mediated vasodilation is impaired in noninsulin-dependent diabetes mellitus. They suggested that the abnormality may be due to increased inactivation of nitric oxide or decreased reactivity of the vascular smooth muscle to nitric oxide (Figure 1-25).

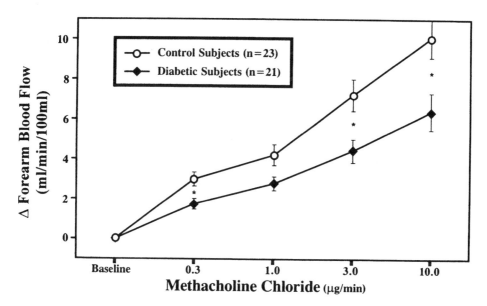

FIGURE 1-25. Forearm blood flow increase from baseline during graded intra-arterial infusion of methacholine chloride in diabetic and nondiabetic subjects. Reproduced with permission from Williams et al.[102]

Sex Differences and Fibrinolysis in Noninsulin-Dependent Diabetes Mellitus

The increase in cardiovascular risks associated with noninsulin-dependent diabetes mellitus is far greater in women than in men. Conventional risk factors do not account for this excess, and attention has focused on the possible contribution of abnormalities of fibrinolysis and coagulation in noninsulin-dependent diabetes mellitus. In the general population, a number of hemostatic factors have been shown to predict the occurrence or progression of CAD. To investigate sex differences in coagulation and fibrinolysis in noninsulin-dependent diabetes mellitus, Mansfield and coinvestigators[103] in Leeds, United Kingdom, measured levels of fibrinogen, factor VIIC, von Willebrand factor, plasminogen activator inhibitor 1 and tPA in 213 subjects (124 men and 89 women) with noninsulin-dependent diabetes mellitus who were not receiving insulin therapy. The women had higher levels of factor VIIC and plasminogen activator inhibitor 1 activity, and these differences remained significant when account was taken of the higher body mass index, glycosylated hemoglobin, and cholesterol levels in women than men. In contrast, levels of fibrinogen, tPA antigen, and von Willebrand factor were no different between women and men, respectively. These results suggested that elevated levels of plasminogen activator inhibitor 1 and factor VIIC may contribute to the increased cardiovascular risks of noninsulin-dependent diabetes mellitus that is particularly marked in women.

Autoantibodies Against Oxidized LDL in Noninsulin-Dependent Diabetes Mellitus

Accelerated atherosclerosis in diabetes has been suggested to be due to an enhanced oxidative modification of LDL. Uusitupa and coinvestigators[104] in Kuopio, Finland, hypothesized that the titers of autoantibodies against oxidized LDL may be increased in patients with noninsulin-dependent diabetes mellitus and that they may contribute to various manifestations of atherosclerosis among such patients. In a 10-year follow-up study of 91 newly diagnosed noninsulin-dependent diabetes mellitus patients and 82 nondiabetic control subjects, autoantibodies against oxidized LDL (expressed as the ratio of autoantibodies against oxidized LDL and native LDL) were measured at baseline and after 10 years. Quantitative ultrasonography to examine the intimal-medial thickness of the common carotid artery (a morphological index of arterial wall injury) and carotid bifurcation was performed at the 10-year examination. The relation of autoantibodies against oxidized LDL to the occurrence of cardiovascular death, fatal and nonfatal AMI, stroke, and any cardiovascular event, as well as to the intimal-medial thickness of the common carotid artery and carotid bifurcation was evaluated. Associations between these autoantibodies and metabolic variables (fasting glucose, glycosylated hemoglobin, insulin, and serum lipids) in noninsulin-dependent diabetes mellitus patients were also examined. Autoantibodies against oxidized LDL did not differ between noninsulin-dependent diabetes mellitus and control subjects. In both groups, the titers of these autoantibodies measured at baseline and after 10 years significantly correlated with each other. The frequency of all cardiovascular events was markedly higher in the noninsulin-dependent diabetes mellitus group than in the control group, but autoantibodies against oxidized LDL had no significant association with any of these events, including cardiovascular mortality. At the 10-year examination, the intimal-medial thicknesses of the common carotid artery and carotid bifurcation were greater in noninsulin-dependent diabetes mellitus patients than in control subjects, but autoantibodies did not show any association with the intimal-medial thicknesses in either the diabetic or control groups. Autoantibodies against oxidized LDL indicate the presence of oxidatively modified LDL *in vitro*, but their titers in the serum do not appear to be associated with excess cardiovascular mortality, morbidity, or intimal-medial thickness of the carotid artery.

Mortality After AMI in Diabetic Patients

Mortality rate after AMI in patients with diabetes is approximately twice that of nondiabetic patients. It is uncertain whether this difference in mortality is due to a lower rate of successful thrombolysis, increased reocclusion after successful thrombolysis, greater ventricular injury, or more adverse angiographic or clinical profile in diabetic patients. Woodfield and colleagues[105] for the Global Utilization of Streptokinase and Tissue Plasminogen Activator for Occluded Coronary Arteries Trial (GUSTO-I) trial evaluated the diabetic cohort (n = 310) in the GUSTO angiographic trial (2431). The diabetic cohort had a significantly higher proportion of female and elderly patients and were more often hypertensive, came to the hospital later, and had more congestive heart failure and a higher number of previous myocardial infarctions and bypass surgery procedures. In patients with and without diabetes, 90-minute patency (TIMI grade 3 flow) rates were 40.3% and 37.6%. Reocclusion rates were 9.2% versus 5.3%. Ejection fraction at 90 minutes after thrombolysis was similar in diabetic and nondiabetic patients. No significant difference in ventricular function was noted at 5- to 7-day follow-up. The 30-day mortality rate was 11.3% in diabetic versus 5.9% in nondiabetic patients. After adjustment for clinical and angiographic variables, diabetes remained an independent determinant of 30-day mortality. These authors concluded that one cannot fully explain the increased risk of diabetes by changes in infarct-related patency or regional and global left ventricular function. Thus, diabetes remained an independent determinant of 30-day mortality after correction for clinical and angiographic variables.

Body Mass Index, Smoking, and Other Risk Factors

Impact of Body Mass Index on Coronary Heart Disease Risk Factors

Increased body weight has been associated with an increased risk of morbidity and mortality from CAD in several populations. Lamon-Fava and associates[106] in Framingham, Massachusetts, studied the distribution of body mass index in men (n = 1566, mean age 49 years) and women (n = 1627; mean age 49 years) participating in the third examination cycle of the Framingham Offspring Study and the association of BMX with known CAD risk factors. In men, BMX increased with age until 50 years, when it reached a plateau. In women, there was a trend toward an increase in body mass index with age up to the 7th decade of life; 72% of men and 42% of women had a BMX greater than 25, the cutoff point for the definition of overweight. In age-adjusted analyses, BMX was significantly and linearly associated with systolic blood pressure, fasting glucose levels, plasma total cholesterol, VLDL cholesterol, and LDL cholesterol levels and was inversely and linearly associated with HDL cholesterol levels in nonsmoking men and women. The association between BMX and apolipoproteins B and A-I was similar to that of LDL and HDL cholesterol, respectively. LDL size was also linearly associated with BMX; subjects with high BMX had smaller LDL particles. Lipoprotein(a) levels were not associated with BMX in this population. Of all these risk factors for CAD, reduced HDL cholesterol levels and hypertension were those most strongly associated with higher BMX in both men and women. Elevated triglyceride levels, small LDL particles, and diabetes in women were also strongly associated with higher BMX values in this population. These results indicated that a higher prevalence of adult Americans are overweight and support the concepts that increased BMX is associated with an adverse effect on all major CAD risk factors. These results emphasize the importance of excess body fat as a public health issue.

Endothelial Function and Smoking

Ichiki and colleagues[107] in Kurume, Japan evaluated whether long-term smoking impairs endothelium-dependent vasodilation by decreasing the availability of nitric oxide. Platelet-derived electrical current induced by collagen was measured with an nitric oxide-selective electrode in 12 smokers and 11 nonsmokers. Collagen-induced intraplatelet cyclic guanosine monophosphate (cGMP) and platelet aggregation were measured in smokers and nonsmokers. S-nitroso-N-acetyl-dl-penicillamine, a direct nitric oxide donor, dose dependently increased in electrical current. Collagen induced platelet aggregation and dose dependently increased electrical current. Collagen-induced electrical current and cGMP was significantly augmented by L-arginine, a precursor of nitric oxide, and attenuated by N^G-monomethyl-L-arginine, an inhibitor of nitric oxide synthesis. Significant correlation was found between collagen-induced electrical current and cGMP. These findings indicate that the change in electrical current reflects nitric oxide release through the L-arginine-nitric oxide pathway in platelets. Collagen-induced electrical current and cGMP were significantly lower in smokers than in nonsmokers. Although L-arginine increased cGMP levels in both smokers and nonsmokers, the level was still lower in smokers. The inhibitory effect of L-arginine on collagen-induced platelet aggregation was lower in smokers than in nonsmokers. These data indicate that platelet-derived nitric oxide release is significantly impaired in long-term smokers, contributing to the augmentation of platelet aggregability.

Smoking impairs the endothelium-dependent relaxation of arteries and veins, with the maximum relaxation saphenous vein rings in response to the calcium ionophore A23187 of being reduced from 53% in nonsmokers to 27% in smokers. Higman and colleagues[108] in London, United Kingdom, investigated whether this endothelial dysfunction was attributable to altered activity or concentration of nitric oxide synthase. The concentration of nitric oxide synthase in saphenous vein endothelium, determined by Western blotting and immunohistochemistry, was not different in nonsmokers and smokers. Nitrite production from vein strips stimulated with A23187 was higher in nonsmokers than in smokers, this difference lacking when vein strips were preincubated in the presence of N^G-monomethyl-L-arginine. Organ-chamber studies to monitor the endothelium-dependent relaxation of vein rings in response to A23187 showed that preincubation of rings from smokers with either L-arginine or superoxide dismutase did not improve the maximum relaxation. In contrast, preincubation of vein rings from smokers with 20 μmol/L tetrahydrobiopterin increased the maximum relaxation from 27% to 51%, p = .01. Preincubation of vein from smokers with tetrahydrobiopterin also significantly increased nitrite in cGMP production in response to stimulation with A23187. The impaired endothelium-dependent relaxation of saphenous vein rings in smokers appeared to be caused by a reduction in the activity of endothelial nitric oxide synthase that was attributable to an inadequate supply of the coenzyme tetrahydrobiopterin.

Heitzer and colleagues[109] in Freiburg, Germany, and Kuopio, Finland, investigated the role of long-term smoking and hypercholesterolemia on endothelial function in relation to plasma levels of autoantibodies against oxidized LDL, which have been implicated in the development of endothelial dysfunction and atherosclerosis. The vascular responses to the endothelium-dependent agent acetylcholine and the endothelium-independent agent sodium nitroprusside were studied in normal control subjects (n = 10), patients with hypercholesterolemia (n = 15), long-term smokers (n = 15), and hypercholesterolemic patients who smoked (n = 15). Drugs were infused into the brachial artery, and forearm blood flow was measured by venous occlusion plethysmography. The forearm blood flow responses to acetylcholine were attenuated in all 3 patient groups compared with normal controls (Figure 1–26). The acetylcholine-induced increase in forearm blood flow was attenuated in patients with hypercholesterolemia who smoked compared with hypercholesterolemic nonsmokers and normocholesterolemic smokers. The response to sodium nitroprusside was the same in all 4 groups. Plasma levels of autoantibody titer against oxidized LDL were inversely related to acetylcholine-induced changes in forearm blood flow. They were substantially increased in the group with both risk factors. Thus, these data suggest that cigarette smoking and hypercholesterolemia synergistically impair endothelial function and that their combined presence is associated with increased plasma levels of autoantibodies against oxidized LDL.

Heitzer and colleagues[110] in Hamburg, Germany, tested the hypothesis that endothelial dysfunction may be a consequence of enhanced degradation

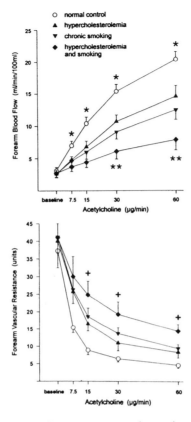

FIGURE 1-26. Plots of forearm blood flow (FBF) (top) and vascular resistance responses (bottom) to acetylcholine in normal subjects (n = 10), hypercholesterolemic patients (n = 15), long-term smokers (n = 15), and patients with hypercholesterolemia who smoked (n = 15). All 3 patient groups had significantly less increase in FBF than did normal subjects (*p<.05). **p<.05 by ANOVA compared with all other groups; †p<.05 vs. all other groups. Data are mean ± SEM. Reproduced with permission from Heitzer et al.[109]

of nitric oxide secondary to formation of oxygen-derived free radicals. Forearm blood flow responses to the endothelium-dependent vasodilator acetylcholine (7.5, 15, 30, and 60 μg/min) and the endothelium-independent vasodilator sodium nitroprusside (1, 3, and 10 μg/min) were measured by venous occlusion plethysmography in 10 control subjects and 10 chronic smokers. Drugs were infused into the brachial artery, and forearm blood flow was measured for each drug before and during concomitant intra-arterial infusion of the antioxidant vitamin C (18 mg/min). In controls, vitamin C had no effect on forearm blood flow in response to acetylcholine and sodium nitroprusside. In contrast, in chronic smokers, the attenuated forearm blood flow responses to acetylcholine were markedly improved by concomitant administration of vitamin C (Figure 1-27), but the vasodilator responses to sodium nitroprusside were not altered. Thus, the present study provides further evidence that the antioxidant vitamin C markedly improves endothelium-dependent responses in chronic smokers.

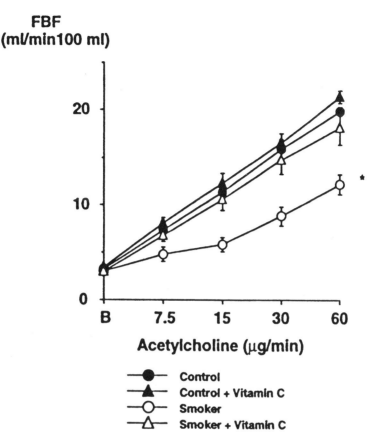

FIGURE 1-27. Mean ± SEM responses of forearm blood flow (FBF) to intra-arterial acetylcholine in control subjects (n = 10) and chronic smokers (n = 10) with and without concomitant administration of vitamin C. Vitamin C treatment markedly improves endothelium-dependent vasodilation to acetylcholine in chronic smokers while having no significant effect on the dose-response curve of control subjects. *Significant difference in the overall dose-response relationship compared with control subjects with and without vitamin C and with smokers with vitamin C. Reproduced with permission from Heitzer et al.[110]

Environmental Smoke and Coronary Heart Disease

Steenland and colleagues[111] conducted the largest study to date evaluating the risk of developing in CAD nonsmokers exposed to environmental tobacco smoke. This prospective study comprised 353,180 females and 126,500 male never-smokers from the American Cancer Society's Cancer Prevention Study II who were enrolled in 1982 and followed through 1989. Analyses focused on subcohorts of 309,599 married pairs and of 135,237 subjects concordant for self-reported exposure and exposure related by each one's spouse. More than 2800 CAD deaths occurred among married pairs; 10% of married men and 28% of married women were married to currently smoking spouses, whereas 10% of men and 32% of women, were married to former smokers. After controlling for many cardiovascular risk factors, the investigators found a 22% higher CAD mortality among never-smoking men married to currently smoking wives than that for men married to wives who never smoked. The corresponding rate ratio for women was 1.10. Never-smokers living with former smokers showed no increased risk. When analyses were restricted to subjects whose environmental tobacco smoke exposure was classified by their own self-report and a spouse's report, the rate ratio was 1.23 for currently exposed men and 1.19 for women. These results are consistent with earlier reports that never-smokers currently exposed to environmental tobacco smoke have approximately 20% higher CAD death rates.

Smoking and Prognosis after AMI

Studies before and during the thrombolytic era have reported similar or lower early mortality after AMI in smokers as compared with nonsmokers. This finding seems contradictory to the numerous epidemiological studies that have clearly shown smoking to be an independent risk factor for atherosclerosis, AMI, and death. Gottlieb and colleagues[112] from Jerusalem, Tel Hashomer, and Hadera, Israel, compared the relation between smoking and the 30-day and 6-month outcome after AMI in an Israeli nationwide survey. The study cohort comprised 999 consecutive patients with an AMI from a prospective nationwide survey during January and February 1994 in all coronary care units operating in Israel. The prognosis of 367 patients (37%) who were smokers (current smokers and those who smoked up to 1 month before admission) was compared with that of 632 nonsmokers (past smokers or those who never smoked). Smokers were an average 10 years younger than nonsmokers and were more frequently men and patients with a family history of coronary heart disease and inferior infarction; smokers less frequently had a history of infarction or angina, hypertension, and diabetes than did nonsmokers. Nonsmokers also had a lower incidence of heart failure on admission during the hospital period. Thrombolytic therapy and aspirin were administered more frequently in smokers than in nonsmokers. The crude 30-day (6.0% vs. 15.7%) and cumulative 6-month (7.9% vs. 21.5%) mortality rates were significantly lower in smokers than nonsmokers, respectively. However, after adjustment for age, baseline characteristics, thrombolytic therapy and invasive coronary procedures, the lower 30-day and 6-month hazard ratios for mortality rate were not significantly different. These authors concluded that the seemingly better prognosis of smokers early after acute myocardial infarction was no longer evident after adjustment for baseline and clinical variables and may be explained by their younger age and a more favorable risk profile. Smokers develop AMI a decade earlier than nonsmokers. Thus, efforts to lower the prevalence of smoking should continue.

Homocysteine

Homocysteine and Risk of Premature Coronary Heart Disease

Gallagher and colleagues[113] in Montreal, Quebec, Canada, examined the hypothesis that the allele that codes for the thermolabile defect of the enzyme methylenetetrahydrofolate reductase increases the risk of CAD as a result of modulating the formation of plasma homocysteine levels. The authors studied 111 patients with clinical and objective investigational evidence of CAD and 105 control subjects. The frequencies of the thermolabile defect in patients and control subjects were measured, and the prevalence of elevated plasma total homocysteine according to genotype was assessed. The frequency of the defective allele was higher in patients than in control subjects. Plasma total homocysteine levels were significantly associated with CAD status, a relationship that matched the strength of the association between disease and homozygous inheritance of the defective enzymes. Thus, these data suggest that homozygotes for the defective allele are at increased risk of premature CAD. Methylenetetrahydrofolate reductase, which modulates basal plasma homocysteine concentration, is folate-dependent, and dietary supplementation or fortification with folic acid may reduce plasma homocysteine levels and consequent risk of CAD.

Case Control Study of MI and Homocysteine

Schmitz and colleagues[114] in Wageningen, The Netherlands, investigated whether a point mutation (C677T) in the gene encoding methylenetetrahydrofolate reductase, an enzyme involved in homocysteine remethylation, influences risk for AMI and plasma levels of homocysteine and whether this effect may be modified by dietary folate intake in 190 patients with MI and 188 control subjects from the Boston Area Health Study. Eligible patients were men and women younger than 76 years of age with a confirmed diagnosis of MI, each matched to a control subject of the same age (within 5 years) and sex without a history of cardiovascular disease. Relevant information on tobacco use, dietary habits, physical activity, folate intake adjusted for total caloric intake, and past medical and family history were obtained from all study subjects. A point mutation (C677T) in the gene encoding methylenetetrahydrofolate reductase has been reported to render the enzyme thermolabile and less active and has been associated with elevated plasma homocysteine levels in homozygous carriers, as well as with an increased risk of premature cardiovascular disease. The relative risk for MI associated with the homozygous carriers was 1.1. Stratification by folate intake values above and below the median did not alter these results. Plasma homocysteine levels were 9.9 ± 2.7 μmol/L in controls, 10.6 ± 3.8 μmol/L in heterozygotes, and 9.1 ± 2.3 μmol/L in homozygotes. Thus, these data demonstrate that homozygosity for the C677T mutation in this largely Caucasian, middle-class United States population is not associated with increase risk for MI, irrespective of folate intake. This mutation may not be a useful marker for increased cardiovascular risk in this and similar populations.

Homocysteine and Risk of MI in United States Physicians

Ma and colleagues[115] in Boston, Massachusetts, assessed the polymorphism in methylenetetrahydrofolate reductase, plasma total homocysteine, and folate using baseline blood levels obtained from 293 Physicians' Health

Study participants who developed MI during 8 years of follow-up and from 290 control subjects. Elevated levels of plasma total homocysteine may result from genetic or nutrient-related disturbances in the transsulfuration or remethylation pathways for homocysteine metabolism. The enzyme 5,10-methylenetetrahydrofolate reductase catalyzes the reduction of 5,10-methylenetetrahydrofolate to 5-methyltetrahydrofolate, the predominant circulatory form of folate, which serves as a methyl donor for remethylation of homocysteine to methionine. The frequency of the 3 genotypes was 47% for homozygous normal; 41% for heterozygous; and 12% for homozygous mutant with a similar disruption among both MI and control subjects. Compared with those with homozygous genotype, the relative risk of MI among those with the heterozygous one was 1.1, and it was 0.8 for the homozygous mutant. None of these differences was statistically significant. However, those with the mutant genotype had an increased mean total plasma homocysteine level compared with those with the normal homozygote genotype, and this difference was most marked among men with low folate levels. Thus, in this population, the methylenetetrahydrofolate reductase polymorphism was associated with higher homocysteine levels but not with an increased risk of MI. The authors speculated that a gene-environment interaction might increase the risk by elevating plasma homocysteine levels further, especially when folate intake is low.

Implications of Low S-Adenosylmethionine

Mild elevation of plasma homocysteine is an independent risk factor for vascular disease. Loehrer and coinvestigators[116] in Basel, Switzerland, studied the role of 5-methyltetrahydrofolate, the folate form directly involved in homocysteine metabolism (in contrast to previous studies, which used total folate measurements), in 70 CAD patients and control subjects. The investigators also measured S-adenosylmethionine, which controls the activity of critical enzymes of homocysteine metabolism. Fasting plasma total homocysteine was elevated in 17% of patients, in accordance with earlier studies. These patients showed lower 5-methyltetrahydrofolate than control subjects, and there was a clear correlation of this relevant form of folate with homocysteine. However, 37% of the normohomocysteinemic patients also revealed similarly low levels of 5-methyltetrahydrofolate, suggesting that a decrease of 5-methyltetrahydrofolate does not necessarily cause hyperhomocysteinemia. S-adenosylmethionine was significantly decreased in patients compared with control subjects, but was not correlated to homocysteine or 5-methyltetrahydrofolate. The correlation between homocysteine and 5-methyltetrahydrofolate that was found in CAD patients, but not in control subjects, confirmed the direct relation between these compounds *in vivo*. (Figure 1-28). The new finding of low S-adenosylmethionine in patients demands further studies, because it might indicate that low levels pose risk and that S-adenosylmethionine might be a protective factor against the development of CAD.

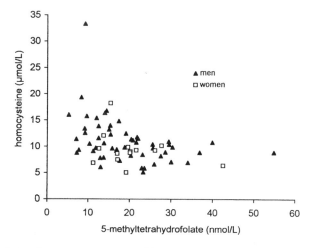

FIGURE 1-28. Relation between 5-MTHF and homocysteine concentrations in plasma in male and female CAD patients. The upper limit of normal homocysteine is 13.3 μmol/L and 12.4 μmol/L in men and women, respectively. Reproduced with permission from Loehrer et al.[116]

Hyperhomocysteinemia as a Risk Factor in End-Stage Renal Disease

Robinson and colleagues[117] evaluated the role of total plasma homocysteine as a risk factor for atherosclerosis or vascular complications of end-stage renal disease. Total fasting plasma homocysteine and other risk factors were documented in 176 dialysis patients, including 97 men and 79 women (mean age, 56 years) (Figure 1-29). Folate, vitamin B_{12}, and pyridoxal phosphate concentrations were also determined. The prevalence of high total homocysteine values was determined by comparison with a normal reference population, and the risk of associated vascular complications by multiple logistic regression. Total homocysteine concentration was higher in patients than in the normal population (27 ± 1.5 vs. 10 ± 1.7 μmol/L). Abnormally high concentrations in control subjects, 16 μmol/L, were seen in 149 patients (85%) with end-stage renal disease. Patients with a homocysteine concentration in the upper 2 quintiles had an independent odds ratio of 2.9 of vascular complications. B vitamin levels were lower in patients with vascular complications than in those without. Vitamin B_6 deficiency was more frequent in patients than in the normal reference population (18% vs. 2%). Thus, a high total plasma homocysteine concentration is an independent risk factor for atherosclerotic complications of end-stage renal disease. It is possible that these patients may benefit from higher doses of B vitamins than are currently given.

Homocysteine in Lower-Limb Atherosclerotic Disease

Elevated plasma homocysteine levels are recognized as an independent risk factor for atherosclerotic disease. It is not known: (1) whether the severity

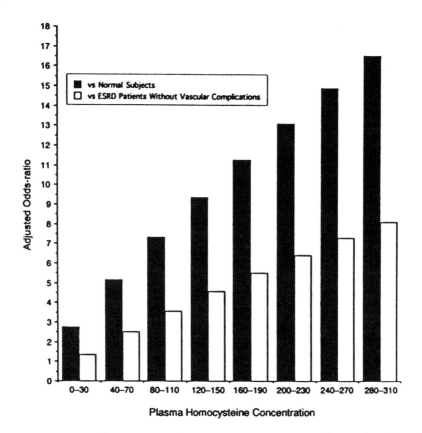

FIGURE 1-29. Odds ratio for increases in homocysteine concentrations for any thromboembolic or atherosclerotic vascular complication, adjusted for age, sex, hypertension, diabetes mellitus, hypercholesterolemia, smoking, and time from first dialysis compared with normal subjects and end-stage renal disease (ESRD) patients without vascular complications. Reproduced with permission from Robinson et al.[117]

of atherosclerotic disease is related to hyperhomocysteinemia or (2) whether any such relation differs between fasting and postmethionine-loading plasma homocysteine level. Therefore, in 171 consecutive patients under 55 years of age with the first symptoms of lower-limb disease, vandenBerg and coinvestigators[118] in Amsterdam, The Netherlands, examined the relation between the severity of atherosclerosis and plasma homocysteine concentration. Severity of atherosclerotic disease was estimated from the prevalence of CAD and cerebral vascular disease and from the angiographic extent of lower-limb disease. Plasma homocysteine was measured after a period of fasting and in response to methionine loading. In multivariate analysis, the prevalence of CAD plus cerebral vascular disease was related to both fasting and post methionine homocysteine levels for the upper quartile versus the lower three quartiles (Figure 1-30). The extent of lower-limb disease was weakly related to the fasting homocysteine level and more strongly related to the postmethionine homocysteine levels. These relations tended to be more pronounced in women than in men. They were independent of age, total serum cholesterol, blood pressure and smoking habit. The investigators concluded that the severity of atherosclerotic

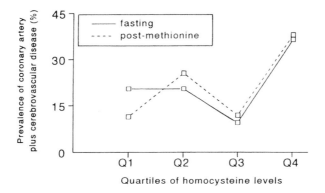

Figure 1-30. Prevalence of coronary artery disease plus cerebrovascular disease across quartiles of fasting and postmethionine homocysteine levels in 171 patients with lower-limb atherosclerotic disease. Reproduced with permission from vanden Berg et al.[118]

disease in young patients with lower-limb atherosclerotic disease is associated with high postmethionine and fasting homocysteine concentrations.

Psychosocial Risk Factors in CAD

Anger and Coronary Heart Disease

Kawachi and colleagues[119] in Boston, Massachusetts, prospectively examined the relationship of anger to the risk of coronary heart disease in the Veterans Administration Normative Aging Study, an ongoing cohort of older (mean age, 61 years) community-dwelling men. A total of 1305 men who were free of diagnosed CAD completed the revised Minnesota Multiphasic Personality Inventory in 1986. Subjects were categorized according to their responses to the Anger Content Scale, which measures the degree to which individuals have problems controlling their anger. During an average of 7 years of follow-up, 110 cases of incident CAD occurred, including 30 cases of nonfatal MI, 20 cases of fatal CAD, and 60 cases of angina pectoris. Compared with men reporting the lowest levels of anger, the multivariate adjusted relative risks among men reporting the highest level of anger were 3.15 for total CAD and 2.66 for combined incident CAD, including angina. A dose-response relation was found between level of anger and overall CAD risk. Thus, these data suggest that high levels of expressed anger may be a risk factor for CAD among older men.

Keltikangas-Järvinen and colleagues[120] in Helsinki, Finland, undertook a study to determine whether psychological factors could incline an individual toward CAD and could, in turn, identify a pattern of pituitary and adrenocortical responses that were associated with the insulin resistance syndrome. The study was performed with 69 normotensive and 21 unmedicated, borderline hypertensive men (age, 30–55 years). Type A behavior, hostility (defined as cynicism, pessimism, and paranoia), vital exhaustion, and anger were the behavioral variables studied. Among these, only the vital exhaustion-anger-out factor identified the neuroendocrine pattern that predicted the insulin resistance syndrome. The neuroendocrine pattern consisted primarily of an adrenal responsiveness to adrenocorticotrophic hormone (ACTH) and, secondarily, of a high mean basal cortisol-to-mean basal ACTH ratio. The contribution of this last variable was, however, slightly questionable. Instead of the traditional coronary prone factors, ie, type A behavior and hostility, the findings emphasized the significance of vital exhaustion and emotional distress. The findings were discussed by the investigators in terms of defeat reaction, hypocortisolemia, and visceral obesity.

Infectious Agents

Chlamydia Pneumoniae *Infection and Coronary Atherosclerosis*

An association between *Chlamydia pneumoniae* infection and coronary atherosclerosis has been suggested, based on increased serologic titers and the detection of bacteria within atherosclerotic tissue. To further test this hypothesis, coronary specimens from 90 symptomatic patients undergoing coronary atherectomy were tested for the presence of *Chlamydia* species using direct immunofluorescence by Muhlestein and colleagues[121] from Salt Lake City, Utah. Control specimens from 24 subjects without atherosclerosis, including 12 specimens from cardiac transplant recipients, were also examined. Atherectomy specimens were definitely positive in 73% and equivocally positive in 6%, resulting in 79% of specimens showing evidence for the presence of *Chlamydia* species within the atherosclerotic tissue. By contrast, only 4% of nonatherosclerotic coronary specimens showed any evidence of *Chlamydia*. These authors concluded that this high incidence of *Chlamydia* only in coronary arteries diseased by atherosclerosis suggests an etiologic role for *Chlamydia* infection in the development of CAD.

Cytomegalovirus Infection and Carotid Intimal Medial Thickening

Nieto and colleagues[122] conducted a case-control study nested within a historical cohort to evaluate a possible role for cytomegalovirus (CMV) and other herpesvirus infections in the development of cardiovascular disease. The case group comprised 150 individuals with elevated carotid intimal-medial thickness measured by B-mode ultrasound at the first 2 examinations of the Atherosclerosis Risk in Communities (ARIC) Study (1987 through 1992). The control group comprised 150 age- and sex-matched individuals with low intimal-medial thickness. Antibody titers for CMV and herpesvirus 1 and 2 were determined in sera obtained in 1974 as part of a community-wide survey conducted in Washington County, Maryland. Case subjects had higher mean CMV antibody titers in 1974 sera than did control subjects, but the difference was not statistically significant when adjusted for other cardiovascular risk factors. There was evidence of a graded relationship between the odds of intimal-medial thickening and the length of CMV antibodies that remained significant after adjustment for the main cardiovascular risk factors (p = .01). The adjusted odds ratio for a high CMV antibody titer compared with a lower one was 5.3. Thus, the results from this population-based cohort study of CMV infection and carotid intimal-medial thickness are compatible with the hypothesis of a causal role of CMV in atherosclerosis in the carotid artery.

Leukocytes

Leukocytes and CAD

Total blood leukocyte count is an independent risk factor for CAD. Few studies, however, have addressed the relation between differential leukocyte counts and CAD. Kawaguchi and associates[123] from Fukuoka, Japan, and Saitama, Japan, investigated the relation of total and differential leukocyte counts to angiographically determined coronary atherosclerosis. The study comprised 486 individuals (335 men, 151 women) who underwent coronary angiography for suspected CAD. Band neutrophil count was significantly positively related to coronary atherosclerosis after adjustments for age, sex, body mass index, cigarettes per day, serum total cholesterol, and hypertension. Although sex- and age-adjusted total blood leukocyte count was significantly positively related to coronary atherosclerosis, this relation did not reach significant levels after adjusting for other risk factors. The positive association with band neutrophil counts was at least as strong as that with serum total cholesterol concentrations. This study indicates that band neutrophil counts serve as an independent risk factor for coronary atherosclerosis.

Because the importance of established risk factors for CAD is unclear in older people, Weijenberg and colleagues[124] in Bilthoven, The Netherlands, investigated the association of white blood cell count with the risk for CAD and all-cause mortality in an elderly cohort that was followed for 5 years. In 1985, complete information on the risk factors of interest was available for 884 randomly selected men (age, 64–84 years) from the Dutch town of Zutphen. Relative risks for each 10^9/L increase in white blood cell count were obtained for the 5-year incidence of and mortality from CAD and all causes. Relative risks were adjusted for age, body mass index, systolic blood pressure, total and HDL cholesterol levels, and cigarette smoking habit. The white blood cell count was 6.7×10^9/L at baseline. An increased white blood cell count was independently associated with mortality due to CAD, and the relative risk amounted to 1.32 (Figure 1-31). For the incidence of CAD, the relative risk was 1.14. These associations were observed regardless of cigarette smoking habit. Regarding all-cause mortality, the relative risk amounted to 1.25. This association was especially noticeable among former smokers and those who had never smoked. In conclusion, during 5 years of follow-up, white blood cell count predicted CAD and

Coronary heart disease mortality

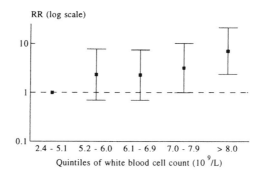

All-cause mortality

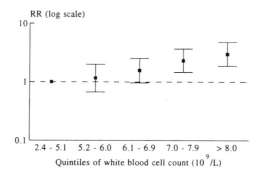

FIGURE 1-31. RRs and 95% CIs for mortality from CHD and from all causes according to quintiles of white blood cell count. Reproduced with permission from Weijenberg et al.[124]

all-cause mortality in elderly men, independent of the conventional risk factors for CAD.

Multiple Risk Factors

Multiple Risk Factor Intervention Trial

The Multiple Risk Factor Interventional Trial[125] assessed the long-term effect of cardiovascular risk factor intervention on CAD, cardiovascular death, and total mortality. During a 7-year active-intervention phase of the trial, 6424 of the men were given dietary recommendations to lower blood cholesterol, antihypertensive drugs to lower blood pressure, and counseling for cigarette smoking cessation. The remaining 6438 men were referred to their usual source of medical care. After 16 years, 370 of the special intervention care and 417 of the other men had died of CAD, representing an 11% lower mortality rate for the special intervention group (Tables 1-13 and 1-14). Results for total mortality followed a similar pattern. For AMI, a subcategory of CAD, the relative difference was 20% (Table 1-14 and Table 1-15). Differences between the 2 groups

TABLE 1-14
Cause of Death for MRFIT SI and UC Men through December 1990

Cause of Death	ICD-9 Code No.	Si, n	UC, n	Relative Difference, %*
All cardiovascular	390–459	507	550	−7.9
Acute myocardial infarction	410	185	232	−20.4†
Other ischemic (coronary) heart disease	411–414, 429.2‡	185	185	−0.1
Cardiac dysrhythmias	427	15	21	−29.0
Hypertensive heart disease	402	10	12	−17.2
Other hypertensive	401, 403–405	6	2	...
Cerebrovascular	430–438	46	44	+5.2
ther cardiovascular disease	...	60	54	+11.0
All noncardiovascular		483	499	−3.3
Neoplastic	140–239	316	321	−1.8
Lip, oral cavity, and pharynx	140–149	5	12	...
Digestive organs and peritoneum	150–159	73	88	−17.2
Colorectal	153–154	28	33	−15.2
Other gastrointestinal	150–152, 155–159	45	55	−18.5
Respiratory and intrathoracic organs	160–165	141	122	+15.2
Lung	162	135	117	+15.0
Other neoplasms	...	97	99	−2.3
Respiratory	460–519	25	31	−19.2
Digestive system	520–579	40	33	+21.0
Accidents, suicides, and homicides	800–999	55	58	−5.1
Other non-cardiovascular disease	...	47	56	−15.9
Cause unknown (death certificate not found)	...	1	1	...
Total	...	991	1050	−5.7

* (RR-1) × 100%, where the RR (relative risk) is estimated from the proportional-hazards regression model.
† p = .02; p>.05 for all other relative differences. Relative difference is not given if there were <10 deaths in either the Si or UC.
‡ In ICD-9, No. 429.2 is cardiovascular disease, unspecified; in ICD-9 this is coded to coronary heart disease, No. 412.4.
Reproduced with permission from the Multiple Risk Factor Interventional Trial.[125]

in mortality rates from AMI, CAD, and all causes were greater during the post-trial follow-up period than during the trial. Thus, the results of the 7-year multifactor intervention program aimed at lowering BP and serum cholesterol and at cigarette smoking cessation among high-risk men provide additional evidence of a long-term continuing mortality benefit from the program.

Diet

Dietary Fiber and Coronary Heart Disease in Finnish Men

Pietinen and colleagues[126] in Helsinki, Finland, used data from the α-Tocopherol, β-Carotene Cancer Prevention Study, a randomized, double-blind,

Table 1-15
Number of Deaths and Death Rates per 1000 Person-years from Baseline
through December 1990* by Cause for 6428 SI and 6438 UC Men

Mortality End Point	SI		UC		Relative Difference, %†	95% CI for Relative Difference
	No. of Deaths	Rate**	No. of Deaths	Rate**		
CHD	370	3.86	417	4.35	−11.4	−23.0 to +1.9
During trial‡	110	2.49	117	2.64	−6.0	−27.5 to +22.0
Posttrial§	260	3.03	300	5.82	−13.5	−26.7 to +2.1
CVD	507	5.29	550	5.74	−7.9	−18.4 to +3.9
During trial‡	143	3.23	144	3.25	−0.7	−21.2 to +25.1
Posttrial§	364	7.05	406	7.88	−10.4	−22.3 to +3.2
Non-CVD	484	5.05	500	5.22	−3.3	−14.7 to +9.5
During trial‡	123	2.78	118	2.67	+4.1	−19.1 to +34.1
Posttrial§	361	6.99	382	7.41	−5.7	−18.3 to +8.9
All Cause	991	10.33	1050	10.96	−5.7	−13.6 to +2.8
During trial‡	266	6.01	262	5.92	+1.5	−14.4 to +20.4
Posttrial§	725	14.03	788	15.29	−8.1	−17.0 to +1.6

* Average time from baseline to 12/31/90 = 15.8 years; average time from baseline to 12/31/90 or death = 14.9 years.

** Deaths per 1000 person-years.

† Defined as (RR-1) × 100; RR estimated from proportional-hazards models.

‡ Average time from baseline to February 28, 1982, or death = 7 years.

§ Average time from March 1, 1982 to December 31, 1990, or death = 8.7 years.
Reproduced with permission from the Multiple Risk Factor Interventional Trial.[125]

placebo-controlled study with daily supplementation of α-tocopherol and/or β-carotene, to test the hypothesis that dietary fiber may reduce the risk of CAD. Among the participants, 21,930 smoking men aged 50 to 69 years who were free of recognized CAD and had completed a validated dietary questionnaire at baseline were followed for 6 years. The authors monitored the incidence of major coronary events, including a combination of first nonfatal MI and CAD-associated death (n = 1399), and mortality from CAD (n = 635). Both of these events had a significant inverse association with dietary fiber, but the association was strongest for coronary death. For men in the highest quintile of dietary fiber intake (median 34.8 g/day), the relative risk for coronary death was 0.69 compared with men in the lowest quintile of intake (median 16 g/day). With an adjustment for known cardiovascular risk factors, intake of saturated fatty acids, β-carotene, vitamin C, and vitamin E did not materially change the result. Water-soluble fiber was more strongly associated with reduced coronary death and water-insoluble fiber, and cereal fiber also had a stronger association than vegetable or fruit fiber. Thus, these data suggest that independent of other risk factors, greater intake of foods rich in fiber may substantially reduce the risk of CAD, and especially coronary death in middle-aged, smoking men.

Mediterranean Diet

Previous studies have suggested that a Mediterranean diet might be cardioprotective against the development of CAD. Although the exact mechanism of this protection is unclear, these diets have increased amounts of ω-3 fatty acids, oleic acid, and antioxidant vitamins. The Lyon Diet Heart[127] study is a secondary prevention trial testing the protective effects of a Mediterranean type of diet. A total of 605 patients (303 controls and 302 study patients) were studied over a mean period of 27 months. Major primary end points (cardiovascular death and nonfatal AMI), secondary end points (including unstable angina, stroke, heart failure and embolism), and minor end points (stable angina, need for myocardial revascularization, postangioplasty restenosis, and thrombophlebitis) were analyzed separately and in combination. When major primary and secondary end points were combined, there were 59 events in control subjects and 14 events in the study patients showing a risk reduction of 76%. When these end points were combined with the minor end points, there were 104 events in control subjects and 68 events in the study patients, giving a risk reduction of 37%. Among the medications, only aspirin appeared to be significantly protective (risk ratio 0.45). These authors concluded that a Mediterranean diet is protective against the development of cardiovascular events.

Fish versus Vegetarian Diet in Tanzanian Villagers

Pauletto and colleagues[128] in Italy explored the effects of fish intake on blood pressure and lipids in 2 groups of Bantu villagers in Tanzania. One group lives on the shores of Lake Nyasa, and their diet includes large amounts of freshwater fish. The other group lives in the nearby hills and consumes a vegetarian diet. A cross-sectional study of 622 fish-consuming villagers and 686 vegetarian villagers was conducted. Anthropometric and self-reported medical history data were collected by one local physician and a medical assistant who also measured blood pressure and took blood samples for measurement of plasma lipids. A dietary questionnaire was administered to 25 families, approximately 15% of the study population in each village. After adjustment for age, sex, and alcohol intake, the fish-consuming group had lower mean blood pressure than the vegetarian group (123/72 vs. 133/76 mm Hg, p<.001). The frequencies of definite and borderline hypertension using World Health Organization (WHO) criteria were lower in the fish-consuming group than in the vegetarian group (2.8 vs. 16.4%). Plasma concentrations of total cholesterol, triglycerides, and lipoprotein(a) were all lower (p<.0001) in the fish-consuming group. The proportions of n-3 polyunsaturated fatty acids in plasma lipids were higher in the fish-consuming group than in the vegetarian group. Thus, these data suggest that consumption of freshwater fish was associated with raised plasma concentrations of n-3 polyunsaturated fatty acids, lower blood pressure, and lower plasma lipid concentrations.

Vitamin Intake in Postmenopausal Women

Kushi and colleagues[129] in Minneapolis, Minnesota, studied 34,486 postmenopausal women with no cardiovascular disease who in early 1986 completed a questionnaire that assessed, among other factors, their intakes of vitamin A, E, and C from food sources and supplements. During approximately 7 years of follow-up ending December 31, 1992, 242 of the women died of coronary heart disease. In analysis adjusted for age and dietary energy intake, vitamin E consumption appeared to be inversely associated with the risk of death from coronary heart disease. This association was particularly striking in the subgroup of 21,809 women who did not consume vitamin supplements; they had a relative risk from lowest to highest quintile of vitamin E intake of 1.0, 0.68, 0.71, 0.42, and 0.42, p for trend = 0.008. After adjustment for other variables, this inverse association remained, with a relative risk from lowest to highest quintile of 1.0, 0.70, 0.76, 0.32, and 0.38, p for trend = 0.004. There was little evidence that the intake of vitamin E from supplements was associated with a decreased risk of death from coronary heart disease, but the effects of high-dose supplementation and the duration of supplemental use could not be definitely addressed. Intake of vitamins A and C did not appear to be associated with the risk of death from coronary heart disease. These data suggest that in postmenopausal women, the intake of vitamin E from food is inversely associated with the risk of death from coronary heart disease and that such women can lower their risk without using vitamin supplements. However, the intake of vitamins A and C was not associated with lower risks of dying from coronary heart disease.

Hormone Replacement Therapy

The Atherosclerosis Risk in Communities Study investigators consisting of Folsom and associates[130] from Minneapolis, Minnesota; Abbott Park, Illinois; and Research Triangle Park, North Carolina, examined nearly 4000 postmenopausal women from 1987 through 1989 and 3 years later to determine changes in plasma lipids occurring with the starting or stopping of hormone replacement therapy. Women who started estrogen plus progestin therapy (n = 74) had decreases of 9.8 mg/dL in LDL cholesterol and 5.8 mg/dL in apolipoprotein B and increases of 1.2 mg/dL in HDL cholesterol, 14 mg/dL in apolipoprotein A-1, and 14 mg/dL in triglycerides. Women who started estrogen alone (n = 149) had similar changes, except for a much larger increase in HDL cholesterol (5.8 mg/dL), principally in HDL-2. Women who stopped hormone therapy (n = 138) had lipid changes opposite to those who started therapy. These results confirm those of the Postmenopausal Estrogen/Progestin Interventions Trial in a community-based longitudinal cohort: women initiating estrogen plus progestin therapy have decreases in LDL cholesterol, but the increase in HDL cholesterol is less than that for starting estrogen alone. In addition, the current study extends findings to apolipoproteins and HDL subfractions.

To characterize the apolipoprotein subfraction specificity of the increase in HDL levels that is induced by oral estrogen and to explore the metabolic mechanisms thereof, Brinton[131] in Winston-Salem, North Carolina, studied 6 healthy postmenopausal women during each of 2 5-week periods of a low-fat diet with and without ethinyl estradiol 0.05 mg/day. With estrogen, HDL levels increased 36%, plasma levels of apolipoprotein A-I increased by 27%, and apolipoprotein A-II levels increased 17%. Apolipoprotein A-I mass in particles that contained apolipoprotein A-I but no apolipoprotein A-II increased 66%, while the sum of apolipoprotein A-I and apolipoprotein A-II mass in particles with both apolipoprotein A-I and apolipoprotein A-II showed only a nonsignificant 14% increase. In radioiodinated protein turnover studies, the production rate of each species changed in proportion to the change in its plasma concentration. Hepatic lipase activity in post-heparin plasma decreased 66% with estrogen, while lipoprotein lipase activity was unchanged. Despite the large decrease in hepatic lipase activity, the fractional catabolic rate of A-I did not decrease, nor was that of the lipoprotein A-I/A-II lessened. Thus, oral estrogen replacement therapy has a novel and potentially antiatherogenic effect: a large and selective increase in lipoprotein A-I levels. The metabolic mechanism of the estrogen-induced increase and lipoprotein A-I concentration appeared to be the increase in its production rate. Although the ability of estrogen to suppress hepatic lipase activity has been confirmed, surprisingly this decrease was not accompanied by any decrease in the fractional catabolic rate of lipoprotein A-I or A-I/A-II. This suggested that hepatic lipase may not play a major role in regulating HDL protein catabolism during suppression of hepatic lipase by estrogen.

To study the responses of serum lipoprotein, apoproteins, and lipoproteins(a) to frequently used hormone replacement therapies, Taskinen and co-workers[132] in Helsinki, Finland, randomly allocated 120 postmenopausal women to receive either transdermal therapy consisting of 28-day cycles with patches that delivered estradiol-17β (50 mg/day) combined with cyclic oral medroxyprogesterone acetate (10 mg/day for 12 days per cycle) or continuous oral estradiol-17β (2 mg/day) together with norethisterone acetate (1 mg/day) for 12 months. Blood samples were taken before and at 6 and 12 months of hormone replacement therapy. Concentrations of serum total, LDL, and HDL cholesterol decreased 14%, 17%, and 9% in the oral hormone replacement therapy group. Respective decreases were 6%, 5%, and 5% in the transdermal group. Serum triglycerides remain unchanged in the oral group, but decreased by 16% in the transdermal group. The investigators observed only trivial changes in serum apolipoprotein B levels. The changes in apolipoprotein A-I levels paralleled those of HDL cholesterol in the oral hormonal replacement therapy group. Concentration of serum lipoprotein(a) decreased by 31% and 16% in the 2 groups. The combination of progestin and transdermal estrogen was not associated with any further change of lipoprotein(a). The decrement in lipoprotein(a) during therapy was possibly associated with baseline lipoprotein(a) level in both groups. Thus, both hormonal replacement therapy regimens were highly effective in lowering elevated lipoprotein(a) levels in postmenopausal women. The divergent responses of LDL and HDL cholesterol in the 2 hormone replacement therapy groups may influence the potential cardioprotective effects of the 2 hormone replacement therapy regimens. Prospective trials are needed to define the long-term effects with respect to CAD risk.

Shahar and colleagues[133] for the Atherosclerosis Risk in Communities Study investigators (ARIC) investigated the relation of current use of replacement hormones to 3 measures of plasma fibrinolytic activity, including tissue-type plasminogen activator (tPA) antigen, plasminogen activator inhibitor-1

(PAI-1) antigen, and D-dimer. The study sample comprised 288 women free of clinical cardiovascular disease who were selected for a case control study of atherosclerosis. One hundred forty-two women with ultrasonographic evidence of carotid intimal-medial thickening and 146 control subjects were evaluated. Twenty percent (59 women) reported concurrent use of replacement hormones. tPA antigen and PAI-1 antigen were significantly correlated with each other, but the D-dimer correlated only weakly with tPA and PAI-1. Current users of replacement hormones had lower mean levels of tPA and PAI-1 antigens, suggesting enhanced fibrinolytic potentials (Figure 1-32). Among the entire sample of women studied, the multivariate-adjusted geometric mean values of tPA antigen were 6.3 and 7.3 ng/mL among current users and nonusers, and the corresponding values for PAI-1 antigen were 6 and 7.5 ng/mL. The results were similar in individuals with atherosclerosis and the control subjects. D-dimer levels were lower in current hormone users than in nonusers, but the differences were not statistically significant. Thus, the use of replacement hormones appears to be associated with enhancement of endogenous fibrinolytic potential.

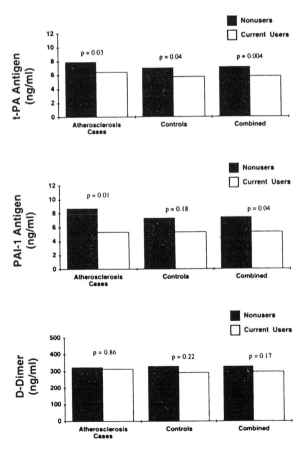

FIGURE 1-32. Geometric mean levels of fibrinolytic factors according to the use of replacement hormones. Reproduced with permission from Shahar et al.[133]

Grodstein and colleagues[134] in Boston, Massachusetts, examined the relation between cardiovascular disease and postmenopausal hormone therapy during up to 16 years of follow-up in 59,337 women from the Nurses' Health Study, who were 30 to 55 years of age at baseline. Information on hormone use was obtained by biennial questionnaires. From 1976 to 1992, the authors documented 770 cases of AMI or death from CAD in this group and 572 strokes. Proportional hazards models were used to calculate relative risks and 95% confidence intervals adjusted for confounding variables. The authors observed a marked decrease in the risk of major CAD among women who took estrogen with progestin, as compared with the risk among women who did not use hormones (multivariate adjusted relative risk, 0.39; 95% confidence interval, 0.19 to 0.78) or estrogen alone (relative risk, 0.60; 95% confidence interval, 0.43 to 0.83). There was no association between stroke and use of combined hormones or estrogen alone. Thus, the addition of progestin does not appear to attenuate the cardioprotective effects of postmenopausal estrogen therapy in young and middle-aged women.

The onset of acute atherothrombotic events (AMI, unstable angina, ischemic stroke) exhibit a circadian pattern that parallels the diurnal pattern of endogenous fibrinolytic activity. Hormone replacement therapy in postmenopausal women has been shown to enhance fibrinolytic capacity by lowering PAI-1 and tPA antigen values. Katz and associates[35] from Washington, D.C., evaluated the impact of 4 weeks of estrogen alone (Premarin 0.625 mg/day) and 2 weeks of estrogen plus progesterone (Provera 2.5 mg/day) on PAI-1 and tPA in 17 postmenopausal women at multiple time points to assess hormone impact on the diurnal pattern of fibrinolytic potential. At baseline, both PAI-1 and tPA exhibited circadian variability. Estrogen alone selectively lowered 8 AM PAI-1 (36 $\pm$ 7 ng/mL at baseline, 20 $\pm$ 4 ng/mL on estrogen vs. baseline). There was no significant change in the 12 PM or 4 PM values, and the diurnal pattern was attenuated. The 8 AM PAI-1 remained low at 17 $\pm$ 4 ng/mL versus baseline with total loss of the circadian rhythm. Estrogen supplementation reduced tPA antigen at all time points, and the diurnal pattern, although blunted, persisted. Addition of progesterone to estrogen did not reverse effects of the estrogen-alone phase of either PAI-1 or tPA values. This hormone-associated reduction of PAI was observed despite increased triglycerides, a known inducer of PAI-1 levels. These observations suggest that hormone replacement therapy may protect postmenopausal women from excess early morning acute ischemic events.

Pharmacological Interactions

Aspirin to Reduce Risk of Cardiac Mortality

Previous studies suggest that aspirin produces a modest decline in cardiac mortality in patients with CAD. Goldstein and colleagues[136] from Bethesda, Maryland, and Rochester, New York, sought to assess the role of aspirin in a precisely defined cohort with CAD receiving current therapy. They evaluated

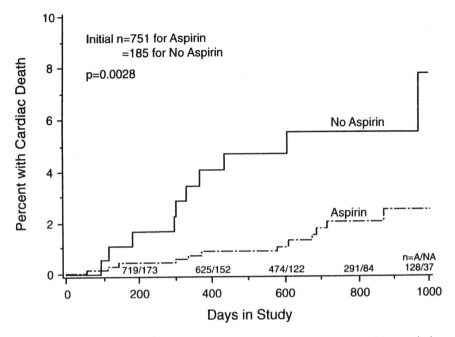

FIGURE 1-33. Kaplan-Meier plot of cardiac mortality for patients using aspirin regularly and those not using aspirin regularly 1 to 6 months after an index coronary event prompting hospitalization (acute myocardial infarction or unstable angina). Reproduced with permission from Goldstein et al.[136]

936 subjects as part of a multicenter study of myocardial ischemia using an average follow-up period of 23 months. At enrollment, 80% of patients took aspirin regularly. Cardiac death rate was markedly reduced as a late outcome (1.6% for aspirin users and 5.4% for nonusers). The difference in mortality rate was particularly prominent after thrombolysis (0.9% for aspirin users and 8.8% for nonusers). These authors concluded that reduction in cardiac deaths among aspirin users is substantially greater than that reported previously and is especially beneficial in patients undergoing thrombolysis (Figure 1-33).

β-Blockers in Diabetes Mellitus and Coronary Artery Disease

The benefit of β-blocker therapy in patients after AMI is well established. The use of β-blockers in the high-risk subgroup of patients with combined diabetes mellitus and CAD remains controversial. From a database of 14,417 patients with CAD who had been screened for participation in the Bezafibrate Infarction Prevention (BIP) study, 2723 (19%) had noninsulin-dependent diabetes mellitus. These patients were analyzed by Jonas and associates[137] for the Bezafibrate Infarction Prevention Study Group in Tel Hashomer, Israel. Baseline characteristics and 3-year mortality were analyzed in patients with diabetes mellitus receiving (n = 911, 33%) and not receiving (n = 1812, 67%) β-blockers. Total mortality during a 3-year follow-up was 7.8% in those receiving

β-blockers compared with 14.0% in those who were not (a 44% reduction). A reduction in cardiac mortality of 42% between the 2 groups was also noted. Three-year survival curves showed significant differences in mortality with increasing divergence. After multiple adjustment, multivariate analysis identified β-blocker therapy as a significant independent contributor to improved survival (relative risk = 0.58). Within the diabetic population, the main benefit associated with β-blocker therapy was observed in older patients, in those with a history of myocardial infarction, those with limited functional capacity, and those at lower risk. Thus, therapy with β-blockers appears to be associated with improved long-term survival in the high-risk subpopulation of patients with diabetes mellitus and CAD.

Calcium Channel Blockers Plus Lipid-Lowering Therapy in the Regression of Atherosclerosis

To date, lipid-lowering therapy appears to be the most effective medical intervention to retard progression of coronary atherosclerosis. Despite promising experimental results, clinical trials completed so far have failed to demonstrate that calcium channel blockers alone influence the evolution of established coronary atherosclerosis. To assess whether the 2 therapies may have an additive or synergistic beneficial effect on human atherosclerosis, Jukema and coinvestigators[138] in Leiden, The Netherlands, reviewed the data of the angiographic Regression Growth Evaluation Statin Study (REGRESS). The statin study was designed to determine the effect of lipid-lowering therapy with pravastatin in symptomatic patients with normal to moderately raised cholesterol levels. Angiographically, with respect to the minimum obstruction diameter in the pravastatin group, patients had on average 0.05 mm less progression if co-treated with calcium channel blockers compared with no calcium channel blocker co-treatment, whereas in the placebo (no pravastatin) group, no effect of calcium channel blocker treatment was observed. With respect to the mean segment diameter, similar, although not significant results were found. With respect to new lesion formation in the pravastatin group, there were 50% fewer patients with new angiographic lesions if co-treated with calcium channel blockers compared with no calcium channel blocker co-treatment, whereas in the placebo group (no pravastatin), no significant effect of calcium channel blocker treatment was observed. No beneficial effects of calcium channel blocker treatment on clinical events were observed. Although REGRESS was not designed to evaluate combination therapy, the results suggested strongly that addition of calcium channel blockers to 3-hydroxy-3-methyl-glutaryl-coenzyme reductase inhibitor therapy (pravastatin) acted synergistically in retarding the progression of established coronary atherosclerosis.

Calcium Antagonists and Mortality in CAD

Recent studies have suggested that the use of short-acting nifedipine may cause an increase in overall mortality in patients with CAD. To further evaluate the potential adverse effects of calcium antagonists, Braun[139] from Tel Aviv, Tel Hashomer, Zrifin, Afula, and Haifa, Israel, obtained mortality data for 11,575 patients who were screened for a secondary prevention trial. Mean follow-up was 3.2 years. The death rate was 8.5% in the calcium antagonist group, compared with 7.2% in the control group. The age-adjusted risk ratio for mortality for calcium blockers was 1.08. After adjustment for the differences between the groups in age and gender, and the prevalence of previous AMI, angina pectoris, hypertension, NYHA functional class, peripheral vascular disease, chronic obstructive pulmonary disease, diabetes, and current smoking, the adjusted risk ratio declined to 0.97. After further adjustment for concomitant medications, the risk ratio was estimated at 0.94. These authors concluded from this analysis that calcium antagonist therapy in patients with chronic CAD did not increase the risk of mortality.

Effect of Coronary Artery Size on the Prevalence of Atherosclerosis

To investigate the effect of coronary artery size on the prevalence of atherosclerosis, Nwasokwa and associates[140] from New Hyde Park, New York, prospectively measured the diameter of the major coronary arteries in 884 consecutive patients referred for coronary arteriography. For each artery, the authors assigned patients to 3 groups: group S (small) and group L (large) with diameters greater than 1 standard deviation smaller and larger, respectively, than the mean; and group A (average), with diameters within 1 standard deviation of the mean. As specified during study design, we compared the frequency of lesions of 50% or greater diameter stenosis in groups S and L for each artery. The authors adjusted for relevant covariates by performing logistic regression on data from all 884 patients with coronary diameter entered as a continuous variable. In group S vs. L, respectively, the frequency of a greater than 50% lesion was 6.5% vs. 2.4% in the left main coronary artery; 61% vs. 36% in the right coronary artery; 58% vs. 41% in the LAD artery, and 47.% vs. 22.% in the left coronary artery. Multivariate analysis showed that coronary diameter was a significant independent predictor of lesions in the right coronary artery, LAD, and left coronary artery and nearly significant in the left main artery. Thus, small coronary artery size may be a risk factor for atherosclerosis (Figure 1-34).

Ultrasound Versus Angiography in the Assessment of Plaque Distribution

Mintz and colleagues[141] in Washington, D.C., compared coronary angiography with intravascular ultrasound to determine the ability of each to assess plaque distribution in 1446 native vessel target lesions in 1349 patients. Angiography and intravascular ultrasound criteria for lesion eccentricity were compared. Angiography demonstrated that 795 of 1446 (55%) of the target lesions were eccentric. However, intravascular ultrasound suggested that only 219 le-

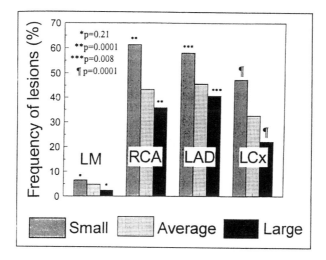

FIGURE 1-34. Effect of coronary artery size on the frequency of lesions ≥50% diameter stenosis in the proximal or midsegment of the left main (LM), right coronary artery (RCA), left anterior descending (LAD), and left circumflex (LCx) coronary arteries. Reproduced with permission from Nwasokwa et al.[140]

sions (15%) had an arc of normal arterial wall within the lesion that would be considered lesion eccentricity. When an eccentricity index of 3.0 or greater was used, intravascular ultrasound classified 659 lesions (46%) as eccentric. The concordance rates of classification were only 48% for lesions containing an arc of normal arterial wall and 54% for lesions with an ultrasound eccentricity index of 3.0 or less. More eccentric lesions had larger lumen cross-sectional areas, smaller plaque and media and external elastic membrane cross-sectional areas, and smaller arcs of calcium, thereby suggesting they may represent less advanced atherosclerotic disease. There was significant discordance between angiography and ultrasound in assessing plaque distribution in this study. Angiography appeared to detect lesion eccentricity more often than did intravascular ultrasound. Markedly eccentric lesions, in which there was an arc of normal vessel wall, were uncommon in this study.

Ultrasound Comparison of Thickness and Distensibility in Carotid Artery and Descending Thoracic Aorta

Early atherosclerotic changes in the carotid artery and thoracic aorta have been examined by high-frequency ultrasound measuring of intimal-medial thickness and stiffness. Whether changes in stiffness and thickness occur in parallel and whether the determinants of stiffness and thickness in the 2 vessels are similar is unknown. To examine the relation between ultrasonographic measures of atherosclerosis in the carotid and the thoracic aorta, 146 patients (age, 20–84 years; mean, 54 years) were studied by both TEE and carotid duplex scanning in this study carried out by Pearson and associates[142] from Columbus, Ohio. From 2-dimensional M-mode recordings of the thoracic aorta and high-frequency B-mode imaging of the common carotid artery, the intimal-medial thickness was measured, along with diastolic and systolic diameters for calculation of stiffness. Interobserver and intraobserver variability of carotid and aortic intimal-medial thickness and diameter were low. There was a good relation between carotid and aortic intimal-medial thickness. Age was the major independent determinant of thickness in both vessels. Carotid and aortic stiffness, as measured by Peterson's elastic modulus, were less closely related. Age was the only independent predictor of stiffness in both vessels. In conclusion, structural ultrasonographic manifestations of early atherosclerosis in the carotid artery and thoracic aorta are closely related. Large population studies measuring only carotid intimal-medial thickness may reflect atherosclerotic changes occurring throughout the vascular bed.

Ultrasound-Assessed Carotid Artery Wall Thickness in Hispanic Populations

Measurements of carotid artery wall thickness are often used as indicators of atherosclerosis. However, few studies have performed these measurements in populations of Mexican origin. Mexicans in Mexico City consume high-carbohydrate diets and have carbohydrate-induced dyslipidemia (high triglycerides and low HDL cholesterol levels) compared with Mexican Americans living in San Antonio, Texas. Therefore, Wei and coworkers[143] in San Antonio, Texas, questioned whether Mexicans in Mexico City also had more atherosclerosis than San Antonio Mexican Americans. Mean maximal anteromedial thickness of the common and internal carotid arteries was measured in 867 patients (age, 35–64 years) (40% men) in 2 Mexican-origin populations, 1 from San Antonio (n = 202) and the other from Mexico City (n = 665). Intimal medial thicknesses in the 2 groups were compared, and their associations with cardiovascular risk factors were analyzed. Old age, male sex, high levels of total cholesterol, low levels of HDL cholesterol, and high systemic blood pressures were positively associated with both common carotid intimal medial thickness and internal carotid intimal medial thickness. Cigarette smoking was significantly associated with internal carotid intimal medial thickness. Common carotid and internal carotid intimal medial thickness in diabetic subjects were higher than in nondiabetic subjects in both men and women. Common carotid intimal medial thickness was thicker in the San Antonio than in the Mexico City subjects after adjustment for cardiovascular risk factors. San Antonio men also had thicker internal carotid intimal medial thickness than did their counterparts in Mexico City, but the reverse was true for women. These results indicated that men had higher intimal medial thickness than women. Common carotid intimal medial thickness was thicker in San Antonio Mexican Americans than in Mexico City residents. The differences in internal carotid intimal medial thickness between San Antonio and Mexico City were inconsistent. Thus, even though Mexico City residents consume higher carbohydrate diets, the data do not support an atherogenic effect of such diets. The investigators concluded that gender differences, as well as geographical influences and their impact on internal carotid intimal medial thickness, deserved further study.

Ultrasound-Assessed Carotid and Femoral Arteries in Familial Hypercholesterolemia

Wendelhag and colleagues[144] in Gothenberg, Sweden, in an ongoing prospective study, evaluated the possibility of measuring plaque size in ultrasound images from carotid and femoral arteries, as well as the potential usefulness of these quantitative plaque measurements. Twenty-five patients with carotid plaques were identified in a group of patients with familial hypercholesterolemia (n = 50), compared with 7 subjects in a low-risk control group (n = 47). Only 20 of the 32 recorded plaques were accessible for quantitative follow-up measurements of area, base link, and thickness, which represented only 21% of all subjects investigated. In contrast, paired observations of intima-media thickness in the common carotid artery were available in 98% and in the carotid bulb in 87% of the subjects investigated. In those with paired observations of plaque area available, the data indicated a close relation between the 2-year change recorded in plaque area and the 2-year change in intima-media thickness measured in a 10-mm long predefined section of the carotid bulb (Figure 1-35). The corresponding relationship between change in plaque area and change in a 10-mm long section of the common carotid artery was r = .38 (p<.05). Quantitative measurements of plaques in the femoral arteries were also performed, but the results from these measurements were, in most cases, not useful. However, measurements of intima-media thickness in a 15-mm long predefined section of the common femoral artery may be performed in a reproducible way in most patients. The usefulness of plaque area measurements in prospective studies of the carotid artery appeared to be limited because plaques available for quantitative measurements were present in only a small portion of subjects. However, reproducible measures of intima-media thickness in a predefined section of a carotid bulb were achievable in most subjects. These data indicated that the changes recorded over time in the carotid bulb closely mirrored changes occurring in the size of atherosclerotic plaques within the carotid artery region. In addition, measurements of intima-media thickness in the common carotid artery complemented measurements performed in the carotid artery bulb in the study of early atherosclerosis.

Transesophageal Echocardiography of the Aorta: Lipid-Lowering in Familial Hypercholesteremia

The thoracic aorta is frequently involved in atherosclerotic lesions associated with familial hypercholesterolemia. Transesophageal echocardiography allows quantitative evaluation of the wall properties of the thoracic aorta. Using TEE, Tomochika and coinvestigators[145] in Yamaguchi, Japan, tested whether atherosclerosis of the thoracic aortic and familial hypercholesterolemia could be improved by cholesterol-lowering therapy. The subjects investigated 22 familial hypercholesterolemic patients and 22 age-matched normal subjects. The descending aorta was divided into 4 longitudinal portions of equal length. Atheromatous lesions of each portion of the descending aorta were scored by char-

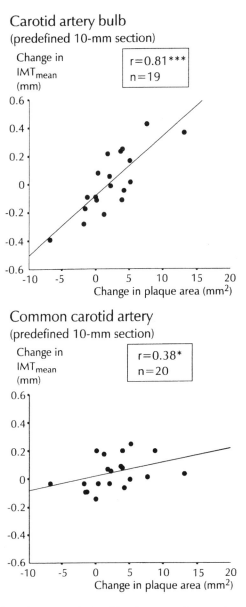

FIGURE 1-35. Scatterplots showing relationships between 2-year change in plaque area and change in mean I-M thickness measured in the carotid bulb (top) and common carotid artery (bottom). Carotid bulb I-M thickness is missing in one patient due to technically inadequate analysis. IMT$_{mean}$ indicates mean I-M thickness. *P<.05; ***P<.001. Reproduced with permission from Wendelhag et al.[144]

acter and extension of the lesion by biplane 2-dimensional TEE. The scores of atheromatous lesions from all 4 portions of the descending aorta were added together to give the total atheromatous score. The investigators also measured instantaneous dimensional changes of the descending aorta in a cardiac cycle by TEE and blood pressure by a cuff method. They calculated the stiffness parameter β (In[SBP/DBP]/[Dmax-Dmin]/Dmin), where SBP is a systolic arteriolar blood pressure, DBP is a diastolic arteriolar blood pressure, Dmax is a maximum aortic dimension during the ejection period, and Dmin is a minimum aortic dimension during the pre-ejection period. The atheromatous score was higher in familial hypercholesterolemic than in normal subjects. The stiffness parameter was also greater in hypercholesterolemic patients, but there were no significant differences in descending aortic dimensions between the groups. In both normal subjects and familial hypercholesterolemic patients, the stiffness parameter correlated with age. In familial hypercholesterolemic patients, stiffness parameter and total atheromatous score correlated well with pretreatment total cholesterol. In 12 of the 22 familial hypercholesterolemic patients, strict cholesterol-lowering therapies with diet and cholesterol-lowering drugs (pravastatin and probucol) were undertaken for 13 months. Cholesterol levels were significantly decreased; this was associated with significant decreases in stiffness parameter and in total atheromatous score. In familial hypercholesterolemic patients, the incidence and severity of morphological and physiological atherosclerosis of the descending aorta were significantly higher than in age-matched normal subjects. A significant regression of atherosclerosis was achieved by strict cholesterol-lowering therapies in relatively young patients with familial hypercholesterolemia.

Transthoracic Echocardiography in Detection of Coronary Atherosclerosis

Petrovic and associates[146] from Indianapolis, Indiana, used transthoracic echocardiography to detect coronary atherosclerosis. Eighty-nine patients undergoing coronary angiography were examined with a broad-band ultrasonic transducer with a frequency between 3 and 5 MHz. A modified short-axis examination was used to identify left main and proximal left anterior descending arteries. The examination was recorded digitally and displayed in a 32-cell, quad screen cine loop. Fifty-six of the 89 patients (63%) had obstructive CAD (ie, at least 1 vessel with 50% obstruction). There were 14 patients with CAD but no vessel had 50% or greater obstruction. Nineteen patients (21%) had angiographically normal arteries. The coronary echograms were judged qualitatively for brightness, uniformity, and persistence (defined as the ability to see segments of the artery walls in more frames than other segments). The length of the coronary artery visualized, the width of the left main coronary artery, and the width of the thickest segment of the coronary artery walls were quantitatively measured. More than 2 cm of the left coronary artery was seen in almost all patients. Segmental changes were noted in 52 of the 56 patients with obstructive CAD, 12 of the 14 patients with nonobstructive CAD, and 3 of the 19 patients with normal arteries. Persistence greatly enhanced the ability to judge the segmental changes. Forty-six patients with obstructive disease had wall thickness of 1.5 mm or greater. Only 6 patients with nonobstructive coronary arteries had this wall thickness, and only 1 normal subject had thick walls. The ultrasonic findings were useful in predicting the presence or absence of coronary atherosclerosis to varying degrees of sensitivity and specificity based on the segmental findings and wall thickness measurements. The results of this study indicate that a transthoracic ultrasonic examination of the proximal left coronary artery could be a clinically valuable tool in the qualitative identification of coronary atherosclerosis.

Ultrafast Computed Tomography in the Detection of Coronary Artery Disease

Budoff and colleagues[147] determined the relations between ultrafast computed tomography (CT) scanning and coronary angiography in 710 symptomatic patients from 6 participating centers to identify the role that ultrafast CT plays in the detection of significant CAD. A multivariate logistic regression model was used to evaluate individual contributions of age, number of calcified vessels, and the calcium score for the probability of angiographically significant CAD. Among 710 patients enrolled, 427 patients had significant angiographic disease, and coronary calcification was detected in 404, providing a sensitivity of 95%. Of the 23 patients without calcification, 19 (83%) had single-

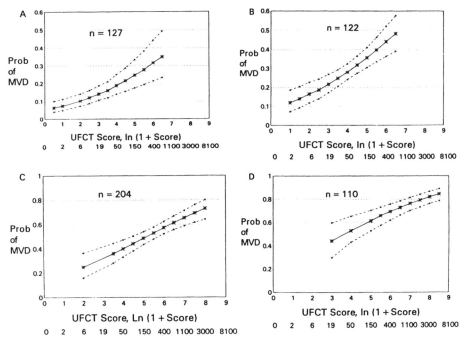

FIGURE 1-36. Natural log of the ultrafast computed tomography (UFCT) score plotted against the probability of angiographic multivessel disease (MVD) for each number of calcified vessels. Dashed lines represent 95% confidence intervals. A, One calcified vessel; B, two calcified vessels; C, three calcified vessels; and D, four calcified vessels. Numbers at the bottom of each panel are approximations of the raw calcium score. Reproduced with permission from Budoff et al.[147]

vessel CAD. Among the 283 patients without angiographically significant disease, 124 had negative ultrafast CT studies for a specificity of 44%. As the log of the calcium score increased, the probability of multivessel CAD also increased (Figure 1-36). Thus, ultrafast CT is a noninvasive, nonexercise-dependent test with a good sensitivity for the detection of CAD, but a lower specificity than might be desirable. The presence of calcification in multiple vessels in younger populations correlates with a higher specificity of obstructive disease, making ultrafast CT scanning a useful diagnostic test.

Imaging Modalities

Cholesterol-Year Score and the Risk of Atherosclerosis

The high concentrations of LDL cholesterol in plasma lead to accelerated atherosclerosis in patients homozygous for familial hypercholesterolemia (FH). Schmidt and associates[148] from Bethesda, Maryland, addressed the hypothesis that lipid deposition in the arterial vasculature and in nonvascular tissues in these patients correlates with both the duration and severity of their hypercholesterolemia. The severity of calcific atherosclerosis was defined by calcification scores and a calcified volume determined by electron beam tomography. The extent of tendinous xanthomatosis was quantitated by computed tomography. A cholesterol-year score was calculated based on the age and the yearly mean serum cholesterol concentration of each patient. Seventeen patients homozygous for FH were followed up. The average total cholesterol concentration in the study group was 780 ± 231 mg/dL (20.2 mmol/L), and the cholesterol-year scores ranged from 2,172 year/dL (56 mmol-year/L) to 32,260 mg-year/dL (834 mmol-year/L). Achilles tendon width and cross-sectional area were best correlated with the cholesterol-year score. In addition, the coronary, ostial, and total calcification atherosclerosis scores all were best correlated with the cholesterol-year score. Calcific atherosclerosis was not observed in these patients until the cholesterol-year score exceeded 10,000 mg-year/dL (260 mmol-year/L). These findings establish a direct association of cholesterol-year with extravascular lipid deposition in tissues of patients with FH. The cholesterol-year score may be useful in defining the risk of atherosclerosis in patients with more common forms of hypercholesterolemia (Table 1-16).

Prognostic Value of Coronary Calcification and Angiographic Stenoses

Coronary artery calcification is an early marker of CAD. Detrano and colleagues[149] in a multicenter study evaluated the prognostic value of coronary calcific deposits and coronary angiography for predicting CAD-related events in patients referred for angiography. Between April 1989 and December 1993, 491 symptomatic patients underwent angiography and electron-beam com-

TABLE 1-16
Patient Characteristics

Patient	Age* (yr) and Sex	Baseline Cholesterol mg/dL (mmol/L)			Cholesterol-Years (mg-yr/dL [mmol-yr/L])	Tendon Xanthoma			
		Total	LDL	HDL		TC/HDL Ratio	Width (mm)	AP (mm)	Area (mm²)
1	3 M	724 (18.7)	672 (17.4)	28 (0.7)	2,172 (56)	26	6	4	26
2	12 M	578 (14.9)	535 (13.8)	32 (0.8)	6,936 (179)	18	19	12	142
3	13 F	906 (23.4)	795 (20.5)	32 (0.8)	11,778 (304)	28	20	12	242
4	15 M	969 (25.0)	641 (16.6)	43 (1.1)	12,606 (326)	23	16	10	10
5	18 M	1,277 (33.0)	1,153 (29.8)	17 (0.4)	16,584 (429)	75	16	9	ND
6	25 F	852 (22.0)	795 (20.5)	24 (0.6)	13,652 (353)	36	30	21	461
7	27 F	612 (15.8)	572 (14.8)	28 (0.7)	9,456 (244)	22	20	10	ND
8	28 M	611 (15.8)	476 (12.3)	26 (0.7)	15,984 (413)	24	23	18	318
9	29 F	488 (12.6)	447 (11.6)	29 (0.7)	12,416 (321)	17	22	11	166
10	31 F	965 (24.9)	879 (22.7)	29 (0.7)	19,648 (508)	33	31	21	560
11	31 F	488 (12.6)	422 (10.9)	27 (0.7)	12,148 (314)	18	20	14	216
12	34 M	711 (18.4)	536 (13.9)	56 (1.4)	18,162 (469)	13	19	11	160
13	35 F	740 (19.1)	534 (13.8)	33 (0.9)	23,170 (599)	22	28	20	300
14	36 M	549 (14.2)	471 (12.2)	33 (0.9)	11,565 (299)	17	19	15	211
15	37 F	713 (18.4)	650 (16.8)	33 (0.9)	19,849 (513)	22	25	16	339
16	48 F	886 (22.9)	815 (21.1)	31 (0.8)	27,540 (712)	29	42	31	1,090
17	53 F	1,187 (30.7)	1,092 (28.2)	40 (1.0)	32,260 (834)	30	41	18	786
Mean	28	780 (20.2)	676 (17.5)	32 (0.8)	15,643 (404)	27	23	15	335
±SD	±13 M	±231 (6.0)	±218 (5.6)	±9 (0.2)	±7,409 (192)	±14	±9	±6	±290

* Age refers to the age when the computerized tomography was performed.

TC/HDL = total cholesterol versus high-density lipoprotein; LDL = low-density lipoprotein; ND = not done.
Reproduced with permission from Detrano et al.[149]

puted tomography. Thirteen CAD-related deaths and 8 nonfatal AMIs occurred during an average follow-up of 30 months. When calcification scores were sorted into quartiles of equal size in an ascending order of calcification, 1 patient in the first quartile had a fatal AMI, 2 in the second quartile, 8 in the third quartile, and 10 in the fourth quartile. Statistical analysis showed that the log calcification score, but not the number of angiographically diseased vessels, significantly predicted the probability of a CAD-related event during follow-up. Thus, CAD-related events in patients undergoing angiography may be predicted by calcification scores, as well as by the number of angiographically affected arteries.

Predictive Value of Computed Tomography of the Coronary Arteries

Arad and colleagues[150] in Roslyn, New York, followed 1173 asymptomatic patients who underwent coronary electron-beam computed tomography between September 1993 and March 1994. During an average follow-up of 19 months, 18 subjects had 26 cardiovascular events, including 1 death, 7 AMIs, 8 CABGs, 9 PTCAs, and 1 nonhemorrhagic stroke. The coronary electron-beam computed tomography estimates the presence of coronary artery atherosclerosis by measuring calcium deposition in the walls of coronary arteries. The electron-beam computed tomography-derived coronary artery calcium score correlates with the severity of underlying CAD in some patients. In this study, the coronary artery calcium score derived from the coronary electron-beam computed tomography demonstrated a close relationship between increasing severity of coronary artery calcium scores and the ability of the electron-beam computed tomography to predict future coronary events. The electron-beam computed tomography had sensitivities of 89%, 89%, and 50%, and specificities of 70%, 82%, and 95%, respectively in association with increasing coronary artery calcification scores. Thus, coronary electron-beam computed tomography predicted future cardiovascular disease events in asymptomatic patients in relation to progressive coronary artery calcification scores.

Coronary Artery Screening by Electron-Beam Computed Tomography: Effect of Lifestyle Behaviors

Wong and associates[151] from Irvine, California, and Torrance, California, evaluated the extent to which cardiovascular risk-reducing behaviors are initiated as a result of knowledge of newly detected CAD, based on test results from noninvasive electron-beam computed tomography. A total of 703 men and women, aged 28 to 84 years, asymptomatic and without prior CAD, who had a baseline electron beam computed tomography coronary artery scan and basic medical history and risk factor information completed a follow-up questionnaire regarding health behaviors practiced since their scan. Baseline calcium scores were significantly higher in those who subsequently reported consulting with a physician, or reported new hospitalization, coronary revascularization, beginning aspirin usage, blood pressure medications, cholesterol-lowering therapy, decreasing dietary fat, losing weight, beginning vitamin E, and worry. Other factors, including reducing time worked, obtaining life insurance, losing employment, increased work absenteeism, increasing exercise, or stopping smoking were not associated with coronary calcium. In logistic regression, after adjusting for age, gender, pre-existing high cholesterol, cigarette smoking, and a positive family history of CAD, the natural log of total calcium score remained associated with new aspirin usage, new cholesterol medication, consulting with a physician, losing weight, decreasing dietary fat, new coronary revascularization, but also new hospitalization and increased worry. The results suggest that potentially important risk-reducing behaviors may be reinforced by the knowledge of a positive coronary artery scan, independent of pre-existing coronary risk factor status.

General Topics

Medial artery calcification is a nonobstructive condition leading to reduced arterial compliance that is commonly considered a nonsignificant finding. The aim of a study by Lehto and coworkers[152] in Kuopio, Finland, was to investigate the predictive value of mean artery calcification in relation to 7-year cardiovascular mortality, CAD events, stroke, and lower extremity amputation in 1059 patients (581 men and 478 women) with noninsulin-dependent diabetes mellitus. At baseline, radiographically detectable mean artery calcification in femoral arteries was found in 439 patients (42%) and intimal-type calcification in 310 diabetic patients (29%). The mean fasting plasma glucose at baseline was somewhat higher in women and the duration of diabetes somewhat longer in patients with mean artery calcification than in those without; otherwise, the presence of mean artery calcification was unrelated to conventional cardiovascular risk factors. During the follow-up, 305 diabetic patients died; 208 from cardiovascular disease, 158 from CAD, and 34 from stroke. Furthermore, 58 noninsulin-dependent diabetes mellitus patients underwent their first lower extremity amputation. Mean artery calcification was a strong predictor of total, cardiovascular, and CAD mortality and it was also a significant predictor of future CAD events (fatal or nonfatal myocardial infarction), stroke and amputation (Figure 1-37). This relation was observed regardless of glycemic control and known duration of noninsulin-dependent diabetes mellitus. Mean artery calcification is a strong marker of future cardiovascular events in noninsulin-dependent diabetes mellitus unrelated to cardiovascular risk factors, supporting the hypothesis that reduced arterial elasticity could lead to clinical manifestations of diabetic microangiopathy.

The aim of this study by Karalis[153] and associates from Philadelphia, Pennsylvania, was to evaluate the risk of performing cardiac catheterization or intra-aortic balloon pump placement in patients with transesophageal echocardiographically detected atherosclerotic aortic debris. Cardiac catheterization was performed in 70 patients with atherosclerotic aortic debris (in 11 via the brachial approach and in 59 via the femoral approach) and in 71 control patients. An embolic event occurred in 10 (17%) of 59 patients with atherosclerotic aortic debris after femoral catheterization compared with 2 (3%) of 71 control patients without atherosclerotic aortic debris. None of the 11 patients with

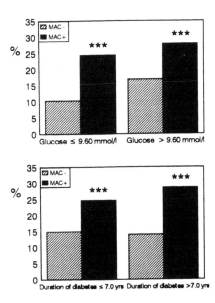

FIGURE 1-37. Bar graphs show presence (+) or absence (−) of MAC at baseline as a predictor of cardiovascular mortality in relation to fasting plasma glucose and duration of diabetes (median values as cutoff points) in patients with NIDDM. ***p<.001. Reproduced with permission from Lehto et al.[152]

atherosclerotic aortic debris who underwent brachial catheterization had an embolic event. An intra-aortic balloon pump was placed in 10 patients with atherosclerotic aortic debris and in 12 control patients. An embolic event related to placement of the intra-aortic balloon pump occurred in 5 (50%) of 10 patients with atherosclerotic aortic debris; no control patient had an embolic event. Patients with mobile atherosclerotic debris were at the highest risk for catheter-related embolism. The strongest clinical predictors of atherosclerotic aortic debris were advanced age and peripheral vascular disease. Transesophageal echocardiographic recognition of atherosclerotic aortic debris identifies patients at high risk of stroke or peripheral embolism after cardiac catheterization or intraaortic balloon pump placement. If the aortic debris is mobile, the risk is particularly high. When atherosclerotic aortic debris is detected, especially if the debris is mobile, substituting brachial for femoral catheterization and avoiding placement of an intra-aortic balloon pump may reduce the risk of embolism.

1. Torzewski J, Oldroyd R, Lachmann P, Fitzsimmons C, Proudfoot D, Bowyer D: Complement-induced release of monocyte chemotactic protein-1 from human smooth muscle cells: A possible initiating event in atherosclerotic lesion formation. Arterioscler Thromb Vasc Biol 1996 (May);16:673–677.
2. Apostolopoulos J, Davenport P, Tipping PG: Interleukin-8 production by macrophages from atheromatous plaques. Arterioscler Thromb Vasc Biol 1996 (August); 16:1007–1012.
3. Wang H, Germain SJ, Benfield PP, Gillies PJ. Gene expression of acyl coenzyme A: cholesterol acyltransferase is upregulated in human monocytes during differentiation and foam cell formation. Arterioscler Thromb Vasc Biol 1996 (June);16: 809–814.
4. Kreuzer J, Denger S, Jahn L, Bader J, Ritter K, VonHodenberg E, Kubler W: LDL stimulates chemotaxis of human monocytes through a cyclooxygenase-dependent pathway. Arterioscler Thromb Vasc Biol 1996 (December);16:1481–1487.
5. Billett MA, Adbeish IS, Alrokayan SAH, Bennett AJ, Marenah CB, White DA: Increased expression of genes for platelet-derived growth factor in circulating mononuclear cells of hypercholesterolemic patients. Arterioscler Thromb Vasc Biol 1996 (March);16:399–406.
6. Nakata A, Miyagawa J, Yamashita S, Nishida M, Tamura R, Yamamori K, Nakamura T, Nozaki S, Kameda-Takemura K, Kawata S, Taniguchi N, Higashiyama S, Matsuzawa Y. Localization of heparin-binding epidermal growth factor-like growth factor in human coronary arteries. Possible roles of HB-EGF in the formation of coronary atherosclerosis. Circulation 1996 (December 1);94:2778–2786.
7. Galea J, Armstrong J, Gadsdon P, Holden H, Francis SE, Holt CM: Interleukin-1β in coronary arteries of patients with ischemic heart disease. Arterioscler Thromb Vasc Biol 1996 (August);16:1000–1006.
8. Naruko T, Ueda M, van der Wal AC, van der Loos CM, Itoh H, Nakao K, Becker AE. C-type natriuretic peptide in human coronary atherosclerotic lesions. Circulation 1996 (December 15);94:3103–3108.
9. Diet F, Pratt RE, Berry GJ, Momose N, Gibbons GH, Dzau VJ: Increased accumulation of tissue ACE in human atherosclerotic coronary artery disease. Circulation 1996 (December 1);94:2756–2767.
10. Bauriedel G, Kandolf R, Schluckebier S, Welsch U: Ultrastructural characteristics of human atherectomy tissue from coronary and lower extremity arterial stenoses. Am J Cardiol 1996 (March 1);77:468–474.
11. Kaartinen M, Penttilä A, Kovanen PT: Mast cells in rupture-prone areas of human coronary atheromas produce and store TNF-α. Circulation 1996 (December 1);94: 2787–2792.

12. Marmur JD, Thiruvikraman SV, Fyfe BS, Guha A, Sharma SK, Ambrose JA, Fallon JT, Nemerson Y, Taubman MB: Identification of active tissue factor in human coronary atheroma. Circulation 1996 (September 15);94:1226–1232.

13. Farb A, Burke AP, Tang AL, Liang Y, Mannan P, Smialek J, Virmani R: Coronary plaque erosion without rupture into a lipid core. A frequent cause of coronary thrombosis in sudden coronary death. Circulation 1996 (April 1);93:1354–1363.

14. Casscells W, Hathorn B, David M, Krabach T, Vaughn WK, McAllister HA, Bearman G, Willerson JT: Thermal detection of cellular infiltrates in living atherosclerotic plaques: Possible implications for plaque rupture and thrombosis. Lancet 1996 (May 25);347:1447–1449.

15. Sakai M, Miyazaki A, Hakamata H, Sato Y, Matsumura T, Kobori S, Shichiri M, Horiuchi S: Lysophosphatidylcholine potentiates the mitogenic activity of modified LDL for human monocyte-derived macrophages. Arterioscler Thromb Vasc Biol 1996 (April);16:600–605.

16. Navazo MDP, Daviet L, Ninio E, McGregor JL: Identification on human CD36 of a domain (155–183) implicated in binding oxidized low-density lipoproteins (OxLDL). Arterioscler Thromb Vasc Biol 1996 (August);16:1033–1039.

17. Jovinge S, Ares MPS, Kallin B, Nielsson J: Human monocytes/macrophages release tumor necrosis factor-alpha in response to oxidized-LDL. Arterioscler Thromb Vasc Biol 1996 (December);16:1573–1579.

18. Sevanian A, Hwang J, Hodis H, Cazzolato G, Avogaro P, Bittolo-Bon G: Contribution of an in vivo oxidized LDL to LDL oxidation and its association with dense LDL sub-populations. Arterioscler Thromb Vasc Biol 1996 (June);16:784–793.

19. Reaven P, Grasse B, Barnett J: Effect of antioxidants alone and in combination with monounsaturated fatty acid-enriched diets on lipoprotein oxidation. Arterioscler Thromb Vasc Biol 1996 (December);16:1465–1472.

20. Thomas SR, Neužil J, Stocker R: Cosupplementation with coenzyme Q prevents the prooxidant effect of α-tocopherol and increases the resistance of LDL to transition metal-dependent oxidation initiation. Arterioscler Thromb Vasc Biol 1996 (May);16:687–696.

21. Mata P, Alonso R, Lopez-Farre A, Ordovas JM, Lahoz C, Garces C, Caramelo C, Codoceo R, Blazquez E, de Oya M: Effect of dietary fat saturation on LDL oxidation and monocyte adhesion to human endothelial cells in vitro. Arterioscler Thromb Vasc Biol 1996 (November);16:1347–1355.

22. Stephens NG, Parsons A, Schofield PM, Kelly F, Cheeseman K, Mitchinson MJ, Brown MJ: Randomised controlled trial of vitamin E in patients with coronary disease: Cambridge Heart Antioxidant Study (CHAOS). Lancet 1996 (March 23); 347:781–786.

23. Azen SP, Qian D, Mack WJ, Sevanian A, Selzer RH, Liu C-R, Liu C-H, Hodis HN: Effect of supplementary antioxidant vitamin intake on carotid arterial wall intima-media thickness in a controlled clinical trial of cholesterol lowering. Circulation 1996 (November 15);94:2369–2372.

24. Bui MN, Sack MN, Moutsatsos G, Lu DY, Katz P, McCown R, Breall JA, Rackley CE: Autoantibody titers to oxidized low density lipoprotein in patients with coronary atherosclerosis. Am Heart J 1996 (April);131:663–667.

25. Mironova M, Virella G, Lopes-Virella MF: Isolation and characterization of human antioxidized LDL autoantibodies. Arterioscler Thromb Vasc Biol 1996 (February); 16:222–229.

26. Zhu W, Roma P, Pirillo A, Pellegatta F, Catapano AL: Human endothelial cells exposed to oxidized LDL express hsp70 only when proliferating. Arterioscler Thromb Vasc Biol 1996 (September);16:1104–1111.

27. Pernow J, Kaijser L, Lundberg JM, Ahlborg G: Comparable potent coronary constrictor effects of endothelin-1 and big endothelin-1 in humans. Circulation 1996 (November 1);94:2077–2082.

28. O'Brien KD, McDonald TO, Chait A, Allen MD, Alpers CE. Neovascular expression of E-selectin, intercellular adhesion molecule-1 and vascular cell adhesion molecule-1 in human atherosclerosis and their relation to intimal leukocyte content. Circulation 1996 (February);93:672–682.

29. Haught WH, Mansour M, Rothlein R, Kishimoto TK, Mainolfi EA, Hendricks JB, Hendricks C, Mehta JL: Alterations in circulating intercellular adhesion molecule-1 and L-selectin: Further evidence for chronic inflammation in ischemic heart disease. Am Heart J 1996 (July);132:1–8.

30. Hackman A, Abe Y, Insull W Jr., Pownall H, Smith L, Dunn K, Gotto AM Jr., Ballantyne CM: Levels of soluble cell adhesion molecules in patients with dyslipidemia. Circulation 1996 (April 1);93:1334–1338.

31. Wolle J, Hill RR, Ferguson E, Devall LJ, Trivedi BK, Newton RS, Saxena U: Selected inhibition of tumor necrosis factor-induced vascular cell adhesion molecule-1 gene expression by a novel flavonoid; Lack of effect on transcription factor NF-kB. Arterioscler Thromb Vasc Biol 1996 (December);16:1501–1508.

32. Marczin N, Antonov A, Papapetropoulos A, Munn DH, Virmani R, Kolodgie FD, Gerrity R, Catravas JD: Monocyte-induced downregulation of nitric oxide synthase in cultured aortic endothelial cells. Arterioscler Thromb Vasc Biol 1996 (September);16:1095–1103.

33. Cooper CJ, Landzberg MJ, Anderson TJ, Charbonneau F, Creager MA, Ganz P, Selwyn AP: Role of nitric oxide in the local regulation of pulmonary vascular resistance in humans. Circulation 1996 (January);93:266–271.

34. Shiode N, Nakayama K, Morishima N, Yamagata T, Matsuura H, Kajiyama G: Nitric oxide production by coronary conductance and resistance vessels in hypercholesterolemia patients. Am Heart J 1996 (June);131:1051–1057.

35. Egashira K, Hirooka Y, Kuga T, Mohri M, Takeshita A: Effects of L-arginine supplementation on endothelium-dependent coronary vasodilation in patients with angina pectoris and normal coronary arteriograms. Circulation 1996 (July 15);94:130–134.

36. Chauhan A, More RS, Mullins PA, Michael GT, Petch MC, Schofield PM: Aging-associated endothelial dysfunction in humans is reversed by L-arginine. J Am Coll Cardiol 1996 (December);28:1796–1804.

37. Levine GN, Frei B, Koulouris SN, Gerhard MD, Keaney JF Jr., Vita JA: Ascorbic acid reverses endothelial vasomotor dysfunction in patients with coronary artery disease. Circulation 1996 (March 15);93:1107–1113.

38. Anderson TJ, Meredith IT, Charbonneau F, Yeung AC, Frei B, Selwyn AP, Ganz P: Endothelium-dependent coronary vasomotion relates to the susceptibility of LDL to oxidation in humans. Circulation 1996 (May 1);93:1647–1650.

39. Vogel RA, Corretti MC, Plotnick GD: Changes in flow-mediated brachial artery vasoactivity with lowering of desirable cholesterol levels in healthy middle-aged men. Am J Cardiol 1996 (January 1);77:37–40.

40. Mancini GBJ, Henry GC, Macaya C, O'Neill BJ, Pucillo AL, Carere RG, Wargovich TJ, Mudra H, Lücher TF, Klibaner MI, Haber HE, Uprichard ACG, Pepine CJ, Pitt B: Angiotensin-converting enzyme inhibition with quinapril improves endothelial vasomotor dysfunction in patients with coronary artery disease. The TREND (Trial on Reversing Endothelial Dysfunction) Study. Circulation 1996 (August 1);94:258–265.

41. Iiyama K, Nagano M, Yo Y, Nagano N, Kamide K, Higaki J, Mikami H, Ogihara T: Impaired endothelial function with essential hypertension assessed by ultrasonography. Am Heart J 1996 (October);132:779–782.

42. Havranek EP, Nademanee K, Grayburn PA, Eichhorn EJ: Endothelium-dependent vasorelaxation is impaired in cocaine arteriopathy. J Am Coll Cardiol 1996 (November 1);28:1168–1174.

43. Pasterkamp G, Borst C, Post MJ, Mali WPTM, Wensing PJW, Gussenhoven EJ, Hillen B: Atherosclerotic arterial remodeling in the superficial femoral artery. Individual variation in local compensatory enlargement response. Circulation 1996 (May 15);93:1818–1825.

44. Cushman M, Psaty BM, Macy E, Bovill EG, Cornell ES, Kuller LH, Tracy RP: Correlates of thrombin markers in an elderly cohort free of clinical cardiovascular disease. Arterioscler Thromb Vasc Biol 1996 (September);16:1163–1169.

45. Scarabin P-Y, Vissac A-M, Krizin J-M, Bourgeat P, Amiral J, Agher R, Guize L: Population correlates of coagulation factor VII: importance of age, sex, and meno-

pausal status as determinants of activated factor VII. Arterioscler Thromb Vasc Biol 1996 (September);16:1170–1176.

46. Cigolini M, Targher G, Andreis IAB, Tonoli M, Agostino G, DeSandre G: Visceral fat accumulation and its relation to plasma hemostatic factors in healthy men. Arterioscler Thromb Vasc Biol 1996 (March);16:368–374.

47. van der Bom JG, Bots ML, van Vliet HHDM, Pols HAP, Hofman A, Grobbee DE: Antithrombin and atherosclerosis in the Rotterdam Study. Arterioscler Thromb Vasc Biol 1996 (July);16:864–867.

48. Freedman JE, Farhat JH, Loscalzo J, Keaney JF Jr. α-Tocopherol inhibits aggregation of human platelets by a protein kinase C-dependent mechanism. Circulation 1996 (November 15);94:2434–2440.

49. Kario K, Matsuo T, Kobayashi H, Asada R, Matsuo M: 'Silent' cerebral infarction is associated with hypercoagulability, endothelial cell damage, and high Lp (a) levels in elderly Japanese. Arterioscler Thromb Vasc Biol 1996 (June);16:734–741.

50. Reverter J-C, Tassies D, Font J, Monoteagudo J, Escolar G, Ingelmo M, Ordinas A: Hypercoagulable state in patients with antiphospholipid syndrome is related to high induced tissue factor expression on monocytes and to low free protein S. Arterioscler Thromb Vasc Biol 1996 (November);16:1319–1326.

51. Lopez-Segura F, Velasco F, Lopez-Miranda J, Castro P, Lopez-Pedrera R, Banco A, Jimenz-Pereperez J, Torres A, Trujillo J, Ordovas JM, Perez-Jimenez F: Monounsaturated fatty acid-enriched diet decreased plasma plasminogen activator inhibitor type I. Arterioscler Thromb Vasc Biol 1996 (January);16:82–88.

52. Svendsen OL, Hassager C, Christiansen C, Nielsen JD, Winther K: Plasminogen activator inhibitor-1, tissue-type plasminogen activator, and fibrinogen: effect of dieting with or without exercise in overweight postmenopausal women. Arterioscler Thromb Vasc Biol 1996 (March);16:381–385.

53. Szczeklik A, Musial J, Undas A, Swadzba J, Gora PF, Piwowarska W, Duplaga M: Inhibition of thrombin generation by aspirin is blunted in hypercholesterolemia. Arterioscler Thromb Vasc Biol. 1996 (August);16:948–954.

54. Halle M, Berg A, Keul J, Baumstark MW: Association between serum fibrinogen concentrations in HDL and LDL subfraction phenotypes in healthy men. Atheroscler Thromb Vasc Biol 1996 (January);16:144–148.

55. Zitoun D, Bara L, Basdevent A, Samama MM: Levels of factor VII(c) associated with decreased tissue factor pathway inhibitor and increased plasminogen activator inhibitor-1 in dyslipidemias. Atheroscler Thromb Vascr Biol 1996 (January); 1:77–81.

56. Silveira A, Karpe F, Johnsson H, Bauer KA, Hamsten A: In vivo demonstration in humans that large postprandial triglyceride-rich lipoproteins activate coagulation factor VII through the intrinsic coagulation pathway. Arterioscler Thromb Vasc Biol 1996 (November);16:1333–1339.

57. Kokawa T, Enjyoji K, Kumeda K, Kamikubo Y, Harada-Shiba M, Koh H, Tsushima M, Yamamoto A, Kato H: Measurement of the free form of TFTI antigen in hyperlipidemia: relationship between free and endothelial cell-associated forms of TFPI. Arterioscler Thromb Vasc Biol 1996 (June);16:802–808.

58. Bröijersen A, Eriksson M, Wiman B, Angelin B, Hjemdahl P: Gemfibrozil treatment of combined hyperlipoproteinemia: No improvement of fibrinolysis despite marked reduction of plasma triglyceride levels. Arterioscler Thromb Vasc Biol 1996 (April);16:511–516.

59. Rothe G, Gabriel H, Kovacs E, Klucken J, Stohr J, Kindermann W, Schmitz G: Peripheral blood mononuclear phagocyte subpopulations as cellular markers in hypercholesterolemia. Arterioscler Thromb Vasc Biol 1996 (December);16: 1437–1447.

60. Jones PJH, Pappu AS, Hatcher L, Li Z-C, Illingworth DR, Connor WE: Dietary cholesterol feeding suppresses human cholesterol synthesis measured by deuterium incorporation and urinary mevalonic acid levels. Arterioscler Thromb Vasc Biol 1996 (October);16:1222–1228.

61. Vega GL, Grundy SM: Hypercholesterolemia with cholesterol-enriched LDL and normal levels of LDL-Apo lipoprotein B: Effects of the Step I Diet and bile acid sequestrants on the cholesterol content of LDL. Arterioscler Thromb Vasc Biol 1996 (April);16:517–522.

62. Campos H, Arnold KS, Balestra ME, Innerarity TL, Krauss RM: Differences in receptor binding of LDL subfractions. Arterioscler Thromb Vasc Biol 1996 (June); 16:794–801.

63. Demuth K, Myara I, Chappey B, Vedie B, Pech-Amsellem MA, Haberland ME, Moatti N: A cytotoxic electronegative LDL subfraction is present in human plasma. Arterioscler Thromb Vasc Biol 1996 (June);16:773–783.

64. Kuivenhoven JA, Stalenhoef AFH, Hill JS, Demacker PNM, Errami A, Kastelein JJP, Pritchard PH: Two novel molecular defects in the LCAT gene are associated with fish eye disease. Arterioscler Thromb Vasc Biol 1996 (February);16:294–303.

65. Benlian P, de Gennes JL, Foubert L, Zhang H, Gagné SE, Hayden M: Premature atherosclerosis in patients with familial chylomicronemia caused by mutations in the lipoprotein lipase gene. N Engl J Med 1996 (September 19);335:848–54.

66. Guérin M, Bruckert E, Dolphin PJ, Turpin G, Chapman MJ: Fenofibrate reduces plasma cholesterol ester transfer from HDL to VLDL and normalizes the atherogenic, dense LDL profile in combined hyperlipidemia. Arterioscler Thromb Vasc Biol 1996 (June);16:763–772.

67. Foger B, Ritsch A, Doblinger A, Wessels H, Patsch JR: Relationship of plasma cholesteryl ester transfer protein to HDL cholesterol: Studies in normotriglyceridemia and moderate hypertriglyceridemia. Arterioscler Thromb Vasc Biol 1996 (December);16:1430–1436.

68. McPherson R, Agnani G, Lau P, Fruchart J-C, Edgar AD, Marcel YL: Role of Lp A-I and Lp A-I/A-II in cholesteryl ester transfer protein-mediated neutral lipid transfer: studies in normal subjects and in hypertriglyceridemic patients before and after fenofibrate therapy. Arterioscler Thromb Vasc Biol 1996 (November); 16:1340–1346.

69. Mowri HO, Patsch JR, Gotto AM, Patsch W: Apolipoprotein A-II influences the substrate properties of human HDL_2 and HDL_3 for hepatic lipase. Arterioscler Thromb Vasc Biol 1996 (June);16:755–762.

70. Nanjee MN, Crouse JR, King JM, Hovorka R, Rees SE, Carson ER, Morgenthaler J-J, Lerch P, Miller NE: Effects of intravenous infusion of lipid-free apo A-I in humans. Arterioscler Thromb Vasc Biol 1996 (September);16:1203–1214.

71. Blangero J, Williams-Blangero S, Mahaney MC, Comuzzie AG, Hixson JE, Samollow PB, Sharp RM, Stern MP, MacCluer JW: Effects of a major gene for apolipoprotein A-I concentration are thyroid hormone dependent in Mexican Americans. Arterioscler Thromb Vasc Biol 1996 (September);16:1177–1183.

72. Nevin DN, Zambon A, Furlong CE, Richter RJ, Humbert R, Hokanson JE, Brunzell JD: Paraoxonase genotypes, lipoprotein lipase activity, and HDL. Arterioscler Thromb Vasc Biol 1996 (October);16:1243–1249.

73. Hau M-F, Smelt AHM, Bindels AJGH, Sijbrands EJG, Van der Laarse A, Onkenhout W, van Duyvenvoorde W, Princen HMG: Effects of fish oil on oxidation resistance of VLDL in hypertriglyceridemic patients. Arterioscler Thromb Vasc Biol 1996 (September);16:1197–1202.

74. Kraft HG, Lingenhel A, Köchl S, Koppichler F, Kronenberg F, Abe A, Mühlberger V, Schönitzer D, Utermann G: Apolipoprotein (a) kringle IV repeat number predicts risk for coronary heart disease. Arterioscler Thromb Vasc Biol 1996 (June); 16:713–719.

75. Carmena R, Lussier-Cacan S, Roy M, Minnich A, Lingenhel A, Kronenberg F, Davignon J: Lp(a) levels in atherosclerotic vascular disease in sample of patients with familial hypercholesterolemia sharing the same gene defect. Arterioscler Thromb Vasc Biol 1996 (January);16:129–136.

76. Assmann G, Schulte H, von Eckardstein A: Hypertriglyceridemia and elevated lipoprotein (a) are risk factors for major coronary events in middle-aged men. Am J Cardiol 1996 (June 1);77:1179–1184.

77. Kinlay S, Dobson AJ, Heller RF, McElduff P, Alexander H, Kickeson J: Risk of primary recurrent myocardial infarction from lipoprotein(a) in men and women. J Am Coll Cardiol 1996 (October);28:870–875.

78. Sunayama S, Daida H, Mokuno H, Miyano H, Yokoi H, Lee YJ, Sakurai H, Yamaguchi H: Lack of increased coronary atherosclerotic risk due to elevated lipoprotein(a) in women ≥55 years of age. Circulation 1996 (September 15);94: 1263–1268.

79. Schreiner PJ, Heiss G, Tyroler HA, Morrisett JD, Davis CE, Smith R: Race and gender differences in the association of Lp (a) with carotid artery wall thickness: The Atherosclerosis Risk in Communities study. Arterioscler Thromb Vasc Biol 1996 (March);16:471–478.

80. Kronenberg F, Trenkwalder E, Dieplinger H, Utermann G: Lipoprotein (a) in stored plasma samples and the ravages of time; Why epidemiological studies might fail. Arterioscler Thromb Vasc Biol 1996 (December);16:1568–1572.

81. Haffner SM, Stern MP, Miettinen H, Robbins D, Howard BV: Apolipoprotein E polymorphism and LDL size in a biethnic population. Arterioscler Thromb Vasc Biol. 1996 (September);16:1184–1188.

82. Wilson PWF, Schaefer EJ, Larson MG, Ordovas JM: Apolipoprotein E alleles and risk of coronary disease: A meta-analysis. Arterioscler Thromb Vasc Biol 1996 (October);16:1250–1255.

83. Kataoka S, Robbins DC, Cowan LD, Go O, Yeh JL, Devereux RB, Fabsitz RR, Lee ET, Welty TK, Howard BV, for the Strong Heart Study Investigators: Apolipoprotein E polymorphism in American Indians and its relation to plasma lipoproteins and diabetes: The Strong Heart Study. Arterioscler Thromb Vasc Biol 1996 (August);16:918–925.

84. Broda G, Davis CE, Pajak A, Williams OD, Rywik SL, Baczyńska E, Folsom AR, Szklo M: Poland and United States collaborative study on cardiovascular epidemiology: A comparison of HDL cholesterol and its subfractions in populations covered by the United States Atherosclerosis Risk in Communities Study and the Polish-MONICA project. Arterioscler Thromb Vasc Biol 1996 (February);16: 339–349.

85. Kroon AA, Aengevaeren WRM, van der Werf T, Uijen GJH, Reiber JHC, Bruschke AVG, Stalenhoef AFH. LDL-Apheresis Atherosclerosis Regression Study (LAARS): Effect of aggressive versus conventional lipid lowering treatment on coronary atherosclerosis. Circulation 1996 (May 15);93:1826–1835.

86. Niebauer J, Hambrecht R, Velich T, Marburger C, Hauer K, Kreuzer J, Zimmermann R, von Hodenberg E, Schlierf G, Schuler G, Kübler W: Predictive value of lipid profile for salutary coronary angiographic changes in patients on a low-fat diet and physical exercise program. Am J Cardiol 1996 (July 15);78:163–167.

87. Mack WJ, Krauss RM, Hodis HN: Lipoprotein subclasses in the Monitored Atherosclerosis Regression Study (MARS): Treatment effects and relation to coronary angiographic progression. Arterioscler Thromb Vasc Biol 1996 (May);16:697–704.

88. Waters D, Lespérance J, Gladstone P, Boccuzzi SJ, Cook T, Hudgin R, Krip G, Higginson L, for the CCAIT Study Group: Effects of cigarette smoking on the angiographic evolution of coronary atherosclerosis. A Canadian Coronary Atherosclerosis Intervention Trial (CCAIT) Substudy. Circulation 1996 (August 15);94: 614–621.

89. Azen SP, Mack WJ, Cashin-Hemphill L, LaBree L, Shircore AM, Selzer RH, Blankenhorn DH, Hodis HN: Progression of coronary artery disease predicts clinical coronary events. Long-term follow-up from the Cholesterol Lowering Atherosclerosis Study. Circulation 1996 (January);93:34–41.

90. Sacks FM, Pfeffer MA, Moye LA, Rouleau JL, Rutherford JD, Cole TG, Brown L, Warnica JW, Arnold JMO, Wun CC, Davis BR, Braunwald E, for the Cholesterol and Recurrent Events Trial Investigators: The effect of pravastatin on coronary events after myocardial infarction in patients with average cholesterol Levels. N Engl J Med 1996 (October);335:1001–1009.

91. de Divitiis M, Rubba P, Di Somma S, Liguori V, Galderisi M, Montefusco S, Car-

reras G, Greco V, Carotenuto A, Iannuzzo G, de Divitiis O: Effects of short-term reduction in serum cholesterol with simvastatin in patients with stable angina pectoris and mild to moderate hypercholesterolemia. Am J Cardiol 1996 (October 1);78:763–768.

92. Prisant LM, Downton M, Watkins LO, Schnaper H, Bradford RH, Chremos AN, Langendörfer A: Efficacy and tolerability of lovastatin in 459 African-Americans with hypercholesterolemia. Am J Cardiol 1996 (August 15);78:420–424.

93. Gidding SS, Liu K, Bild DE, Flack J, Gardin J, Ruth KJ, Oberman A: Prevalence and identification of abnormal lipoprotein levels in a biracial population aged 23 to 35 years (The CARDIA Study). Am J Cardiol 1996 (August 1);78:304–308.

94. Ashraf T, Hay JW, Pitt B, Wittels E, Crouse J, Davidson M, Furberg CD, Radican L: Cost-effectiveness of pravastatin in secondary prevention of coronary artery disease. Am J Cardiol 1996 (August 15);78:409–414.

95. Mitchell BD, Kammerer CM, Mahaney MC, Blangero J, Comuzzie AG, Atwood LD, Haffner SM, Stern MP, MacCluer JW: Genetic analysis of the insulin resistant syndrome: Pleiotropic effects of genes influencing insulin levels on lipoprotein and obesity measures. Arterioscler Thromb Vasc Biol 1996 (February);16:281–288.

96. Howard G, O'Leary DH, Zaccaro D, Haffner S, Rewers M, Hamman R, Selby JV, Saad MF, Savage P, Bergman, for the IRAS Investigators: Insulin sensitivity and atherosclerosis. Circulation 1996 (May 15);93:1809–1817.

97. Eliasson B, Taskinen M-R, Smith U: Long-term use of nicotine gum is associated with hyperinsulinemia and insulin resistance. Circulation 1996 (September 1);94:878–881.

98. Mäkimattila S, Virkamäki A, Groop P-H, Cockcroft J, Utriainen T, Fagerudd J, Yki-Järvinen H: Chronic hyperglycemia impairs endothelial function and insulin sensitivity via different mechanisms in insulin-dependent diabetes mellitus. Circulation 1996 (September 15);94:1276–1282.

99. Lambert J, Aarsen M, Donker AJM, Stehouwer CDA: Endothelium-dependent and-independent vasodilation of large arteries in normoalbuminuric insulin-dependent diabetes mellitus. Arterioscler Thromb Vasc Biol 1996 (May);16:705–711.

100. Clarkson P, Celermajer DS, Donald AE, Sampson M, Sorensen KE, Adams M, Yue DK, Betteridge J, Deanfield JE: Impaired vascular reactivity in insulin-dependent diabetes mellitus is related to disease duration and low density lipoprotein cholesterol levels. J Am Coll Cardiol 1996 (September);28:573–579.

101. Lloyd CE, Kuller LH, Ellis D, Becker DJ, Wing RR, Orchard TJ: Coronary artery disease in insulin dependent diabetes mellitus: Gender differences in risk factors, but not risk. Arterioscler Thromb Vasc Biol 1996 (June);16:720–726.

102. Williams SB, Cucso JA, Roddy AM, Johnstone MT, Creager MA: Impaired nitric oxide-mediated vasodilation in patients with non-insulin-dependent diabetes mellitus. J Am Coll Cardiol 1996 (March 1);27:567–574.

103. Mansfield MW, Haywood DM, Grant PJ: Sex differences in coagulation and fibrinolysis in white subjects with noninsulin dependent diabetes mellitus. Atheroscler Thromb Vasc Biol 1996 (January);16:160–164.

104. Uusitupa MIJ, Niskanen L, Luoma J, Vilja P, Mercuri M, Rauramaa R, Ylä Herttuala S: Autoantibodies against oxidized LDL do not predict atherosclerotic vascular disease in non-insulin-dependent diabetes mellitus. Arterioscler Thromb Vasc Biol 1996 (October);16:1236–1242.

105. Woodfield SL, Lundergan CF, Reiner JS, Greenhouse SW, Thompson MA, Rohrbeck SC, Deychak Y, Simoons ML, Califf RM, Topol EJ, Ross AM: Angiographic findings and outcome in diabetic patients treated with thrombolytic therapy for acute myocardial infarction: The GUSTO-I Experience. J Am Coll Cardiol 1996 (December);28:1661–1669.

106. Lamon-Fava S, Wilson PWF, Schaefer EJ: Impact of body mass index on coronary heart disease risk factors in men and women: The Framingham Offspring Study. Arterioscler Thromb Vasc Biol 1996 (December);16:1509–1515.

107. Ichiki K, Ikeda H, Haramaki N, Ueno T, Imaizumi T: Long-term smoking impairs platelet-derived nitric oxide release. Circulation 1996 (December 15);94: 3109–3114.

108. Higman DJ, Strachan AMJ, Buttery L, Hicks RCJ, Springall DR, Greenhalgh RM, Powell JT: Smoking impairs the activity of endothelial nitric oxide synthase and saphenous vein. Arterioscler Thromb Vasc Biol 1996 (April);16:546–552.

109. Heitzer T, Ylä-Herttuala S, Luoma J, Kurz S, Münzel T, Just H, Olschewski M, Drexler H: Cigarette smoking potentiates endothelial dysfunction of forearm resistance vessels in patients with hypercholesterolemia: Role of oxidized LDL. Circulation 1996 (April 1);93:1346–1353.

110. Heitzer T, Just H, Münzel T: Antioxidant vitamin C improves endothelial dysfunction in chronic smokers. Circulation 1996 (July 1);94:6–9.

111. Steenland K, Thun M, Lally C, Heath C Jr: Environmental tobacco smoke and coronary heart disease in the American Cancer Society CPS-II cohort. Circulation 1996 (August 15);94:622–628.

112. Gottlieb S, Boyko V, Zahger D, Balkin J, Hod H, Pelled B, Stern S, Behar S: Smoking and prognosis after acute myocardial infarction in the thrombolytic era (Israeli Thrombolytic National Survey). J Am Coll Cardiol 1996 (November 15); 28:1506–1513.

113. Gallagher PM, Meleady R, Shields DC, Tan KS, McMaster D, Rozen R, Evans A, Graham IM, Whitehead AS: Homocysteine and risk of premature coronary heart disease. Evidence for a common gene mutation. Circulation 1996 (November 1); 94:2154–2158.

114. Schmitz C, Lindpaintner K, Verhoef P, Gaziano JM, Buring J: Genetic polymorphism of methylenetetrahydrofolate reductase and myocardial infarction. A case-control study. Circulation 1996 (October 15);94:1812–1814.

115. Ma J, Stampfer MJ, Hennekens CH, Frosst P, Selhub J, Horsford J, Malinow R, Willett WC, Rozen R: Methylenetetrahydrofolate reductase polymorphism, plasma folate, homocysteine, and risk of myocardial infarction in United States physicians. Circulation 1996 (November 15);94:2410–2416.

116. Loehrer FMT, Angst CP, Haefeli WE, Jordan PP, Ritz R, Fowler B: Low whole blood S-Adenosyl methionine in correlation between 5-methyltetrahydrofolate and homocysteine in coronary artery disease. Arterioscler Thromb Vasc Biol 1996 (June);16:727–733.

117. Robinson K, Gupta A, Dennis V, Arheart K, Chaudhary D, Green R, Vigo P, Mayer EL, Selhub J, Kutner M, Jacobsen DW: Hyperhomocysteinemia confers an independent increased risk of atherosclerosis in end-stage renal disease and is closely linked to plasma folate and pyridoxine concentrations. Circulation 1996 (December 1);94:2743–2748.

118. vandenBerg M, Stehouwer CDA, Bierdrager E, Rauwerda JA: Plasma homocysteine and severity of atherosclerosis in a young patient with lower limb atherosclerotic disease. Arterioscler Thromb Vasc Biol 1996 (January);16:165–171.

119. Kawachi I, Sparrow D, Spiro A III, Vokonas P, Weiss ST: A prospective study of anger and coronary heart disease. The Normative Aging Study. Circulation 1996 (November 1);94:2090–2095.

120. Keltikangas-Järvinen L, Räikkönen K, Hautanen A, Adlercreutz H: Vital exhaustion, anger expression, and pituitary and adrenocortical hormones: Implications for the insulin resistance syndrome. Arterioscler Thromb Vasc Biol 1996 (February);16:275–280.

121. Muhlestein JB, Hammond EH, Carlquist JF, Radicke E, Thomson MJ, Karagounis LA, Woods ML, Anderson JL: Increased incidence of *Chlamydia* species within the coronary arteries of patients with symptomatic atherosclerotic versus other forms of cardiovascular disease. J Am Coll Cardiol 1996 (June);27:1555–1561.

122. Nieto FJ, Adam E, Sorlie P, Farzadegan H, Melnick JL, Comstock GW, Szklo M: Cohort study of cytomegalovirus infection as a risk factor for carotid intimal-medial thickening, a measure of subclinical atherosclerosis. Circulation 1996 (September 1);94:922–927.

123. Kawaguchi H, Mori T, Kawano T, Kono S, Sasaki J, Arakawa K: Band neutrophil count and the presence and severity of coronary atherosclerosis. Am Heart J 1996 (July);132:9–12.

124. Weijenberg MP, Feskens EJM, Kromhout D: White blood cell count and the risk of coronary heart disease and all-cause mortality in elderly men. Arterioscler Thromb Vasc Biol 1996 (April);16:499–503.

125. The Multiple Risk Factor Intervention Trial Group: Mortality after 16 years for participants randomized to the Multiple Risk Factor Intervention Trial. Circulation 1996 (September 1);94:946–951.

126. Pietinen P, Rimm EB, Korhonen P, Hartman AM, Willett WC, Albanes D, Virtamo J: Intake of dietary fiber and risk of coronary heart disease in a cohort of Finnish men. The Alpha-Tocopherol, Beta-Carotene Cancer Prevention Study. Circulation 1996 (December 1);94:2720–2727.

127. de Lorgeril M, Salen P, Martin J-L, Mamelle N, Monjaud I, Touboul P, Delaye J: Effect of a Mediterranean type of diet on the rate of cardiovascular complications in patients with coronary artery disease: Insights into the cardioprotective effect of certain nutrients. J Am Coll Cardiol 1996 (November 1);28:1103–1108.

128. Pauletto P, Puato M, Caroli MG, Casiglia E, Munhambo AE, Cazzolato G, Bon BG, Angeli MT, Galli C, Pessina AC: Blood pressure and atherogenic lipoprotein profiles of fish-diet and vegetarian villagers in Tanzania: The Lugalawa Study. Lancet 1996 (September 21);348:784–788.

129. Kushi LH, Folsom AR, Prineas RJ, Mink PJ, Wu Y, Bostick RM: Dietary antioxidant vitamins and death from coronary heart disease in postmenopausal women. N Engl J Med 1996 (May 2);334:1156–1162.

130. Folsom AR, McGovern PG, Nabulsi AA, Shahar E, Kahn ESB, Winkhart SP, White AD for the Atherosclerosis Risk in Communities Study Investigators: Changes in plasma lipids and lipoproteins associated with starting or stopping postmenopausal hormone replacement therapy. Am Heart J 1996 (November);132:952–958.

131. Brinton EA: Oral estrogen replacement therapy in postmenopausal women selectively raises levels and production rates of lipoprotein A-I and lowers hepatic lipase activity without lowering the fractional catabolic rate. Arterioscler Thromb Vasc Biol 1996 (March);16:431–440.

132. Taskinen M-R, Puolakka J, Pyörälä T, Luotola H, Björn M, Kääriäinen J, Lahdenperä S, Ehnholm C: Hormone replacement therapy lowers plasma Lp(a) concentrations: Comparison of cyclic transdermal and continuous estrogen-progestin regimens. Arterioscler Thromb Vasc Biol 1996 (October);16:1215–1221.

133. Shahar E, Folsom AR, Salomaa VV, Stinson VL, McGovern PG, Shimakawa T, Chambless LE, Wu KK, for the Atherosclerosis Risk in Communities (ARIC) Study Investigators: Relation of hormone-replacement therapy to measures of plasma fibrinolytic activity. Circulation 1996 (June 1);93:1970–1975.

134. Grodstein F, Stampfer MJ, Manson JE, Colditz GA, Willett WC, Rosner B, Speizer FE, Hennekens CH: Postmenopausal estrogen and progestin use and the risk of cardiovascular disease. N Engl J Med 1996 (August 15);335:453–461.

135. Katz RJ, Hsia J, Walker P, Jacobs H, Kessler C: Effects of hormone replacement therapy on the circadian pattern of atherothrombotic risk factors. Am J Cardiol (October 15) 1996;78:876–880.

136. Goldstein RE, Andrews M, Hall WJ, Moss AJ: Marked reduction in long-term cardiac deaths with aspirin after a coronary event. J Am Coll Cardiol (August);28:326–330.

137. Jonas M, Reicher-Reiss H, Boyko V, Shotan A, Mandelzweig L, Goldbourt U, Behar S, for the Bezafibrate Infarction Prevention (BIP) Study Group: Usefulness of beta-blocker therapy in patients with non-insulin-dependent diabetes mellitus and coronary artery disease. Am J Cardiol 1996 (June 15);77:1273–1277.

138. Jukema JW, Zwinderman AH, van Boven AJ, Reiber JHC, Van der Laarse A, Lie KI, Bruschke AVG, REGRESS Study Group: Evidence for a synergistic effect of calcium channel blockers with lipid-lowering therapy in retarding progression of coronary atherosclerosis in symptomatic patients with normal to moderately raised cholesterol levels. Arterioscler Thromb Vasc Biol 1996 (March);16:425–430.

139. Braun S, Boyko V, Behar S, Reicher H, Shotan A, Schlesinger Z, Rosenfeld T, Palant A, Friedensohn A, Laniado S, Goldbourt U: Calcium antagonists and mortality in patients with coronary artery disease: A cohort study of 11,575 patients. J Am Coll Cardiol 1996 (July);28:7–11.

140. Nwasokwa ON, Weiss M, Gladstone C, Bodenheimer MM: Effect of coronary artery size on the prevalence of atherosclerosis. Am J Cardiol 1996 (October 1);78:741–746.

141. Mintz GS, Popma JJ, Pichard AD, Kent KM, Satler LF, Chuang YC, DeFalco RA, Leon MB: Limitations of angiography in the assessment of plaque distribution in coronary artery disease. A systematic study of target lesion eccentricity in 1446 lesions. Circulation 1996 (March 1);93:924–931.

142. Pearson AC, Peterson JW, Orsinelli DA, Guo R, Boudoulas H. Comparison of thickness and distensibility in the carotid artery and descending thoracic aorta: In vivo ultrasound assessment. Am Heart J 1996 (April);131:655–662.

143. Wei M, Gonzalez C, Haffner SM, O'Leary DH, Stern MP: Ultrasonographically assessed maximum carotid artery wall thickness in Mexico City residents and Mexican-Americans living in San Antonio, Texas: association with diabetes and cardiovascular risk factors. Arterioscler Thromb Vasc Biol 1996 (November);16:1388–1392.

144. Wendelhag I, Wiklund O, Wikstrand J: On quantifying plaque size and intima-media thickness in carotid and femoral arteries: comments on results from a prospective ultrasound study in patients with familial hypercholesterolemia. Arterioscler Thromb Vasc Biol 1996 (July);16:843–850.

145. Tomochika Y, Okuda F, Tanaka N, Wasaki Y, Tokisawa I, Aoyagi S, Morikuni C, Ono S, Okada K, Matsuzaki M: Improvement of atherosclerosis and stiffness of the thoracic descending aorta with cholesterol-lowering therapies in familial hypercholesterolemia. Arterioscler Thromb Vasc Biol 1996 (August);16:955–962.

146. Petrovic O, Elsner GB, Wilensky RL, Swanson ST, Feigenbaum H: Transthoracic echocardiographic detection of coronary atherosclerosis. Am J Cardiol 1996 (March 15);77:569–574.

147. Budoff MJ, Georgiou D, Brody A, Agatston AS, Kennedy J, Wolfkiel C, Stanford W, Shields P, Lewis RJ, Janowitz WR, Rich S, Brundage BH. Ultrafast computed tomography as a diagnostic modality in the detection of coronary artery disease. A multicenter study. Circulation 1996 (March 1);93:898–904.

148. Schmidt HHJ, Hill S, Makariou EV, Feuerstein IM, Dugi KA, Hoeg JM: Relation of cholesterol-year score to severity of calcific atherosclerosis and tissue deposition in homozygous familial hypercholesterolemia. Am J Cardiol 1996 (March 15);77:575–580.

149. Detrano R, Hsiai T, Wang S, Puentes G, Fallavollita J, Shields P, Stanford W, Wolfkiel C, Georgiou D, Budoff M, Reed J: Prognostic value of coronary calcification and angiographic stenoses in patients undergoing coronary angiography. J Am Coll Cardiol 1996 (February);27:285–290.

150. Arad Y, Spadaro LA, Goodman K, Lledo-Perez A, Sherman S, Lerner G, Guerci AD: Predictive value of electron beam computed tomography of the coronary arteries: 19-month follow-up of 1173 asymptomatic subjects. Circulation 1996 (June 1);93:1951–1953.

151. Wong ND, Detrano RC, Diamond G, Rezayat C, Mahmoudi R, Chong EC, Tang W, Puentes G, Kang X, Abrahamson D: Does coronary artery screening by electron beam computed tomography motivate potentially beneficial lifestyle behaviors? Am J Cardiol (December 1) 1996;78:1220–1223.

152. Lehto S, Niskanen L, Suhonen M, Rönnemaa T, Laakso M: Medial artery calcification: a neglected harbinger of cardiovascular complications in noninsulin-dependent diabetes mellitus. Arterioscler Thromb Vasc Biol 1996 (August);16:978–983.

153. Karalis DG, Quinn V, Victor MF, Ross JJ, Polansky M, Spratt KA, Chandrasekaran K: Risk of catheter-related emboli in patients with atherosclerotic debris in the thoracic aorta. Am Heart J 1996 (June);131:1149–1155.

2

Coronary Artery Disease

Coronary Artery Disease

Cost-Effectiveness of Coronary Care Unit Versus Intermediate Care Unit (for Patients with Chest Pain)

Tosteson and colleagues[1] in Boston, Massachusetts; Hanover, New Hampshire; and San Francisco, California, used clinical and resource utilization data from 12,139 emergency department patients with acute chest pain in a decision-analytic model to identify cost-effective guidelines for admission to the coronary care unit as compared with an intermediate care unit for initially uncomplicated patients without other indications for intensive care. Probability of clinical complications and death were derived from data on age-specific subsets of the population. Resource utilization estimates were based on cost data from a subset of 901 patients and length of stay data for the entire cohort. Survival benefit associated with initial triage to the coronary care unit instead of an intermediate care unit was assumed to be 15%. In the baseline analysis for 55- to 64-year-old patients, the probability of acute myocardial infarction of (AMI) at which the coronary care unit had an incremental cost-effectiveness below $50,000 per year of life saved was 29%. Triage to the coronary care unit was more cost effective in the elderly patients because their higher early complication rate more than offset their shorter life expectancy. Thus, the analysis indicates that the coronary care unit should be reserved for patients with a moderate (21% or more depending on the patient's age) probability of AMI unless the patients need intensive care for other reasons. The clinical data suggest that only patients with electrocardiographic changes of ischemia or AMI not known to be old have a probability of AMI this high. Intermediate care units are appropriate for patients whose risks are not high enough for a coronary care unit to be cost effective, but too high for other alternatives to be recommended for safety and effectiveness.

Electrocardiogram Abnormalities in American Indians

As part of the Strong Heart Study Assessment of prevalent cardiovascular disease in middle-aged to elderly American Indians, Oopik and associates[2] from 4 United States medical centers assessed the prevalence of major Minnesota code electrocardiographic abnormalities in 4531 participants aged 45 to 74 years (59% women) in selected tribal communities in Arizona, South and North Dakota, and Oklahoma. The overall prevalence of major electrocardiographic abnormalities was lowest in Arizona participants, (eg, definite electrocardiographic AMI in 0.3% vs. 1.8% in the other centers), although nearly two thirds of them had diabetes. One or more major electrocardiographic abnormalities occurred in progressively more women (10.4% to 21.2%) and men (13.3% to 32%) from 45 to 54, 55 to 64, and 65 to 74-year age groups, with the latter prevalence rates exceeding those in predominately white age peers in the Cardiovascular Health Study. Diabetes in women, but not in men, and hypertension in both genders showed positive associations with prevalence rates of major electrocardiographic abnormalities compatible with coronary artery disease (CAD) or hypertensive cardiac hypertrophy. Hypercholesterolemia was not associated with electrocardiographic abnormalities except for definite AMI in women. In conclusion, major electrocardiographic abnormalities are common in middle-aged to elderly American Indians, consistent with recent documentation of higher cardiovascular mortality in this population than in similar-aged United States whites.

ST-T Wave Changes as a Marker of CAD

The prognostic and clinical importance of ST-T wave changes in men with no other manifestations of CAD is still unclear. Sigurdsson and colleagues[3] from Reykjavik and Hafnarffordur, Iceland, and Göteborg, Sweden, evaluated 9139 men born in the years 1907 to 1934 and followed up for 4 to 24 years. The prevalence of silent ST-T changes among men without overt CAD was strongly influenced by age, increasing from 2% at age 40 years to 30% at age 80 years. Men with ST-T changes were older, had higher serum triglyceride levels, worse glucose tolerance, higher blood pressure, and enlarged heart or left ventricular hypertrophy and more often took antihypertensive medication, digitalis or diuretics. These authors concluded that silent ST-T changes that appear ischemic are probably both a marker of silent CAD and hypertension, and are independent predictors of reduced survival.

Papillary Muscle Rupture

Moursi and colleagues,[4] attempted to find additional or more definite diagnostic echocardiographic features of papillary muscle rupture, especially for patients in whom the ruptured head may not prolapse into the left atrium. They analyzed intraoperative transesophageal echocardiograms in 21 consecutive patients with papillary muscle rupture: 20 involved the left ventricle (LV); and 1 involved the right ventricle (RV), which was confirmed at surgery. In 7 (35%) of 20 patients with LV papillary muscle rupture, the ruptured head did not appear to prolapse into the LA. In these patients, examination of the LV proved useful in that abnormal, large amplitude erratic motion of 1 to 5 cm in 17 patients and 0.5 cm in 1 patient of a large echo density in the LV consistent with the ruptured head was noted in 18 (90%) of these patients (Figure 2-1). This included all 7 patients with nonprolapse of the ruptured papillary muscle

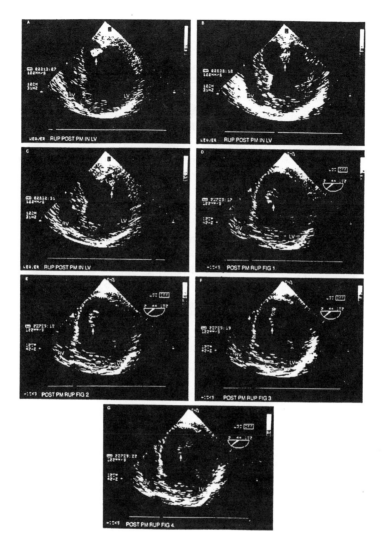

Figure 2-1. Transesophageal echocardiographic (TEE) examination in left ventricular papillary muscle (PM) rupture. A, B, and C and D, E, F, and G represent transgastric views in 2 different patients, who demonstrated erratic motion of the ruptured PM head (arrows) in the left ventricle (LV). In both patients, the ruptured head, which involved the posterior PM, did not prolapse into the left atrium. L, liver; RV, right ventricle. Reproduced with permission from Moursi et al.[4]

head into the left atrium (LA). Less prominent erratic motion or flutter of the papillary muscles still attached to the left ventricular wall was noted, but was less sensitive in the diagnosis of papillary muscle rupture. The one patient with right ventricular papillary muscle rupture showed erratic motion as well as prolapse of the ruptured head into the right atrium (RA). Transesophageal echocardiographic evaluation of the LV is useful in the diagnosis of papillary muscle rupture, especially in those patients in whom the ruptured head does not prolapse into the LA.

Nitrate Tolerance

Pizzulli and associates[5] from Bonn, Germany, investigated whether captopril is able to potentiate vasodilation and prevent tolerance to a 48-hour infusion of nitroglycerin. Twenty-six patients were randomly assigned to a 7-day regimen of captopril (50 mg/day) or placebo. The hemodynamic response to a 0.8 mg sublingual nitroglycerin dose was assessed by measuring mean arterial pressure, mean pulmonary artery (PA) pressure, PA wedge pressure, RA pressure, and cardiac output, and calculating systemic and pulmonary vascular resistances. The parameters were obtained serially at baseline and 1 to 10 minutes after the sublingual nitroglycerin application (day 1). Then intravenous nitroglycerin was started and maintained for 48 hours (1.5 μg/kg/min), and the hemodynamic study was repeated (day 3). There was no difference between the captopril and the placebo groups at day 1 (baseline values and response to sublingual nitroglycerin). After the 48-hour infusion, there was a complete loss of the nitroglycerin effects in the placebo group (day 1 vs. day 3), whereas there was still evidence of a persistent vasodilatation in the captopril group (day 1 vs. day 3). The response to sublingual nitroglycerin on day 3 was markedly attenuated in the placebo group only. It was concluded that captopril does not increase the vasodilatory response to nitroglycerin, but is able to prevent developing nitrate tolerance in arterial and venous circulation.

Cardioesophageal Reflex

Several previous studies have shown that esophageal acid stimulation can reduce coronary blood flow in patients with syndrome X. Chauhan and colleagues[6] from Cambridge, England, evaluated this potential cardioesophageal reflex in 14 patients with angiographically documented significant CAD and in 18 heart transplant recipients. Hydrochloric acid (0.1 mol/L) and 0.9% saline solution were infused in random, double-blind manner (60 mL over 5 minutes) into the distal esophagus. Coronary blood flow measurements were obtained by an intracoronary Doppler catheter positioned in the proximal LAD. Coronary blood flow was significantly reduced by esophageal acid stimulation in the group with CAD (70.4 mL/min to 46 mL/min). There was no difference in the blood flow during saline infusion. Coronary blood flow in the heart transplant group was not affected by either solution. These authors concluded that esophageal acid stimulation can cause anginal attacks and significantly reduce coronary blood flow in patients with CAD. The lack of any significant effect in heart transplant recipients with heart denervation suggests a neural reflex.

Risk Stratification for CAD

Prognostic Value of SPECT

Hachamovitch and colleagues[7] in Los Angeles, California, evaluated the incremental prognostic value, the role of risk stratification, and the impact on patient management of myocardial perfusion single-photon emission computed tomography (SPECT) in a population of patients without prior MI, catheterization, or revascularization. They examined 2200 consecutive patients who at the time of their dual-isotope SPECT had not undergone catheterization, coronary artery bypass grafting (CABG) or percutaneous transluminal coronary angioplasty (PTCA), and had no known history of previous AMI. Follow-up was performed at a mean of 566 days for hard events, including cardiac death and AMI for referral to cardiac catheterization or CABG within 60 days after nuclear testing. Clinical, exercise, and nuclear models using pre-exercise tolerance test, postexercise tolerance test, and nuclear information were observed with a stepwise Cox proportional hazards model and receiver-operating characteristic curve analysis. These observations revealed that nuclear testing added incremental prognostic value after inclusion of the most predictive clinical and exercise variables (Figure 2-2). Multiple logistic regression analysis revealed that scan information contributed 95% of the information regarding referral to catheterization, with further additional information provided by presenting symptoms and exercise-induced ischemia. Referral rates to early catheterization and revascularization paralleled the hard event rates in all scan categories with very low referral rates in patients with normal scans and significant increases in referral rates as a function of worsening scan results. Thus, in a patient population with no evidence of previous CAD at overall risk, myocardial perfusion SPECT adds incremental prognostic information and risk-stratifies patients even after clinical and exercise information is known.

^{201}Tl Tomography versus Dobutamine Echocardiography

In a study by Perrone-Filardi and associates[8], 40 patients with CAD underwent rest-4-hour-24-hour thallium-201 tomography and dobutamine echocardiography (5 to 10 μg/kg/min infusion rates). Late redistribution occurred in 46 (21%) of 219 persistent defects at 4 hours as studied by thallium scintigraphy. Contractile reserve was more frequently present in segments with normal thallium-201 uptake (59%), completely reversible defects (53%), or mild-to-moderate defects at 4 hours (56%) compared with severe defects (14%). Among 105 hypokinetic segments, 99 (94%) were viable by thallium-201, and 88 (84%) showed contractile reserve. However, in 155 akinetic segments, 119 (77%) were viable by thallium-201, but only 34 (22%) had contractile reserve (Figure 2-3). Concordance between thallium-201 and dobutamine was 82% in hypokinetic segments, but 43% in akinetic segments. In 109 revascularized segments, positive accuracy for functional recovery was 72% for thallium and 92% for dobutamine, whereas negative accuracy was 100% and 65%, respectively. Sensitivity was 100% for thallium-201 and 79% for dobutamine. Thus, late redistribution occurs in one-fifth of persistent defects at 4 hours, and it does not correlate to systolic function or contractile reserve. Dobutamine and thallium-201 provide concordant information in the majority of hypokinetic segments, whereas concordance is low in akinetic segments. Dobutamine demonstrates higher positive accuracy and sensitivity in predicting recovery of dysfunctional segments, whereas thallium-201 shows higher negative predictive accuracy, but reduced positive accuracy.

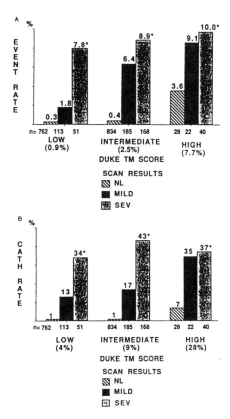

FIGURE 2-2. **A,** Duke treadmill (TM) score category and scan result vs. hard event rates. Rates of hard (MI or cardiac death) events over the follow-up period in patients in low, intermediate, and high Duke treadmill score categories with normal (NL), mildly abnormal (MILD), and severely abnormal (SEV) scans. Parentheses under Duke treadmill subgroups show hard event rates in these groups. *p<.05 across scan results. **B,** Duke treadmill (TM) score category and scan result vs. rate of referral to catheterization. Rates of referral to early catheterization (within 60 days after nuclear testing) in patients in low, intermediate, and high Duke treadmill score categories with normal (NL), mildly abnormal (MILD), and severely abnormal (SEV) scans. Parentheses under Duke treadmill subgroups show hard event rates in these groups. *p<.05 across scan results. Reproduced with permission from Hachamovitch et al.[7]

Impaired Fatty Acid Uptake in Ischemic Myocardium by ^{201}Tl Reinjection

Iodine 123-labeled 15-iodophenyl-3-methyl-pentadecanoic acid has been proposed as a potential myocardial fatty acid probe. Matsunari and associates[9] from Fukui and Kanazawa, Japan, studied iodine 123-labeled 15-iodophenyl-3-methyl-pentadecanoic acid uptake in ischemic myocardium identified by thallium reinjection. Fifty-five patients with CAD who had persistent defects on standard exercise-redistribution thallium imaging were investigated. Patients underwent exercise-redistribution-reinjection thallium and resting iodine 123-labeled 15-iodophenyl-3-methyl-pentadecanoic acid imaging. Iodine 123-labeled 15-iodophenyl-3-methyl-pentadecanoic acid uptake less than that seen

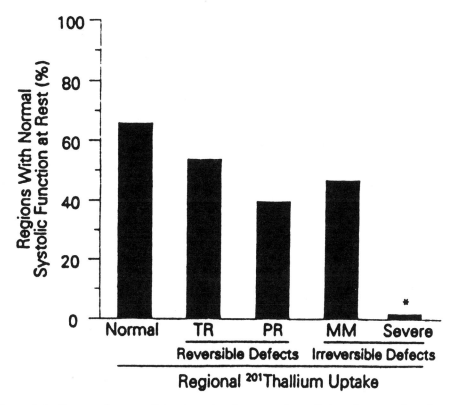

FIGURE 2-3. Percent of myocardial regions showing normal systolic function at rest by echocardiography in relation to regional rest-4-hour redistribution ^{201}Tl uptake. MM indicates mild to moderate persistent ^{201}Tl defects at 4 hours; PR, partially reversible ^{201}Tl defects; and TR, completely reversible ^{201}Tl defects. *p<.01 compared with all other groups. Reproduced with permission from Perrone-Filardi et al.[8]

with thallium on reinjection imaging was observed in 105 (82%) of 128 myocardial segments with new fill-in after thallium reinjection and in 87 (37%) of 238 segments with reversible thallium defects. In contrast, only 32 (19%) of 166 segments with no fill-in showed discordantly decreased iodine 123-labeled 15-iodophenyl-3-methyl-pentadecanoic acid uptake. Quantitative analysis showed reduction in iodine 123-labeled 15-iodophenyl-3-methyl-pentadecanoic acid activity, compared with differential uptake of thallium, an index of resting myocardial perfusion, especially in the area of fill-in (54% ± 15% vs. 76% ± 12% of peak). These observations are consistent with impaired fatty acid uptake in ischemic myocardium, particularly in the area of fill-in after thallium reinjection.

Cardiovascular Performance in Healthy Older Men

Schulman et al.[10] undertook a study to test cardiovascular performance in healthy, older men with a broad range of fitness levels. In this study 10 sedentary men, age 60 years, who were carefully screened to exclude cardiac disease underwent exercise training for 24 to 32 weeks, and 8 age-matched endurance-trained men stopped their exercise training for 12 weeks. All underwent treadmill exercise, rest, and maximal cycle exercise upright gated blood pool scintigraphy at baseline and after the lifestyle intervention. Before the intervention, the treadmill maximum rate of oxygen consumption was 49 and 32 mL·kg^{-1}·min^{-1} in the endurance-trained men and the sedentary men. Although heart rate did not differ between groups during upright cycle exercise at exhaustion, cardiac index, stroke volume index, LVEF, and LV contractility index (systolic blood pressure/end-systolic volume index) were significantly higher, and end-systolic volume index, diastolic blood pressure, and total systemic vascular resistance were lower in the exercise trained individuals. After the partial deconditioning of the exercise-trained men, Vo$_2$max fell to 42 mL·kg^{-1}·min^{-1} and training of sedentary increased Vo$_2$max. Training of seden-

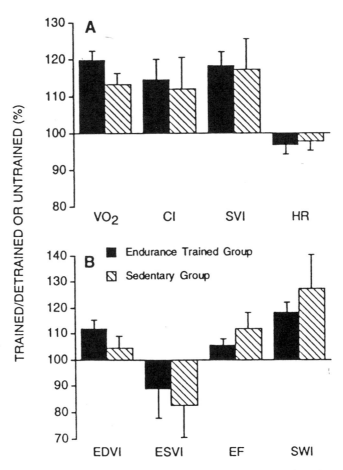

Figure 2-4. Training effect on cardiovascular measures at the maximal work rate assessed as the absolute difference between the relatively more and less conditioned states. Reproduced with permission from Schulman et al.[10]

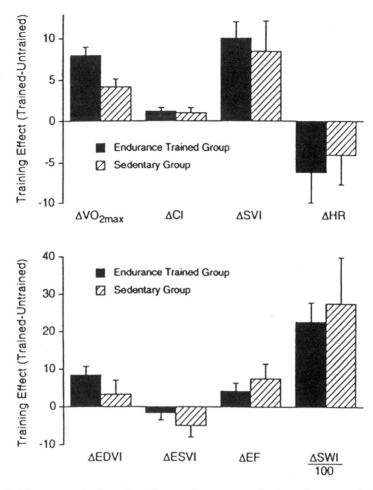

FIGURE 2-5. VO_2max and selected cardiovascular measures in the sedentary and endurance-trained groups. Data for each individual within groups at the greater relative level of conditioning (trained) are expressed relative to the lesser level of conditioning (detrained or untrained) in each group, and the data are averaged. None of the average ratios depicted in the figure differed between groups. Reproduced with permission from Schulman et al.[10]

tary men had effects on cardiovascular function that were similar in magnitude but directionally opposite those of detraining endurance-trained men. All initial differences in cardiovascular performance at peak work rate between sedentary and endurance-trained groups were abolished with the intervention. A broad range of fitness levels was encountered before and after change in training status; cardiac index, stroke volume index, end-systolic volume index, LVEF, and left ventricular contractility index were all linearly correlated with maximal oxygen consumption. Thus, exercise training or detraining of older men results in changes in left ventricular performance that are qualitatively and quantitatively similar regardless of the initial level of fitness before the intervention (Figures 2-4 and 2-5).

Exercise Thallium Tomography in Individuals at Risk for CAD

Blumenthal and colleagues[11] in Baltimore, Maryland, undertook exercise thallium scintigraphy in 264 asymptomatic individuals of less than 60 years of age who had a sibling with documented CAD before age 60. Despite an average age of only 46 years at the time of screening, 19 of the 264 siblings developed clinical evidence of CAD, including sudden death in 1, AMI in 10, and CABG in 8 over a mean of 6 years of follow-up (range 1 to 9 years). Abnormal thallium-201 scans were observed in 29% of men and 9% of women, whereas abnormal exercise electrocardiograms occurred in 12% and 5%, respectively. Among men 45 years of age or older, 45% had an abnormal exercise electrocardiogram thallium scan, or both. In contrast, only 3% of women younger than 45 years of age had an abnormal test at rest. The abnormal exercise ECGs and thallium-201 scans were both predictive of future clinical CAD, but the thallium scan was associated with a higher relative risk. After adjustment for age, sex, and exercise electrocardiographic result, the relative risk of developing clinical CAD was 4.7 for an abnormal scan. Siblings with a concordant abnormal exercise electrocardiogram and thallium scan had a relative risk of 14.5. These siblings were all men older than 45 years of age at the time of screening, and they had a high incidence of clinical CAD subsequently (6 of 12, 50%). Thus, exercise thallium scintigraphy appears to be useful in the risk assessment of asymptomatic siblings of patients with premature CAD, especially in male siblings 45 years of age and older (Figure 2-6).

Stress Echocardiography to Predict the Site of Future MI

The severity and extent of stress-induced dyssynergy are strong predictors of subsequent cardiac events. However, it is less clear whether high-grade ste-

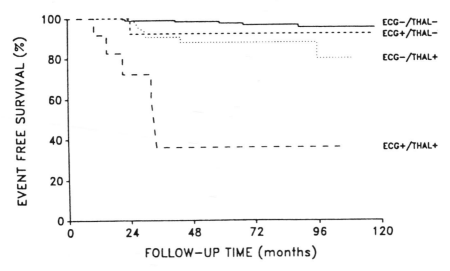

FIGURE 2-6. Kaplan-Meier survival curves for each combination of exercise test results (normal electrocardiogram and thallium scan, only electrocardiogram abnormal, only thallium scan abnormal, or both electrocardiogram and thallium scan abnormal). Curves are drawn until the end of follow-up for each group. Reproduced with permission from Blumenthal et al.[11]

notic lesions are associated with the site of future coronary occlusions. Varga and colleagues[12] from Pisa, Italy, evaluated 70 patients from the data bank of the stress cardiography multicenter trial who had a stress echocardiogram, a spontaneously occurring infarction, and a follow-up rest echocardiogram. A complete ischemia-infarction mismatch (infarct-related dysfunction in a patient with negative stress test) occurred in 29 patients (41%). A partial mismatch (ischemic dysfunction in a territory different from the infarct area) occurred in 9 patients (13%). A match (ischemia-related and infarct-related dyssynergy involving the same region) occurred in 32 patients (46%). The average time interval between the stress examination and the infarction was 144 days. These authors concluded that induced ischemia inconsistently identifies the site of future infarction. The majority of spontaneous coronary occlusions leading to AMI are unheralded by induced ischemia. However, most AMIs occurring within 1 year of stress testing are in the area identified as ischemic during testing.

Risk Factors Associated with CAD

Platelet Glycoprotein Receptor Polymorphism as a Risk Factor for Coronary Thrombosis

Weiss and colleagues[13] in Baltimore, Maryland, investigated the relation between a particular polymorphism, PI^{A2} of the gene-encoding glycoprotein IIIa, and acute coronary syndromes by conducting a case-control study of 71 case patients with AMI or unstable angina in 68 inpatient controls without known heart disease. The groups were matched for age, race, and sex. Two methods for determining the PI^{A} genotype were used, including dot blot hybridization and allele-specific restriction digestion. The prevalence of PI^{A2} was 2 times higher among the case patients than among the controls (39% vs. 19%, p = .01). In a subgroup of patients whose disease began before the age of 60 years, the prevalence of PI^{A2} was 50%, a value that was 3.6 times that among control subjects under 60 years of age. In subjects with PI^{A2} polymorphism, the odds ratio for having a coronary event was 2.8 (95% confidence interval, 1.2 to 6.4). In patients less than 60 years of age at the onset of disease, the odds ratio was 6.2 (95% confidence interval, 1.8 to 22.4). These data suggest a strong association between the PI^{A2} polymorphism of the glycoprotein IIIa gene and acute coronary thrombosis; this association appears to be strongest in patients who had coronary events before the age of 60 years.

Angiotensin-Converting Enzyme Genotype—Increased Risk for Coronary Events

Angiotensin-converting enzyme is a key component of the renin-angiotensin system that plays an important role in cardiovascular regulation. An association between the angiotensin-converting enzyme insertion-deletion, polymorphism, and increased coronary risk has been found in some studies, but not in others. To explore this further in an Australian white population, Wang and colleagues[14] in Sydney, Australia, compared the angiotensin-converting enzyme genotype distribution in 550 patients aged 37 to 65 years with CAD documented by angiography with a genotype distribution in 404 healthy school children aged 6 to 13 years. The investigators also explored the associations in the patients between the angiotensin-converting enzyme I/D polymorphism and a history of AMI and CAD severity assessed by the number of major coronary arteries with more than 50% luminal obstructions and by the Green Lane coronary score. The frequencies of angiotensin-converting enzyme genotype in the CAD patients were 0.24 for I/I, 0.40 for I/D, and 0.37 for D/D genotypes. This distribution with an excess of the D/D genotype was significantly different from that in school children, in whom the genotype distribution was in the Hardy-Weinberg equilibrium. There was also a significant excess of D/D genotype among patients with a history of AMI, and there was the same D/D excess in the subgroup of children with two or more grandparents who had CAD. The investigators found no association between the angiotensin-converting enzyme polymorphism and the number of significantly stenosed coronary arteries. The investigators concluded that D/D genotype is a significant predictor for CAD events in the Australian white population, but is not a marker for angiographically assessed CAD severity. The angiotensin-converting enzyme genotype-associated increased risk for coronary events may be mediated more by angiotensin II-induced coronary vasoconstriction than by an increase in injury-related smooth muscle cell proliferation in the coronary vasculature.

Detection and Prognostic Implications for CAD in Exercise Testing

Exercise Testing

Pharmacological stress echocardiography has changed over the years from low- to high-dose regimens and now uses atropine. Pingitore and colleagues[15] from Pisa, Italy, evaluated variations of stress echocardiographic tests in 360 patients with a chest pain syndrome in 13 different echocardiographic laboratories. Dobutamine (up to 40 μg/kg body weight/min) plus atropine (up to 1 mg over 4 hours) and dipyridamole (up to .84 mg/kg/min over 10 hours) plus atropine (up to 1 mg over 4 hours) stress echocardiography was performed on different days in random order and within 1 week. No major complications occurred during either test. Diagnostic accuracy was assessed in a subset of 110 patients with no obvious asynergy who underwent coronary angiography independently of test results and within 1 week of testing. Sensitivity for detection of CAD was 84% for dobutamine-atropine and 82% for dipyridamole-atropine stress echocardiography with a specificity of 89% for dobutamine-atropine and 94% for dipyridamole-atropine stress echocardiography. These authors concluded that these 2 tests are safe and feasible, although submaximal studies are more frequent with dobutamine. The 2 stresses have comparable accuracy in the detection of angiographic CAD, although dobutamine was marginally more sensitive and dipyridamole marginally more specific.

Inotropic stress during graded dobutamine infusion has evolved as an alternative form of pharmacological stress in conjunction with perfusion and functional imaging for evaluation of patients with CAD. The prognostic value of technetium-99m (Tc-[99]m) sestamibi SPECT imaging in patients undergoing dobutamine stress testing for the detection of CAD is unclear. Accordingly, Senior and associates[16] from Harrow, Middlesex, United Kingdom, performed SPECT imaging at rest and during stress in 61 patients undergoing coronary arteriography for evaluation of chest pain on the basis of symptoms and treadmill exercise electrocardiography. The patients were followed for ± 11 months (2 to 33) during which 2 died, 2 had AMI, 13 developed unstable angina, and 3 had CHF. Univariate Cox regression analysis revealed that those with reversible defects (95%) and defects in multiple vascular territories (80%) on SPECT had a greater number of cardiac events (59%) compared with those without (34%). When multivariate analysis was performed using clinical, exercise testing, and SPECT variables, the independent predictors of cardiac events were a history of myocardial infarction, number of reversible segments, and presence of defects in multiple vascular territories. In summary, dobutamine stress Tc-[99m] sestamibi SPECT is a powerful predictor of future cardiac events in patients undergoing coronary arteriography for evaluation of chest pain and may be used to stratify patients for further intervention.

Among 23,059 patients who underwent exercise myocardial tomography in a 10-year period by Zuo-Xiang He and associates[17] from Houston, Texas, there were 817 (3.5%) with a strongly positive exercise electrocardiogram and normal myocardial tomogram. Among these, 52 patients had no conditions known to be associated with a false-positive exercise electrocardiogram and no previous coronary revascularization, and underwent coronary angiography. Of the 32 patients with significant coronary stenoses, 50% had 1-vessel disease and only 22% had 3-vessel disease. Among 55 stenosed arteries, 56% were of moderate severity (50% to 74%), whereas only 9% had subtotal or total occlusion (95% to 100%). There was a significant gender difference in the prevalence of significant coronary stenoses (80% in male vs. 24% in female patients). A strongly positive exercise electrocardiogram coupled with normal exercise myocardial tomograms is a rare clinical finding. In women, this finding is usually associated with normal coronary arteries, whereas in men it often denotes CAD, usually of mild-to-moderate degree.

The presence of myocardial perfusion abnormalities is generally accepted to suggest underlying CAD. In previous animal studies, myocardial contrast echocardiography has been shown to be useful in delineating areas at risk after coronary occlusions. Meza and associates[18] from New Orleans, Louisiana, compared the presence or absence, size, and location of perfusion defects detected in human beings by myocardial contrast echocardiography and sestamibi SPECT. Regional wall motion was qualitatively assessed in the parasternal and apical views of a resting 2-dimensional echocardiogram. Coronary angiography was performed in all patients, and myocardial contrast echocardiography was performed with 2 mL of intracoronary sonicated meglumine (Nycomed). A cine loop of the digitized contrast echocardiograms was used to analyze perfusion defects. Gated SPECT resting images in standard views were obtained after technetium ^{99m} sestamibi (20 mCi) was administered. Visually perceived perfusion defects were established at 30% of maximal counts at end diastole. Perfusion defects by both techniques were planimetered, assigned to 1 of 3 perfusion artery territories, and expressed as a percentage of the perfusion territory studied. Comparison was made by linear regression analysis. Forty-one patients were studied. Perfusion defects were observed in 12 (29%) patients by myocardial contrast echocardiography, 19 (46%) patients by SPECT, and 11 (27%) patients by both techniques. No perfusion defects were detected by myocardial contrast echocardiography in 29 (70%) patients, by SPECT in 22 (53%) patients, or by either technique in 21 (51%) patients. The 2 techniques agreed in 78% of the patients. In 67 matching orthogonal views suitable for comparison between the 2 techniques, an 82% concordance for the presence or absence of defects was observed. The location of the defects matched in 86% of the cases. A significant correlation between these techniques was observed in assessing the size of perfusion defects. In conclusion, these results suggest that myocardial contrast echocardiography and sestamibi SPECT are comparable techniques for detecting severely underperfused myocardium in human beings.

Estimating left ventricular wall stress has recognized applications, but formulas for global stress cannot be applied to ischemic ventricles. A mathematic method for estimating regional stress in infarcted ventricles has been described. The hypothesis tested by Ginzton and associates[19] from Torrance, California, was that exercise-induced ischemia increases end-systolic wall stress. Subcostal 4-chamber echocardiograms were recorded at rest and during peak symptom-limited exercise in 19 controls and 41 patients with chest pain undergoing coronary arteriography. Centerline regional wall motion and regional end-systolic wall stress were measured at rest and at peak exercise. The normal controls had increased wall motion with exercise, but wall stress remained low. All 32 of the patients with CAD (≥50 diameter narrowing) had wall motion abnormalities with exercise, but the sensitivity of identifying right coronary artery obstructions was poor. Patients with CAD had higher regional stress at peak exercise than did the controls. The sensitivity of identifying lesions in all 3 coronary arteries (0.95 to 1.0) was better than that for wall motion. The specificity of wall stress needs to be tested in a larger population. Exercise-induced ischemia causes increased regional end-systolic wall stress that reflects its distribution in patients with CAD. These changes can be measured noninvasively during exercise echocardiography.

Lauer and colleagues[20] in Cleveland, Ohio, conducted a prospective investigation to evaluate the prognostic implications of exercise heart rate responses in a population-based sample from the Framingham Offspring Study involving 1575 male participants with a mean age of 43 years. The participants were free of CAD and were not taking β-blockers. All underwent submaximal exercise testing. Heart rate response was assessed in three ways: 1) failure to achieve 85% of the age-predicted maximum heart rate; 2) the actual increase in heart rate from rest to peak exercise; and 3) the ratio of heart rate to metabolic reserve used by stage 2 of exercise. Proportional hazards analyses were used to evaluate the associations of heart rate responses with all-cause mortality and with CAD incidence during 8 years of follow-up. Failure to achieve target heart rate occurred in 327 (21%) of the subjects. During follow-up, there were

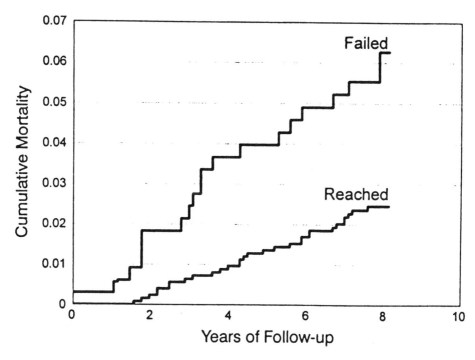

FIGURE 2-7. Kaplan-Meier plot of cumulative mortality according to ability to achieve target heart rate. Inability to achieve target heart rate includes effects of factors other than inherent chronotropic response. Reproduced with permission from Lauer et al.[20]

55 deaths, with 14 caused by CAD, and 95 cases of CAD. Failure to achieve target heart rate, a smaller increase in heart rate with exercise, and the chronotropic response index were predictive of total mortality and CAD incidence (Figure 2-7). Failure to achieve target heart rate remained predictive of CAD incidence even after adjusting for age, ST segment response, physical activity, and traditional CAD risk factors. After adjusting for the same factors, the increase in exercise heart rate remained inversely predictive of total mortality and CAD incidence. The chronotropic response index was predictive of total mortality and CAD incidence after adjusting for age and risk factors. Thus, an attenuated heart rate response to exercise, itself a manifestation of chronotropic incompetence, is predictive of increased mortality and CAD incidence.

Barthélémy and colleagues[21] conducted a prospective study in 236 consecutive male patients, to evaluate a global muscle fatigue parameter, the blood lactate level achieved at maximal exercise, as a method of distinguishing between diseased and nondiseased coronary status. None of the patients had had previous AMI or referral for the diagnosis of CAD. None of the patients had cardiomyopathy, severe congestive heart failure (CHF), or valvular heart disease. Blood lactate concentration at maximal exercise was measured, as well as other classic exercise-derived variables. Correlations between variables and CAD status as assessed by coronary arteriography were described using receiver operating characteristic curves and logistic regression analysis. The first 4 most powerful variables were lactate level, maximal power output, exercise duration, and percentage of maximal predicted heart rate, which directly represented global functional capacity. For variables, values were shown of 0.77, 0.77, 0.76, and 0.74, respectively, by the receiver operating characteristic curve analysis. Mean blood lactate level at peak exercise reached 7.68 mmol/L in the 153 patients with disease and 10.6 in the 83 patients without disease, and these differences were highly significant. After adjustment for other variables, blood lactate level remained a significant predictor of CAD by logistic regression analysis. Global muscle fatigue as assessed by lactate levels in the blood at maximal exercise appears to be a powerful distinguisher of pressure and absence of significant CAD.

Krittayaphong and associates[22] from Chapel Hill, North Carolina, examined the relation between anginal symptoms and ischemic indexes during ischemia on exercise testing and daily activities in 76 patients (59 men and 17 women, mean age 61 years). All had documented CAD and exercise-induced myocardial ischemia. All patients underwent upright bicycle exercise testing and 48-hour ambulatory electrocardiographic monitoring. Angina was reported in 28 patients (37%) during exercise-induced ischemia. A total of 287 ischemic episodes was detected from 44 patients (58%) during ambulatory electrocardiographic monitoring. There was a mean number of 7.4 episodes and a mean total duration of 75 min/48 hours. There were no differences in the prevalence and the magnitude of ambulatory ischemia between patients with and without angina during exercise testing. Among the 44 patients who had ischemia during both tests, 50% with angina during exercise testing had symptomatic ischemia during ambulatory electrocardiographic monitoring, compared with 14% with silent ischemia during exercise testing. Ninety-two percent of ischemic episodes were preceded by an increase in heart rate of more than 10 beats/min. There was a strong positive correlation ($r = 0.70$) between HR at onset of 1 mm ST depression (ischemic threshold) during exercise testing and during ambulatory electrocardiographic monitoring. The authors concluded that: 1) patients with exercise-induced angina have significantly more symptoms during ambulatory ischemia; 2) ischemic threshold during exercise testing and daily life are positively correlated; and 3) myocardial oxygen demand increases in the development of ambulatory ischemia.

Ambrosio and colleagues[23] investigated whether stunning may result from effort angina in patients with CAD. Patients with CAD had exercise testing combined with quantitative measurements of contractile function for up to 240 minutes after exercise. Contractile function was determined by either measurement of regional ejection fraction (EF) using radionuclide angiography ($n = 17$, group A) or by computer-assisted measurement of systolic wall thickening ($n = 14$, group B). In the latter group, myocardial perfusion was also evaluated by ^{99m}Tc-sestamibi tomographic imaging. Angina resulted in marked contractile dysfunction. Hemodynamic and electrocardiographic changes caused by ischemia were promptly normalized. Furthermore, no perfusion defects could be detected in group B patients 30 minutes after exercise, yet contractile function remained impaired well after the cessation of exercise. Thirty minutes into recovery, regional EF of previously ischemic areas was still 83% ± 4.6% of baseline in group A. In group B patients, systolic thickening of previously ischemic segments was significantly impaired 60 minutes after exercise, averaging 34% ± 2.8% versus 41% ± 2.7% at baseline. Contractile impairment was reversible as the functioning of previously ischemic segments normalized between 60 and 120 minutes after recovery (Figure 2-8). Thus, prolonged but reversible impairment of regional function occurs in patients after exercise-induced angina in the absence of perfusion abnormalities, suggesting that myocardial stunning may occur after effort angina in patients with CAD.

Repeated short episodes of coronary occlusion in experimental animals and in humans during balloon angioplasty cause myocardial preconditioning. Maybaum and associates[24] from Jerusalem, Israel, examined whether myocardial ischemia induced by repeated exercise testing can reduce the extent of the ischemia induced by subsequent exercise test. Twenty-six patients with positive stress tests underwent 3 treadmill exercise tests at 30-minute intervals. Two additional tests were performed on each of the previous 2 days in order to eliminate and/or reduce the training effect. All 3 exercise tests were of similar work load. In spite of that, total ischemic time was markedly shortened from 633 to 399 seconds, as well as the recovery time from 259 to 126 seconds, between the first and the second tests. There was no further improvement on the third test. Time to 1-mm ST depression was prolonged from 487 to 593 seconds, and double product at 1-mm ST depression was increased in the second test from 20,322 to 22,325 mm Hg/second, implying a higher ischemic threshold. An improvement in at least 1 ischemic parameter was observed in 96% of patients, and improvement in 2 or more ischemic parameters was observed in 76% of the patients. Improvement in ischemic parameters develops during repeated exercise-induced ischemia in most patients. The authors suggested that this phenomenon, which was previously known as "warm up," is the clinical counterpart of myocardial preconditioning, which develops not only during ischemia caused by reduction in coronary flow, but also during demanding induced ischemia.

Although the accuracy of dobutamine stress echocardiography for detecting CAD has been established, its role in determining prognosis is less defined. Marcovitz and associates[25] from Ann Arbor, Michigan, evaluated the prognostic significance of dobutamine stress echocardiography in patients with known or suspected CAD. Follow-up was obtained on 291 patients an average of 15 months after clinically indicated dobutamine stress echocardiography. Studies were stratified with respect to resting and inducible wall motion abnormalities into 1 of 4 responses: normal, ischemic, fixed, and mixed. Hard end points of nonfatal myocardial infarction and cardiac death were tabulated for outcome. Statistically significant differences in the incidence of hard cardiac end points were noted for 2 of 4 echocardiographic responses. A normal dobutamine stress echocardiogram was associated with a statistically lower likelihood of a hard cardiac event than was an echocardiogram with resting or inducible abnormalities. Dobutamine stress echocardiography with a mixed response (resting abnormality with additional inducible ischemia) was associated with a higher likelihood of cardiac events by multivariate analysis. By multiple logistic regression analysis of dobutamine response, age, and cardiac risk factors, only a mixed response on dobutamine stress echocardiography was independently associated with the occurrence of a hard cardiac event in the follow-up period. In addition, LV dysfunction on the resting echocardiogram was associated with a worse prognosis in patients with major noncardiac disease. We conclude that dobutamine response is an independent predictor of cardiac events compared

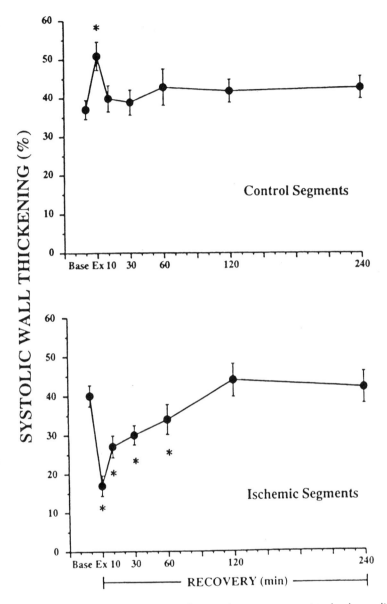

FIGURE 2-8. Time course of systolic wall thickening (by computer-assisted echocardiography) in 14 patients with stable angina measured at baseline (Base), immediately after symptom-limited exercise stress test (Ex), and at various time points into recovery after exercise. For this analysis, segments showing ≥15% decrease in thickening with exercise in each patient were identified and considered ischemic segments. Systolic wall thickening data for the ischemic segments from all patients were then averaged together (bottom). Data for the control segments represent the average of the remaining segments of each patient pooled together (top). *p<.05 vs. baseline. Reproduced with permission from Ambrosio et al.[23]

with traditional risk factor analysis and that dobutamine-stress echocardiography can identify high- and low-risk subsets of patients with known or suspected CAD.

Increasing numbers of women are undergoing noninvasive stress testing for CAD evaluation. Limited information is available regarding the presence, magnitude, and importance of gender-related differences in exercise ventriculography among the heterogeneous population of patients referred for noninvasive stress testing. This study was carried out by Merz and associates[26] from Los Angeles, California; Jerusalem, Israel; and New York, New York. Patients referred for exercise radionuclide ventriculography between 1979 and 1986 were evaluated, including 175 patients with a low likelihood of CAD, 59 patients with angiographically normal coronary arteries, and 419 patients with CAD. Overall, women demonstrated higher resting left ventricular ejection fraction (LVEF) and lower change in LVEF response to exercise compared with men. Although LV response to exercise correlated with the underlying severity of CAD in both women and men, fewer women demonstrated a 5% or greater change in LVEF despite a lower prevalence of multivessel CAD. It was concluded that gender-related differences in LV response to exercise are present in a wide range of patients referred for testing.

Myocardial Viability

Comparison of Techniques to Predict Functional Recovery after Revascularization

One of the difficult problems in managing patients with CAD is determining the presence and extent of ischemic but viable myocardium because this information may greatly influence decisions regarding revascularization. Bax and colleagues[27] from Amsterdam and Rotterdam, The Netherlands, compared 3 different techniques to predict functional recovery after revascularization. The techniques included fluorine-18 (F-18), fluorodeoxyglucose in combination with SPECT, thallium-201 reinjection, and low-dose dobutamine echocardiography. Seventeen patients who had a mean LVEF of 36% were studied by the 3 techniques. Regional and global ventricular function were evaluated before and 3 months after revascularization. The sensitivities for F-18 fluorodeoxyglucose/thallium-201, thallium-201 reinjection, and low-dose dobutamine echocardiography to assess recovery of function were 89%, 93%, and 85%, respectively. Specificities were 77%, 43%, and 63%, respectively. Stepwise logistic regression indicated that F-18 fluorodeoxyglucose/thallium-201 was the best predictor. In hypokinetic segments, the combination of F-18 fluorodeoxyglucose/thallium-201 and low-dose dobutamine echocardiography was the best predictor. Global function improved (LVEF increased more than 5%) in 6 patients and remained unchanged in 11. All 3 techniques correctly identified 5 of 6 patients with improvement. F-18 fluorodeoxyglucose/thallium-201 identified all patients without improvement; low-dose dobutamine echocardiography identified 9 of 11 without improvement; and thallium-201 reinjection identified 6 of 11 patients without improvement. These authors concluded that F-18 fluorodeoxyglucose/thallium-201 SPECT was superior to the other techniques in assessing functional recovery. In hypokinetic segments, integration of metabolic and functional data is necessary for optimal prediction of improvement of regional function.

Positron Emission Tomography for Assessment of Myocardial Kinetics

vom Dahl and colleagues[28] in Ann Arbor, Michigan, compared myocardial rubidium-82 chloride kinetics assessed by dynamic positron emission tomography as a marker for tissue viability with regional fluorine-18 (F-18) fluorodeoxyglucose uptake in patients with CAD. Twenty-seven patients with angiographically proven CAD and 5 with a low likelihood for CAD underwent dynamic positron emission tomography under resting conditions using rubidium-82 and fluorodeoxyglucose. Both image sequences served as input data for a semiautomated regional analysis program. This program generated polar maps representing rubidium-82 tissue half-life and fluorodeoxyglucose utilization. Myocardial tissue viability was visually determined from static rubidium-82 and fluorodeoxyglucose images. Regions were categorized as normal, ischemically compromised, and scar tissue. In normal subjects, rubidium-82 tissue half-life was homogeneous throughout the left ventricle. In patients with CAD, differences between rubidium-82 tissue half-life in normal and scar tissue were highly significant. Fluorodeoxyglucose uptake in these 2 tissue groups was 78% and 40%, respectively. Ischemically compromised tissue with reduced perfusion but maintained fluorodeoxyglucose uptake displayed a rubidium-82 half-life of 75 seconds, indicating active cellular tracer retention, which was different from that found with scar tissue (Figure 2-9). Overall agreement of tissue categorization as either viable or scar was 86% between rubidium-82 kinetics and fluorodeoxyglucose utilization. In a subgroup of 11 patients with all 3 tissue types within 1 image, rubidium-82 tissue half-life discriminated between normal, ischemic, and scar tissue. This study demonstrates a significant relationship between cell membrane integrity as assessed by dynamic rubidium-82 positron emission tomography imaging and myocardial glucose utilization as markers for tissue viability. In myocardial regions with reduced perfusion, rubidium-82 kinetics were different in compromised but metabolically active and irreversibly injured myocardium.

Glucose Uptake in Dysfunctional but Viable Myocardium

Mäki and colleagues[29] in Turku, Finland, evaluated the regulation of glucose uptake in dysfunctional but viable myocardium in 7 patients with an occluded major coronary artery but no previous AMI. These individuals were studied twice with 2-[^{18}F]fluoro-2-deoxy-D-glucose positron emission tomography, including once in the fasting state and once during hyperinsulinemic euglycemic clamping. Myocardial blood flow was measured with [^{15}O]H$_2$O,

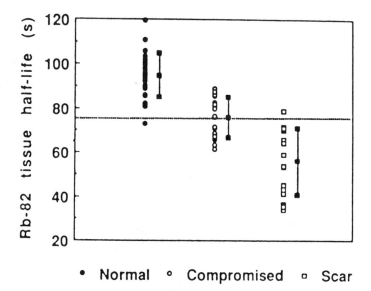

• **Normal**   ◦ **Compromised**   ▫ **Scar**

FIGURE 2-9. Plot shows individual rubidium-82 chloride (Rb-82) tissue half-lives for normal, compromised, and scar tissue displayed together with values for mean ± SD. Dotted line represents the physical half-life of Rb-82 (76 seconds). A measured half-life above this line represents active myocardial retention of Rb-82; half-life below the dotted line indicates accelerated Rb-82 washout from tissue. Reproduced with permission from vom Dahl et al.[28]

and the myocardial region beyond an occluded artery that showed stable wall motion abnormality was considered to represent chronically dysfunctional but viable tissue. Six of the patients were later revascularized, and wall motion recovery was detected in the corresponding regions, which confirmed their viability. Slightly reduced myocardial blood flow was detected in the dysfunctional regions. In the fasting state, glucose uptake was slightly increased in the dysfunctional regions compared with normal myocardium; during insulin clamping, a striking increase in glucose uptake by insulin was obtained in both the dysfunctional and the normal regions (Figure 2-10, 2-11, and 2-12). Thus, these data indicate that glucose uptake may be strikingly increased by insulin in chronically dysfunctional but viable myocardium.

Myocardial Hibernation and Stunning

There are little data on the ultrastructure and cytoskeleton of cardiomyocytes in myocardial hibernation. Schwarz and colleagues[30] from Aachen and Bad Nauheim, Germany, and Seattle, Washington, evaluated 24 patients with regional wall motion abnormalities to address this question. The combination of regional wall motion abnormalities with relatively normal radionuclide scans and fluorine-18 (f-18) fluorodeoxyglucose uptake on positron emission tomography identified hibernating myocardium, which was then evaluated by transmural biopsies taken during CABG from the center of the hypocontractile area of the anterior wall. Results showed varying signs of mild-to-severe degen-

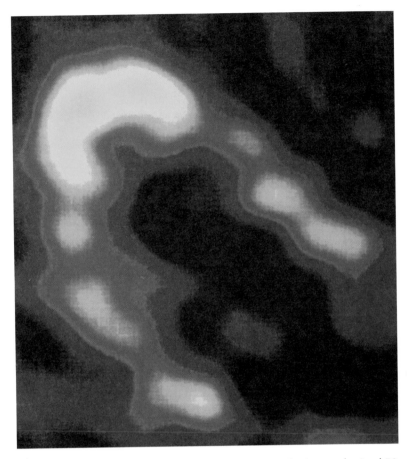

FIGURE 2-10. Transaxial 10-minute positron emission tomography image obtained 50 minutes after [^{18}F]fluoro-2-deoxy-D glucose injection in the fasting state. Increased [^{18}F]fluoro-2-deoxy-D glucose uptake is seen in the dyskinetic anterior wall. Reproduced with permission from Mäki et al.[29]

erative changes and fibrosis. Immunohistochemical analysis demonstrated disruption of the cytoskeletal proteins titin and α-actinin. Wall motion abnormality showed postoperative improvement. These authors concluded that long-term hypoperfusion causes different degrees of morphological alterations leading to degeneration. Preoperative analysis of regional contractility and perfusion metabolism imaging did not distinguish the severity of morphological alterations or the functional outcome after revascularization.

The mechanism by which dobutamine increases the contraction of chronically dysfunctional myocardium and its effects on metabolism is still unknown. The aim of this study by Indolfi and associates[31] from Naples, Italy, was to assess regional myocardial metabolism at rest and during an intracoronary dobutamine infusion in patients with hibernating myocardium. Eleven asymptomatic patients with single proximal stenosis of the left anterior descending (LAD) coronary artery and persistent left ventricular dysfunction at rest (undergoing percutaneous transluminal coronary angioplasty [PTCA]) were studied prospectively. Regional left ventricular function was assessed by

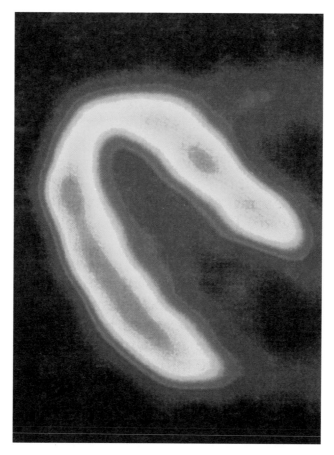

FIGURE 2-11. Transaxial 10-minute positron emission tomography image obtained 50 minutes after [^{18}F]fluoro-2-deoxy-D glucose injection during insulin clamping (same patient and comparable slice as in Fig. 2-10. Reproduced with permission from Mäki et al.[29]

2-dimensional echocardiography, and regional perfusion was assessed by thallium-201 SPECT. Great cardiac vein and aortic blood samples were obtained for measurements of lactate and plasma free fatty acid concentrations. Inotropic challenge, obtained by using intracoronary dobutamine infusion, increases regional left ventricular function. However, the arteriovenous lactate difference was 0.206 ± 0.070 mmol/L at, rest and it decreased to 0.018 ± 0.069 mmol/L at 4 minutes of dobutamine infusion and 0.066 ± 0.068 mmol/L at 10 minutes of dobutamine infusion. Thus the hibernating myocardium does not produce lactate at rest. However, when regional contraction is stimulated, dobutamine-induced inotropic challenge may cause a perfusion-contraction mismatch with an activation of anaerobic glycolysis.

With positron emission tomography, the resting flow abnormalities underlying reversible left ventricular dysfunction in 17 patients with chronic CAD were delineated by Conversano and associates[32] from St. Louis, Missouri. The level of flow in reversibly dysfunctional segments (those demonstrating improvement after revascularization) was markedly variable, ranging from 0.32 to 1.25 mL/gm/min. In 20 of these segments flow was preserved, whereas in

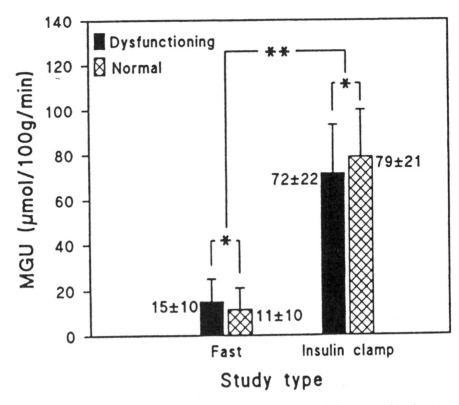

Figure 2-12. Myocardial glucose uptake in the fasting state and during insulin clamping in dysfunctional and normal segments. *p<.05; **p ≤ .001. Reproduced with permission from Mäki et al.[29]

12 segments flow was reduced, when compared with that in age-matched controls. Preservation of flow was associated with preservation of myocardial oxygen consumption and no alterations in myocardial substrate use. In contrast, a reduction in flow resulted in a decrease of myocardial oxygen consumption and an increase in myocardial glucose use. Thus, resting reversible left ventricular dysfunction in patients with chronic CAD can reflect a diversity of resting flow abnormalities. Moreover, myocardial perfusion at rest is frequently within normal limits, suggesting that the reversible mechanical dysfunction in these patients is attributable to intermittent myocardial stunning and not hibernation.

Gerber and colleagues[33] in Brussels and Louvain-la-Neuve, Belgium, designed a study to test whether unselected patients with chronic left ventricular dysfunction and a prior AMI have altered resting myocardial perfusion. Dynamic positron emission tomographic images with [13N]ammonia and [18F]fluorodeoxyglucose were used to assess myocardial perfusion, and glucose uptake was performed in 39 surgical CABG bypass patients who had chronic anterior wall dysfunction after AMI. Left ventricular function was evaluated by echocardiography before (at rest and during low-dose dobutamine infusion) and 5 months after CABG. At follow-up, left ventricular wall motion was improved in 24 patients and unchanged in 15. Before CABG, absolute myocardial blood flow was higher in reversible compared with persistently dysfunctional segments (Figure 2-13). In segments with reversible left ventricular dysfunction, values of myocardial blood flow were similar to those in the remote segments of the same patients or in anterior segments of normal volunteers. During glucose clamp, the [^{18}F]fluorodeoxyglucose uptake was higher, but myocardial glucose uptake was not different in reversibly injured compared with persistently dysfunctional segments (Figure 2-14). A flow-metabolism mismatch was present in 18 of 24 reversibly injured, but absent in 10 of 15 persistently dysfunctional left ventricular segments. With dobutamine, left ventricular wall motion improved in 17 of 24 reversibly dysfunctional segments, but did not change in 13 of 15 segments with persistent left ventricular dysfunction. Thus, this study indicates that chronic but reversible ischemic left ventricular dysfunction is associated with almost normal resting myocardial perfusion, with maintained [^{18}F]fluorodeoxyglucose uptake, and with recruitable inotropic reserve. The data support the hypothesis that chronic hibernation is not the consequence of a permanent reduction of transmural myocardial perfusion at rest.

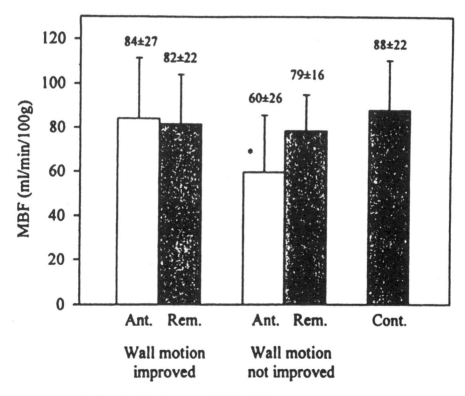

FIGURE 2-13. Absolute levels of myocardial blood flow among remote normal and dysfunctional segments in patients with and without postoperative functional improvement and in normal volunteers. *p<.01 vs. remote (Rem.) of the same patients, vs. anterior (Ant.) of patients with improved function, and vs. control (Cont.) subjects. Reproduced with permission from Gerber et al.[33]

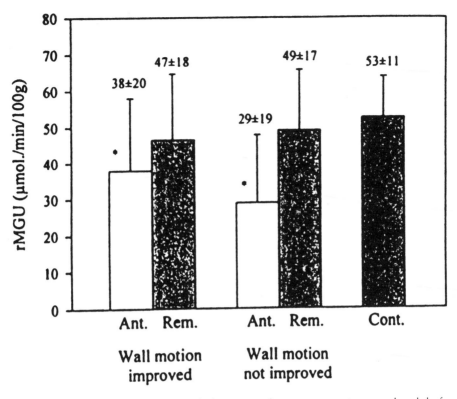

FIGURE 2-14. Absolute levels of regional glucose uptake among remote normal and dysfunctional segments in patients with and without postoperative functional improvement and in normal volunteers. *p<.01 vs. remote of the same patients and vs. control subjects. Abbreviations as in Fig. 2-13. Reproduced with permission from Gerber et al.[33]

Coronary Blood Flow

Gibson and colleagues[34] for the TIMI 4 Study Group developed and evaluated an objective coronary flow grade to supplement the previously developed TIMI flow grade, which is limited by its subjective and categorical nature. In normal patients and patients with AMI in the TIMI 4 study, the number of cineframes needed for dye to reach standardized distal landmarks was counted to assess objectively an index of coronary blood flow as a continuous variable. The TIMI frame-counting method was reproducible with a mean absolute difference between 2 injections of 4.7 frames in 85 studies. In 78 consecutive normal coronary arteries, the LAD TIMI frame count of 36 fames was 1.7 times longer than the mean of the right coronary artery (20 counts) and circumflex (22 counts). Thus, the longer LAD frame count was corrected by dividing by 1.7 to derive the corrected TIMI frame count. The mean corrected TIMI frame count in culprit arteries 90 minutes after thrombolytic therapy followed a continuous unimodal distribution with a mean value of 39 frames, which improved to 32 frames within 18 to 36 hours after therapy. There was no correlation between improvements in corrected TIMI frame counts and changes in minimal luminal diameter. The mean 90-minute corrected TIMI frame count among nonculprit arteries was significantly higher than that for arteries with normal flow in the absence of AMI, but improved to that of normal arteries by 1 day after thrombolysis. Thus, the corrected TIMI frame count method is a simple, reproducible, objective, and quantitative index of coronary flow that allows standardization of TIMI flow grades and facilitates comparisons of angiographic end points between trials (Figure 2-15).

Hundley and colleagues[35] in Dallas, Texas, used phase-contrast MRI (MRI) to measure coronary arterial flow in 12 subjects (7 men and 5 women; age range, 44 to 67 years) in the LAD or 1 of its diagonal branches at rest and after administration of adenosine. Immediately thereafter, intracoronary Doppler velocity and flow measurements were made during cardiac catheterization at rest and after administration of adenosine. For the 12 patients, the correlation between MRI and invasive measurements of coronary arterial flow and arterial

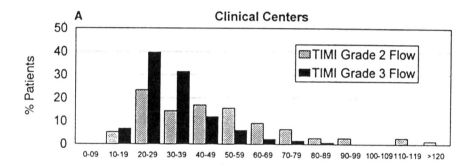

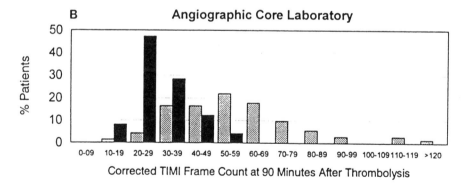

FIGURE 2-15. A, When clinical centers interpreted TIMI flow grade, there was a large degree of overlap in the distribution of the CTFC for TIMI grade 2 vs. TIMI grade 3 flow. **B,** For the angiographic core laboratory, overlap was also present but appeared to be reduced compared with the clinical centers. This is demonstrated by the fact that among culprit lesions classified as having TIMI grade 2 flow, the corrected TIMI flow count (CTFC) was <30 (ie, flow was actually fast) in 22 (28.6%) of 77 culprit lesions assessed by the clinical center, which was significantly higher than the 4 (5.5%) of 73 culprits assessed by the core laboratory (p = .003). Likewise, among culprit lesions classified as having TIMI grade 3 flow, the CTFC was >60 (ie, flow was actually slow) in 6 (4.4%) of 134 culprits assessed by the clinical center, compared with none (0%) of 148 culprits assessed by the core laboratory (p = .03). Reproduced with permission from Gibson et al.[34]

flow reserve was excellent: coronary flow$_{MRI}$ (mL/min) = 0.85 × coronary flow-$_{IDV}$ (mL/min) + 17 (mL/min), r = .89 and coronary flow reserve$_{MRI}$ = 0.79 × coronary velocity reserve$_{IDV}$ + 0.34, r = .89. For the range of coronary arterial flows measured by MRI, the limit of agreement between MRI and cardiac catheterization measurements of flow was −13 mL/min; for the range of coronary reserves measured by MRI, the limit of agreement between the 2 techniques was 0.1 ± 0.4. Thus, cine velocity-encoded phase-contrast MRI can noninvasively measure absolute coronary arterial flow in the LAD in humans (Figure 2-16). Moreover, it can detect pharmacologically induced changes in coronary arterial flow and may reliably distinguish between those subjects with normal and abnormal coronary flow reserve.

To evaluate coronary flow dynamics after direct PTCA and to define the determinants of flow-velocity variables in the infarct artery, Nakamura and associates[36] from Tokyo, Japan, measured coronary flow velocity in 36 infarct arteries and 64 normal coronary arteries by using a Doppler guide wire. Flow-velocity variables in the infarct arteries did not return to normal even after successful direct angioplasty, and phasic coronary flow in infarct arteries varied considerably. Normal phasic flow was calculated as the ratio of diastolic to systolic flow ratio of greater than or equal to mean diastolic to systolic flow ratio −1 standard deviation in normal coronary arteries. Infarct-related arteries were divided into 2 groups: normal diastolic to systolic flow ratio (n = 28) and low diastolic to systolic flow ratio (n = 8). Reduced diastolic peak

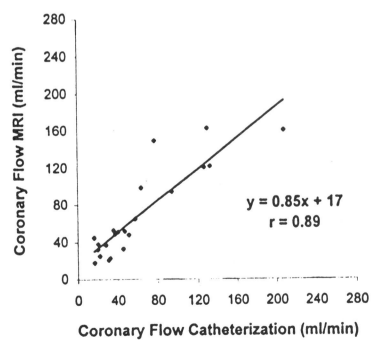

Figure 2-16. Catheterization (*x* axis) and phase contrast (PC)-MRI (*y* axis) measurements of coronary arterial flow for the 12 subjects. For each subject, 2 data points are displayed: baseline and after intravenous infusion of adenosine. The regression line (solid line) and equation are shown. Reproduced with permission from Hundley et al.[35]

velocity with a relative preservation of systolic velocity contributed to a low diastolic to systolic flow ratio. Angiographic slow flow and late recanalization were significantly related to low diastolic to systolic flow ratio. Thus the extent of disturbed microcirculation can be evaluated by assessing phasic flow after direct PTCA for AMI.

Nakamura and associates[37] from Tokyo, Japan, investigated the safety and limitations of the Doppler guidewire for continuous monitoring of coronary flow velocity outside the catheterization laboratory in 17 patients with AMI. After direct angioplasty, patients were taken to the coronary care unit with the Doppler guidewire positioned within the artery. Flow velocity was continuously monitored. Heparin was titrated to an active clotting time of greater than 200 seconds. Clinical outcome and angiographic analyses were evaluated. Flow velocity monitoring was conducted with an 88% success rate and lasted for 16 ± 5 hours. Monitoring failed in 2 of the 4 right coronary artery cases. Small amounts of thrombus were seen adhering to the Doppler guidewire at the end of monitoring. No complications were related to the procedure. No deterioration of angiographic findings was observed. This preliminary study confirmed the safety of the Doppler guidewire for continuous monitoring of coronary flow in patients with AMI.

The functional importance and protective nature of the coronary collateral circulation has been well established. There are few data, however, regarding the phasic nature and absolute velocities of collateral flow in patients. The aim of this study by Tron and associates[38] from St. Louis, Missouri, was to characterize and quantify ipsilateral coronary collateral blood flow velocity in patients during PTCA. Coronary collateral flow velocity was measured in 49 patients during PTCA. Angiographic collateral filling was categorized by the Rentrop grading scale (0 to 3) and by anatomic pathway (epicardial, intramyocardial, or unknown [acutely recruited]). Collateral blood flow velocity was measured with a Doppler-tipped guidewire placed distal to the balloon occlusion in the collateralized vessel. Collateral flow velocity was characterized as predominantly systolic or diastolic, and phasic flow patterns were defined as biphasic (both systolic and diastolic), monophasic (only systolic or diastolic), or bidirectional (antegrade and retrograde velocity). Twenty-three (47%) patients had biphasic flow; 17 (35%) patients had monophasic flow; and 9 (18%) patients had bidirectional flow. Thirty-six (73%) of 49 patients had predominantly systolic flow signals. Epicardial collateral pathways had the highest total flow velocity integral, at 15.0 ± 7.0 (vs. intramyocardial [8.4 ± 5.7] and acutely recruitable [5.4 ± 2.1]). There were no differences in flow velocity integrals among the Rentrop angiographic grades of collateral filling. These data establish 3 patterns of coronary collateral blood flow and demonstrate that the majority of collateral flow in the ipsilateral receiving vessel occurs during systole. The measurement of coronary collateral flow velocity provides a unique means to study the effects of pharmacological or mechanical interventions on human collateral blood flow.

Nitzsche and colleagues[39] in Los Angeles, California, tested the hypothesis that [^{13}N]ammonia positron emission tomography provides good estimates of myocardial blood flow comparable to those obtained with the [^{15}O]water technique. A total of 30 pairs of positron emission tomographic flow measurements were performed in 30 healthy volunteers. Fifteen volunteers were studied

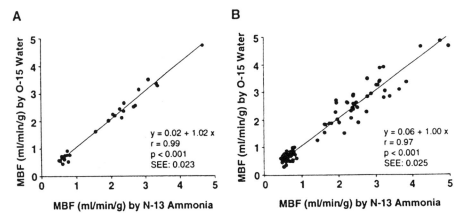

FIGURE 2-17. A, Comparison of mean estimates of myocardial blood flow (MBF) by [^{13}N]ammonia and by [^{15}O]water. There is a significant linear correlation between estimates of MBF (n = 30) by [^{13}N]ammonia and by [^{15}O]water for flow ranging from 0.45 to 4.75 mL/min^{-1}/g^{-1}. Slope of regression line is 1.02. **B,** Comparison of regional estimates of MBF by [^{13}N]ammonia and by [^{15}O]water. There is a significant linear correlation between regional estimates of MBF (n = 90) by [^{13}N]ammonia and by [^{15}O]water, with flow ranging from 0.45 to 4.74 mL/min^{-1}/g^{-1}. Slow of regression line is 1.00. Reproduced with permission from Nitzsche et al.[39]

at rest and 15 during adenosine-induced hyperemia. Estimates of average and of regional myocardial blood flow by the [^{13}N]ammonia and the [^{15}O]water approaches correlated closely (Figure 2-17). At rest, mean myocardial blood flow was 0.64 mL·min^{-1}·g^{-1} for [^{13}N]ammonia and 0.66 mL·min^{-1}·g^{-1} for the [^{15}O]water. For adenosine-induced hyperemia, mean blood flow was 2.6 mL·min^{-1}·g^{-1} for the [^{13}N]ammonia and 2.7 mL·min^{-1}·g^{-1} for the [^{15}O]water. Thus, these 2 approaches provide comparable estimates of myocardial blood flow in humans that support the utility of [^{13}N]ammonia method in estimates of human myocardial blood flow.

Stable Angina

Histomorphological Analysis of Atherosclerotic Plaques

Angioscopic observations in coronary artery vessels have been helpful in better understanding the pathogenesis of acute ischemic syndromes. Thieme and colleagues[40] from Berlin, Germany, compared angioscopic findings in patients with different coronary syndromes with atherosclerotic material retrieved by directional coronary atherectomy. Angioscopy and directional coronary atherectomy were performed in 26 patients with stable, angina and 37 patients with unstable angina. Patients with unstable angina had predominantly yellow lesions (89%). In patients with stable angina, gray-white (43%) or yellow (57%) lesions were similarly distributed. Ruptured yellow plaques and red or pink thrombi were identified in 11% of patients with stable angina and 39% of patients with unstable angina or early postmyocardial infarction angina. Histologically, gray-white lesions represented fibrous plaque without degeneration in 64% of patients and with degeneration in 36% of patients. Gray-yellow lesions were associated predominantly with degenerative plaque (64%) and to a lesser extent with fibrous plaque (14%) or atheroma (14%). Deep yellow and yellow-red lesions represented either atheromas (53%) or degenerated plaque (42%). This study provided further information about coronary syndromes by providing histomorphologic data. The authors concluded that yellow plaque is closely related to degenerated plaque or atheroma and is associated with unstable coronary syndromes.

Fibrinolytic Factors and Risk of MI

Juhan-Vague and colleagues[41] in Marseille, France, on behalf of the ECAT Study Group, conducted a prospective multicenter study of 3043 patients with angina pectoris followed for 2 years. They obtained baseline measurements, including 10 fibrinolytic variables, to examine the risk of myocardial infarction and sudden death in these patients. The data were presented before and after adjustment for clusters of confounding variables that are markers of different mechanisms: insulin resistance, including body mass index; serum triglyceride concentration; HDL cholesterol; inflammation, including fibrinogen and C-reactive protein; and endothelial cell damage, as evidenced by the presence of circulating von Willebrand factor. An increased incidence of events was associated with higher baseline concentrations of tissue plasminogen activator (tPA) antigen, plasminogen activator inhibitor-1 activity (PAI-1), and PAI-1 antigen. The associations of PAI-1 activity and PAI-1 antigen with the risk of events disappeared after adjustment for variables reflecting insulin resistance, but they were not affected by other adjustments. The tPA antigen was affected to a similar extent by adjustment for variables reflecting insulin resistance, inflammation, or endothelial damage, but the risk association disappeared only after combined adjustments. Thus, these data suggest that a prognostic role of PAI-1 in predicting coronary events is related to insulin resistance, whereas that of tPA antigen may be explained by its relationship with different mechanisms, including insulin resistance, inflammation, and endothelial cell damage.

Plasma Fibrinogen, tPA Antigen, Plasma Activator Inhibitor, and C-Reactive Protein in Healthy Volunteers and Angina Patients

de Maat and coinvestigators[42] in Leiden, The Netherlands, compared interindividual and intraindividual variability at the plasma levels of fibrinogen, tissue type plasminogen activator (tPA) antigen, plasminogen activator inhibitor activity, and C-reactive protein in 10 young healthy individuals and 26 patients with stable angina pectoris with high risk for cardiovascular disease. For each of the 4 parameters, the contribution of the intraindividual variation to the total variance for the healthy volunteers and angina pectoris patients, respectively, were smaller than the contribution from the interindividual variation. These results indicate that single sampling is efficient to assess an individual level of tPA antigen and plasminogen activator inhibitor activity, whereas duplicate sampling for fibrinogen and triplicate sampling for C-reactive protein are recommended. In an epidemiological study, the sample sizes (based on the variances found in the transverse part of the study) needed to detect a 15% difference between the 2 groups were as follows: 31 and 40 for fibrinogen, 568 and 146 for tPA, 603 and 119 for plasminogen activator inhibitor activity, and 1490 and 2263 for C-reactive protein in healthy volunteers and patients with angina pectoris, respectively. Additionally, the investigators studied the contribution of genetic polymorphisms of β-fibrinogen and plasminogen activator inhibitor activity genes to intraindividual and interindividual variations. Fibrinogen genotypes were associated with plasma fibrinogen levels in the volunteers, but not in the angina pectoris patients. No effects of fibrinogen or plasminogen activator inhibitor polymorphisms on intraindividual variation were observed in either healthy individuals or angina pectoris patients. In this study, intraindividual variations in plasma levels of the cardiovascular risk indicators fibrinogen, tPA antigen, plasminogen activator inhibitor activity, and C-reactive protein were small when compared with the interindividual variation in healthy young volunteers and patients with stable angina pectoris.

Metoprolol and Nifedipine Versus Monotherapy (IMAGE Study)

Combination antianginal therapy with a β-blocking agent and a dihydropyridine calcium antagonist has been shown to have combined benefit in reducing anginal episodes. Previous studies, however, did not clearly sort out whether this anti-ischemic effect was a group benefit or also an individual benefit. Savonitto and colleagues[43] in a multicenter study (IMAGE) evaluated 280 patients with stable angina pectoris who were enrolled in a double-blind trial in 25 European centers. Patients were randomized to metoprolol controlled release, 200 mg a day, or nifedipine retard, 20 mg twice daily, for 6 weeks. Placebo or the alternative drug was then added for a further 4 weeks, and exercise tests were performed at weeks 0, 6, and 10. At week 6, both metoprolol and nifedipine increased the mean exercise time to 1-mm ST segment depression. Metoprolol was more effective than nifedipine. At week 10, the groups randomly assigned to combination therapy had a further increase in time to 1-mm ST segment depression. However, analysis in individual patients revealed that only 11% of patients having nifedipine added to metoprolol and 29% of patients having metoprolol added to nifedipine showed an increase in exercise tolerance that was greater than the 90th percentile of the distribution of changes observed in the corresponding monotherapy and placebo groups. Thus, these authors concluded that the mean additive anti-ischemic effects showed by combination therapy with metoprolol and nifedipine in patients with stable angina pectoris are not the result of an additive effect in individual patients, but rather can be attributed to the recruitment by the second drug of patients not responding well to monotherapy.

Total Ischemic Burden Bisoprolol Study

Transient ischemia on an ambulatory electrocardiogram appears to have adverse prognostic implications in stable angina. It is unclear whether medical treatment can change that prognosis. von Arnim and colleagues[44] for the Total Ischemic Burden Bisoprolol Study (TIBBS) examined cardiac event rates in relation to transient ischemia and its treatment. This was an 8-week, randomized, controlled comparison of the effects of bisoprolol and nifedipine on transient ischemic episodes in patients with stable angina pectoris. There was a relation between the number of episodes of ischemia and adverse events. Hard events (death, acute myocardial infarction, hospital admission for unstable angina pectoris) were more frequent in patients with 2 or more ischemic episodes (12.1% vs. 4.7%). Patients with a 100% reduction in ischemic episodes during the TIBBS trial had a 17.5% event rate at 1 year compared with 32.3% of patients who did not completely respond to therapy. Patients receiving bisoprolol had a lower event rate (22.1%) than did patients randomized to nifedipine (33.1%). These authors concluded that in patients with stable angina pectoris, frequent episodes of transient ischemia is a marker for an increased event rate. A 100% response to medical treatment reduces the event rate (Figure 2-18).

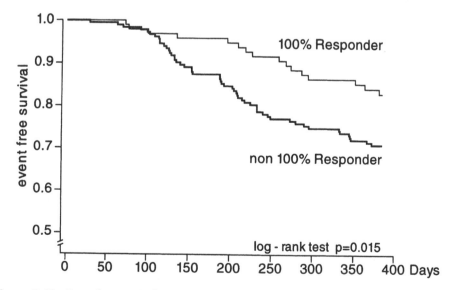

FIGURE 2-18. Event-free survival in 283 patients treated in the TIBBS trial. A 100% reduction of transient ischemic episodes (top curve) was achieved in 97 patients who had a reduced risk of subsequent events over the non-100% risk responders (bottom curve, 186 patients). Reproduced with permission from von Arnim.[44]

Myocardial Ischemia

Protocol to Rule Out Ischemia in the Emergency Room

Patients with a missed diagnosis of AMI in the emergency room have a high mortality rate. However, providing routine hospital care to low-risk patients may not be time- or cost-effective. Gomez and colleagues[45] from Salt Lake City, Utah, entered 100 low-risk patients either to an emergency department-based rapid rule out protocol or to routine hospital care. Patients receiving routine care were managed by their attending physicians. The rapid protocol included serum enzyme testing at 0, 3, 6, and 9 hours; serial electrocardiograms with continuous ST segment monitoring; and, if results were negative, a predischarge graded exercise test. Myocardial infarction or unstable angina occurred in 6% of patients within 30 days; no diagnoses were missed. By intention to treat analysis, the hospital stay was shorter and charges were lower for the rapid protocol as compared with routine care. These authors concluded that in low-risk patients who present to an emergency room with chest pain, a rapid rule out protocol is safe and more cost-effective than routine hospital care.

Circadian Variation of Ambulatory Ischemia

Krantz and colleagues[46] assessed: 1) the effects of exogenous activity triggers at different times of the day, and 2) the contribution of an endogenous circadian vulnerability for ambulatory ischemia. Sixty-three stable CAD patients underwent ambulatory electrocardiographic monitoring and completed a structured diary assessing physical and mental activities. During 2519 hours of observation, a morning increase in ischemia coincided with increases in physical and mental activities, and an evening decrease in ischemia coincided with a decline in activities. During the morning, ischemic (versus ischemic-free periods) were more likely to occur with high levels of physical activity. High levels of physical activity triggered ischemia to a lesser but still significant extent in the afternoon, but not in the evening. High levels of mental activity triggered ischemia significantly during the morning and evening, but not in the afternoon. When a residualized score procedure was used to correct ischemic time for each patient's simultaneously measured activities, for hourly heart rates, or for activity-related heart rate fluctuations, the circadian variation in ischemia was still observed with a peak at 6 AM each day. A significant increase in ischemia occurred immediately after awakening, but activity-adjusted increases in morning ischemia persisted for 2 hours after awakening. Thus, exogenous factors, including physical and mental activities, are most powerful as triggers of ischemia during the morning hours, and the postural

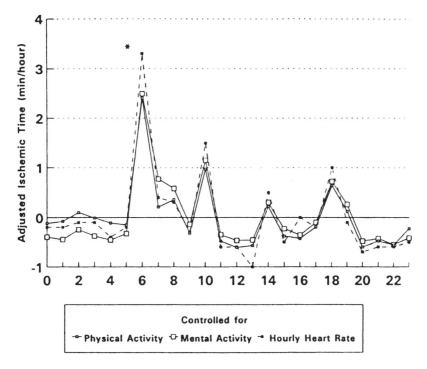

FIGURE 2-19. Diurnal variation of ischemia, corrected for activity levels and for hourly heart rate. Data represent residualized scores, with separate curves displayed for physical and mental activity-adjusted and heart rate-adjusted estimates of predicted ischemic time for each hour of the day. Values below zero indicate that ischemic time was shorter than expected on the basis of concurrent activity level or heart rate. Analyses showed a significant diurnal fluctuation of the physical (p<.01) and mental (p<.01) activity-adjusted ischemic time and HR-adjusted ischemic time (p<.01). *Increase p<.05 vs. previous hour for each of the three curves. Reproduced with permission from Krantz et al.[46]

change after awakening contributes to the morning increase in ischemia (Figure 2-19).

Patient Characteristics and Daily Activity

Cardiac ischemia during daily life activities, detected by ambulatory electrocardiographic ambulatory monitoring, has been associated with increased risk for adverse outcomes. Because daily life myocardial ischemia is usually asymptomatic, prevalence and descriptive data of patients with asymptomatic cardiac ischemia (ACI) are not well defined. Pepine and associates[47] for the Asymptomatic Cardiac Ischemia Pilot Data Bank, a study group from multiple medical centers, investigated patients screened for asymptomatic myocardial ischemia by 48-hour ambulatory electrocardiographic monitoring to identify factors associated with ACI. A total of 1820 patients with myocardial ischemia on a screening stress test and known or suspected CAD underwent ambulatory electrocardiographic monitoring. Their mean age was 61 years, range 33 to 89; 83% were men, and 81% were white. On ambulatory electrocardiographic monitoring, ACI occurred in 897 patients (49%). There was a modest trend between increasing age and ACI prevalence. Increased risk for ACI was observed in patients reporting angina 6 weeks before screening (odds ratio 1.38). There was a positive association between increases in heart rate during daily life and ACI prevalence. No daily, monthly, or seasonal variation in ACI prevalence was found, although ACI was more prevalent in northern than in southern sites. In this group of clinically stable patients, selected on the basis of high risk for CAD, the prevalence of ACI was higher than expected from previous reports. Several readily available clinical characteristics (ie, advanced age, recent angina, increased heart rate change with daily activity) were associated with significantly increased probability of ACI.

Asymptomatic Cardiac Ischemia Pilot (ACIP) Study: Exercise Versus Ambulatory Ischemia

Stone and colleagues[48] for the Asymptomatic Cardiac Ischemia Pilot (ACIP) study investigated whether the presence and frequency of asymptomatic ischemic episodes recorded during ambulatory electrocardiographic monitoring might be predicted on the basis of clinical characteristics or exercise treadmill test performance in patients with stable CAD. They also noted whether the estimate of ischemia severity was similar between the 2 tests. Patients screened for ACIP were selected for this analysis if data were available from 48-hour ambulatory electrocardiographic monitoring, as well as from an exercise treadmill test during which the patient developed ST segment depression of 1 mm or greater. Exercise electrocardiographic data were available for 143 of the 910 patients without ischemic episodes and for 659 of the 910 patients with ischemic episodes during ambulatory electrocardiographic monitoring. Angina was more frequent among patients with ambulatory ischemic episodes than among patients without such ischemia. Patients with ambulatory electrocardiographic ischemia had a consistently more marked ischemic response on the exercise treadmill test than did patients without ambulatory electrocardiographic evidence of ischemia. The likelihood of having ambulatory electrocardiographic patients likely to have evidence of ischemia could be predicted on the basis of exercise treadmill tolerance performance characteristics. However, the correlation coefficients between the severity of ischemia estimated by the 2 tests were small. Thus, there are significant relationships between ischemia detected by ambulatory electrocardiographic monitoring and by exercise treadmill test, but the relations are limited, suggesting that the 2 tests are not redundant in the characterization of patients with CAD.

ACIP Study: Comparison of Subgroups

Pratt and associates[49] for the ACIP Study Group Investigators prepared a report focusing on the subset of 235 patients who received randomly assigned medical therapy to treat angina and suppress myocardial ischemia detected on ambulatory electrocardiography: 121 patients received the sequence of atenolol and nifedipine, and 114 received diltiazem and isosorbide dinitrate. After 12 weeks of therapy, the primary end point (absence of ambulatory electrocardiographic ischemia and no clinical events) was reached in 47% of atenolol/nifedipine versus 31% of diltiazem/isosorbide dinitrate-treated patients. A trend to increased exercise time to ST depression was seen in the atenolol and nifedipine versus diltiazem and isosorbide dinitrate regimens (median treadmill duration, 5.8 vs 4.8 minutes). However, when adjusted for baseline imbalances in ambulatory electrocardiographic ischemia, the 2 medical combinations were similar in suppression of ambulatory electrocardiographic ischemia. In both medication regimens, an association between mean heart rate and ischemia on ambulatory electrocardiography after 12 weeks of treatment was observed so that patients on either regimen with a mean heart rate greater than 80 beats/min had ischemia detectable almost twice as often as those with a mean heart rate less than 70 beats/min (Figure 2-20).

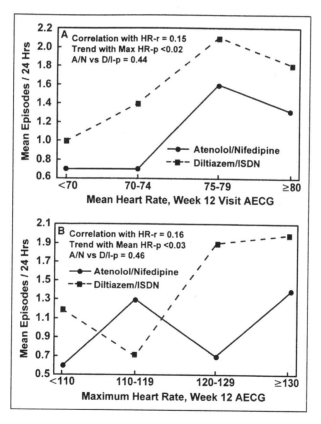

FIGURE 2-20. Relation of mean (**A**) and maximal (Max) (**B**) heart rate (HR) to the mean number of ischemic episodes on ambulatory electrocardiography (AECG) at 12 weeks by medication regimen. Reproduced with permission from Pratt et al.[49]

Hyperinsulinemia as an Independent Risk Factor for Ischemic Heart Disease

Després and colleagues[50] in Montreal, Canada, collected blood samples from 2103 men from the suburbs of Quebec City, Canada, who were 45 to 76 years of age and who did not have ischemic heart disease. A first ischemic event, including angina pectoris, AMI, or death from CAD occurred in 114 men between 1985 and 1990. Each case patient was matched for age, body mass index, smoking habits, and alcohol consumption with a control selected from among the 1989 men who remained free of ischemic heart disease during follow-up. After excluding men with diabetes, the authors compared fasting plasma insulin and lipoprotein concentrations in 91 case patients and 105 controls. Fasting insulin concentrations at baseline were 18% higher in the case patients than in the controls ($p < .001$). Logistic-regression analysis showed that the insulin concentration remained associated with ischemic heart disease with an odds ratio for ischemic heart disease with each increase of 1 SD in the insulin concentration, 1.7 after adjustment for systolic blood pressure, use of medications, and family history of ischemic heart disease. Further adjustment by multivariate analysis for plasma triglycerides, apolipoprotein B, LDL cholesterol, and HDL cholesterol concentrations did not diminish the association between the insulin concentration and the risk of ischemic heart disease (odds ratio, 1.6; 95% confidence interval, 1.1 to 2.3). Thus, high fasting insulin concentrations appear to be an independent predictor of ischemic heart disease in men.

β-Blocker Therapy

Myocardial ischemia appears to increase the risk in every subset of patients with CAD. Madjlessi-Simon and colleagues[51] from Paris, France, evaluated the prevalence and significance of transient myocardial ischemia in the presence of *β*-adrenergic blockade in patients with CAD. Three hundred thirteen patients with documented CAD and *β*-blocker therapy with (n = 84) or without (n = 229) transient ischemia on ambulatory electrocardiographic monitoring were followed up for an average of 21 months for cardiac events. The number of coronary stenoses did not differ significantly between the 2 groups. *β*-Blocker therapy was discontinued more frequently during follow-up in the group without transient ischemia (25% vs. 14%). PTCA and CABG were significantly more frequent in the group with ischemia. Transient ischemia was associated with a higher cumulative probability of adverse events. In the group with transient ischemia, the relative hazard of cardiac events was increased 3-fold when *β*-blocker therapy was interrupted. These authors concluded that the occurrence of transient ischemia, despite *β*-blocker therapy, identifies a high-risk group of patients with CAD. Similarly, the interruption of *β*-blocker therapy in this group increases the risk of adverse cardiac events.

Circadian Pattern of Ischemic Activity in Women

The circadian variation in ischemic activity, myocardial infarction, and sudden cardiac death in patients with CAD was established primarily using male patients. Mulcahy and colleagues[52] from Bethesda, Maryland evaluated 31 women to see if there was a similar and significant circadian variation in women. Forty-five men were also evaluated with 48 hours of ambulatory ST segment monitoring. A significant circadian variation was found both in men and women with a trough at night and a peak during activity hours. The majority of ischemic episodes had a heart rate increase in the 5 minutes before ischemia. These authors concluded that women with CAD have a circadian pattern of ischemic activity similar to that in men. The primary factor appears to be an increase in the heart rate, presumably reflecting an increase in myocardial oxygen demand.

Effect of Aspirin on Mortality in Women

The benefit of aspirin therapy among women with CAD is not well established. Previous studies have shown conflicting results among women. Harpaz and associates[53] for the Israeli BIP Study Group analyzed data from 2418 women with CAD screened for participation in the ongoing Bezafibrate Infarction Prevention (BIP) Study: 45% reported aspirin therapy. Baseline characteristics were similar in both groups. Cardiovascular mortality at 3.1 ± 0.9 years of follow-up was 2.7% in the aspirin-treated group versus 5.1% in the nonaspirin-treated group. All cause mortality was 5.1% and 9.1%, respectively. Treatment with aspirin emerged as an independent predictor of reduced cardiovascular and all cause mortality after multiple adjustment for possible confounders such as age, history of AMI, systemic hypertension, diabetes mellitus, peripheral vascular disease, current smoker, New York Heart Association classification, and concomitant treatment with digitalis. Women who benefited the most from aspirin therapy were older, diabetic, symptomatic, or had a previous AMI. Thus, treatment with aspirin was associated with reduced mortality among women with CAD. This study suggests that women with CAD should be treated with aspirin, unless specific contraindications exist.

Pravastatin Versus Conventional Treatment

van Boven and colleagues[54] in Groningen, The Netherlands, evaluated the effects of pravastatin given as 40 mg/day on transient myocardial ischemia in a 2-year prospective randomized placebo-controlled study in 768 male patients with stable angina pectoris, documented CAD, and serum cholesterol values between 155 and 310 mg/dL. Forty-eight-hour ambulatory electrocardiograms with continuous ST-segment analysis were obtained. During the trial, patients received routine antianginal treatment. As detected by ambulatory electrocardiography, transient myocardial ischemia was present at baseline in 28% of the patients randomly assigned to receive pravastatin, and it was present after treatment in 19%. In the placebo group, it was found in 20% at baseline and in

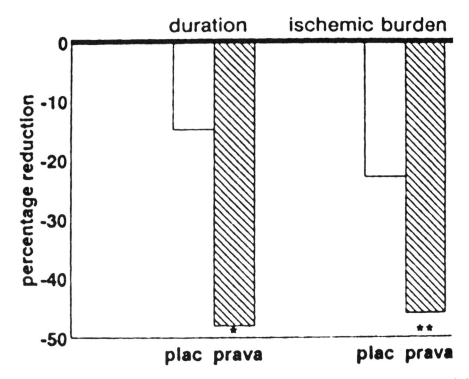

FIGURE 2-21. Diagram of the percentage reduction in components of transient myocardial ischemia during the study in placebo patients (plac, open bars) and in pravastatin-treated patients (prava, hatched bars). *p = .017 and **p = .0058. Reproduced with permission from van Boven et al.[54]

23% of patients after treatment (Figure 2-21). Episodes of myocardial ischemia decreased by 1.2 episodes with pravastatin and by 0.5 with placebo. While taking pravastatin, the duration of ischemia decreased from 80 ± 12 minutes to 42 ± 10 minutes, but there was no significant change with placebo. The total ischemic burden decreased from 41 ± 5 to 22 ± 5 mm/min in the pravastatin-treated group, but it did not change significantly in the placebo-treated group. After adjustment for independent risk factors for the development of myocardial ischemia, the effect of pravastatin on the reduction of risk for ischemia remained statistically significant. Thus, this study suggests that in men with documented CAD and optimal antianginal therapy, pravastatin reduces transient myocardial ischemia.

Effect of Exercise Testing

It has been suggested that the myocardium is able to recruit endogenous protective mechanisms in response to repeated ischemia and reperfusion. Ylitalo and associates[55] from Oulu, Finland, studied whether this is manifested in patients with CAD in the form of fewer signs of myocardial ischemia during the second of 2 successive exercise tests and whether any relations exist between ischemia adaptation and findings at cardiac catheterization. Twenty-one patients with typical angina pectoris symptoms underwent 2 repeated bicycle exercise tests with identical protocols, followed by cardiac catheterization and coronary angiography the following day. The first exercise test was discontinued whenever a 2-mm ST depression in the electrocardiogram was achieved or further exercise was limited by symptoms. The second exercise test was performed after disappearance of the symptoms or ST depression or both. Kaplan-Meler survival analysis for the appearance of a 1-mm ST depression demonstrated improved ischemia tolerance during the second test, when the required time for its appearance was significantly longer (6.5 ± 0.8 minutes vs. 4.5 ± 0.5 minutes). The maximal intensity of anginal pain was lower during the second exercise (2.2 ± 1.0 minutes vs. 0.7 ± 0.3 minutes), and the time required for disappearance of the ST depression was shorter after this exercise (3.0 ± 0.8 minutes vs. 6.2 ± 0.9 minutes), with a similar tendency in the disappearance of angina. The rate-pressure product on the appearance of a 1-mm ST depression was significantly higher during the second test (17,990 ± 1210 mm Hg × min^{-1} vs. 15,960 ± 869 mm Hg × min^{-1}). Eighteen of the patients had 3-vessel disease, as evidenced by coronary angiography, and the change in the time required for the appearance of a 1-mm ST depression in the repeated exercise tests was inversely correlated with the severity of the LAD coronary artery obstruction and LV end-diastolic pressure. No significant correlation with the degree of collateral vessels was found. It was concluded that most patients with extensive CAD are able to increase their tolerance of ischemia during repeated dynamic exercise and that increased vasodilation and oxygen delivery are the major mechanisms for this warm-up phenomenon. Conversely, collaterals visible in routine resting angiography do not predict the degree of adaptation to ischemia during repeated dynamic exercise.

Variant Angina, Spastic Angina

Multivessel Spasm with Normal Coronaries

Although the prognosis of variant angina without significant stenosis is generally good, there is a high incidence of multivessel spasm, which is generally an adverse prognostic factor. Onaka and colleagues[56] from Takatsuki, Japan, evaluated 122 patients with suspected variant or unstable angina who underwent 24-hour 12-lead electrocardiographic recording and analysis to evaluate the clinical manifestations of ischemic episodes. Thirty of these patients had variant angina with normal or near normal coronary arteries; of those, 22 experienced anginal attacks with ST segment elevation during monitoring and were evaluated. There were 138 episodes of transient ST segment elevation and 13 episodes of ST depression. Three different patterns of spasm were observed: migratory spasm in different sites, spasm sequentially affecting 2 different sites, and simultaneous spasm at more than 1 site. The duration of ST segment elevation was much longer in patients with sequential and simultaneous spasm than in those with single vessel spasm, and arrhythmias were more frequent during the 2 types of multivessel spasm. The authors concluded that multivessel spasm produces more ischemia than does single-vessel spasm or migratory multivessel spasm, and may have adverse prognostic significance.

Microvascular Dysfunction in Syndrome X

In addition to coronary vascular abnormalities, patients with syndrome X and variant angina often have systemic vascular symptoms. To determine whether these patients exhibit a generalized abnormality of vasoreactivity, Bøtker and associates[57] from Aarhus, Denmark, used high-resolution ultrasound to compare flow responses and endothelial function in the brachial artery in 3 groups: 21 patients with syndrome X, 15 patients with variant angina, and 20 control patients who were healthy. Arterial diameter was measured at rest, after reactive hyperemia (endothelium-dependent flow-mediated vasodilation), and after sublingual glyceryl trinitrate (endothelium-independent vasodilation). The magnitude of hyperemic flow response was measured after transient forearm occlusion. Flow-mediated dilation in the brachial artery did not differ among patients with syndrome X, variant angina, and controls (2.7% ± 2.3%, 3.8% ± 3.5%, and 4.2% ± 3.0%). Endothelium-independent vasodilation in the brachial artery was similar in the 3 groups (16.0% ± 7.2%, 12.7% ± 4.6%, and 14.8% ± 4.9%). Despite a considerable overlap, reactive hyperemia was lower in patients with syndrome X than in patients with variant angina and controls (342% ± 86% vs. 466% ± 184% and 452 ± 104%). These findings indicate that a substantial proportion of patients with syndrome X have a systemic microvascular abnormality, whereas variant angina is predominantly a segmental disorder of conduit vessels.

Vitamin E Deficiency

Miwa and colleagues[58] in Toyama, Japan, measured vitamin E levels by high-performance liquid chromatography in normolipidemic subjects, including 29 patients with active variant angina (group 1), 13 patients with an inactive stage of variant angina without anginal attacks during the prior 6 months (group 2), 32 patients with a significant (>75%) coronary stenosis and stable effort angina (group 3), and 30 patients without coronary artery disease (group 4). Total lipid levels in blood were calculated as total cholesterol plus triglyceride levels. The plasma α-tocopherol levels, as well as α-tocopherol/lipids, were significantly lower in group 1 than in groups 2 through 4. Vitamin E levels were not significantly different between group 1 patients with and without a significant organic stenosis. In group 1 patients, both α- and γ-tocopherol levels were significantly elevated after a 6-month or longer angina-free period. The α-tocopherol levels in the LDL fraction were significantly lower in group 1 than in group 4. Plasma α-tocopherol levels were significantly correlated with those in the LDL fractions. In 6 patients still having anginal attacks while receiving calcium channel blockers, the addition of vitamin E acetate (300 mg/day) significantly elevated plasma α-tocopherol levels and inhibited the occurrence of angina. These data suggest that plasma vitamin E levels are significantly lower in patients with active variant angina than in those without coronary spasm.

Nitric Oxide Deficiency

Kugiyama and colleagues[59] from Kumamoto City, Japan, determined whether nitric oxide release is deficient in coronary arteries of patients with coronary vasospasm. N^G-monomethyl-L-arginine (L-NMMA), an inhibitor of nitric oxide synthase, was infused into coronary arteries in 21 patients with coronary vasospastic angina and in 28 control patients. Coronary spasm was induced by intracoronary injection of acetylcholine and was documented angiographically in all patients. L-NMMA dose-dependently decreased basal luminal diameter of coronary arteries in control patients, whereas it had no effect on basal diameter of the spasm arteries in patients with coronary vasospasm (Figure 2-22). L-NMMA abolished the dilator response to acetylcholine and enhanced constrictor response to acetylcholine in control arteries, but it had no effect on the constrictor response to acetylcholine in arteries in patients with coronary vasospasm. Intracoronary infusion of L-arginine did not affect the diameter of the spasm or control arteries. The dilator response to nitroglycerin was increased markedly in the spasm arteries compared with control arteries, but the response to diltiazem did not differ between them (Figure 2-23). Thus, there appears to be a deficiency in endothelial nitric oxide activity in coronary arteries of patients with vasospasm, which may lead to the supersensi-

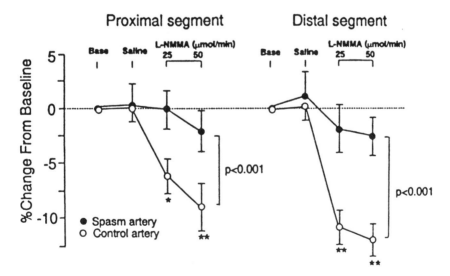

FIGURE 2-22. Percent change (mean ± SEM) of coronary luminal diameter of spasm (●) and control (○) arteries from baseline values at the proximal and distal segments after intracoronary infusion of saline and L-NMMA in patients with coronary spastic angina and in control patients (protocol 1). The probability value refers to the comparison of the 2 curves by two-way ANOVA for repeated measures. *p<.05 and **p<.01 compared with the respective saline values. Reproduced with permission from Kugiyama et al.[59]

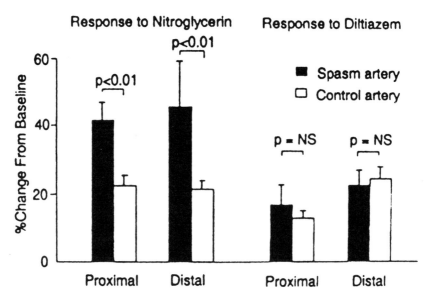

FIGURE 2-23. Percent change (mean ± SEM) of coronary luminal diameter of spasm (solid bars) and control (open bars) arteries from baseline values at the proximal and distal segments in response to nitroglycerin and diltiazem in patients with coronary spastic angina and in control patients (protocol 1). Reproduced with permission from Kugiyama et al.[59]

tivity of the artery to the vasodilator effect of nitroglycerin and to the vasoconstrictor effect of acetylcholine.

Unstable Angina Pectoris

Correlation Between Clinical and Morphological Findings

De Servi and associates[60] from Pavia, Italy, did a study to provide the hypothesis that the discrepant findings in published reports on the prevalence of thrombus in unstable angina depend on the inclusion of different clinical subsets in the various studies. The authors correlated the clinical characteristics of patients included under the label of unstable angina with the morphologic features assessed by coronary angiography and intravascular ultrasound, and with histopathologic findings of atherectomy specimens. Fifty-eight patients with unstable angina (class B of the Braunwald classification) undergoing coronary arteriography followed by either coronary angioplasty (n = 20) or directional coronary atherectomy (n = 38) were studied. Fifteen patients were in class IB, and 43 were in class II to IIIB. Among these 43 patients with angina at rest, 28 had ST segment elevation during pain, 15 had ST segment depression, and 26 developed negative T waves on the baseline electrocardiogram as a result of prolonged or repeated episodes of resting chest pain. Intravascular ultrasound examination of the culprit lesion was performed in 43 patients before the interventional procedure, and histopathologic analysis of atherectomy

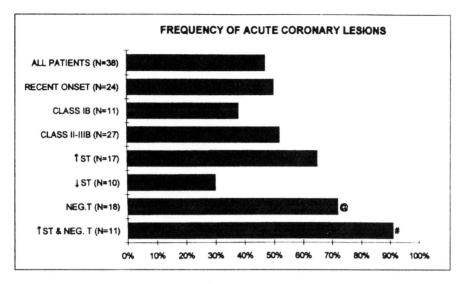

FIGURE 2-24. Frequency of acute coronary lesions (thrombus or intraplaque hemorrhage, or both) by histology in subsets of patients with unstable angina. Patients with negative T waves (NEG. T) and combined negative T waves on the baseline electrocardiogram and ST segment elevation (↑ST) during pain had a significantly higher incidence of acute coronary lesions. @p = .005; #p = .001. Reproduced with permission from De Servi et al.[60]

specimens was performed in 38 patients. Complex lesion morphology by angiography was observed in 31 patients (53%) without any significant relation to various clinical subsets. Patients in Braunwald class IB had more calcific plaques than did patients in class II to IIIB. Among patients with angina at rest, those with negative T waves on the baseline electrocardiogram, as well as those with transient ST elevation during pain, had a significantly higher incidence of noncalcific lesions. Analysis of atherectomy specimens revealed acute coronary lesions (thrombus and/or intraplaque hemorrhage) in 18 patients (47%). The incidence of acute coronary lesions was significantly higher in patients with than without negative T waves on the baseline electrocardiogram, and increased further when negative T waves were combined with ST elevation during pain. Multivariate analysis revealed that the presence of negative T waves on the baseline electrocardiogram was the only explanatory variable related to the presence of acute coronary lesions by histology. Patient subsets included in the broad spectrum of unstable angina have different morphological features and incidence of acute coronary lesions by histology. These data provide an explanation for the discrepant findings in published reports on the relevance of thrombus formation in the pathogenesis of unstable angina (Figure 2-24, Table 2-1).

Troponin-T and the Risk of Coronary Events

Lindahl and colleagues[61] from Uppsala, Sweden, have evaluated 976 patients participating in a randomized study of low molecular weight heparin in

TABLE 2-1
Angiographic Analysis of the Culprit Lesion (58 patients)

	Complex Morphology (No. of pts.)	Noncomplex Morphology (No. of pts.)
All patients (n = 58)	31	27
Recent onset (n = 40)	23	17
Class IB (n = 15)	9	6
Class II-IIIB (n = 43)	22	21
↑ST (n = 28)	14	14
↓ST (n = 15)	8	7
Neg. T waves (n = 26)	16	10
↑ST & Neg. T Waves (n = 17)	9	8

Neg. T Waves = negative T waves on baseline electrocardiogram; ↑ST = ST elevation during pain; ↓ST = ST depression during pain.
Reproduced with permission from De Servi et al.[60]

patients with unstable coronary heart disease who were followed for 5 months after their index episode. The risk of cardiac events increased with increasing maximal levels of troponin T obtained during the first 24 hours after hospital admission (Figure 2-25). The lowest quintile (<0.06 μg/L) constituted a low-risk group; the second quintile (0.06 to 0.18 μg/L) an intermediate-risk group; and the 3 highest quintiles (≥0.18 μg/L) a high-risk group with 4%, 11%, and 16% risk of either AMI or cardiac death, respectively. In a multivariate analysis, troponin T level, age, hypertension, number of antianginal drugs used, and

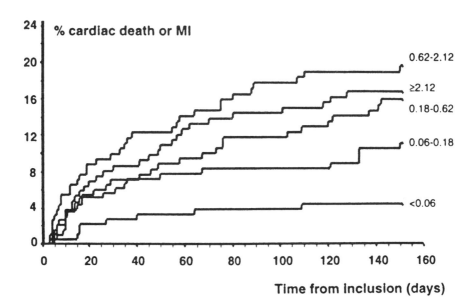

FIGURE 2-25. Cumulative risk and time of occurrence of cardiac death or myocardial infarction in groups based on quintiles of maximal tn-T levels (μg/L). The number of patients in each group (lowest through highest) was 187, 201, 190, 191, and 194, respectively. Pooled log rank p<.0001. Reproduced with permission from Lindahl et al.[61]

electrocardiographic changes at rest were identified as independent prognostic variables for AMI or cardiac death. Prognostic value of troponin T was independent of the classification of index event into unstable angina or AMI. Thus, these data indicate that troponin T determination provides important insight as regards the early risk for AMI or death in patients with unstable angina.

Temporal Relation Between Ischemic Episodes and Coagulation System

Biasucci and colleagues[62] in Rome, Italy, investigated the temporal relation between ischemic episodes and activation of the coagulation system in patients with unstable angina. Thrombin-antithrombin III and prothrombin fragment 1 + 2 levels were measured in 13 patients during spontaneous ischemic episodes at the onset of chest discomfort, and 5 and 15 minutes, and 1 hour later to evaluate the time course of the activation of the coagulation system associated with the development of ischemia. These same variables were measured in 28 patients with unstable angina on admission to the hospital and every 6 hours for 24 hours and daily for 3 days thereafter to assess their temporal relation with ischemic episodes. In the first protocol, thrombin-anti-

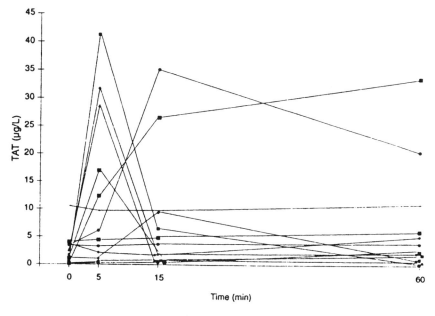

FIGURE 2-26. Time course of individual thrombin-antithrombin III (TAT) levels during spontaneous ischemia (protocol A). At time 0, all but 1 patient had normal TAT levels; at 5 minutes, values had increased in 6 patients, in 4 of whom it represented the peak value (median, 22.8 μg/L and range, 6.1 to 41.3 for the 6 patients; median, 6.1 and range, 0.3 to 41.3 for all 13 patients). In 2 other patients, the peak was reached at 15 minutes, at which time 3 patients continued to have elevated levels. In all but 2 patients, TAT levels returned to baseline at 1 hour; in 1 patient, levels increased further, and in another, TAT levels increased slightly only at 1 hour. Reproduced with permission from Biasucci et al.[62]

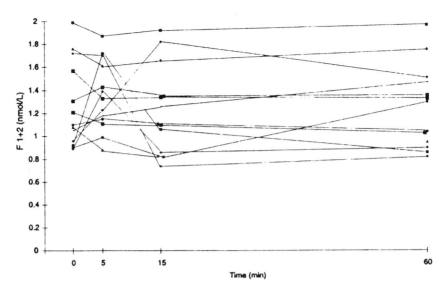

Figure 2-27. Time course of individual F_{1+2} levels during spontaneous ischemia (protocol A), p=NS. There is not a clear increase in F_{1+2} during the study. F_{1+2} was elevated in 5 patients at time 0, in 7 at 5 minutes (peak median value), in 5 at 15 minutes, and after 1 hour in 7 patients. Reproduced with permission from Biasucci et al.[62]

thrombin III and prothrombin fragment 1 + 2 were elevated in 10 of 13 patients (77%) in at least 1 sample. The median value of thrombin-antithrombin III showed a peak at 5 minutes and return to baseline within 15 minutes consistent with its plasma half-life of 5 minutes, whereas the median value of the prothrombin fragment 1 + 2 showed no significant changes (Figures 2-26 and 2-27). In the second protocol, activation of the clotting system was found in 10 of the 33 samples (30%) temporally related to ischemia and also in 23 of 150 (15%) of those not temporally related to ischemia. Thus, this study demonstrates that patients with active unstable angina develop frequent bursts of thrombin production not necessarily associated with ischemic episodes, and some ischemic episodes are not associated with systemic evidence of thrombin activation.

Increased Levels of B-Natriuretic Peptide

This study by Kikuta and colleagues[63] from Kumamoto, Japan, and Kyoto, Japan, was designed to examine the plasma levels of B-type or brain natriuretic peptide, as well as A-type or atrial natriuretic peptide in patients with unstable angina as compared with those in patients with stable exertional angina and control subjects. These investigators measured the plasma levels of brain natriuretic peptide and atrial natriuretic peptide in 33 patients with unstable angina, 20 patients with stable exertional angina, and 20 control subjects. The plasma levels of brain natriuretic peptide were significantly increased in patients with unstable angina compared with those in patients with stable exertional angina and control subjects, respectively (40 ± 29 pg/mL vs. 15 ± 8.0 pg/mL; and 40 ± 29 pg/mL vs. 10 ± 6.4 pg/mL; respectively). Conversely, there was no significant difference in the plasma levels of atrial natriuretic peptide among the 3 groups. Furthermore, in patients with unstable angina, the plasma levels of brain natriuretic peptide decreased significantly after medical treatment (from 40 ± 29 pg/mL to 16 ± 11 pg/mL), whereas the plasma levels of atrial natriuretic peptide did not change. It was concluded that the plasma levels of brain natriuretic peptide are increased in the majority of patients with unstable angina and that the increased levels decrease toward normal after treatment.

Plasma Protein Acute Phase Response

Liuzzo and colleagues[64] in Rome, Italy, determined whether ischemia-reperfusion injury causes elevated levels of C-reactive protein, which have been associated with an unfavorable clinical outcome in patients with unstable angina. They studied the temporal relation between plasma levels of C-reactive protein and ischemic episodes in 48 patients with unstable angina and 20 control patients with active variant angina in whom severe myocardial ischemia was caused by occlusive coronary artery spasm. Blood samples were obtained on admission and subsequently at 24, 48, 72, and 96 hours. All patients had Holter monitoring for the first 24 hours and remained in the coronary care unit under electrocardiographic monitoring until completion of the study. On admission, C-reactive protein was significantly higher in individuals with unstable angina than in those with variant angina (Figure 2-28). In unstable angina 70 ischemic episodes were observed, and in variant angina 192 ischemic episodes were observed during Holter monitoring. The plasma concentration of C-reactive protein did not increase in either group during the 96 hours of study, even in patients who had episodes of ischemia lasting more than 10 minutes. Thus, normal levels of C-reactive protein in individuals with variant angina and the failure of C-reactive protein values to increase in those with unstable angina indicate that transient myocardial ischemia, within the range of duration observed, does not cause a detectable acute-phase response.

Elevated Fibroblast Growth Factor

Fujita and colleagues[65] in Kyoto, Japan, hypothesized that angiogenic growth factors are produced by cardiac tissue, and because they are diffusible, they may be concentrated in pericardial fluids and increased in amounts by myocardial ischemia. To test this hypothesis, they used an enzyme-linked immunosorbent assay to measure the concentrations of basic fibroblast growth factor and vascular endothelial growth factor in pericardial fluids of 12 patients with unstable angina (group 1) and of 8 patients with nonischemic heart disease (group 2). The levels of protein in pericardial fluids were comparable between the 2 groups, but the concentration of basic fibroblast growth factor in the pericardial fluids in patients in group 1 was significantly higher than that in patients in group 2 (Figure 2-29). The amount of basic fibroblast growth

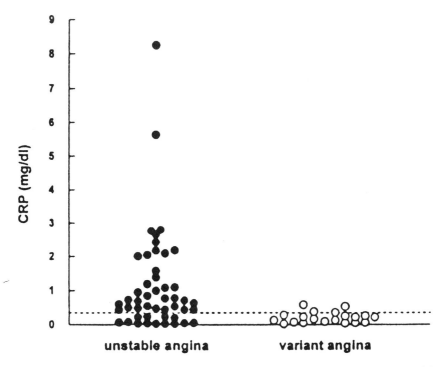

Figure 2-28. C-reactive protein (CRP) concentration in individual patients. Left, unstable angina (●); right, variant angina (○). CRP is <0.3 mg/dL in 90% of healthy subjects, shown by broken line. Reproduced with permission from Liuzzo et al.[64]

factor per milligram of protein was also higher in group 1 than in group 2. The concentration of vascular endothelial growth factor was not significantly different. These data suggest that basic fibroblast growth factor may play an important role in mediating collateral coronary artery growth in humans.

Macrophages, Smooth Muscle Cells, and Tissue Factor

Moreno and colleagues[66] in New York City, New York, and Boston, Massachusetts, identified the cellular correlations of tissue factor in patients with unstable angina. Tissue from 50 coronary specimens (1560 pieces) from patients with unstable angina and 15 specimens from patients with stable angina were analyzed. Total and segmental areas were identified with trichrome staining. Macrophages, smooth muscle cells, and tissue factor were identified by immunostaining. Tissue factor content was larger in unstable angina (42% ± 3%) than in stable angina (18% ± 4%) (p=.0001). Macrophage content was also larger in unstable angina (16% ± 2%) than in stable angina (5% ± 2%) (p=.002). The percentage of tissue factor located in cellular areas was larger in coronary samples from patients with unstable angina (67% ± 8%) than in samples from patients with stable angina (40% ± 5%). Multiple linear stepwise regression analysis showed that coronary tissue factor content correlated sig-

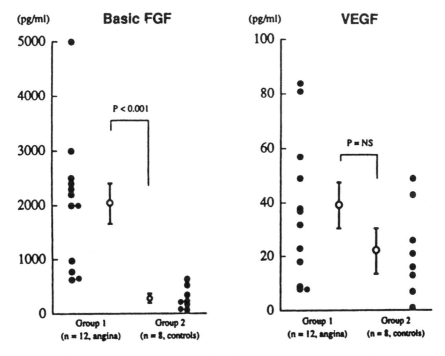

FIGURE 2-29. Concentrations of basic FGF (fibroblast growth factor) and VEGF (vascular endothelial growth factor) in pericardial fluids from patients with unstable angina (group 1) and nonischemic heart disease (group 2). Error bars indicate ± SEM. Reproduced with permission from Fujita et al.[65]

nificantly with macrophages and smooth muscle cells only in tissue from patients with unstable angina and that there was a strong relationship between tissue factor content and macrophages in the atheromatous gruel (r=.98, p<.0001). Thus, tissue factor content is increased in the atherosclerotic lesions in patients with unstable angina and correlates with areas of macrophages and smooth muscle cells, suggesting cell-mediated thrombogenicity in patients with acute coronary syndromes.

Neutrophil Platelet Adhesion

Ott and colleagues[67] obtained systemic venous blood samples from 25 patients with stable angina pectoris and 25 patients with unstable angina. Neutrophil activation and neutrophil-platelet adhesion were evaluated by 2-color flow cytometry. Patients with unstable angina showed a significant increase in neutrophil-based platelet adhesion compared with patients with stable angina (Figure 2-30). Systemic neutrophil activation was found in patients with unstable angina compared with those with stable angina. Markers of neutrophil activation were related to the extent of neutrophil-platelet adhesion. *In vitro* studies revealed that binding of purified platelet membranes to control neutrophils caused a dose-dependent increase in the surface expression of CD11b, a de-

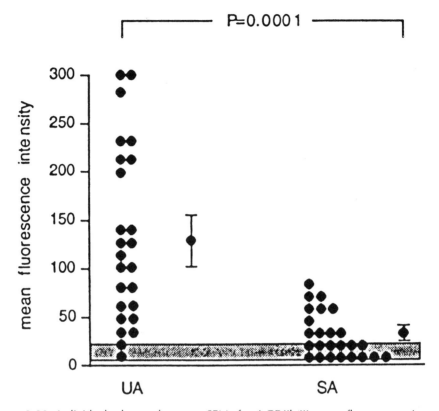

Figure 2-30. Individual values and mean ± SEM of anti-GP IIb/IIIa mean fluorescence intensity of neutrophils from patients with unstable angina (UA) and those with stable angina (SA). The gray bar represents the interquartile range of healthy control subjects. Reproduced with permission from Ott et al.[67]

crease in surface L-selectin, and the release of superoxide anions. Thus, this study demonstrates that increased neutrophil-platelet adhesion may contribute to neutrophil activation in patients with unstable angina.

Glycoprotein IIb/IIIa Antagonism: Randomized Trial

Théroux and colleagues[68] evaluated the potential of lamifiban, a novel nonpeptide antagonist of platelet glycoprotein IIb/IIIa receptors in the management of patients with unstable angina. In a prospective, dose-ranging, double-blind study, 365 patients with unstable angina were randomized to an infusion of 1, 2, 4, or 5 μg/min of lamifiban or of placebo. Treatment was administered for 72 to 120 hours. Outcome events were measured during the infusion period and after 1 month. Additional aspirin was administered to all patients and heparin to 28% of them. Lamifiban, when all doses were combined, reduced the risk of death, nonfatal AMI, or the need for urgent CABG or PTCA during the infusion period from 8% to 3% (p = .04) (Figure 2-31). The rates were 2.5%, 4.9%, 3%, and 2% with increasing doses. At 1 month, death or AMI occurred in 8% of patients with placebo and 2.5% of patients with the 2 highest doses (p = .03). The highest dose of lamifiban prevented the need for an urgent intervention. Lamifiban dose-dependently inhibited platelet aggregation. Bleeding times were more prolonged with platelet inhibition of greater than 80%. Major, but not life-threatening nor intracranial, bleeding occurred in 0.8% of patients with placebo and 3% with lamifiban. Thus, the nonpeptide platelet glycoprotein IIb/IIIa antagonist lamifiban protected patients with unstable angina from severe ischemic events during the 3- to 5-day infusion and reduced the incidence of death and AMI at 1 month, suggesting a possible role for therapy of similar patients with inhibitors of platelet glycoprotein IIb/IIIa receptors.

Schulman and colleagues[69] evaluated the effect of integrelin, which inhibits the platelet fibrinogen receptor glycoprotein IIb/IIIa, in 227 patients with unstable angina to determine its potential protective effects. Patients received intravenous heparin and standard anti-ischemic therapy and were randomly assigned to receive oral aspirin and placebo integrelin; placebo aspirin and low-dose integrelin (45 μg/kg bolus followed by a 0.5 μg/kg/min continuous infusion); or placebo aspirin and high-dose integrelin (90 μg/kg bolus followed by 1 μg/kg/min constant infusion). Integrelin was continued for 24 to 72 hours

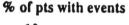

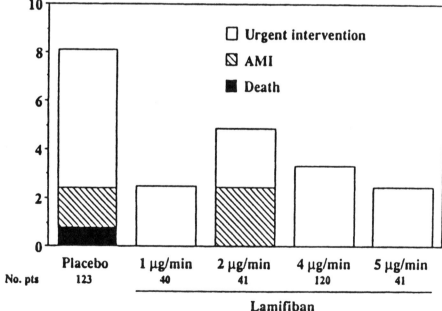

FIGURE 2-31. Incidence of events during study drug infusion in the 5 study groups. No death and no myocardial infarction occurred with the doses of 4 and 5 μg/min. The highest dose of lamifiban, in addition, prevented recurrent ischemia requiring an urgent intervention. AMI, acute myocardial infarction; pts, patients. Reproduced with permission from Théroux et al.[68]

and Holter monitoring was also performed. On Holter monitoring, patients randomly assigned to high-dose integrelin experienced 0.24 ± 0.11 ischemic episodes (mean ± standard error of the mean) lasting 8.4 ± 5.3 minutes over 24 hours of study drug infusion. Patients randomly assigned to aspirin experienced a greater number (1.0 ± 0.33) and longer duration (26 ± 9.8 minutes) of ischemic episodes than did the high-dose integrelin group (Figure 2-32). There was no evidence of rebound ischemia after withdrawal of the drug. In 46 patients, platelet aggregation was rapidly inhibited by integrelin in a dose-dependent fashion. The number of clinical events was small, and there were no bleeding differences in the 3 groups. Thus, intravenous integrelin is well tolerated, is a potent reversible inhibitor of platelet aggregation, and when added to full dose heparin, reduces the number and duration of Holter ischemic events in patients with unstable angina as compared with the events seen in patients treated with aspirin.

Restenosis after Coronary Intervention

Moreno and colleagues[70] tested the hypothesis that primary lesions associated with restenosis after coronary atherectomy have more macrophages and smooth muscle cells than do primary lesions not associated with restenosis. Fifty patients with unstable angina were identified. Total and segmental areas were quantified on trichrome-stained sections of coronary atherectomy tissue. Macrophages and smooth muscle cells were identified by immunohistochemical staining. Restenosis, defined as greater than 50% stenosis diameter by quantitative cineangiography, was present in 30 patients. The remaining 20 patients had less than 50% stenosis. The percentages of smooth muscle cell areas were similar in specimens from patients with and without restenosis (57% ± 5% and 52% ± 6%). Macrophage-rich areas were larger in plaque tissue from patients with restenosis (20% ± 2%) than in tissue from patients without restenosis (9% ± 2%) (p = .0007). Multiple, stepwise logistic regression analysis identified macrophages as the only independent predictor for restenosis (p = .006). Macrophages are increased in coronary atherectomy tissue from primary lesions that lead to restenosis, suggesting a possible role for macrophages in this process (Figure 2-33).

Interleukin-6 Levels

Biasucci and colleagues[71] in Rome, Italy, and Pomezia, Italy, measured levels of interleukin-6 in 38 patients with unstable angina at the time of their hospital admission to the coronary care unit and in 29 patients with stable angina. In the same groups of patients, they also measured C-reactive protein. Interleukin-6 was detectable in 23 (61%) of 38 patients with unstable angina, but in only 6 (21%) of 29 with stable angina (p<.01) (Figure 2-34). Interleukin-6 levels were undetectable in healthy volunteers. Median interleukin-6 levels were 5.3 pg/mL in patients with unstable angina, but were below the level of detection of the assay in patients with stable angina. A significant correlation

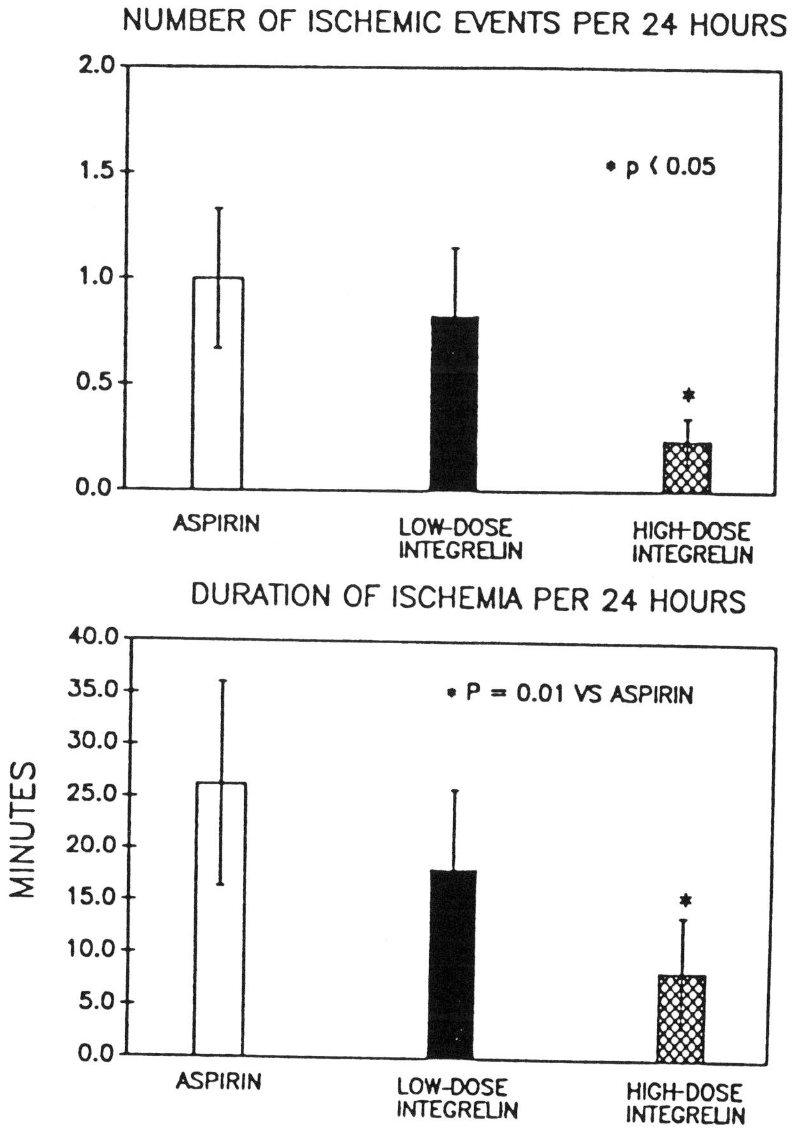

NUMBER OF ISCHEMIC EVENTS PER 24 HOURS

DURATION OF ISCHEMIA PER 24 HOURS

FIGURE 2-32. **Top:** Number of ischemic episodes per 24 hours on Holter monitoring for the 3 groups of patients in the efficacy analysis. Patients randomized to high-dose intravenous integrelin had significantly fewer episodes of Holter ischemia than did the aspirin group. Values are mean ± SEM. **Bottom:** Duration of ischemia per 24 hours on Holter monitoring for the 3 groups of patients in the efficacy analysis. The duration of Holter ischemia was significantly less in patients randomized to high-dose integrelin than it was with aspirin therapy. Values are mean ± SEM. Reproduced with permission from Schulman et al.[69]

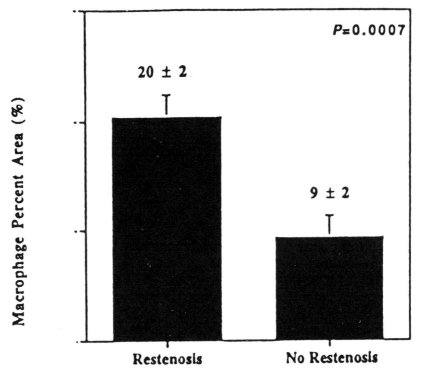

FIGURE 2-33. Increased percent area (mean ± SEM) of macrophages in tissue from primary coronary lesions of patients who developed restenosis vs. tissue from patients without restenosis at follow-up angiography 4 months after successful DCA. Reproduced with permission from Moreno et al.[70]

was observed between interleukin-6 and C-reactive protein levels. Thus, this study demonstrates that increased levels of interleukin-6 are common in patients with unstable angina, they correlate with C-reactive protein, and they suggest a role for the cytokine pathway in the production of inflammation in patients with unstable angina.

Thrombin Activity and Early Outcome

Ardissino and colleagues[72] in Milan, Italy, prospectively determined plasma concentrations in 24-hour urinary excretion of fibrinopeptide A in 150 patients with unstable angina. All patients had 24-hour Holter monitoring and urine collections. A blood sample was taken and coronary arteriography was performed. Patients were followed for the development of cardiac events, including death and myocardial infarction until they had CABG or were discharged from the hospital. Fibrinopeptide A plasma levels and 24-hour urinary excretion were found to be abnormally elevated in 50% and 45% of the patients, respectively. During hospitalization, 11 patients had AMI and 2 patients died. Kaplan-Meier analysis demonstrated a significantly higher probability of devel-

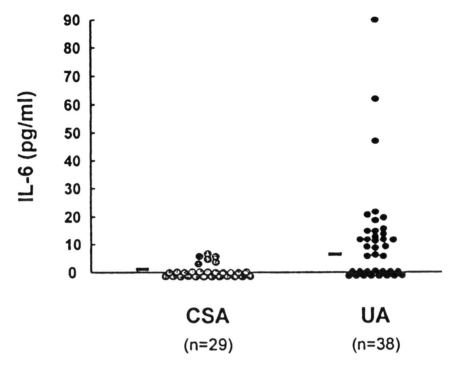

FIGURE 2-34. Levels of IL-6 (in picograms per milliliter) in patients with chronic stable angina (CSA) and in patients with unstable angina (UA). In CSA, levels of IL-6 were detectable in only 6 of 29 patients, and the median value was <3 pg/mL. Conversely, in UA patients, levels of IL-6 were detectable in 23 of 38 patients (p<.01 vs. CSA), and the levels ranged from 0 to 90 pg/mL (median value, 5.25 pg/mL; p<.01 vs. CSA). Reproduced with permission from Biasucci et al.[71]

oping cardiac events in patients with abnormal plasma levels of fibrinopeptide A than in those with normal levels (Figure 2-35). There was no difference in outcome between patients with normal and those with abnormal 24-hour urinary excretion. Cox regression analysis showed that the only variables independently related to an early unfavorable outcome were: 1) the presence of persistent ischemia during a 24-hour Holter monitoring; 2) intracoronary thrombosis at angiography; and 3) abnormal fibrinopeptide A plasma levels (Figure 2-36). Thus, patients with unstable angina pectoris and abnormal fibrinopeptide A levels are at increased risk for an early unfavorable outcome.

Nitric Oxide Inhibition of Continuing Platelet Activation

Platelet activation and thrombus formation within the coronary artery are major factors in AMI and unstable angina, and continuing platelet activation is associated with an adverse prognosis. Langford and coinvestigators[73] in London, United Kingdom, assessed platelet activation by using flow cytometry to measure platelet surface expression of P-selectin and glycoprotein IIb/IIIa in 20 patients with AMI and in 20 with unstable angina, all of whom were

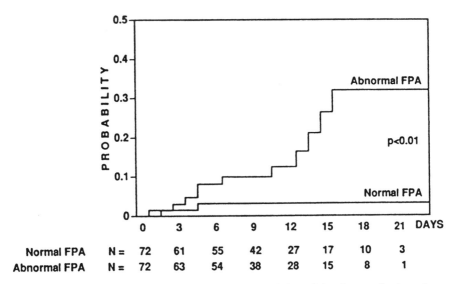

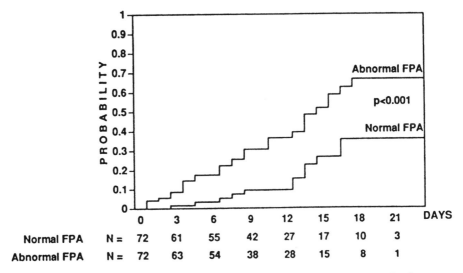

FIGURE 2-35. Kaplan-Meier curves comparing the probability of developing death or Q-wave or non-Q-wave myocardial infarction during hospitalization in patients with normal and abnormal fibrinopeptide A (FPA) plasma levels. Reproduced with permission from Ardissino et al.[72]

FIGURE 2-36. Kaplan-Meier curves comparing the probability of developing death, Q-wave or non-Q-wave myocardial infarction, or the need for emergency coronary revascularization during hospitalization in patients with normal and abnormal fibrinopeptide A (FPA) plasma levels. Reproduced with permission from Ardissino et al.[72]

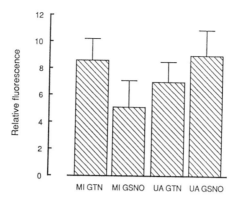

FIGURE 2-37. Bar graph showing fall in platelet surface expression of GPIIb/IIIa, which was reduced in both AMI (MI) and UA patients after intravenous infusion of GTN or GSNO. Data are mean ± SEM. Reproduced with permission from Langford et al.[73]

treated with aspirin. Platelet studies were repeated after the infusion of a nitric oxide donor (glyceryl trinitrate or S-nitrosoglutathione) that produced a fall in mean arteriolar pressure of no more than 10 mm Hg. P-selectin was expressed on 2.5% of platelets from AMI patients and on 2.3% of platelets from unstable angina patients, compared with 1% of platelets from 20 controlled volunteers without angina. Glycoprotein IIb/IIIa expression was 101 arbitrary units of relative fluorescence in AMI and 100 in unstable angina, compared with 88 in control subjects. In both AMI and unstable angina, S-nitrosoglutathione reduced P-selectin and glycoprotein IIb/IIIa expression, as did glyceryl trinitrate (Figure 2-37). In 3 of 20 patients receiving glyceryl trinitrate, the lowest dose was not tolerated because of headache or hypotension. These findings show that platelet activation persists in AMI and unstable angina despite aspirin treatment and that this can be inhibited by using glyceryl trinitrate or S-nitrosoglutathione. S-nitrosoglutathione is better tolerated at the doses required.

AMI

Chronobiology of Occurrence (CAST Study)

The onset of AMI has been shown to occur in a reproducible pattern with a peak in mid-morning and a secondary peak in late afternoon and early evening. More detailed information on the timing of this catastrophic event may provide important pathophysiological information. Using the database from the Holter Registry of the Cardiac Arrhythmia Suppression Trial (CAST) (n = 22,516), Peters and associates[74] for the CAST Investigators obtained the day of the week, the month, and season of the onset of AMI and correlated this information with demographic characteristics. The pattern of the day of onset for the entire population was significantly nonuniform, with a Monday

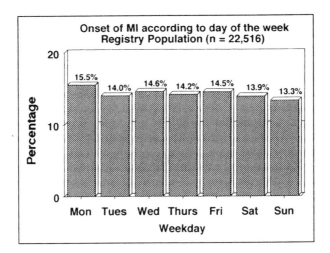

FIGURE 2-38. The day of onset of symptoms of acute myocardial infarction (MI) for the entire Cardiac Arrhythmia Suppression Trial registry population. The pattern is significantly nonuniform (p<.0001) with a Monday peak and a weekend nadir. Reproduced with permission from Peters et al.[74]

peak and a weekend nadir (Figure 2-38). The pattern was observed in most of the examined subgroups. Analysis of seasonal data revealed nonuniform distribution with a peak in winter and autumn (Figure 2-39). The authors concluded that AMI is not a random event but occurs in definite patterns related to the day of the week and the season of the year. These patterns were observed in a wide variety of patient subgroups and appear to be related to climate, occupation, and other factors.

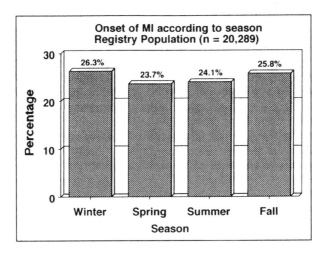

FIGURE 2-39. The seasonal distribution of onset of myocardial infarction (MI) for the Cardiac Arrhythmia Suppression Trial registry population. The distribution is significantly nonuniform (p<.001) with a peak in winter and autumn and a trough in spring and summer. Reproduced with permission from Peters et al.[74]

Seasonal Pattern of Occurrence

Identification of specific patterns in the timing of the onset of AMI is of importance because it implies that there are triggers external to the atherosclerotic plaque. From death certificate data, some investigators have noted a seasonal pattern in the death rate from AMI. Ornato and colleagues[75] for the participants in the National Registry of Myocardial Infarction evaluated whether the rate of hospital admission for AMI varied seasonally. Cases were submitted to the National Registry of Myocardial Infarction by 138 high-volume core hospitals over a 3-year period (December 21, 1990 through December 20, 1993). A total of 83,541 cases of AMI were reported to the registry during the study period. Approximately 10% more such cases were entered into the registry in winter or spring than in summer. The same trends were seen in both northern and southern states, men and women, patients younger than 70 years versus older than 70 years, and those with Q wave versus non-Q wave AMI. These authors concluded that there is a seasonal pattern to the reporting rate of cases of AMI in this registry base. This observation further supports the hypothesis that acute cardiovascular events may be triggered by events that are external to the atherosclerotic plaque.

Pathophysiology of Plaque Rupture

Atherosclerotic plaque rupture may occur when regions of weakened extracellular matrix are subjected to increased mechanical stresses. Because collagen is a major determinant of extracellular matrix strength, enzymes that degrade collagen may play an important role of destabilizing the atherosclerotic lesion. To test the hypothesis that matrix metalloproteinase 1, which initiates degradation of fibrillar collagens, co-localizes with increased stress in the fibrous cap of the atherosclerotic lesion, 12 unruptured human coronary lesions were studied by Lee and colleagues[76] in Boston, Massachusetts. Finite element analysis was used to determine the distribution of stress in the lesion, with estimates of material properties from previous measurements of human tissue. A computerized image analysis system was used to determine the distribution of immunoreactive matrix metalloproteinase 1 within the fibrous tissue of the lesion. There was a significant correlation between immunoreactive matrix metalloproteinase 1 and circumferential tensile stress in the fibrous cap within a given lesion. (Figure 2-40). Within a given lesion, the highest stress region had a 2-fold greater matrix metalloproteinase 1 expression than did the lower stress regions. In unruptured human atherosclerotic coronary lesions, overexpression of matrix metalloproteinase 1 is associated with increased circumferential stress in the fibrous plaque. Degradation and weakening of the collagenous extracellular matrix at these critical high-stress regions may play a role in the pathogenesis of plaque rupture and acute ischemic syndrome.

Determination of TIMI Flow Grade by Doppler

Kern and colleagues[77] attempted to compare different TIMI angiographic flow grades (flow grades based on results of the Thrombolysis In Myocardial

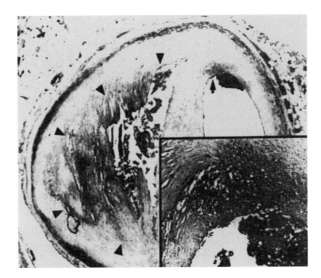

FIGURE 2-40. Digital image of histological section of moderately stenotic atherosclerotic lesion in a native coronary artery stained by the immunoperoxidase technique using antibodies to MMP-1 (magnification × 16). Inset, Higher-power image of region of lesion with MMP-1 overexpression (red-brown color), marked by dark arrows (magnification × 100). The Spearman correlation coefficient for this specimen was .59. Reproduced with permission from Lee et al.[76]

Infarction trial) with intracoronary blood flow velocity using Doppler guide-wires during primary or rescue PTCA in 41 patients with AMI. The coronary flow velocity measured by the Doppler catheter was compared with a TIMI grade and cineframes-to-opacification count. Prior to PTCA, 34 patients had TIMI grade 0 or 1, 5 had TIMI grade 2, and 2 had TIMI grade 3 flow in the infarct-related artery. Flow velocity was similar among patients with TIMI grades 0, 1, or 2, but was lower than in those with TIMI grade 3 flow (Figure 2-41). After PTCA, 1 patient had TIMI grade 1, 5 had TIMI 2, and 35 had TIMI 3 flow. Poststenotic flow velocity increased from 6.6 to 20 cm/s. TIMI grade 3 flow increased to 21.8 ± 10.9 cm/s after PTCA. Although post-PTCA flow velocity correlated with angiographic cineframes-to-opacification count, there was a large overlap with TIMI grades of 2 or less that had low flow velocity (Figure 2-42). Nine of 11 clinical events, including unstable angina and need for CABG occurred in patients with low coronary flow velocity. Thus, determination of flow velocity after reperfusion may enhance patient characterization and provide the physiological rationale for clinical variations after reperfusion therapy.

Length of Hospital Stay

Hospital length of stay is an important contributor to the cost of cardiac care. Every and colleagues.[78] from Seattle, Washington, and Stanford, California, sought to identify current trends in length of stay in patients with acute myocardial infarction. They evaluated length of stay in 11,932 patients with acute myocardial infarction admitted to 19 Seattle area hospitals between 1988

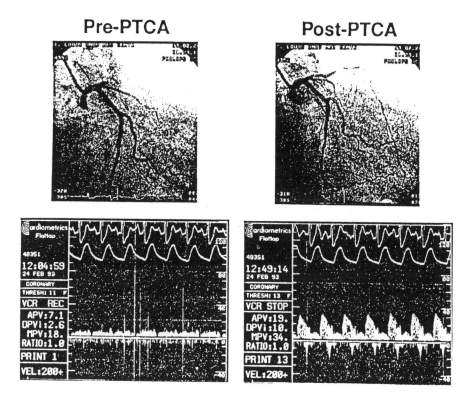

FIGURE 2-41. Coronary angiography (**top**) and corresponding poststenotic flow velocity spectra (**bottom**) before and after angioplasty of a proximal LAD coronary artery during acute anterior MI. Flow velocity panels display (from top to bottom) electrocardiogram, aortic pressure, and velocity spectra (velocity scale 0 to 160 cm/s full scale). Bottom left, average peak velocity (APV) before angioplasty for TIMI flow grade 0 or 1 was 7.1 cm/s; bottom right, after angioplasty, APV for TIMI flow grade 3 was 19 cm/s with normal phasic pattern. PTCA, percutaneous transluminal coronary angioplasty; DPVi, diastolic peak velocity integral; MPV, maximal peak velocity. Reproduced with permission from Kern et al.[77]

and 1994. Length of hospital stay decreased from 8.5 to 6.0 days during the study period. None of the measured variables, such as clinical characteristics or use of angioplasty explained the 29% reduction in length of stay that occurred between 1988 and 1994. They concluded that unmeasured economic and administrative factors played important roles in influencing the hospital length of stay.

Risk Factors for AMI

Depression

Barefoot and colleagues[79] in Durham, North Carolina, evaluated whether depression plays a role in the initial development of CAD among 409 men and

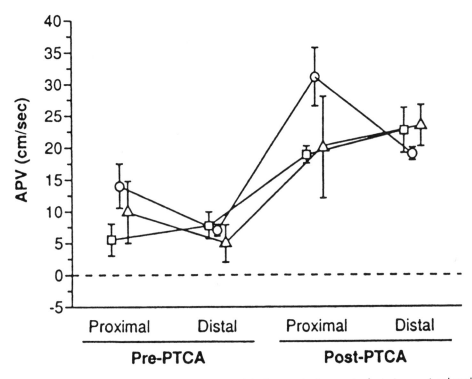

FIGURE 2-42. Average peak velocity (APV, cm/s) before and after angioplasty in proximal and poststenotic (distal) target vessel regions. PTCA, percutaneous transluminal coronary angioplasty; ○, left anterior descending artery; △, circumflex artery; □, right coronary artery. Reproduced with permission from Kern et al.[77]

321 women who were residents of Glostrup, Denmark, born in 1914. Physical and psychological examinations in 1964 and 1974 established baseline risk factors and disease status and their level of depressive symptomatology. Initial AMI was observed in 122 participants. There were 290 deaths during follow-up, which ended in 1991. A 2 standard deviation difference in depression score was associated with the relative risks of 1.71 for AMI and 1.6 for death from all causes. These findings were unchanged after the authors' controlled for risk factors and signs of disease at baseline. There were no sex differences in the impact of these variables on risk of AMI and death. Thus, these data suggest that high levels of depressive symptomatology are associated with increased risk of MI and death.

Natural Disasters (Northridge Earthquake)

On January 17, 1994, at 4:30 AM, southern California was shocked by a magnitude 6.7 earthquake resulting in "the strongest ground motion ever recorded in an urban setting in North America." The Northridge Earthquake caused the greatest financial losses from any natural disaster in the United States. Casualties included more than 29 deaths and 7000 injuries as a direct

TABLE 2-2
**Coronary Care Unit Admissions and Related In-Hospital Mortality
Before and After the Earthquake**

	Before Earthquake (January 10–16, 1994)	After Earthquake (January 17–23, 1994)
Admission (% of total admission)		
Myocardial infarction	149 (13%)	201 (17%)*
Unstable angina	261 (24%)	280 (23%)
Total coronary care unit admissions	1,102 (100%)	1,201 (100%)
Mortality (% of admission)		
Myocardial infarction	10 (7%)	13 (6%)
Unstable angina	3 (1%)	0 (0%)
Total coronary care unit admissions	67 (6%)	63 (5%)

* $p=0.02$ by Cochran-Mantel-Haenszel statistic controlling for hospital.

Numbers within parentheses refer to percentage of total admissions.

Reproduced with permission from Leor et al.[80]

result of the earthquake. The week after the earthquake was characterized by thousands of aftershocks; 20,000 people remained homeless and thousands of homes remained without electricity, gas, and water. The Northridge Earthquake afforded an opportunity to investigate the possible relation between extensive environmental disaster and the risk of acute coronary events. Leor and associates[80] from Los Angeles, California, therefore investigated the impact of this stressful event on the incidence of acute coronary events. One month after the earthquake, the authors mailed a questionnaire to 189 hospitals in southern California. The questionnaire evaluated the number of admissions with AMI or unstable angina, total coronary care unit admissions, and related in-hospital mortality during the week before (January 10–16, 1994) and the week after the earthquake (January 17–23, 1994). One hundred and nine hospitals responded to the questionnaire. Twenty-nine hospitals did not have an active coronary care unit at the time of the earthquake. One coronary care unit refused to participate in the study. Of the remaining 79 coronary care units, the authors excluded 7 because they were completely or temporarily closed after the earthquake or provided incomplete data. Thus, the final analysis was performed in 72 coronary care units. The average of admissions per coronary care unit increased from 15 ± 13 in the week before the earthquake to 17 ± 13 in the week after the earthquake (Table 2-2). There was a 35% increase in the number of admissions with AMI after the earthquake (from 149 to 201). Admissions with AMI as a percent of total coronary care admissions increased from 13% to 17%. For unstable angina, the difference between the week before and after was not significant.

Triggering MI by Sexual Activity

Muller and colleagues[81] in Boston, Massachusetts, determined the relative risks of nonfatal AMI triggered by sexual activity among the general population and in patients with prior CAD. Relative risks and effect modification were calculated by the case-crossover method. The case-crossover method is a new epidemiological technique designed to quantify the transient change in risk after exposure to a potential disease trigger. A total of 1774 patients with AMI were interviewed in 45 hospitals throughout the United States. Data were gathered on potential triggers of AMI occurring immediately prior to the event and during the previous year. Results are presented for the 858 patients who were sexually active in the year prior to the AMI, with special attention to 273 patients who had CAD prior to their index MI and the effect of regular exertion on risk. Among 858 patients, 79 (9%) reported sexual activity in the 24 hours preceding AMI and 27 (3%) reported sexual activity in the 2 hours preceding symptoms of AMI. The relative risk of AMI occurring in the 2 hours after sexual activity was 2.5. The relative risk of triggering onset of AMI among patients with a history of prior angina or prior MI was not greater than that observed in those without prior cardiac disease. Sexual activity was a likely contributor to the onset of AMI in only 0.9% of cases, and regular exertion was associated with decreasing risk. Thus, sexual activity can trigger the onset of AMI. However, the relative risk is low, approximately 1 chance in 1 million for a healthy individual. The relative risk is not increased in patients with a prior history of cardiac disease, and regular exercise appears to prevent this relation.

Diagnosis and Early Testing in AMI

Serum Creatine Kinase and MB Fraction Elevations

Müllner and associates[82] from Vienna, Austria, described the course of serum creatine kinase (CK) and its MB fraction in patients surviving cardiac arrest, and they identified factors influencing CK and CK-MB release. Data concerning cardiopulmonary resuscitation, collected within a period of 33 months, were evaluated retrospectively and compared with laboratory blood investigations collected prospectively in 107 adult patients surviving a witnessed cardiac arrest. CK and CK-MB were elevated in more than 75% of the patients within 24 hours. Release of CK and CK-MB was mainly associated with electrocardiographic evidence of AMI, cumulative energy administered during defibrillation, and duration of chest trauma by compression. The CK-MB/CK ratio was elevated in 32% of the patients. Of patients with electrocardiographic evidence of AMI, only 49% had an elevated CK-MB/CK ratio. In conclusion, the elevation in serum CK and CK-MB fraction in patients after nontraumatic cardiac arrest is a frequent finding, and it is associated with ischemic myocardial injury, as well as physical trauma to the chest. This should be considered when interpreting the course of CK and CK-MB fraction for the diagnosis of AMI.

Electrocardiography to Predict Infarct-Related Artery

Midgette and associates[83] from several United States medical centers developed a scoring system to predict the artery responsible for AMI using ST-segment and T-wave changes on the initial electrocardiogram from 228 patients (development set) with symptoms compatible with AMI. This scoring system was tested in a similar group of 223 patients (test set) from the Thrombolysis and Angioplasty in Myocardial Infarction (TAMI-5) Trial. Using stepwise logistic regression, the authors were able to accurately predict LAD, right, or left coronary artery as the infarct-related artery by using 2 variables: (1) the summation of the ST-segment elevation in leads V_1 to V_4, and (2) the summation of the T-wave negativity in leads I, aVL, and V_5. In the development set, these 2 variables demonstrated respective sensitivity and specificity of 98% and 90% for LAD lesions, 82% and 85% for right coronary narrowings, and 82% and 84% for left coronary narrowings. In the test set, the sensitivity and specificity were 97% and 95% for LAD lesions, 85% and 86% for right coronary artery lesions, and 73% and 60% for left coronary artery lesions. Information easily obtained on the electrocardiogram can accurately predict the likelihood of the LAD, right, or left coronary artery as the infarct-related artery. This may be useful in the decision to administer thrombolytic treatment.

Electrocardiography: Correlation with Infarct Size and Long-Term Prognosis

Previous studies have shown an association between distortion of the terminal portion of the QRS (QRS [+]) pattern: emergence of the J point of 50% or greater of the R wave in leads with qR configuration, or disappearance of the S wave in leads with an Rs configuration) on admission and in-hospital mortality in AMI. The mechanism for this association, however, is not known. Birnbaum and associates[84] for the TIMI 4 Investigators assessed the relation between QRS (+) pattern and coronary angiographic findings, infarct size, and long-term prognosis in the Thrombolysis In Myocardial Infarction 4 trial. Patients were allocated into 2 groups based on the presence (QRS [+], n=85) or absence (QRS[−], n=293) of QRS distortion. The QRS (+) patients were older (mean ± SD: 61.1 ± 10.6 vs. 57.5 ± 10.6 years), had more anterior AMI (49% vs. 37%), and less previous angina (42% vs. 54%). QRS (+) patients had larger infarct size as assessed by creatine kinase release over 24 hours (209 ± 147 vs. 155 ± 129), and predischarge sestamibi (MIBI) defect (17.9 ± 15.9% vs. 11.2 ± 13.4%). One-year mortality (18% vs. 6%) was higher and the weighted end point of death, reinfarction, heart failure, or LVEF <40% (0.33 ± 0.37 vs. 0.24 ± 0.32) tended to be higher in the anterior AMI patients with QRS (+). No difference in clinical outcome was found in patients with nonanterior AMI. These findings suggest that this simple electrocardiographic definition of presence of QRS (+) pattern on admission may provide an early estimation of infarct size and long-term prognosis, especially in anterior AMI (Figures 2-43–2-45) (Table 2-3).

Electrocardiography: ST Segment Depression in Risk Stratification

Precordial ST segment depression has been associated with a poor prognosis in patients with inferior myocardial infarction. Peterson and colleagues

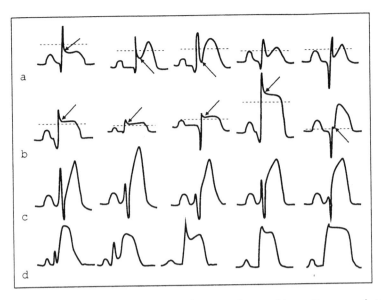

FIGURE 2-43. Illustrations of electrocardiographic complexes without *(lines a and c)* and with *(lines b and d)* terminal QRS distortion. Terminal QRS distortion (QRS[+]) is defined as emergence of the J point ≥50% of the R-wave amplitude in leads with qR configuration or disappearance of the S wave in leads with an R_5 configuration. To be included in the QRS(+) group, at least 2 adjacent leads demonstrated terminal QRS distortion. Line a: QR complexes with QRS(−) pattern. Despite different degree of ST-segment elevation, in all complexes the J point *(arrow)* emerges below 50% of the R-wave amplitude *(dashed line)*. Line b: QR complexes with QRS(+) pattern. In all complexes, the J point emerges above 50% of the R-wave amplitude. Line c: RS complexes with QRS(−) configuration (leads V_1 to V_3). In all complexes the S wave is preserved (compared with line d). Line d: complexes in leads usually demonstrating RS pattern (V_1 to V_3) with QRS(+) pattern showing different magnitude of ST-segment elevation. However, in all complexes S wave disappeared. Reproduced with permission from Birnbaum et al.[84]

TABLE 2-3
Clinical Outcome of Patients with Versus Without Distortion of the Terminal Portion of the QRS

In-Hospital End Points	QRS (+) Group (n=85) No. (%)	QRS (−) Group (n=293) No. (%)	p Value
In-hospital mortality	5 (6)	10 (3)	0.31
Severe CHF/shock	1 (1)	4 (1)	0.89
Recurrent ischemic pain	14 (21)*	59 (28)*	0.26
Reinfarction	5 (6)	16 (5)	0.881
Death/reinfarction/CHF/LVEF <40%	26 (31)	62 (21)	0.070
Weighted end point for death/reinfarction/ CHF/LVEF <40% (mean ± SD)	0.21±0.33	0.14±0.28	0.06
Q-wave infarction	62 (74)*	168 (61)*	0.03
One yr mortality	9 (11)	16 (6)	0.09

CHF = congestive heart failure; LVEF = left ventricular ejection fraction.

* Total number value is lower in these categories.

Reproduced with permission from Birnbaum et al.[84]

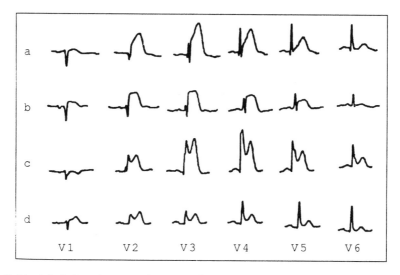

FIGURE 2-44. Admission electrocardiograms of 4 patients with anterior wall acute myocardial infarction (recorded at a paper speed of 25 mm/s; sensitivity: 1 mV = 10 mm). Examples *a* and *b* are of QRS(−) pattern. Despite having a high degree of ST segment elevation, the S waves in leads V_2 and V_3 are preserved and the J points emerge below 50% of the R waves. Examples *c* and *d* are of QRS(+) pattern. Despite having a different magnitude of ST segment elevation, in both examples the S waves in leads V_2 and V_3 disappeared, and in example *c* the J points in leads V_2 and V_3 emerge at greater than 50% of the R-wave height. Reproduced with permission from Birnbaum et al.[84]

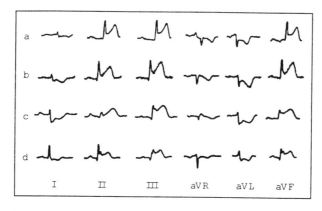

FIGURE 2-45. Admission electrocardiograms of 4 patients with inferior wall acute myocardial infarction (recorded at a paper speed of 25 mm/s; sensitivity: 1 mV = 10 mm). Examples *a* and *b* are of QRS(−) pattern. The J points in leads II, III, and aVF emerge at <50% of the R-wave height. Examples *c* and *d* are of QRS(+) pattern, because the J points in leads III and aVF emerge at greater than 50% of the R-wave height. Reproduced with permission from Birnbaum et al.[84]

from Durham, North Carolina; Cleveland, Ohio; Ann Arbor, Michigan; and Rotterdam, The Netherlands, sought to evaluate the quantitative prognostic significance of precordial ST segment depression in patients with an inferior AMI. They examined the clinical and angiographic outcomes of 16,521 patients with an inferior AMI who underwent thrombolysis in the GUSTO-I study. Patients with precordial ST segment depression had larger infarctions, more post-infarction complications, and a higher mortality than did those without precordial segment depression (4.7% vs. 3.2% of 30 days; 5.0% vs. 3.4% at 1 year). The magnitude of precordial ST segment depression (sum of leads V_1 to V_6) added significant independent prognostic information after adjustment for clinical risk factors. The risk of 30-day mortality increased by 36% for every 0.5 mV of precordial ST segment depression. These authors concluded that assessment of the magnitude of precordial ST segment depression is useful for acute risk stratification in patients with an inferior AMI.

Early Diagnosis by Echocardiographic Stress Tests

Schröder and associates[86] from Berlin, Germany, assessed and compared the diagnostic potential of submaximal exercise, transesophageal atrial pacing, dipyridamole, and dobutamine-atropine stress echocardiography tests shortly after AMI in 121 study patients. In those patients, 325 digital echocardiographic tests were attempted 10 to 11 days after AMI, including the following: 83 submaximal exercise tests; 121 high-dose dipyridamole echocardiography tests (DET); 69 transesophageal atrial pacing tests (<150 beats per minute), and 52 dobutamine tests, starting at 10 μg/kg per minute and increasing stepwise to 40 μg/kg per minute. In the dobutamine tests, atropine was co-administered in 12 patients (dobutamine-atropine stress echocardiography [DASE]. Results were correlated to a coronary artery diameter stenosis of 50% or greater as determined by quantitative angiography. Feasibility to perform submaximal exercise echocardiography, atrial pacing echocardiography, DET, and DASE was 89%, 52%, 98%, and 88%, respectively. Atrial pacing was not tolerated by 18 patients and was refused by 6 (9%). Severe, but not life-threatening, side effects included hypotension in DET (2%) and tachyarrhythmias in DASE (6%). Test positivity in multivessel disease with submaximal exercise, DET, and DASE was 55%, 93%, and 90%, respectively, and in 1-vessel disease 47%, 65%, 71%, and for atrial pacing, 82%, respectively. The authors concluded that submaximal exercise has limited sensitivity and atrial pacing, limited feasibility. The pharmacologic stressors provide a useful, safe diagnostic approach: DET with slightly lower sensitivity in 1-vessel disease, and DASE with insignificantly less feasibility.

Echocardiography and Thallium Scintigraphy to Assess Myocardial Viability

Spontaneous improvement of contraction and perfusion occurs after AMI. The relative merit of low-dose dobutamine stress echocardiography and rest-redistribution thallium scintigraphy after recent AMI has not been evaluated. Elhendy and associates[87] from Rotterdam, The Netherlands, studied 30 patients at 7 ± 3 days after AMI with low-dose dobutamine stress echocardiography (5 to 10 μg/kg/min) and rest-redistribution thallium scintigraphy SPECT. Viability was defined as improvement of wall thickening at low-dose dobutamine stress echocardiography in the presence of redistribution or a defect with uptake greater than or equal to 50% of peak activity at rest-redistribution thallium scintigraphy. Baseline echocardiography and rest-redistribution thallium scintigraphy were repeated after 3 months. Of 112 dyssynergic segments, viability was detected in 60 (54%) by rest-redistribution thallium scintigraphy and in 39 (35%) by low-dose dobutamine stress echocardiography. Spontaneous improvement of function was detected in 35 (31%) segments. In the same regions, thallium uptake increased significantly. The sensitivity, specificity, and accuracy of low-dose dobutamine stress echocardiography for predicting late improvement of wall motion were 77%, 84%, and 82%, respectively. Specificity and accuracy of low-dose dobutamine stress echocardiography were higher than rest-redistribution thallium scintigraphy. It was concluded that a myocardial viability pattern after AMI is more frequently detected by rest-redistribution thallium scintigraphy than by low-dose dobutamine stress echocardiography. Both techniques are equally sensitive, but low-dose dobutamine stress echocardiography is a more specific predictor of spontaneous recovery of regional left ventricular function.

Ultrasonic Backscatter (In Old MI)

The purpose of this study by Naito and associates[88] from Suita, Japan, and Osaka, Japan, was to clarify whether the abnormalities in integrated backscatter may be used to assess myocardial viability in patients with old myocardial infarction. Integrated backscatter parameters were compared with conventional radionuclide and echocardiographic estimates of myocardial viability. Two myocardial integrated backscatter parameters, the magnitude of cyclic variation in integrated backscatter, and the myocardial integrated backscatter, calibrated with the power of Doppler signals from the blood along the same ultrasound beam (calibrated myocardial integrated backscatter), were measured in 21 normal persons and in 33 patients with old anteroseptal myocardial infarction. Calibrated myocardial integrated backscatter was higher and the magnitude of cyclic variation in integrated backscatter was lower in the infarct septum than in the normal septum. Percent thallium uptake, as assessed in scintigraphic images taken at rest or after reinjection, correlated well with the calibrated myocardial integrated backscatter and more weakly but significantly with the magnitude of cyclic variation in integrated backscatter in 16 of 33 patients. The measurement of calibrated myocardial integrated backscatter, in addition to the magnitude of cyclic variation of integrated backscatter, may be valuable in the noninvasive assessment of myocardial viability.

Cost-Effectiveness of Routine Angiography

Coronary angiography is indicated for many patients after AMI. There are a number of subgroups of AMI patients, however, for whom the indication for coronary angiography is not well established. Kuntz and associates[89] developed a decision-analytic model for AMI in representative patient subgroups based on relevant clinical characteristics. The model estimates quality-adjusted life expectancy and direct lifetime costs for two strategies: coronary angiography and treatment guided by its results versus initial medical therapy without angiography. Decision-tree chance node probabilities were estimated with the use of pooled data from randomized clinical trials and other relevant literature, costs were estimated with the use of the Medicare Part A database, and quality-of-life adjustments were derived from a survey of 1051 patients who had had a recent AMI. In their analysis, incremental cost-effectiveness ratios for coronary angiography and treatment guided by its result, compared with initial medical therapy without angiography, ranged between $17,000 and more than $1 million per quality-adjusted year of life gained. Patient subgroups with severe postinfarction angina or a strongly positive exercise tolerance test typically had cost-effectiveness ratios of less than $50,000 per quality-adjusted year of life gained. In addition, most patient subgroups with a prior AMI had cost-effectiveness ratios of less than $50,000 per quality-adjusted year of life gained, even with a negative ETT result. In many patient subgroups after AMI, the cost-effectiveness of routine coronary angiography and treatment guided by its results compares favorably with other treatment strategies for coronary heart disease (Table 2-4).

Prognostic Indicators for AMI

Age

Køber and associates[90] from multiple centers on behalf of the TRACE Study Group assessed the importance of CHF and LV systolic dysfunction after an AMI on long-term mortality in different age groups. A total of 7001 consecutive enzyme-confirmed AMIs (6676 patients) were screened for entry into the TRAndolapril Cardiac Evaluation (TRACE) study. Medical history, echocardiographic estimation of LV systolic function determined as wall motion index, infarct complications, and survival were documented for all patients. To study the importance of CHF and wall motion index independent of age, we performed Cox proportional-hazard models in 4 different age strata (less than or equal to 55 years, 56 to 65 years, 66 to 75 years, and more than 75 years). Patients in these strata had 1-year mortality rates of 5%, 11%, 21%, and 32%, respectively. Three-year mortality rates were 11%, 20%, 34%, and 55%, respectively. The risk ratios (and 95% confidence limits) associated with CHF in the same 4 age strata were 1.9 (1.3 to 2.9), 2.8 (2.1 to 3.7), 1.8 (1.5 to 2.2), and 1.8 (1.5 to 2.2), respectively. The risk ratios associated with decreasing wall motion index were 6.5 (3.6 to 11.4), 3.3 (2.3 to 4.6), 2.7 (2.2 to 3.4), and 2.1 (1.7 to 2.6), respectively. In absolute percentages, there was an excess 3-year mortality

TABLE 2-4
Incremental Quality-Adjusted Life Expectancy, Cost, and Cost-Effectiveness Ratios for Routine Coronary Angiography Compared With Initial MEDS: Strongly Positive ETT Result and Prior AMI

Age/Gender	No CHF			CHF		
	ΔQALE	ΔCost	ΔC/ΔE*	ΔQALE	ΔCost	ΔC/ΔE*
Mild postinfarction angina, ETT**, LVEF 0.20–0.49, and prior AMI						
Men						
35–44 y	1.16	15 200	18 300	1.05	15 700	20 100
45–54 y	1.47	19 000	16 900	1.18	19 500	20 700
55–64 y	1.32	20 600	19 300	0.90	20 600	27500
65–74 y	1.07	23 300	25 800	0.61	23 000	43 300
75–84 y	0.92	29 600	35 800	0.40	28 000	77 500
Women						
35–44 y	0.58	11 600	32 300	0.48	11 700	37 700
45–54 y	0.92	15 600	24 400	0.77	16 000	29 400
55–64 y	1.29	18 200	18 400	0.93	18 700	24 900
65–74 y	1.03	20 800	24 300	0.60	20 600	40 400
75–84 y	1.25	30 800	28 200	0.52	28 600	61 900
Mild postinfarction angina, ETT**, LVEF ≥ 0.50, and prior AMI						
Men						
35–44 y	0.76	11 700	23 100	0.78	12 200	22 400
45–54 y	1.18	15 300	18 100	1.12	15 900	19 000
55–64 y	1.28	17 200	17 800	1.08	17 700	20 800
65–74 y	1.32	20 500	19 400	0.94	20 700	26 600
75–84 y	1.56	29 300	21 800	0.91	28 100	34 800
Women						
35–44 y	0.28	8 700	52 800	0.27	8 900	55 600
45–54 y	0.56	11 800	33 000	0.54	12 200	34 500
55–64 y	1.06	14 900	18 500	0.95	15 400	21 100
65–74 y	1.10	17 400	20 100	0.61	17 700	26 900
75–84 y	1.99	30 600	18 300	1.20	29 100	26 300

QALE indicates quality-adjusted life expectancy; ΔC/ΔE, incremental cost-effectiveness ratio; and ETT**, exercise tolerance test result with ≥2-mm ST segment depression.
* Life-years and costs are discounted at 3% per year.
Reproduced with permission from Kuntz et al.[89]

associated with CHF in the 4 age strata of 14%, 24%, 25%, and 28%, respectively. The absolute excess in 3-year mortality associated with LV systolic dysfunction in the 4 age strata was 15%, 19%, 25%, and 21%, respectively. Thus, the relative importance of LV systolic dysfunction and CHF diminished with increasing age. However, the absolute excess mortality associated with CHF and LV systolic dysfunction was more pronounced in the elderly than in the young (Figure 2-46).

Smoking, Serum Lipids, and Gender Differences

Njølstad and colleagues[91] in Tromsø, Norway, evaluated the associations between smoking, serum lipids, blood pressure, and MI in a population-based

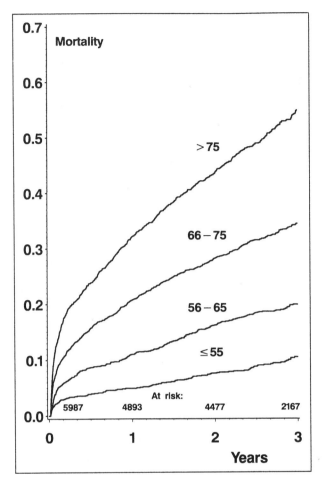

FIGURE 2-46. Long-term mortality of patients according to age. The patients were alive at day 6 after acute myocardial infarction and were divided into 4 groups: ≤55 years, 56 to 65 years, 66 to 75 years, and >75 years. Reproduced with permission from Køber et al.[90]

prospective study of 11,843 men and women aged 35 to 52 years at entry. During a 12-year period, 495 cases of first MI among men and 103 cases among women were identified. The incidence of MI was 4.6 times higher among men. The incidence was increased 6-fold in women and 3-fold in men who smoked at least 20 cigarettes per day compared with never-smokers, and the rate in female heavy smokers exceeded that of never-smoking men. Multivariate analysis identified current smoking as a stronger risk factor in women than in men. Among those under 45 years of age at entry, the smoking-related sex difference was more pronounced (Table 2-5). Serum total cholesterol, HDL cholesterol, and systolic blood pressure were also highly significant predictors in both sexes. Thus, these data indicate that smoking is a stronger risk factor for MI in middle-aged women than in men. Relative risks associated with serum lipids and blood pressure were similar despite large sex differences in MI incidence rates.

TABLE 2-5
Age-Adjusted Incidence Rates of Myocardial Infarction per 1000 Person-Years, Relative Risk, and 95% Confidence Interval According to Serum HDL Cholesterol and Smoking Status by Sex: The Finnmark Study, 1977–1989

HDL Cholesterol, mmol/L	Daily Smoking							
	Yes				No			
	Cases, n	Rate per 1000	Relative Risk*	95% CI	Cases, n	Rate per 1000	Relative Risk*	95% CI
	Men							
<1.00	104	13.00	1.00	ref	36	7.73	1.00	ref
1.00–1.49	208	8.91	0.77	0.60–0.97	79	4.69	0.70	0.47–1.05
1.50†	43	4.74	0.43	0.30–0.61	25	3.20	0.46	0.27–0.77
p, test for trend			.0001					.0029
	Women							
<1.00	8	4.75	1.00	ref	2	1.57	1.00	ref
1.00–1.49	42	2.93	0.72	0.33–1.56	20	1.22	1.13	0.25–5.07
1.50†	23	1.83	0.46	0.20–1.06	8	0.38	0.37	0.07–1.84
p, test for trend			.0337					.0171

CI indicates confidence interval.

* Relative risk adjusted for age, systolic blood pressure, serum total cholesterol, ethnic group, treated hypertension, angina pectoris, and diabetes.

Reproduced with permission from Njølstad et al.[91]

Gender

Detection of myocardial ischemia after an acute coronary event predicts subsequent cardiac events. Gender-related aspects in the prevalence and prognostic significance of myocardial ischemia detection after an acute coronary event, however, have not been reported. Moriel and associates[92] for The Multicenter Myocardial Ischemia Research Group from multiple medical centers performed noninvasive tests including resting 12-lead electrocardiogram, 24-hour ambulatory electrocardiography, exercise electrocardiography, and thallium-201 stress scintigraphy in 936 stable patients (224 women and 712 men) 1 to 6 months (average 2.7) after an acute coronary event (i.e., AMI or unstable angina). Primary end points during an average follow-up of 23 months included cardiac death, nonfatal AMI, and unstable angina, whereas restricted end points included cardiac death and nonfatal AMI. Ischemia detection was significantly less frequent among women than among men on 24-hour ambulatory electrocardiography, exercise electrocardiography, and thallium-201 stress scintigraphy. Primary end points occurred in 19.2% of women and in 19% of men, and restricted end points occurred in 5.8% of women and in 8% of men. Cox analyses revealed that gender and its interaction with each of the ischemia tests did not contribute to the prediction of the primary or restricted end points. The authors concluded that in stable patients 1 to 6 months after an acute coronary event, ischemia detection by noninvasive tests was significantly less prevalent in women than in men. However, subsequent cardiac event rates in

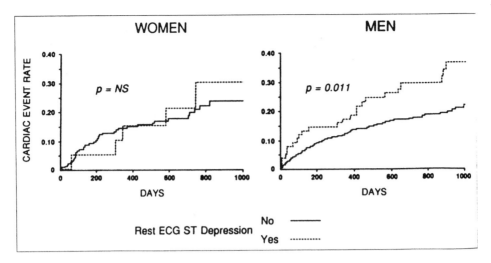

FIGURE 2-47. The unadjusted time-dependent associations (Kaplan-Meier curve) between 12-lead resting electrocardiogram (ECG), ST depression, and cardiac event by gender. Reproduced with permission from Moriel et al.[92]

women were similar to those observed in men, and there was no gender-ischemia detection interaction regarding subsequent events (Figures 2-47–2-50).

Both hyperestrogenemia and hypotestosteronemia have been reported in association with AMI in men. It was previously observed that the serum testosterone concentration correlated negatively with the degree of CAD in men who had never had a known AMI. Phillips and coinvestigators[93] in New York, New York, investigated the relation of sex hormone levels to the thrombotic component of AMI by comparing these levels in 18 men with a history of AMI and

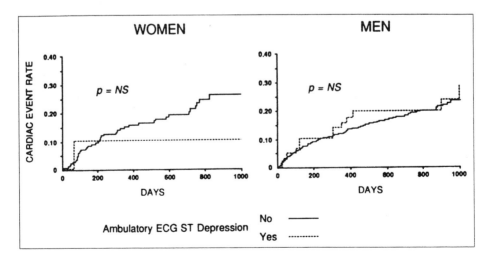

FIGURE 2-48. The unadjusted time-dependent associations (Kaplan-Meier curve) between an ischemic response during 24-hour ambulatory electrocardiogram (ECG) and cardiac event by gender. Reproduced with permission from Moriel et al.[92]

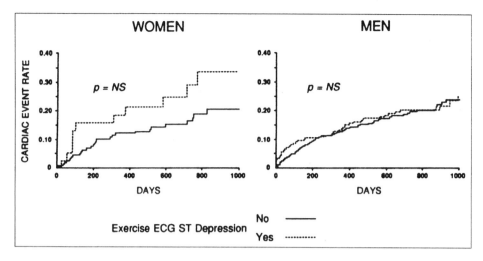

FIGURE 2-49. The unadjusted time-dependent associations (Kaplan-Meier curve) between an ischemic response during exercise electrocardiogram (ECG) and cardiac event by gender. Reproduced with permission from Moriel et al.[92]

50 men with no history of AMI; for both groups, the degree of CAD was in the same range. The mean degree of CAD, age, and body mass index in these 2 groups was not significantly different. The mean serum estradiol level in the men with a history of AMI was higher than that in the men who had no history of AMI. The mean levels of testosterone, free testosterone, sex hormones-binding globulin, insulin, dehydroepiandrosterone sulfate, cholesterol, HDL cholesterol, and systolic and diastolic blood pressure did not differ significantly. Estradiol was the only measured variable that showed a significant relationship

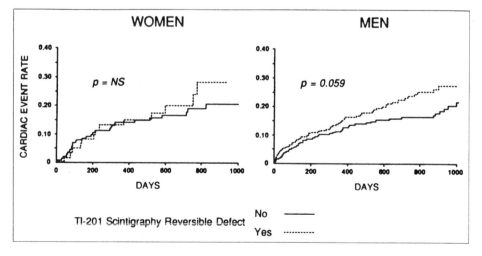

FIGURE 2-50. The unadjusted time-dependent associations (Kaplan-Meier curve) between reversible defect on thallium (Tl)-201 stress scintigraphy and cardiac event by gender. Reproduced with permission from Moriel et al.[92]

to AMI by multivariant logistic regression. These findings suggest that hyperestrogenemia may be related to the thrombosis of AMI.

Heart Rate Variability

Singh and colleagues[94] in Toronto, Canada; Edmonton, Canada; and Washington, D.C., examined heart rate variability and ST segment analysis on 48-hour Holter tapes in 204 patients as part of an ST monitoring substudy of the Global Utilization of Streptokinase and TPA for Occluded Arteries (GUSTO) Trial. Both time-domain measures of the average normal RR interval for all 5-minute segments of a 24-hour ECG recording and percent differences between adjacent normal RR intervals greater than 50 msec computed over the entire 24-hour electrocardiographic recording and frequency-domain measures of low-frequency, high-frequency, and low frequency/high frequency ratio were assessed on days 1 and 2 after AMI. Coronary angiography performed within the first 24 hours was available in 75% of the patients. All heart rate variability measures decreased between days 1 and 2 except the low-frequency/high-frequency ratio. There was no difference in heart rate variability among groups assigned to 1 of 4 different thrombolytic treatment strategies, including streptokinase and subcutaneous heparin, streptokinase and intravenous heparin, accelerated tPA, and combined streptokinase and tPA. Heart rate variability measures were lower in anterior than in nonanterior MIs and increased with TIMI grade 3 flow and better LVEFs (Figure 2-51). An inverse correlation between the duration of ST shift and frequency domain measures was observed. Lower low-frequency/high-frequency ratio by 24 hours after AMI was seen in those who ultimately died at 30 days. Thus, changes in heart rate variability occur early after thrombolysis and appear to be of prognostic value. Heart rate variability measures were improved in patients with better LVEF and greater angio-

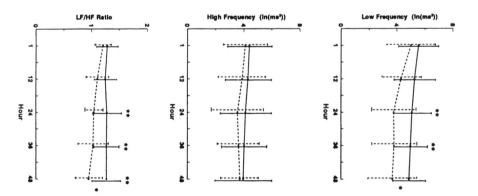

FIGURE 2-51. Mean hourly measures of heart rate variability (LF, HF, LF/HR ratio) during the first 48 hours in patients surviving (solid line) and not surviving (dashed line) at 30 days. *p = .02 for 2 way ANOVA with repeated measures for LF and p = .002 for LF/HF ratio. **p<.01 for Student's t test with Bonferroni correction (based on 5 comparisons). Reproduced with permission from Singh et al.[94]

graphic patency suggesting a possible mechanism for the enhanced survival observed with TIMI grade 3 flow in this study.

No-Reflow Phenomenon

Ito and colleagues[95] in Osaka, Japan, evaluated the prognostic importance of the no-reflow phenomenon studying complications, left ventricular morphology, and in-hospital survival after AMI. The study population consisted of 126 patients with first anterior AMI. All patients received coronary reflow within 24 hours of onset of symptoms and underwent myocardial contrast echocardiography before and shortly after coronary reflow with an intracoronary injection of sonicated microbubbles. From the contrast reperfusion patterns, patients could be divided into 2 groups: those with myocardial contrast echocardiography no reflow (47 patients), and those with myocardial contrast echocardiography reflow (79 patients). There was no difference in the frequency of arrhythmia or coronary events between the 2 groups. Pericardial effusion and early CHF were observed more frequently in patients with myocardial contrast echocardiography no reflow than in those with myocardial contrast echocardiography reflow (26% vs. 4%). CHF tended to be more prolonged in those with myocardial contrast echocardiography no reflow; 3 patients in this group died of CHF and low output state. LV end-diastolic volume increased in patients with myocardial contrast echocardiography no reflow, whereas it decreased in those with myocardial contrast echocardiography reflow (Figure 2-52). Thus, these data indicate that relatively large myocardial contrast echocardiography no-reflow phenomenon at coronary reflow after temporary coronary occlusion identifies the risk of left ventricular remodeling in individual patients with anterior wall AMI.

Plasma Fibrinogen Levels

Becker and associates[96] for the TIMI III investigators from multiple medical centers studied the prognostic value of fibrinogen, an acute-phase protein directly involved in thrombotic processes, by serially measuring its level in 1473 patients with unstable angina in non-Q-wave AMI. Participants were from the Thrombolysis in Myocardial Infarction (TIMI) IIIB trial. Overall, no association was found between baseline (pretreatment) fibrinogen and in-hospital AMI and death; however, patients with spontaneous ischemia and the combined unsatisfactory outcome of death, AMI, and spontaneous ischemia had higher fibrinogen concentrations than did those without these events. This association was confined to patients with unstable angina. A baseline fibrinogen concentration of 300 mg/dL or greater was associated with a modest trend toward an increased risk of death, myocardial infarction, or spontaneous ischemia (odds ratio, 1.61; 95% confidence interval, 1.02 to 2.52). Elevation of fibrinogen, a readily measurable acute-phase protein, at the time of hospital admission is associated with coronary ischemic events and a poor clinical outcome in patients with unstable angina (Figure 2-53).

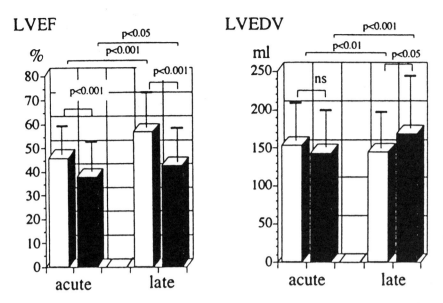

FIGURE 2-52. Bar graphs showing the temporal changes in left ventricular ejection fraction (left; LVEF [%]) and end-diastolic volume (right; LVEDV[mL]) from the early to late stage in patients with and without the no reflow phenomenon assessed by myocardial contrast echocardiography (MCE). Patients with MCE no reflow (solid bar) showed a little functional improvement, whereas patients with MCE reflow (open bar) showed significant temporal improvement in ventricular function. Ventricular function was significantly better in patients with MCE reflow than those with MCE no reflow. LVEDV increased in the late stage in patients with MCE no reflow and decreased in patients with MCE reflow. Therefore, late-stage LVEDV was significantly greater in patients with MCE no reflow than those with MCE reflow. Values are expressed as mean ± SD. Reproduced with permission from Ito et al.[95]

Behague and colleagues[97] from the ECTIM Study Group evaluated the β fibrinogen gene in relation to plasma fibrinogen and to the severity of CAD in patients with AMI in the ECTIM study (Figure 2-54). Ten polymorphisms of the β fibrinogen gene, including 5 new polymorphisms identified by single-strand conformation polymorphism analysis and 1 polymorphism in the 3′ flanking region of the α fibrinogen gene, were investigated in 565 patients with AMI and 668 control individuals. The polymorphisms were in tight linkage disequilibrium, and the genotype frequencies were similar in patients with AMI and control subjects. In the multivariate analysis, only 2 polymorphisms, β Hae III and β-854, were independently associated with plasma fibrinogen. A significant association between β fibrinogen polymorphisms and plasma fibrinogen was present in smokers but not in nonsmokers. In patients of French descent who had MIs, the number of coronary arteries with more than 50% stenosis was estimated by angiography and used as a criterion for the severity of CAD. Presence of the less frequent allele of the β Bcl I and of other polymorphisms was positively associated with the severity of CAD. Thus, genetic variants of the β fibrinogen gene are associated with an increased plasma level of fibrinogen, especially in smokers. The association with CAD appears to be the consequence of an increased risk of MI in patients with severe CAD who carried a predisposing β fibrinogen genotype.

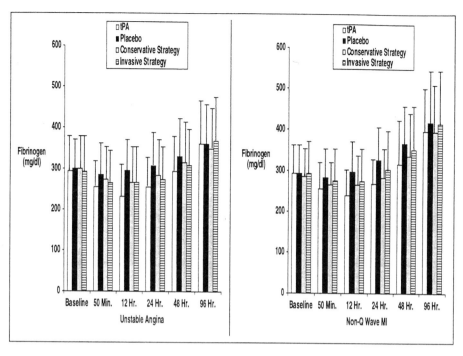

Figure 2-53. Mean fibrinogen values at the 6 sampling times according to treatment (tissue plasminogen activator [tPA] vs placebo), strategy (invasive vs conservative), and diagnosis (unstable angina vs non-Q-wave myocardial infarction [MI]). A decrease was observed within 50 minutes of enrollment that was most pronounced in patients given tPA. Levels increased after 24 hours and exceeded baseline values by 96 hours in all patient groups. Reproduced with permission from Becker et al.[96]

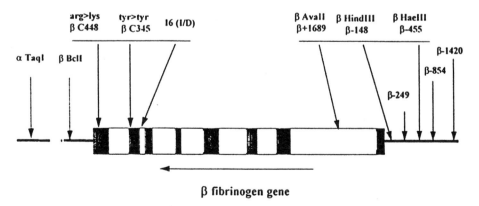

β fibrinogen gene

Figure 2-54. Schematic representation of the β fibrinogen gene and location of the polymorphisms investigated in the ECTIM study. Wide black bars, exons; wide white bars, introns; thin black bars, flanking regions. Reproduced with permission from Behague et al.[97]

Plasma Adrenomedullin

Adrenomedullin has a potent vasodilating effect comparable to that of calcitonin gene-related peptide. To investigate the pathophysiologic role of endogenous adrenomedullin, Kobayashi and associates[98] from Miyazaki, Japan, sequentially determined the plasma adrenomedullin level in 15 consecutive patients with AMI. Plasma adrenomedullin was higher immediately after the onset of AMI and decreased gradually. Plasma levels during the 3-week period after the AMI were higher in AMI patients than in 15 healthy control individuals; higher levels were observed in patients with CHF than in patients without CHF throughout the period of the study. Plasma adrenomedullin was positively correlated with PA wedge pressure, PA pressure, RA pressure, and heart rate in the early stage of AMI. These findings suggest that the elevation of plasma adrenomedullin is related to the retention of body fluid volume, the enhancement of sympathetic activity, and the elevation of pressure in pulmonary vascular beds. Adrenomedullin may act against excessive vasoconstrictors increased in AMI.

Serum Lipoprotein(a) and Spontaneous Intermittent Coronary Occlusion

Haider and colleagues[99] assessed the relation of thrombotic occlusion of the infarct-related artery occurring intermittently in the early, evolving phase of AMI with serum or plasma concentrations of cholesterol, triglyceride, lipoprotein(a), and coagulation and fibrinolytic factors as measured in venous blood before the initiation of thrombolytic therapy. Thirty-two patients with AMI, including 23 men and 9 women, ages 30 to 70 years, received intermittent recombinant tPA within 6 hours of symptom onset. Continuous electrocardiographic ST segment recording demonstrated intermittent occlusion of the infarct-related artery in 12 patients (group 1) before the start of thrombolytic therapy and persistent occlusion in 20 patients (group 2). Groups 1 and 2 were similar in age, sex, race, duration of symptoms, blood sample collection time, location of the infarct-related artery, and extent of CAD. The serum and plasma level of thrombin-antithrombin III complex was 10.9 μg/L^{-1} as compared with 6.8 μg/L^{-1} in groups 1 and 2, respectively. The serum level of lipoprotein(a) was 34 mg/dL versus 11.5 mg/dL in groups 1 and 2, respectively. The levels of other factors were similar in both groups. Thus, the phenomenon of spontaneous intermittent closure and reopening of coronary arteries early during AMI in humans is associated with a higher level of lipoprotein(a) and with a marker of thrombin generation, suggesting that lipoprotein(a) and thrombin may be closely related to coronary patency in these patients.

Prospective Study of Triglyceride Level and LDL Particle Diameter and Risk of MI

Stampfer and colleagues[100] in Boston, Massachusetts, tested the hypothesis that a predominance of small, dense LDL particles and elevated triglyceride levels are independent risk factors for AMI. They performed a prospective cohort study using the nested case-control study method. Blood samples were collected at baseline from 14,916 men, aged 40 to 84 years, in the Physicians' Health Study. The primary end point was the development of AMI during 7 years of follow-up. Cases (n=266) had a significantly smaller LDL diameter than did controls (n = 308) matched on age and smoking. Cases also had higher median triglyceride levels (168 vs. 132 mg/dL, p<.001). The LDL diameter had an inverse correlation with triglyceride level (r = 0.71), and a high direct correlation with HDL cholesterol. The authors observed a significant multiplicative interaction between serum triglyceride and total cholesterol levels. After simultaneous adjustment for lipids and a variety of cardiac risk factors, LDL particle diameter was no longer a statistically significant risk indicator, with a relative risk of 1.09. However, serum triglyceride levels remained significant. The association between serum triglyceride level and AMI risk appeared linear across the distribution. Men in the highest quintile had a risk approximately 2.5 times that of those in the lowest quintile. Triglyceride level, but not HDL level, also remained significant. These data indicate that nonfasting triglyceride levels appear to be a strong and independent predictor of future AMI, especially when the total serum cholesterol is also elevated. LDL particle diameter is associated with the risk of AMI, but not after adjustment for serum triglyceride level. Increased triglyceride level, small LDL particle diameter, and decreased HDL levels appear to reflect underlying metabolic perturbations with adverse consequences for risk of MI. Elevated serum triglycerides may help to identify high-risk individuals.

Troponin T Concentrations

Stubbs and colleagues[101] in London, United Kingdom, tested the prognostic significance of increases in troponin T in 240 patients admitted with AMI who were followed prospectively for a median of 3 years. The prognostic significance of the admission troponin T concentration greater than or equal to 0.2 ng/mL for subsequent cardiac death and/or reinfarction was assessed and compared with other variables in a regression model. Any detectable troponin T on admission was associated with a worse prognosis on follow-up. The admission concentration of 0.2 ng/mL or greater was associated with a higher risk of subsequent cardiac death and death or nonfatal reinfarction (Figure 2-55). The excess risk was seen primarily in patients with admission electrocardiographic ST segment elevation. In a stepwise regression model for cardiac death or nonfatal reinfarction, troponin T was superior to that of other variables entered in both myocardial infarction subgroups. Thus, the presence of troponin T on admission in patients with AMI defines a subgroup at increased risk of subsequent cardiac events, especially in patients with ST segment elevation.

Plasma Brain Natriuretic Peptide (in Predicting Survival)

Various neurohumoral levels have prognostic implications in patients with CHF. Arakawa and colleagues[102] from Morioka, Japan, evaluated whether

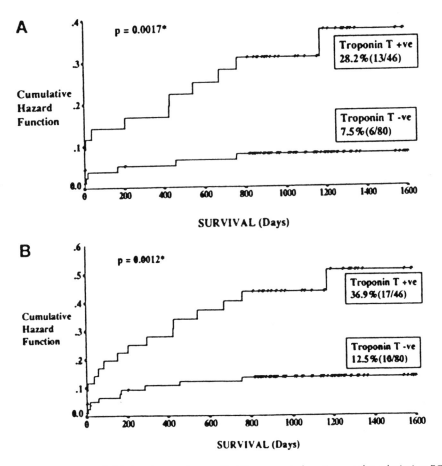

FIGURE 2-55. Myocardial infarction patients with ST-segment elevation on the admission ECG. Kaplan-Meier cumulative hazard survival curves according to admission TnT status. **A,** End point, cardiac death as first event. **B,** End point, cardiac death or myocardial reinfarction as first event. *Log rank statistic. +ve indicates positive; −ve, negative. Reproduced with permission from Stubbs et al.[101]

plasma brain natriuretic peptide BNP levels can predict prognosis after AMI. Plasma BNP and atrial natriuretic peptide (ANP) levels were measured in 70 patients with AMI on admission and on day 2 after the onset of AMI. The mean follow-up period was 18 months. Plasma BNP levels, but not ANP levels, correlated with hemodynamic variables. Patients with plasma BNP levels higher than the median level, both on admission and on day 2, had significantly higher mortality rates than did those with submedian levels. However, only the plasma ANP level obtained immediately after admission was significantly related to survival. These authors concluded that increased plasma BNP concentrations are a powerful noninvasive predictor of poor prognosis.

Omland and colleagues[103] in Boston, Massachusetts, obtained venous blood samples for measurement of ANP, the N-terminal fragment of the ANP prohormone (N-ANP), and BNP on day 3 after symptom onset in 131 patients with documented AMI. LVEF was determined by echocardiography in a sub-

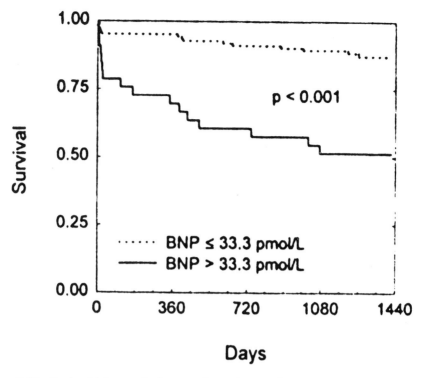

FIGURE 2-56. Kaplan-Meier survival curves for patients with AMI subdivided into 2 groups according to the 75th percentile concentration of BNP in plasma (33.3 pmol/L). Reproduced with permission from Omland et al.[103]

sample of 79 patients. Twenty-eight cardiovascular and 3 noncardiovascular deaths occurred during the follow-up period of 1293 days. All 3 peptides proved to be powerful predictors of cardiovascular mortality. In a multivariate model, plasma BNP, but not ANP or N-ANP, provided additional prognostic information beyond what is provided by measurement of LVEF (Figure 2-56). Logistic regression analysis showed that ANP and N-ANP, but not BNP, was significantly associated with LVEF of 45% or higher.

Programmed Ventricular Stimulation in Predicting Sudden Death

Zoni-Berisso and associates[104] from Genoa, Italy, assessed the prognostic value of the response to programmed ventricular stimulation in selected post-AMI patients identified at risk of sudden death and spontaneous sustained VT (arrhythmic events) by noninvasive, highly sensitive testing. They prospectively studied 286 consecutive patients and followed them for 12 months: 103 patients (group 1) with either LVEF of greater than or equal to 40%, or ventricular late potentials, or spontaneous complex ventricular arrhythmias, were considered at risk of late arrhythmic events and were eligible for programmed ventricular stimulation; the remaining 183 patients (group 2) were discharged without any further evaluation. [Electrophysiological study was performed 11 to 20 days after AMI, utilizing up to 2 extrastimuli and rapid ventricular burst pacing]. At the end of the follow-up period, 10 patients in group 1, and 2 in group 2 died of cardiac causes; in addition, 10 patients in group 1, and 1 in group 2 had arrhythmic events. Sustained monomorphic VT was the only inducible arrhythmia related either to cardiac death or to arrhythmic events. It was induced in 11 patients (3 died suddenly, and 3 had spontaneous VT). Multivariate analysis showed that such arrhythmia was the strongest independent predictor of arrhythmic events. In the entire study population, it allowed identification of patients at risk, with a sensitivity, specificity, and positive predictive value of 55%, 99%, and 67%, respectively. The authors concluded that programmed ventricular stimulation performed in selected post-AMI patients, utilizing a moderately aggressive stimulation protocol, is a specific but less sensitive procedure for predicting arrhythmic events. The induction of sustained monomorphic VT allows the accurate identification of patients who may profit by prophylactic antiarrhythmic therapy.

Complications of AMI

Angina Pectoris

Angina pectoris before and after AMI was evaluated by Brand and associates[105] from Framingham, Massachusetts, in a sample of 729 men and women from a general population in whom AMI developed during a 36-year period of follow-up. The relation of angina pectoris to subsequent CAD events and mortality after initial AMI was analyzed by proportional hazards regression models and was adjusted for covariates (age, sex, blood pressure, serum cholesterol, body mass index, glucose intolerance, cigarette smoking, and antihypertensive medications) obtained from routine blennial examinations preceding the initial AMI. Comparisons of the influence of angina were made between pre-AMI angina, post-AMI angina, and absence of angina pectoris. The sample had 484 men and 245 women (mean ages, 63 and 69, respectively) who survived at least 30 days after AMI. The initial AMI was clinically unrecognized in 165 (34%) men and 115 (47%) women. Data on covariates were complete for 622 individuals, among whom 30% had pre-AMI angina, 18% had post-AMI angina, and 52% did not have angina pectoris. Angina was half as common in persons with unrecognized AMI as in those with clinically recognized AMI. During an average of 8.7 years of follow-up, 57% of individuals developed subsequent CAD events, including recognized and unrecognized AMI, CHF, and CAD death, and 74% died. Patients with pre-AMI angina or post-AMI angina adjusted for accompanying risk factors had an increased risk for subsequent CAD events compared with patients without angina pectoris. Neither pre-AMI nor post-AMI angina was associated with excess overall mortality.

Cardiac Rupture

Although cardiac rupture is the second most common cause of death after left ventricular failure in AMI, no diagnosis has ever been made before an episode of clinical compromise, and no significant predictive factors have been described. This study by Ueda and associates[106] from Tochigi, Japan, was designed to determine whether high serum C-reactive protein levels could predict the incidence of subacute cardiac rupture after AMI. Nine consecutive patients with cardiac rupture were compared retrospectively with 28 consecutive control patients without rupture after AMI. In the rupture group, peak serum C-reactive protein levels increased rapidly and markedly after infarction, reaching more than 20 mg/dL on day 2, and persisted at higher levels than those in the control group. However, the time course and levels of serum creatine phosphokinase were not significantly different between the 2 groups. High serum C-reactive protein levels (>20 mg/dL) had a high diagnostic sensitivity (89%) and specificity (96%) for cardiac rupture. Patients with persistently high serum C-reactive protein levels, particularly above 20 mg/dL, might have high probability of occurrence of subacute cardiac rupture after AMI.

Figueras and associates[107] assessed the reliability of electromechanical dissociation in diagnosing acute left ventricular free wall rupture in 479 consecutive patients with AMI. Electromechanical dissociation was the mechanism of death in 193 patients: 140 without heart failure (group A, 74%), and 53 with heart failure (group B, 26%). Autopsies performed on 121 patients with electromechanical dissociation showed left ventricular free wall rupture in 81 (95%) of 85 from group A and in 7 (17%) of 36 from group B. Of the 106 patients without electromechanical dissociation (group C) autopsied, 5 (4.7%) had left ventricular free wall rupture. Excluding the 8 patients with associated septal rupture, left ventricular free wall rupture occurred in 79 (95%) of 83 patients from group A, 4 (12%) of 33 from group B, and 2 (1.9%) of 103 from group C. Predictive accuracy of electromechanical dissociation for LV free wall rupture was 95% in group A, but only 17% in group B. Moreover, in 13 consecutive cases with a first AMI without heart failure and electromechanical dissociation, emergency surgery revealed left ventricular free wall rupture in all. Thus electromechanical dissociation has a highly predictive accuracy in diagnosing left ventricular free wall rupture in patients with a first AMI without overt heart failure.

Ventricular Tachyarrhythmias

Huikuri and colleagues[108] of Oulu, Finland, tested the hypothesis that alterations in RR-interval dynamics occur before the spontaneous onset of ventricular tachyarrhythmias, including VT. Ambulatory electrocardiographic recordings from 15 patients with prior AMI who had spontaneous episodes of sustained VT during the recording and VT inducible by programmed electrical stimulation were analyzed by plotting each RR interval of a single beat as a function of the previous one. Plots were also generated for 30 post-MI patients who had no history of spontaneous VT and no inducible VT and 30 age-matched subjects without heart disease. The MI control subjects and the VT group were matched with respect to age and severity of underlying heart disease. All of the healthy subjects and MI control individuals showed plots characterized by an increased next-interval difference for long RR intervals relative to short ones. All of the VT patients had abnormal plots, including 9 with a complex pattern, 3 ball-shaped, and 3 torpedo-shaped. Quantitative analysis of the plots showed the standard deviation of the long RR-interval variability to be smaller in all VT patients (52 ± 14 msec) than in MI control subjects (110 ± 24 msec) or the normal subjects (123 ± 38 msec), but the standard deviation of the instantaneous beat-to-beat variability did not differ between the groups. The complex plots were caused by periods of alternating sinus intervals resulting in an increased standard deviation 1/standard deviation 2 ratio in the VT group. This ratio increased during the 1-hour period preceding the onset of 27 spontaneous VT episodes compared with the 24-hour average ratio. These data suggest that reduced long-term RR interval variability, associated with episodes of beat-to-beat sinus alternans, is a very specific sign of a propensity for spontaneous onset of VT, suggesting that abnormal beat-to-beat heart-rate dynamics reflect a transient electrical instability favoring the onset of VT in patients with prior MI (Figure 2-57).

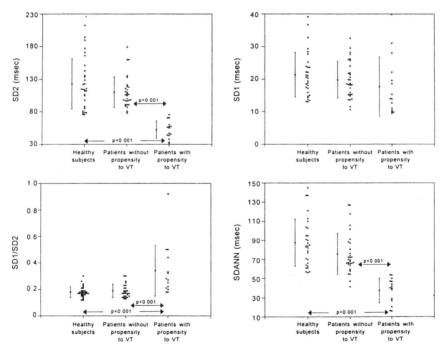

FIGURE 2-57. Individual and mean values (±SD) for the quantitative analyses of Poincaré plots (diagram in which each RR interval of a tachogram is plotted as a function of the previous RR interval for a predetermined segment length) and SDANN (a time domain measure of heart rate variability) in healthy subjects and postinfarction patients with and without a propensity for ventricular tachyarrhythmias. SD1 indicates SD of instantaneous beat-to-beat RR-interval variability; SD2, SD of long-term continuous RR-interval variability. Reproduced with permission from Haikuri et al.[108]

Mitral Regurgitation

In this study by Van Dantzig and associates[109] from Amsterdam, The Netherlands, the pathogenesis of MR (MR) was determined by quantitative echocardiography in 188 patients with AMI within 48 hours after admission. By using color Doppler, MR was classified as significant (grade 3 to 4) or trivial (grades 0 to 2). Left ventricular function (global and regional), volume, and shape, as well as mitral valvular features, were measured and analyzed by stepwise logistic regression. Significant MR occurred in 25 (13%) patients. Univariately, recurrent infarction, left ventricular dilatation and sphericity, inferoposterolateral asynergy, mitral annular dilatation, and mitral leaflet restriction were associated with significant MR. In regression analysis, only recurrent infarction, left ventricular sphericity index, and inferoposterolateral asynergy were independently associated with significant MR, whereas none of the mitral valvular features examined had an independent association. In conclusion, changes in left ventricular shape and regional function and not mitral valvular changes are prime determinants of significant MR after AMI.

Lack of Ventricular Remodeling (in Non-Q wave MI)

Irimpen and associates[110] from New Orleans, Louisiana, prospectively examined 45 patients with serial echocardiography to measure left ventricular end-diastolic volume index within 1 week and at 6 weeks after AMI. Left ventricular volume increased in patients with Q-wave AMI but not in those with non-Q AMI or in control patients without recent infarction. Peak creatine phosphokinase levels were greater in patients with Q-wave AMI than in those with no Q-wave AMI. There was a strong correlation between the change in the LV end-diastolic index and the peak creatine phosphokinase level. After correcting for infarct size, there was still a difference between the 2 groups. These data indicate that ventricular remodeling does not occur in non-Q-wave as opposed to Q-wave infarcts, and this may be related both to the limited amount of myocardial necrosis and to the nontransmural extent of the necrosis.

Vagal Reflexes and Patency of the Infarct-Related Artery

Mortara and colleagues[111] in Pavia, Italy, tested the hypothesis that patency of the infarct-related artery may enhance vagal reflexes, a factor known to affect electrical stability of the infarcted myocardium. They analyzed angiographic data in 359 of 1284 post-AMI patients enrolled in a multicenter prospective study within 8 weeks after the index MI. Patients underwent baroreflex sensitivity assessment by the phenylephrine method. The baroreflex sensitivity of the entire population averaged 8 msec/mm Hg and was significantly related to age, but not to LVEF. One, 2, and 3-vessel CAD were present in 138, 96, and 99 patients, respectively, while no coronary stenosis was found in 26. Infarct-related artery (IRA) patency was documented in 234 patients (65%), while in

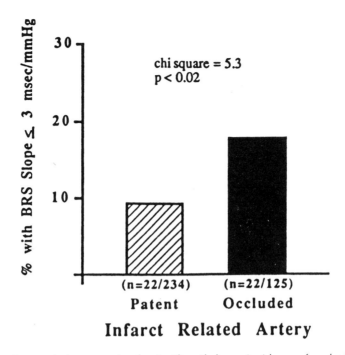

FIGURE 2-58. Bar graph demonstrating the significantly lower incidence of markedly depressed BRS slope (≤3 msec/mm Hg) in patients with patent IRAs compared with patients with occluded IRAs. Reproduced with permission from Mortara et al.[111]

the remaining 125 (35%), the artery remained occluded. Patients with occluded IRAs had more extensive CAD, including 2- and 3-vessel disease (71% vs. 46%) and more depressed LVEF (48% versus 53%). Patency of the IRA was associated with higher baroreflex sensitivity values and with a lower incidence of markedly depressed baroreflex sensitivity, a condition shown to be associated with increased risk of mortality post-MI (Figure 2-58). The association between IRA patency and baroreflex sensitivity was more evident in patients with anterior than inferior MIs. Multivariate regression analysis showed that the age of the patient and patency of the IRA were the major independent determinants of baroreflex sensitivity, whereas LVEF was weakly related to baroreflex sensitivity and only when analyzed as a categorized variable. Thus, the presence of an open IRA is associated with a higher baroreflex sensitivity, and this effect is largely independent of the limitation of infarct size by infarct artery patency.

Mortality in AMI

Mortality

Le Feuvre and associates[112] from Hamilton, Canada, studied mortality from in-hospital AMI and at 1 year from 3 selected 1-year periods in a stable population during a 13-year period, beginning in 1979 and continuing into the thrombolytic era. The purpose of the study was to detect any changes occurring in conjunction with the introduction of new therapies. Every patient with AMI from the geographically defined stable community (Hamilton, Canada) in 3 1-year periods (1979 to 1980, 1986 to 1987, and 1991 to 1992) was identified and clinically characterized by standardized criteria. Subsequent in-hospital and 1-year survival were ascertained prospectively. The 3 cohorts were similar in prognostic factors. Mean age was progressively greater over the study period from 63 years in 1979 to 1980, to 67 years in 1991 to 1992. In-hospital mortality rates did not change from 1979 to 1980 (17%) and 1986 to 1987 (16%). However, from 1986 to 1987 and 1991 to 1992, in-hospital mortality decreased from 16% to 9%, and 1-year mortality decreased from 26% to 19% (Figure 2-59). For patients who survived the hospital phase of AMI, 1-year mortality did not change and was between 11% and 12% in each of the 3 study periods. From 1986 to 1987 and from 1991 to 1992, the use of thrombolytic therapy increased from 5% to 44% of patients. The acute use of aspirin increased from 30% to 88%, and the acute use of β blockers increased from 19% to 48% of patients. The observed increase in use of these agents could account for half of the actual mortality reduction observed. This prospective population-based survey demonstrates improved in-hospital survival after AMI associated with increased use of established effective therapies between 1987 and 1992. The 1-year mortality of hospital survivors of AMI was unchanged throughout the period of study, remaining at 11% and 12%.

A number of therapeutic interventions have recently changed the prognosis of patients with AMI. Rouleau and colleagues[113] in a multicenter data analysis evaluated all patients younger than 75 years of age presenting with an AMI between July 1, 1990, and June 30, 1992, at 9 Canadian hospitals. A total of 3178 patients were recruited. In-hospital mortality rate of patients younger than 75 years of age was 8.4%, and that at 1 year after hospital discharge was 5.3%. Female patients had a 2-fold greater risk of in-hospital death.

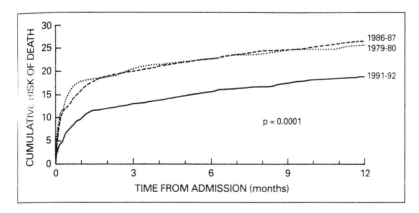

FIGURE 2-59. Kaplan-Meier curves showing cumulative mortality in the year following hospital admission for acute myocardial infarction in Hamilton, Ontario, for the years 1979 to 1980, 1986 to 1987, and 1991 to 1992. Reproduced with permission from Le Feuvre et al.[112]

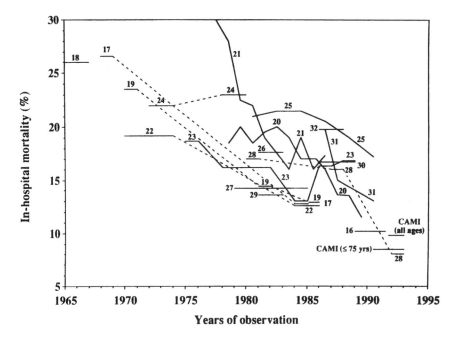

FIGURE 2-60. Evolution of in-hospital mortality following AMI since 1965. Bars represent the time period of patient recruitment for each study. The numbers indicate the reference article in the original publication. CAMI, Canadian Assessment of Myocardial Infarction. Reproduced with permission from Rouleau et al.[113]

These authors concluded that 1-year mortality after AMI continues to decrease (Figure 2-60).

This study by Gheorghiade and associates[114] from Chicago, Illinois, and Detroit, Michigan, examined the profile and management of AMI in patients hospitalized in the coronary care unit of Henry Ford Hospital to determine risk factors or treatments that best explained a decline in in-hospital mortality rates. During the 1980s and 1990s, many therapeutic advances occurred in management of AMI. Overall and in-hospital mortality were observed also to decline, but little is known about the relation of newer treatments to clinical outcome. The study population consisted of 1798 patients with a confirmed diagnosis of AMI. Of these, 982 consecutive patients were hospitalized in the coronary care unit of Henry Ford Hospital from January 1981 through December 1984 and compared with the 816 consecutive patients hospitalized from January 1990 through October 1992. Data on baseline demographics, initial clinical features, in-hospital management, and in-hospital outcome were compared for the 2 groups. Logistic regression was used to define independent predictors of the improved outcome of the 2 groups. Demographic features of the earlier group were similar to those of the later cohort, with the exception of a greater incidence of diabetes and hypertension and a lesser incidence of angina and prior heart failure. The occurrence of non-Q wave AMI increased from 27% in the earlier group to 39% in the later group, whereas the magnitude of peak creatine kinase elevation in serum was higher in the later group. Medical management differed significantly, with increased use of aspirin, thrombolytics, heparin, warfarin, nitrates, and β-blockers and decreased use of antiarrhythmic agents, digoxin, and vasopressors in the later group. Coronary revascularization was performed during hospitalization in 6.4% of the earlier group of patients and in 32% of the later group. In-hospital mortality was 15% in the earlier group and 7.4% in the later group. Multivariate logistic regression analysis showed that the difference in mortality between the 2 groups was best accounted for by increased use of β-blockers, PTCA, and thrombolytics; decreased incidence of cardiogenic shock and asystole; and decreased use of lidocaine. In conclusion, the presentation and in-hospital management of patients with AMI has changed from the early 1980s to the early 1990s. The improved hospital mortality rate may be associated with both the expanded use of effective therapies and a more favorable in-hospital course, although these are not mutually exclusive.

AMI—Miscellaneous

BCL-2 Protein and Bax Related to Myocyte Death in Humans after MI

Misao and colleagues[115] in Gifu, Japan, conducted an immunohistochemically study of 37 autopsied hearts, including 15 with AMI, 12 with old MI, and 10 with no infarction (normal hearts) as controls, with antibodies to bcl-2 and Bax. The ratio of bcl-2 protein, an inhibitor of apoptosis or programmed cell death, to Bax protein, an inducer of apoptosis, determines survival or death after an apoptotic stimulus. The authors hypothesized that bcl-2 or Bax expression is induced by ischemia and that it may be related to myocyte death in human hearts. In this study, there were no myocytes with positive bcl-2 immunoreactivity in the controls or hearts with old MI. However, myocytes with positive bcl-2 immunoreactivity were found in 9 of 15 hearts (60%) with acute MI. The bcl-2 in these hearts was localized in salvaged areas surrounding the infarcted areas. Myocytes with slightly positive Bax immunoreactivity were observed in the control hearts. In the salvaged myocytes surrounding the infarcted tissues, Bax was overexpressed in 2 of 15 hearts (13%) with acute MI, but in 10 of 12 hearts (83%) with old MI (Figure 2-61). Thus, this study suggests that bcl-2 protein is induced in salvaged myocytes in the acute stages of MI, but Bax protein is overexpressed in hearts with old MIs. The expression of bcl-2 and the overexpression of Bax may be important pathophysiologically in the protection or development of cell death in human myocytes with prolonged myocardial ischemia.

Exercise Tolerance in Patients with Recent MI

To investigate the influence of intrinsic limb vasodilator capacity on exercise performance, limb reactive hyperemic flows and their relation to exercise capacity during upright bicycle exercise were examined in 52 patients with

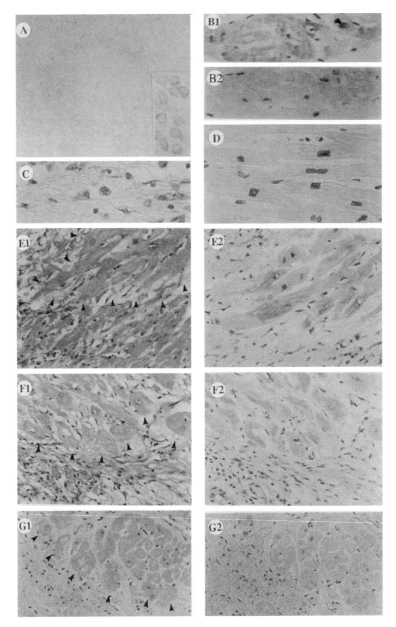

FIGURE 2-61. Immunohistochemical findings of bcl-2 protein. **A,** bcl-2 immunohistochemical staining of human lymph nodes as a positive control. Most cells within the interfollicular regions of lymph node showed dark-brown positive immunoreactive staining against monoclonal antihuman bcl-2 protein antibody. In contrast, the majority of cells within the germinal center were negative (magnification, ×40). **Bottom right,** High-power magnification of the interfollicular regions (×400). In this specimen, counterstaining with hematoxylin to identify the nucleus was not done because of clear observation of positive bcl-2 immunoreactivity in the lymphocytes. **B1,** bcl-2 immunohistochemical staining of salvaged tissues surrounding the infarcted areas in a heart with acute infarction. Dark-brown bcl-2 positive immunoreactivity is seen in the salvaged myocytes (×200). **B2,** A serial section of B1 incubated with antihuman bcl-2 antibody preabsorbed with excess bcl-2. The positive immunoreactivity of B1 disappeared (×200). **C,** bcl-2 immunohistochemical staining of inflammatory cells infiltrating the

recent myocardial infarction in this study by Hattori and associates[116] from Osaka, Japan. Reactive hyperemic flow was measured in the forearm and the calf by venous occlusive plethysmography after 5 minutes of arterial occlusion. Calf reactive hyperemic flow correlated significantly with cardiac output, systemic vascular resistance, and oxygen consumption at peak exercise, whereas flow in the forearm did not. In patients with preserved exercise capacity (group 1, n = 20) compared with those with exercise impairment (group 2, n = 32), calf reactive hyperemic flow was significantly augmented, but forearm flow was similar in the 2 groups. There were no significant differences in hemodynamic parameters at rest between the 2 groups. At peak exercise, however, cardiac output was lower and systemic vascular resistance was higher in group 2 than in group 1, whereas arterial blood pressure was maintained identically in the 2 groups. Thus, intrinsic calf but not forearm vasodilator capacity was linked to exercise hemodynamic responses and exercise capacity in patients with recent myocardial infarction. In addition, reduced calf vasodilation and concomitant enhanced vascular tone seemed to be useful for preserving arterial blood pressure in decreased cardiac output response to exercise in patients with exercise impairment.

General Treatment for AMI

Differences by Sex, Age, and Other Factors

Oka and associates[117] from Palo Alto, California, examined the temporal trends in the use of angiography following revascularization procedures for AMI in 2021 hospitalized men and in 995 women aged 30 to 74 years who participated in the Stanford Five-City Project during the years 1986 to 1992. The sample included hospitalized patients who received a discharge diagnosis code of 410 through 414 and met study criteria for either a definite or possible AMI. Incident and recurrent AMI occurring in the years 1986 through 1992

---

infarcted tissue. Dark-brown bcl-2 positive immunoreactivity is evident in some inflammatory mononuclear cells ($\times 400$). **D,** bcl-2 immunohistochemical staining of a normal control heart. There is no evidence of positive immunoreactivity ($\times 400$). **E1,** Hematoxylin and eosin staining in the early stage of acute infarction and salvaged cardiac tissue obtained from patient 4. Bottom half, infarcted tissue. Top half surrounded by arrowheads, salvaged tissue ($\times 200$). **E2,** bcl-2 immunohistochemical staining of a serial section of E1. Dark-brown positive bcl-2 immunoreactivity is evident in the cytoplasm of salvaged myocytes. However, infarcted (dead) myocytes show negative immunoreactivity ($\times 200$). **F1,** Hematoxylin and eosin staining in the late stage (granulation) of acute infarction and salvaged cardiac tissue obtained from patient 14. Bottom half, infarcted tissue. Top half surrounded by arrowheads, salvaged tissue ($\times 200$). **F2,** bcl-2 immunohistochemical staining of a serial section of F1. Dark-brown positive immunoreactivity is evident in the cytoplasm of salvaged myocytes ($\times 200$). **G1,** Hematoxylin and eosin staining of old infarction and salvaged cardiac tissue. Bottom half, infarcted tissue. Top half surrounded by arrowheads, salvaged tissue ($\times 200$). **G2,** bcl-2 immunohistochemical staining of a serial section of G1. Positive immunoreactivity is absent in the cytoplasm of salvaged myocytes ($\times 200$). Reproduced with permission from Misao et al.[115]

were included, but only the first event in this period for each patient. The authors performed stepwise multiple logistic regression analysis to determine the probability of: 1) receiving coronary angiography, 2) revascularization by either CABG or PTCA among those with angiograms, and 3) thrombolytic therapy. Age, year of procedure, disease severity, and time between symptom onset and medical treatment were included as covariates. After adjustment of these factors, women were less likely than men to undergo angiography but were equally likely to undergo revascularization. Age and disease severity were inverse predictors of coronary angiography, but not of revascularization. Age, severity, and time delay between onset of symptoms and medical therapy were inverse predictors of thrombolysis; time delay was significantly greater in women than in men and averaged more than 6 hours in both sexes. The likelihood of receiving angiography, revascularization, and thrombolysis increased sharply over the study period.

Kudenchuk and associates[118] for the Myocardial Infarction Triage and Intervention Project Investigators compared the presentation (symptoms and signs), treatment, and outcome of 1097 consecutive patients (851 men and 246 women) from the Myocardial Infarction Triage and Intervention (MITI) Project Registry with confirmed acute myocardial infarction (AMI). All patients were initially evaluated in the prehospital setting, met clinical criteria for possible thrombolysis, and were followed throughout their hospital course. Women were, on average, older than men and had a higher prevalence of known cardiovascular risk factors, including systemic hypertension and congestive heart failure. The presentation of AMI with respect to symptoms, delay, and hemodynamic and electrocardiographic findings was, for the most part, indistinguishable between men and women. Women appeared "undertreated" early in the course of AMI and were half as likely as men to undergo acute catheterization, angioplasty, thrombolysis, or coronary bypass surgery (odds ratio, 0.5). The risk for hospital mortality in women was almost twice that for men (odds ratio,

TABLE 2-6
Presenting Symptoms and Signs in Men and Women with Acute Myocardial Infarction

Symptom or Sign	All	Men	Women
Chest pain	1,086 (99%)	841 (99%)	245 (99.6%)
Dyspnea	557 (51%)	434 (51%)	123 (50%)
Diapharesis	793 (72%)	621 (73%)	172 (70%)
Nausea	601 (55%)	451 (53%)	150 (61%)
Epigastric discomfort	109 (10%)	94 (11%)	15 (6%)
Clinical shock*	16 (1.5%)	14 (2%)	2 (1%)
Duration of symptoms (min)†	67 ± 121	65 ± 115	75 ± 139
Systolic blood pressure (mm Hg)	136 ± 27	137 ± 26	136 ± 28
Diastolic blood pressure (mm Hg)	84 ± 14	86 ± 16	82 ± 16
Heart rate (beats/min)	74 ± 21	74 ± 20	75 ± 24

* Clinical shock with heart rate >120 beats per minute and systolic blood pressure <100 mm Hg on hospital arrival.

† Time period from symptom onset until medical assistance summoned.

There were no significant differences between men and women except for diastolic blood pressure ($p=0.001$).

Reproduced with permission from Kudenchuk et al.[118]

TABLE 2-7
Electrocardiographic Findings

Electrocardiogram	All	Men	Women
ST elevation of acute injury	679 (62%)	529 (62%)	150 (61%)
Inferior only	295 (43%)	224 (26%)	71 (29%)
Anterior only	126 (19%)	99 (12%)	27 (11%)
Lateral only	23 (3%)	15 (2%)	8 (3%)
Anterolateral	157 (23%)	132 (16%)	25 (10%)
Inferolateral	45 (7%)	32 (4%)	13 (5%)
Anterior and inferior	19 (3%)	16 (2%)	3 (1%)
T wave peaking	10 (1%)	9 (1%)	1 (0.5%)
ST depression			
Without ST elevation	128 (12%)	97 (11%)	31 (13%)
With accompanying ST elevation	511 (47%)	388 (46%)	123 (50%)
T wave inversion			
Without ST elevation	216 (20%)	164 (19%)	52 (21%)
With accompanying ST elevation	617 (56%)	473 (56%)	144 (59%)
Q waves	242 (22%)	210 (25%)	32 (13%)
Atrial fibrillation	31 (3%)	23 (3%)	8 (3%)
Intraventricular conduction abnormalities	257 (23%)	218 (26%)	39 (16%)

There were no significant differences between men and women except for Q waves ($p=0.0001$) and intraventricular conduction abnormalities ($p=0.002$).
Reproduced with permission from Kudenchuk et al.[118]

1.95). Hospital mortality after AMI was also independently predicted by older age, early evidence of hemodynamic instability, and an intraventricular conduction abnormality on the initial electrocardiogram. Although similar in its presentation, AMI in women is not as aggressively treated, and results in a less favorable outcome than in men. Gender, as well as nongender-specific risk factors, is important in assessing risk and the likelihood of early intervention after AMI (Tables 2-6–2-9).

TABLE 2-8
Treatment

Treatment	Total n	Men	Women	p Value*
Intravenous thrombolysis	623 (57%)	490 (57%)	133 (54%)	NS
Within 6 hrs of admission	613 (56%)	486 (57%)	127 (52%)	0.12
Prehospital thrombolysis	164 (15%)	135 (20%)	29 (17%)	NS
Cardiac catheterization	815 (74%)	649 (76%)	166 (67%)	0.005
Within 6 hrs of admission	259 (24%)	217 (28%)	42 (20%)	0.01
Coronary angioplasty	356 (33%)	284 (33%)	72 (29%)	NS
Within 6 hrs of admission	153 (14%)	127 (15%)	26 (11%)	0.07
Revascularization surgery	157 (14%)	129 (15%)	28 (11%)	0.16
Within 48 hrs of admission	49 (4%)	42 (5%)	6 (2%)	0.07
Any acute† intervention	777 (71%)	624 (73%)	153 (62%)	0.001

* Comparing women with men.

† Intravenous thrombolysis, cardiac catheterization, or angioplasty within 6 hours of hospital admission, or revascularization surgery within 48 hours of hospital admission.
Reproduced with permission from Kudenchuk et al.[118]

TABLE 2-9

Multivariate Predictors of Acute Cardiac Procedures (cardiac catheterization, coronary angioplasty, or intravenous thrombolytic therapy within 6 hours of hospital admission, or coronary revascularization surgery [CABG] within 48 hours of hospital admission)

Predictor	Odds Ratio (95% CI)	p Value
Female gender	0.5 (0.3-0.7)	0.0018
Age*	0.58 (0.57-0.59)	<0.0001
Symptom duration†	0.98 (0.97-0.98)	0.001
Heart rate‡	0.85 (0.84-0.86)	0.0003
CABG history	0.5 (0.3-0.8)	0.009
ST elevation	15.8 (10.7-22.9)	<0.0001

* Per decade increase in age; † per 10 minutes increase; ‡ per 10 beats per minute increase in heart rate. CI = confidence interval.
Reproduced with permission from Kudenchuk et al.[118]

Oral Anticoagulants

Treatment with oral anticoagulant therapy always entails a risk of bleeding. The optimal intensity required to prevent the occurrence of bleeding or thromboembolism is uncertain. Azar and colleagues[119] from Rotterdam, Leiden, The Netherlands, attempted to determine the optimal intensity of anticoagulant therapy in patients after AMI. The study population included 3404 patients enrolled in the ASPECT (ASPECT, Anticoagulants in the Secondary Prevention of Events in Coronary Thrombosis) trial. Major bleeding occurred in 0.8/100 patient-years and thromboembolic complications in 5.7/100 patient-years. If equal weight is given to hemorrhagic and thromboembolic complications, their studies show that the optimal intensity of long-term anticoagulant therapy for AMI patients lies between 2.0 and 4.0 INR, with a trend to suggest an optimal intensity of 3.0 to 4.0.

Antioxidant Vitamins

In a randomized, double-blind, placebo-controlled trial, Singh and associates[120] from Moradabad, India, compared the effects of combined treatment with the antioxidant vitamins A (50,000 IU/day), C (1000 mg/day), E (400 mg/day), and β-carotene (25 mg/day) for 28 days in 125 patients with suspected AMI. There were 63 patients in the intervention group and 62 in the placebo group. After treatment with antioxidants, the mean infarct size (creatine kinase and creatine kinase-MB gram equivalents) was significantly less in the antioxidant group than in the placebo group. Serum glutamic-oxaloacetic transaminase decreased by 45.6 IU/dL in the antioxidant group versus 25.8 IU/dL in the placebo group. Cardiac enzyme lactate dehydrogenase increased slightly (88.6 IU/dL) in the antioxidant group compared with that in the placebo group (166.5 IU/dL). QRS score in the electrocardiogram was significantly less in the antioxidant than in the placebo group. The increases in plasma levels of vitamins were higher in the antioxidant group than in the placebo group: vitamin A increased by 0.36 and 0.12 μmol/L, vitamin C increased by 12.6 and 4.2 μmol/L, plasma levels of vitamin E increased by 8.8 and 2.2 μmol/L, and β-carotene increased by 0.28 and 0.06 μmol/L. Serum lipid peroxides decreased by 1.22 pmol/mL in the antioxidant and 0.22 pmol/mL in the placebo group. Angina pectoris, total arrhythmias, and poor left ventricular function occurred less often in the antioxidant group. Cardiac end points were significantly less in the antioxidant group (20.6% vs. 30.6%, respectively). These results suggest that combined treatment with antioxidant vitamins A, E, C, and β-carotene in patients with recent AMI may be protective against cardiac necrosis and oxidative stress, and could be beneficial in preventing complications and cardiac event rate in such patients.

Calcium Angatonists

A multicenter, double-blind, randomized, placebo-controlled trial was conducted by Rengo and the Calcium Antagonist Reinfarction Italian Study (CRIS)[121] to assess the effects of verapamil on total mortality, cardiac mortality, reinfarction, and angina after an AMI. All patients, aged 30–75 years, consecutively admitted for AMI between 1985 and 1987 to the participating centers, and without contraindications to verapamil or history of severe CHF were enrolled. Seven to 21 days (mean 13.8) after myocardial infarction, 531 patients were randomly assigned to verapamil retard (360 mg/day), and 542 patients were randomly assigned to placebo. At baseline, the 2 groups of patients had similar characteristics. The mean age was 55.5 years; 91% were men. During a mean follow-up of 23.5 months, 5.5% of the patients died. No differences between verapamil and placebo were observed in total mortality (n = 30 and 29, respectively) and cardiac death (n = 21 and 22, respectively). The verapamil group had nonsignificant lower reinfarction rates (n = 39 vs. 49). The number of patients developing angina was significantly less in the verapamil group (n = 100 vs. 132, RR = 0.8). There were no differences in discontinuation of therapy caused by adverse reactions. This trial showed no effect of verapamil on mortality. The lower reinfarction rates found in the verapamil group are in agreement with the results of other studies.

In the last decade, several clinical trials in patients with or recovering from AMI have evaluated the effect of calcium antagonists on prognosis. Results have been disparate, with evidence of possible harm, no effect, or some benefit, depending on the agent used. Zuanetti and associates[122] from multiple centers, on behalf of the GISSI Investigators, evaluated how the evidence from these trials has influenced the pattern of prescriptions for calcium antagonists, and they assessed the important determinants of use of calcium antagonists after AMI. The authors retrospectively analyzed the prescription of calcium antagonists at discharge in all patients recovering from AMI enrolled in 3 large randomized clinical trials (Gruppo Italiano per lo Studio della Sopravvivenza nell'Infartol [GISSI-1], GISSI-2, and GISSI-3) over the last 10 years. A progressive decrease in prescriptions for calcium antagonists was evident, from 47.2% in GISSI-1, to 35.1% in GISSI-2, to 19.0% in GISSI-3. The presence of post-AMI angina, history of hypertension, and occurrence of reinfarction were associated

TABLE 2-10
Prescription of Calcium Antagonists at Discharge for Secondary Prevention After AMI

		GISSI-2 (n = 4,739)	GISSI-3 (n = 7,887)
Overall		26.1%	10.3%
Men/women		26.2/25.4	9.9/12.4
Age (yr)	≤70/>70	26.1/25.8	9.7/12.6
Previous AMI	Yes/no	29.0/25.7	14.3/10.0
Killip class at entry	1/>1	26.1/26.1	10.1/12.7
Site of AMI	Anterior/other	24.8/26.9	8.2/11.3
Type of AMI	Q/non-Q	25.4/30.1	9.4/14.3
Left ventricular dysfunction at discharge	Yes/no	21.4/27.0	9.6/10.5
Ventricular premature complexes (>10/h) during Holter	Yes/no	27.0/24.0	11.5/9.2
β blockers at discharge	Yes/no	9.8/31.4	5.1/12.5
Digitalis at discharge	Yes/no	18.0/26.9	11.3/10.3
Antiarrhythmics at discharge	Yes/no	22.6/26.5	10.3/10.4

Reproduced with permission from Zuanetti et al.[122]

with a higher usage of calcium antagonists, whereas the use of β blockers at discharge was a major independent negative determinant. Use of calcium antagonists for secondary prevention after AMI (ie, without specific clinical indications for their use) decreased by approximately 60% (from 26.1% to 10.3%). The data indicate that the usage of calcium antagonists in GISSI studies has been strongly affected by the results of other large multicenter trials evaluating calcium antagonists. These agents are now prescribed in patients after AMI almost exclusively in the presence of specific indications such as systemic hypertension or angina (Table 2-10).

Effect of Sotalol on Mortality

Waldo and the The Survival With Oral d-Sotalol Trial (SWORD) investigators[123] sought to determine whether d-sotalol, a potassium channel blocker with no clinically significant β-blocking activity, reduces all-cause mortality in patients with left ventricular dysfunction after AMI. Patients with an LVEF of 40% or less and either a recent (6–42 days) MI or symptomatic CHF with a remote (>42 days) AMI were randomly assigned to receive d-sotalol (100 mg increased to 200 mg twice daily, if tolerated) or matching placebo. The trial was discontinued after 3121 of the planned 6400 patients had been recruited. Among 1549 patients given d-sotalol, there were 78 deaths (5%) compared with 48 deaths (3%) among the 1572 patients assigned placebo (p=0.006). Presumed arrhythmic deaths accounted for the increased mortality. The effect was greater in patients with an LVEF of 31% to 40% than in those with lower (≤30%) LVEFs (relative risk 4.0 vs. 1.2, p=0.007). These data suggest that the administration of d-sotalol may be associated with increased mortality in patients with left ventricular dysfunction after AMI. Thus, the prophylactic use of a specific potassium-channel blocker does not reduce mortality and may be associated with increased mortality in high-risk patients after AMI.

β-*Blockers*

β-Blockers reduce infarct size and improve survival after AMI. Post-AMI angiotensin-converting enzyme inhibition also improves survival and may attenuate LV dilatation. Bonarjee and associates[124] from Stavanger, Norway; Copenhagen, Denmark; Gothenburg Sweden; Stockholm, Sweden; and Blue Bell, Pennsylvania, evaluated the effect of early enalapril treatment on left ventricular volumes and EF in patients on concomitant *β*-blockade after AMI. Intravenous enalaprilat or placebo was administered within 24 hours after AMI and was continued orally for 6 months. Left ventricular volumes were assessed by echocardiography, 3 ± 2 days, 1 and 6 months after AMI. Change in left ventricular diastolic volume during the first month was attenuated with enalapril (2.7 vs. placebo 6.5 mL/m^2 change), and significantly lower left ventricular diastolic and systolic volumes were observed with enalapril treatment compared with placebo at 1 month (enalapril 47/24 vs. placebo 53/29 mL/m^2) and at 6 months (enalapril 48/25 vs. placebo 54/30 mL/m^2). EF was also significantly higher 1 month after AMI in these patients (enalapril 50% vs placebo 46%). These data demonstrate that early enalapril treatment attenuates left ventricular volume expansion and maintains lower left ventricular volumes and higher EF in patients receiving concurrent *β*-blockade after AMI. A possible additive effect of combined therapy should be prospectively evaluated.

Lisinopril

In the GISSI-3 trial[125] 6-week treatment with lisinopril revealed an early benefit on the remodeling process. The GISSI group evaluated the potential benefit over 6 months using a combined end point of mortality and severe left ventricular dysfunction. In the study, 19,394 patients with AMI were randomly assigned within 24 hours of onset of symptoms to a 6-week treatment course of oral lisinopril or open control and, according to a 2 × 2 factorial design, to glyceryl trinitrate or open control. Treatments were stopped after 6 weeks in the absence of specific indications, and the patients were followed-up for 6 months. At 6 months, there was an 18% mortality or severe ventricular dysfunction in the lisinopril group compared with a 19.3% mortality for those randomized to no lisinopril. No difference was found between patients with and without glyceryl trinitrate therapy. These authors concluded that the early benefit of lisinopril seemed to continue through the first 6 months after randomization, even after treatment withdrawal.

Thrombolysis

Early Thrombolytic Treatment in AMI—Meta-Analysis

Boersma and colleagues[126] in Rotterdam, The Netherlands, determined the relation between treatment delay with thrombolytic intervention and short-term mortality up to 35 days using tabulated data from all randomized trials of at least 100 patients. Twenty-two trials including 50,246 patients that compared fibrinolytic therapy with placebo or control reported between 1983 and 1993 were used to make these evaluations and to determine specifically whether additional gain can be achieved from thrombolytic therapy with very early treatment. Analysis of the data revealed that the benefit of fibrinolytic therapy was 65 lives saved per 1000 treated patients in the 0–1, 1–2, 2–3, and 3–6 hour intervals, respectively. Proportional mortality reduction was significantly higher in patients treated within 2 hours compared with those treated later (44% versus 20%). The relation between treatment delay and mortality reduction per 1000 treated patients was expressed best by nonlinear regression equation. Thus, the data obtained in this study demonstrate that the beneficial effect of fibrinolytic therapy is substantially higher in patients presenting within 2 hours after symptom onset compared to those presenting later.

Reperfusion Strategies and Aspirin

In order to improve the morbidity and mortality associated with AMI, new research has been focused on adjuvant agents that may improve outcomes following coronary thrombolysis. O'Connor and associates[127] for the DUCCS-II, The Duke University Clinical Cardiology Group Study-II). Investigators enrolled 162 patients with AMI in a randomized trial comparing front-loaded tPA plus weight-adjusted heparin with anisoylated plasminogen streptokinase activator complex (APSAC) without heparin, as well as standard-dose (325 mg) and low-dose (81 mg) aspirin. The primary end point was an in-hospital morbidity profile; secondary end points were clinical and angiographic patency and hemorrhagic events. Selected sites performed an electrocardiographic substudy to determine the time to 50% ST-segment recovery and the time to steady state. Although the trial was terminated when the Global Utilization of Streptokinase and tPA for Occluded Coronary Arteries-I (GUSTO-I) trial showed that tPA had a significant mortality advantage over streptokinase, important trends were evident. Patients given tPA and heparin were better anticoagulated, yet APSAC-treated patients had more bleeding complications. The primary end point favored tPA (25.4% vs. 31.3%), and the secondary end points were similar in both groups. In the electrocardiographic substudy, the tPA group achieved both 50% ST-segment recovery and steady-state recovery sooner than the APSAC group. Patients taking low-dose aspirin had lower in-hospital mortality and less recurrent ischemia but more strokes than did the standard-dose aspirin group. Thus, this trial demonstrated trends favoring front-loaded tPA with weight-adjusted heparin over APSAC without heparin in the treatment of AMI. The use of low-dose aspirin did not appear to impose a loss of protection from adverse events, nor did standard-dose aspirin increase serious bleeding (Figure 2-62).

Randomized Trials of Intravenous Heparin

Glick and associates[128] from Tel Aviv, Israel, examined whether extending the anticoagulation effect of heparin by low-molecular-weight heparin (clex-

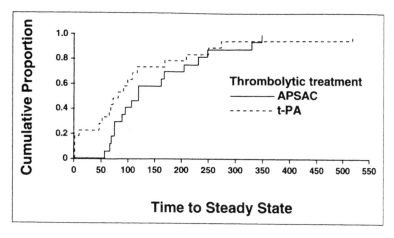

FIGURE 2-62. Cumulative distribution plot. The median time to steady state was 40 minutes faster in patients receiving t-PA with heparin than in patients randomized to APSAC without heparin. Reproduced with permission from O'Connor et al.[127]

ane) in patients with AMI can prevent recurrent myocardial ischemic events after treatment with streptokinase. On the fifth day after AMI and after heparin therapy cessation, 103 patients were randomly assigned to either treatment with low-molecular-weight heparin (40 mg subcutaneously per day for 25 days, n = 43) or control (no treatment, n = 60). All patients were followed carefully for 6 months after the infarction date. A total of 32 patients (31%) sustained a cardiac event during the 6-month observation period. There were 12 patients (20%) with reinfarction in the control group versus 2 patients (4.6%) in the low-molecular-weight heparin group during the first 30 days of the study. One additional patient sustained reinfarction at 3 months of follow-up in the control group, which yielded a total of 13 patients (21.6%) sustaining reinfarction in the control group and 2 patients (4.6%) in the low-molecular-weight heparin group during 6 months of follow-up. Angina pectoris after AMI was diagnosed in 13 control patients (21.6%) and in 4 low-molecular-weight heparin-treated patients (9.3%) during the study period. No major bleeding events were reported in either low-molecular-weight heparin-treated or control patients. Among patients with a recently diagnosed AMI treated by streptokinase, extending the anticoagulant effect of heparin by continuous treatment with low-molecular-weight heparin for 25 days may prevent recurrent coronary events for at least 1 month.

Intravenous heparin is routinely given after thrombolytic therapy for patients with AMI in the United States and in some, but by no means all, other countries. Several trials have documented improved infarct-artery patency in patients treated with heparin; none was large enough, however, to assess the effect of heparin on clinical outcomes. Mahaffey and associates[129] from Durham, North Carolina; Oxford, United Kingdom; Metairie, Louisiana; and Brussels, Belgium, performed a systematic overview of the 6 randomized control trials (1735 patients) to summarize the available data concerning the risks and benefits of intravenous heparin versus no heparin after thrombolytic therapy.

Mortality before hospital discharge was 5.1% for patients allocated to intravenous heparin, compared with 5.6% for controls (relative risk reduction, 9%; odds ratio, 0.91; 95% confidence interval, 0.59–1.39). Similar rates of recurrent ischemia and reinfarction were observed among those allocated to heparin therapy or control. The rates of total stroke, intracranial hemorrhage, and severe bleeding were similar in patients allocated to heparin; however, the risk of any severity of bleeding was significantly higher (22.7% vs. 16.2%; odds ratio, 1.55: 95% confidence interval, 1.21–1.98). There was no significant difference in the observed effects of heparin between patients receiving tissue-type plasminogen activator and those receiving streptokinase or anisoylated plasminogen streptokinase activator complex, or between patients who did and did not receive aspirin. This overview emphasizes that insufficient clinical data are available to support or to refute the routine use of intravenous heparin therapy after thrombolysis. It is not known if these findings are due to lack of statistical power, inappropriate levels of anticoagulation, or lack of benefit of intravenous heparin. Large randomized studies of heparin (and of newer antithrombotic regimens) are needed to establish the role of such therapy (Figures 2-63 and 2-64).

tPA Versus Streptokinase and Heparin

Califf and colleagues and the GUSTO Investigators[130] evaluated vital status at 1 year in the patients who were alive at 30 days after entry into the thrombolytic regimen that compared 4 different thrombolytic regimens. In the GUSTO

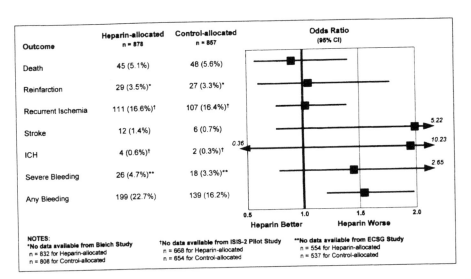

FIGURE 2-63. Odds ratios and 95% confidence intervals (CI) for intravenous heparin compared with no heparin for major clinical outcome events for all trials. ECSG = European Cooperative Study Group; ICH = intracranial hemorrhage; ISIS-2 = International Study of Infarct Survival-2; Severe Bleeding = bleeding associated with hemodynamic compromise or requiring blood transfusion. Reproduced with permission from Mahaffey et al.[129]

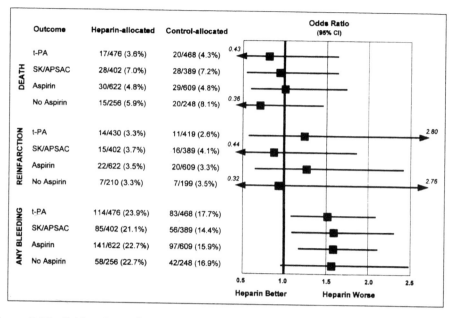

FIGURE 2-64. Odds ratios and 95% confidence intervals (CI) for intravenous heparin compared with no heparin for selected major clinical outcome events subdivided by type of treatment. APSAC = anisoylated plasminogen streptokinase activator complex; SK = streptokinase; t-PA = tissue-type plasminogen activator. Reproduced with permission from Mahaffey et al.[129]

trial, patients treated with accelerated tPA had a lower 30-day mortality rate (6.3%) than did those treated with the other regimens (7.3%, combined streptokinase groups). Final follow-up was 96% of the patients worldwide. One-year mortality rates remained in favor of accelerated tPA (9%) over streptokinase with subcutaneous heparin (10%, p = .011) and streptokinase with intravenous heparin (10.1%, p = .009) (Figure 2-65). Combination therapy had an intermediate 1-year mortality (9.9%), and this outcome was not statistically different from that with streptokinase but was marginally different from that with accelerated tPA (p = .05). Thus, the 1-year results demonstrated a savings of 10 lives per 1000 patients treated with accelerated tPA versus streptokinase and either subcutaneous or intravenous heparin.

Heparin versus Hirudin

The GUSTO investigators[131] compared the clinical efficacy of a potent, direct thrombin inhibitor, recombinant hirudin, with that of heparin, an indirect antithrombin in patients with unstable angina or AMI. At 373 hospitals in 13 countries, 12,142 patients with acute coronary syndromes were randomized to 72 hours of therapy with either intravenous heparin or hirudin. Patients were stratified according to the presence of ST segment elevation on the baseline electrocardiogram (4131 patients) or its absence (8011 patients), with the latter characteristic considered to indicate unstable angina or non-Q wave AMI.

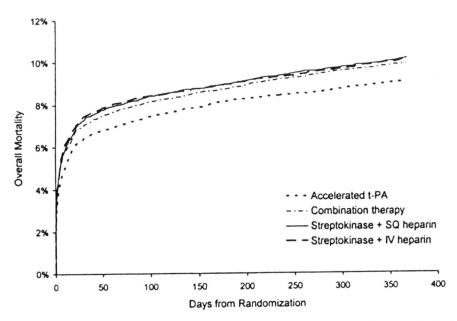

FIGURE 2-65. Overall 1-year mortality in the Global Utilization of Streptokinase and tPA for Occluded Coronary Arteries (GUSTO-I) trial by treatment assignment. SQ, subcutaneous; tPA, tPA: combination therapy, streptokinase and tPA with intravenous (IV) heparin. Reproduced with permission from Califf et al.[130]

At 24 hours, the risk of death or AMI was significantly lower in the group assigned to hirudin therapy than in the group assigned to heparin (1.3% vs. 2.1%, p = .001). The primary end point of death or nonfatal AMI or reinfarction at 30 days was reached in 9.8% of the heparin group, as compared with 8.9% of the hirudin group. The predominant effect of hirudin was on AMI or reinfarction and was not influenced by ST segment status. There was no significant difference in the incidence of serious or life-threatening bleeding complications, but hirudin therapy was associated with a higher incidence of moderate bleeding (8.8% vs. 7.7%, p = .03). Thus, for treatment of acute coronary diseases, recombinant hirudin provided a small advantage as compared with heparin, principally related to a reduction in the risk of AMI.

Antman and the TIMI 9B Investigators[132] evaluated whether the direct antithrombin hirudin is more effective than an indirect-acting antithrombin, heparin, as adjunctive therapy for thrombolysis in patients with AMI. Three thousand and two patients with AMI were treated with aspirin and either accelerated tPA or streptokinase. They were randomized within 12 hours of symptoms to receive either intravenous heparin (5000 U bolus followed by an infusion of 1000 U/h) or hirudin (0.1 mg/kg bolus followed by infusion of 0.1 mg/kg/hr). The infusions of both antithrombins were titrated to a targeted aPTT of 55 to 85 seconds and were administered for 96 hours. Patients randomly assigned to hirudin were more likely to have a partial thromboplastin time measurement in the target range (p < .0001). The primary end point of death, recurrent AMI, or development of severe CHF or cardiogenic shock by 30 days occurred in 11.9% of the 1491 patients in the heparin group and 12.9% of the

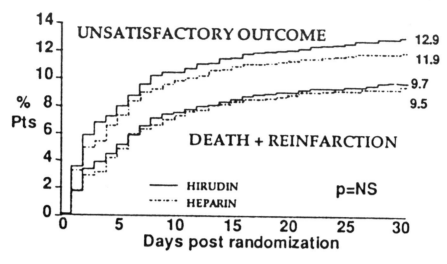

FIGURE 2-66. Time to development of unsatisfactory outcome. Kaplan-Meier plot of time to occurrence of any element of the unsatisfactory outcome composite end point in the heparin (broken line) and hirudin (solid line) groups. No difference in the timing of events was observed (p = NS by log rank test). Similarly, no difference was seen in the rate of occurrence of the sum of death and recurrent infarction. Reproduced with permission from Antman et al.[132]

1511 patients in the hirudin group (Figure 2-66). Subgroup analyses did not reveal any profile of patients who benefited more from one or the other anti-thrombins. The rate of major hemorrhage was similar in the heparin (5%) and hirudin (5%) groups, as was the incidence of intracranial hemorrhage (0.9% in the heparin and 0.4% in the hirudin-treated patients). Thus, heparin and hirudin have an equal effect as adjunctive therapy to tPA and streptokinase in preventing unsatisfactory outcome in patients with AMI. Similar rates of major bleeding were observed for patients in the heparin and hirudin groups.

Urokinase

Patients with severe and chronic refractory angina in end-stage CAD have few options available to them. Leschke and colleagues[133] from Dusseldorf, Germany, evaluated 2 low-dose regimens of urokinase administered over a prolonged time period to evaluate its effects on clinical symptoms and objective measures of myocardial ischemia. Ninety-eight patients with chronic refractory end-stage CAD were randomly assigned to group A receiving 50,000 IU or group B receiving 500,000 IU of urokinase as an intravenous bolus injection 3 times a week over a period of 12 weeks. After 12 weeks of treatment, anginal symptoms were significantly reduced in the second group by 70%, compared with 24% in the first group. Fibrinogen decreased by 3% in group A and by 33% in group B. Plasma viscosity and red blood cell aggregation were reduced by 6.4% and 19.9%. Objective measurements of myocardial ischemia were significantly improved only in group B. These authors concluded that long-term intermittent urokinase therapy in a dose of 3 times 500,000 IU/week is an effective anti-ischemic and antianginal approach for patients with refractory angina pectoris and end-stage CAD.

Reteplase Versus Alteplase

Bode and colleagues[134] in the RAPID II study determined whether a double-bolus regimen of reteplase, a recently developed deletion mutant of wild-type tPA, improves 90-minute coronary artery patency rates achieved with the most successful standard regimen, an accelerated front-loaded regimen of tPA (alteplase). The therapeutic benefit of thrombolytic therapy has been shown to correlate directly with completeness and speed of reperfusion in the infarct-related coronary artery, TIMI grade 3 flow. Three hundred and twenty-four patients with AMI were randomly assigned to receive either a 10-plus-10 megaunit double-bolus of reteplase or front-loaded alteplase, along with intravenous aspirin and heparin. The primary end point of "patency at 90 minutes, graded according to the TIMI classification" was centrally assessed in a blinded fashion. Infarct-related coronary artery patency (TIMI grade 2 or 3) and complete patency (TIMI grade 3) at 90 minutes after the start of thrombolytic therapy were significantly higher in the reteplase-treated patients (TIMI grade 2 or 3: 83% vs. 73% for front-loaded alteplase-treated patients, $p = 0.03$; and TIMI grade 3 flow: 59.9% versus 45%, $p = .01$), respectively (Figure 2-67). At 60 minutes, the incidence of both patency and complete patency was also significantly

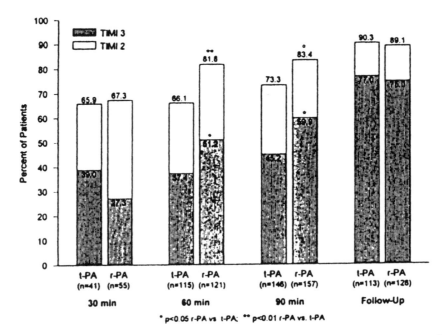

FIGURE 2-67. Patency rates at different time points achieved with alteplase (t-PA) and reteplase (r-PA). Reproduced with permission from Bode et al.[134]

higher in reteplase-treated patients (TIMI 3 grade flow was 51% vs. 37%, p<.03 at 60 minutes in the reteplase and alteplase-treated patients, respectively). Reteplase-treated patients required fewer acute additional coronary interventions (14% vs. 27%, p<.01), and 35-day mortality was 4% for reteplase and 8% for alteplase. There were no significant differences in bleeding requiring a transfusion between the 2 forms of therapy (12% vs. 10%, respectively) or hemorrhagic stroke (1% vs. 2%). Thus, reteplase when given as a double bolus of 10 plus 10 megaunits to patients with AMI achieves significantly higher rates of early reperfusion of the infarct-related coronary artery and requires significantly fewer acute coronary interventions than does front-loaded alteplase without an apparent increased risk of complications.

Circadian Variations of Onset of AMI and Efficacy of Thrombolytic Therapy

Previous studies have demonstrated a peak of AMI in the early morning hours and in some studies a secondary peak incidence in the evening. Kono and colleagues[135] from Takatsuki, Japan, evaluated the circadian variation of resistance to thrombolysis in 608 Japanese patients with an AMI. Two hundred forty-four were treated with thrombolysis within 12 hours of the onset of symptoms. TIMI grade 0, 1, or 2 flow was defined as resistance to thrombolysis, and patency was evaluated at 60 minutes after the initiation of thrombolytic therapy. Both the onset of AMI and resistance to thrombolysis showed circadian variations with early morning and late evening peaks. Resistance to thrombolysis showed a phased difference of about 2 hours earlier than the infarction incidence. The variation in resistance to thrombolysis was also independent of the types of thrombolytic agents used. These authors concluded that the circadian variation of resistance to thrombolysis may have clinical implications for adjustment of treatment.

Time from Symptom Onset to Treatment and Outcomes

In general, studies have shown that the earlier thrombolysis is applied after AMI, the greater the benefit, but the relative benefits of various thrombolytic agents with earlier administration are less certain. Newby and colleagues[136] in the multicenter GUSTO-I trial evaluated 3 time variables: symptom onset to treatment; symptom onset to hospital arrival; and hospital arrival to treatment, in relation to clinical outcomes and relative 30-day mortality benefit with tPA and streptokinase. Female, elderly, diabetic, and hypertensive patients have longer delays at all stages. Previous infarction or CABG was an additional risk factor for treatment delay. Earlier thrombolysis was associated with a lower mortality rate (<2 hours, 5.5%; >4 hours, 9%), but no additional relative benefit resulted from earlier treatment with tPA versus streptokinase. Longer presentation and treatment delays were both associated with increased mortality rate. As time to treatment increased, the incidence of recurrent ischemia or reinfarction decreased, but the rates of shock, CHF, and stroke increased. These authors concluded that earlier treatment resulted in better outcomes regardless of the thrombolytic agent used. Elderly, female, and diabetic patients were treated later, adding to their already substantial risk.

Symptom Duration as a Predictor for Infarct Size after Therapy

Raitt and colleagues[137] in Seattle, Washington, quantitated the relation between final myocardial infarct size and the duration of symptoms before initiation of thrombolytic therapy in patients treated within 6 hours of symptom onset with AMI. Patient data from 4 studies of thrombolytic therapy were combined for analysis: the Western Washington Randomized Trial of Intracoronary Streptokinase in Acute Myocardial Infarction, the Western Washington Intravenous Streptokinase in Acute Myocardial Infarction Trial, the Western Washington Myocardial Infarction Registry, the Emergency Department Tissue Plasminogen Activator Treatment Study, and the Myocardial Infarction Triage and Intervention Trial. All patients presented within 6 hours of symptom onset, had ST elevation on ECG, and had no contraindications to thrombolytic therapy. Patients were randomly assigned to thrombolysis with streptokinase or standard therapy with thrombolysis in the 2 older studies and in 2 more recent trials, recombinant tPA was used in all patients. Findings from patients in the 4 prospective randomized trials of thrombolytic therapy were combined for analysis. The study population consisted of 432 patients presenting within 6 hours of onset of symptoms of first AMI who met electrocardiographic criteria that allowed estimation of myocardial area at risk before treatment with thrombolytic therapy and who had thallium-201 myocardial infarct size measurements performed several weeks after AMI. Univariate and multivariate analysis showed that final infarct size was dependent on the duration of symptoms before initiation of therapy. For each 30-minute increase in symptom duration before thrombolytic therapy, there was an increase in infarct size of 1% of the myocardium (Figure 2-68). Final infarct size in patients treated 4 to 6 hours after symptom onset was indistinguishable from that in patients who did not receive thrombolytic therapy. Thus, these data suggest that for patients treated within 4 to 6 hours of the onset of symptoms after AMI, there is a progressive decline in the extent of myocardium salvaged as the duration of symptoms before therapy increases.

Prognosis in Non-Q Wave Infarction

Prior to the thrombolytic era, patients with non-Q wave as compared with Q wave myocardial infarction were thought to have a higher rate of reinfarction and death between hospital discharge and 1 year such that the overall prognosis at 1 year was similar for the 2 groups. Langer and colleagues[138] in the multicen-

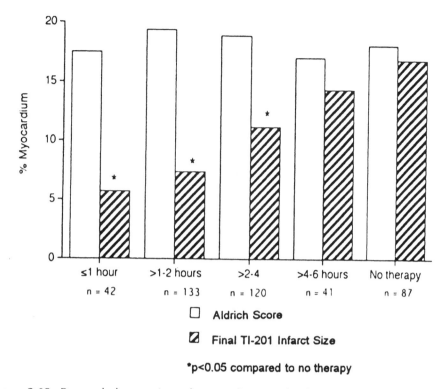

FIGURE 2-68. Bar graph shows estimated myocardium at risk (Aldrich score) and final myocardial infarct size, expressed as a percent of the myocardium, for patients with acute myocardial infarction treated with thrombolytic therapy at various time intervals after the onset of symptoms, as well as for patients who did not receive thrombolytic therapy. Duration of symptoms before therapy was a significant predictor of final infarct size (p<.0001 by ANOVA). There was no difference in final infarct size between patients treated more than 4 hours after symptom onset and those who did not receive thrombolytic therapy. The number of patients from which the determinations were calculated is shown. Reproduced with permission from Raitt et al.[137]

ter LATE (Late Assessment of Thrombolytic Efficacy) trial randomized patients with either tPA or matching placebo 6 to 24 hours after the onset of chest pain. Among 5711 participants, 4759 had a confirmed AMI, including 1309 with a non-Q wave infarction at hospital discharge. Regardless of treatment assignment, patients with non-Q wave versus Q wave infarction had a lower mortality rate (13.3% vs. 17.1%) and a similar 1-year reinfarction rate (8.6% vs. 7.9%). Patients with ST elevation who were treated with tPA versus placebo within 3 hours after hospital admission had a lower mortality rate at 1 year (15.8% vs. 19.6%) than did those treated after 3 hours (17.6% vs. 13.0%). Patients presenting initially with ST depression of greater than 2 mm had significant benefit from treatment with tPA with respect to 1-year mortality (20.1% versus 31.9%). These authors concluded that patients with a non-Q wave AMI constitute a heterogenous group of patients. Patients with a non-Q wave infarction receiving thrombolytic therapy have a better prognosis than do those given placebo. Late administration of thrombolytic therapy (after 6 hours) may also be beneficial in patients presenting with ST depression greater than 2 mm, and confirmed myocardial infarction.

aPTT, Patient Characteristics, and Outcome

Granger and colleagues[139] in the Global Utilization of Streptokinase and Tissue Plasminogen Activator for Occluded Coronary Arteries (GUSTO-I) trial examined the aPTT (aPTT) in 29,656 patients, evaluating the relationship between the aPTTs and patient characteristics and clinical outcomes. In this study, intravenous heparin was used after thrombolytic therapy. Intravenous heparin was administered as a 5000 U bolus followed by an initial infusion of 1000 U/hour with dose adjustment to achieve a target aPTT of 60 to 85 seconds. aPTTs were collected 6, 12, and 24 hours after thrombolytic administration. Higher aPTT at 24 hours was strongly related to lower patient weight, as well as older age, female sex, and lack of cigarette smoking (Figure 2-69). At 12 hours, the aPTT associated with the lowest 30-day mortality, stroke, and bleeding rates was 50 to 70 seconds (Figures 2-70 and 2-71). There was a direct relation between the aPTT and the risk of subsequent reinfarction. There was a clustering of reinfarction in the first 10 hours after discontinuation of intravenous heparin. aPTTs higher than 70 seconds were associated with higher likelihood of mortality, stroke, bleeding, and reinfarction. The authors suggest that physicians should consider the aPTT range of 50 to 70 seconds as optimal with intravenous therapy after thrombolytic therapy.

Systemic Anticoagulation—Relation to Clinical Events

Although coronary thrombosis is thought to play a pivotal role in the pathogenesis of unstable angina and non-Q wave AMI, and antithrombotic therapy

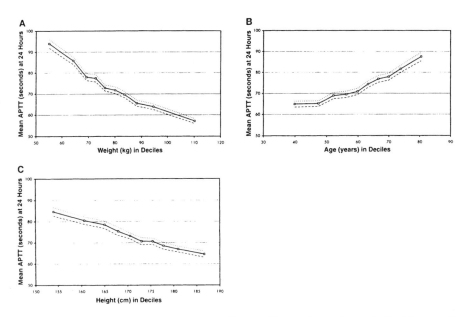

FIGURE 2-69. Mean aPTTs (aPTT) 24 hours after enrollment for patients divided into deciles according to weight (A), age (B), and height (C) for patients assigned to intravenous heparin who had 24-hour aPTTs recorded. Dotted lines represent 95% confidence intervals. Reproduced with permission from Granger et al.[139]

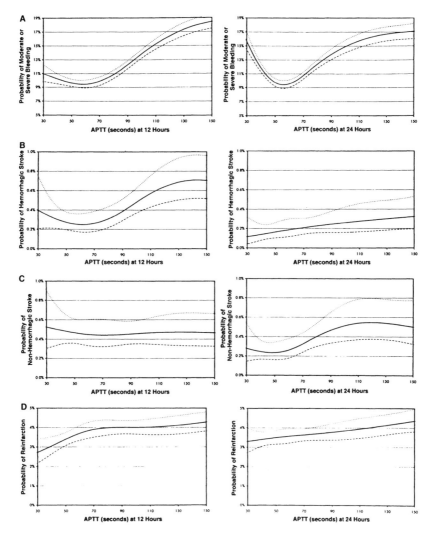

Figure 2-70. Activated partial thromboplastin times (aPTT) vs. probability of moderate or severe bleeding **(A)**, hemorrhagic stroke **(B)**, nonhemorrhagic stroke **(C)**, and reinfarction **(D)** at 12 (left) and 24 (right) hours after enrollment. Dotted lines represent 95% confidence intervals. Reproduced with permission from Granger et al.[139]

is a mainstay in the early management of these patients, the relation between measures of systemic anticoagulation and clinical events has not been clearly defined. In the Thrombolysis in Myocardial Infarction III trial carried out by Becker and associates[140] from Worcester, Massachusetts; Boston, Massachusetts; Burlington, Vermont; and Baltimore, Maryland, 1473 patients with ischemic chest pain at rest evaluated within 24 hours of symptom onset were randomized to: 1) tPA or placebo, and 2) an early invasive or an early conservative strategy. All patients received a full complement of anti-ischemic medication, aspirin, and continuous intravenous heparin titrated to an activated partial thromboplastin time (aPTT) of 1.5 to 2.0 times control for 72 to 96 hours.

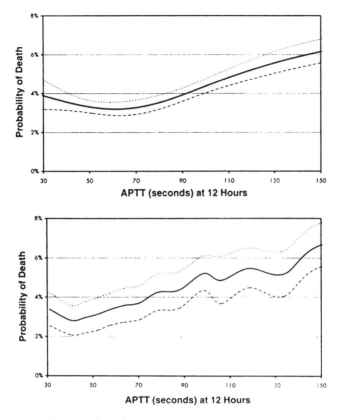

FIGURE 2-71. Activated partial thromboplastin time (aPTT) vs. probability of 30-day mortality for patients assigned to intravenous heparin unadjusted (top) and adjusted (bottom) for prognostically important baseline clinical characteristics. Dotted lines represent 95% confidence intervals. Reproduced with permission from Granger et al.[139]

The median aPTT in all study groups exceeded the minimum threshold (45 seconds) by 24 hours and remained within the designated range during the protocol-directed heparin infusion. No differences in median aPTT values for the 72- to 96-hour study period were observed between groups. Median 12-hour heparin concentrations were >0.2 U/mL in all groups; however, values less than 0.2 U/mL were common thereafter, particularly in tPA-treated patients. Time-dependent covariate analyses failed to identify statistically significant differences in either aPTT or heparin levels between patients with in-hospital clinical events (spontaneous ischemia, AMI, or death) and those without events. Furthermore, early clinical events occurred in a similar percentage of patients with optimal anticoagulation (all aPTT >60 seconds, all heparin levels >0.2 U/mL), and those with aPTT or heparin levels below these thresholds. Aggressive (high-intensity) anticoagulation with heparin to achieve aPTTs greater than 2.0 times control did not appear to offer additional clinical benefit to lower levels (1.5 to 2.0 times control) among patients with unstable angina and non-Q wave AMI receiving intravenous heparin and oral aspirin. Therefore, the optimal level of anticoagulation in this common clinical setting is between

45 and 60 seconds when heparin is included in the treatment strategy. Direct plasma heparin measurement does not offer an advantage to routine aPTT monitoring. The occurrence of spontaneous ischemia, AMI, and death in spite of antiischemic therapy and optimal anticoagulation (as it is currently defined) with heparin supports ongoing efforts to develop more effective antithrombotic agents.

Procoagulant Markers in Predicting Outcome

Thrombin activity is increased in the setting of AMI and has been shown to increase further after the administration of thrombolytic therapy for AMI. This increase in thrombin activity may play an important role in the 15% to 25% rate of failure to achieve initial reperfusion and in the 5% to 15% rate of early reocclusion after initially successful thrombolysis. To investigate potential mechanisms of thrombin formation *in vivo*, to understand better the balance of coagulation and fibrinolysis during treatment with recombinant tissue-type plasminogen activator (rtPA), and to investigate the role of hemostatic markers as predictors of clinical events, Scharfstein and associates[141] for the TIMI-5 Investigators measured 3 markers of procoagulant activity: fibrinopeptide A (FPA), thrombin-antithrombin III complexes (TAT) and prothrombin fragment 1.2 (F1.2), and a marker of fibrinogenolytic activity (Bβ1-42) in patients enrolled in the Thrombolysis in Myocardial Infarction (TIMI)-5 study. This trial was a randomized, dose-ranging, pilot trial of hirudin versus heparin as adjunctive antithrombotic therapy, with rtPA administered to patients with AMI. Correlation of markers at 1 hour with clinical outcomes revealed that increased FPA and TAT levels were associated with increased mortality and TIMI grades 0, 1, or 2 flow at 90 minutes; increased F1.2 levels were associated with TIMI grade 0 or 1 flow at 90 minutes; and increased levels of all 3 procoagulant markers were associated with hemorrhagic events. Late (12 to 24 hours) increases in F1.2, TAT, and Bβ1-42 may be predictive of recurrent ischemia. These results suggest that selected markers of procoagulant and fibrinogenolytic activity may be useful in predicting clinical outcomes in patients treated with thrombolytic therapy for AMI.

Infarct Expansion and Late Ventricular Remodeling

Popović and associates[142] from Belgrade, Yugoslavia, and Cleveland, Ohio, investigated the impact of thrombolysis on AMI expansion and subsequent left ventricular remodeling in patients with anterior wall AMI. The authors evaluated 51 consecutive patients (24 treated with thrombolysis) with anterior AMI by 2-dimensional echocardiography in the following sequence: days 1, 2, 3, and 7 after 3 and 6 weeks, and after 3, 6, and 12 months. Left ventricular end-diastolic and end-systolic volume indexes were determined from apical 2- and 4-chamber views using Simpson's biplane formula. Infarct and total left

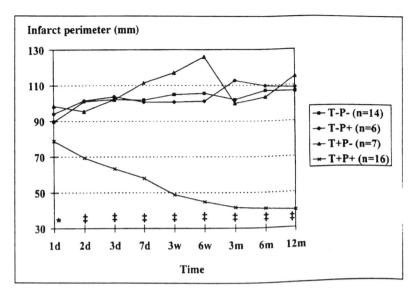

Figure 2-72. Combined impact of thrombolysis (T) and infarct-related artery patency (P) on infarct perimeter. *p<.05; ‡p<.001 between T+P+ patients vs. all other subgroups. Reproduced with permission from Popović et al.[142]

ventricular perimeters were determined in the same views and their ratio expressed as infarct percentage. Infarct expansion was defined as: 1) an increase in infarct percentage and total perimeter greater than 5% on days 2 to 3 in either of the views, or 2) initial infarct percentage greater than 50% with an increase in total perimeter greater than 5% on days 2 to 3. Coronary angiography was performed in 43 patients before discharge, and patency of the infarct-related artery was assessed using TIMI trial criteria. Infarct expansion was detected in 23 patients. Infarct perimeter steadily decreased in patients with patent versus occluded infarct-related arteries. Furthermore, by logistic regression, thrombolysis and patency of the infarct-related artery were strong negative predictors of expansion, whereas initial infarct perimeter was directly associated with subsequent expansion. End-systolic volume index was higher in patients with expansion from day 1 throughout the end of the study, and end-diastolic volume index was higher in these patients from day 2 through 12 months. Thus thrombolysis, initial infarct size, and infarct-related artery patency are major predictors of infarct expansion after anterior wall AMI (Figures 2-72 and 2-73).

Electrocardiographic Changes as Predictors of Stabilization

Bär and associates[143] from Maastricht, The Netherlands, and Mainz, Germany, assessed sequential electrocardiograms from admission to 36 hours in 358 patients with AMI from the Pro-urokinase in Myocardial Infarction trial. The electrocardiogram also was examined at discharge in 69 of 358 patients.

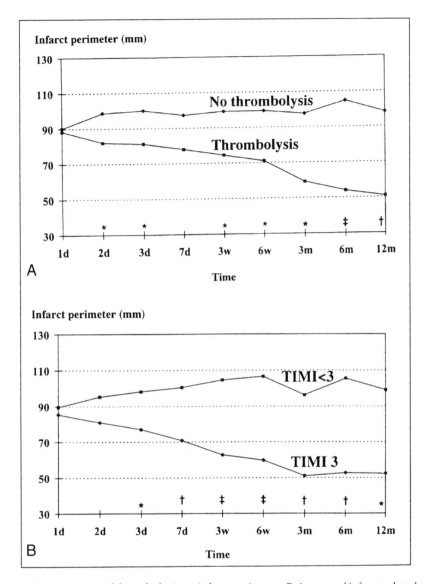

FIGURE 2-73. A, impact of thrombolysis on infarct perimeter. **B,** impact of infarct-related artery patency on infarct perimeter. *p<.05; †p<.01; ‡p<.001. d = day; m = month; w = week; TIM-I = Thrombolysis in Myocardial infarction trial. Reproduced with permission from Popovic et al.[142]

Patients underwent acute angiography, after which angioplasty was performed in most patients with impaired flow. The sum of the ST segment deviation and Q- and R-wave voltages, and the QRS score were calculated and used for further evaluation. Development of Q waves, loss of R waves, and QRS score were completed within the first 9 hours after onset of AMI and remained stable thereafter. Reperfused patients had earlier stabilization and less severe electrocardiographic abnormalities than did nonreperfused patients. ST segment elevation had already stabilized after 5 hours, was unchanged at 36 hours, and had significantly decreased at discharge. No significant electrocardiographic and clinical outcome differences were found between the Thrombolysis in Myocardial Infarction trial (TIMI) 2 and TIMI 3 patients. A 23.3% gain in electrocardiographic-estimated infarct size was found in the reperfusion group, compared with a 12.0% gain in the nonreperfusion group. In summary, as early as 9 hours after onset of AMI, QRS changes were already complete. Thereafter, QRS morphology was stable. Thus, a QRS-based estimation of infarct size can be made as early as 9 hours after AMI. A similar electrocardiographic outcome for patients with TIMI 2 and 3 flow was found, which was significantly different from patients with TIMI 0 to 1 flow.

Q waves as Predictors of Left Ventricular Dysfunction

Although the natural history of regional LV dysfunction after Q wave and non-Q wave AMI was well defined in the prethrombolytic era, the functional and structural implications of the absence of Q waves after thrombolysis are less clear. In this study by Isselbacher and associates[144] from Boston, Massachusetts, echocardiography was performed within 48 hours of admission (entry) in 86 patients treated with thrombolysis for their first AMI. The extent of abnormal wall motion (square centimeters) and left ventricular endocardial surface area index were quantified by using a previously validated echocardiographic endocardial surface-mapping technique. Electrocardiography performed at 48 hours after thrombolysis was used to classify patients into groups with (Q: n = 70) and without (non-Q; n = 16) Q waves. All patients in the Q group had regional LV dysfunction on initial echocardiogram compared with 69% of those in the non-Q group. When the patients in the non-Q group without abnormal wall motion were excluded from analysis, there was no significant difference in the extent of abnormal wall motion between the Q and non-Q groups. Among those patients with abnormal wall motion on entry, follow-up echocardiography at 6 to 12 weeks demonstrated a significant reduction in extent of abnormal wall motion for both the Q and non-Q groups. However, the fractional change in abnormal wall motion was significantly greater in the non-Q than in the Q group (-0.74 ± 0.28 vs. -0.29 ± 44) with a trend toward less abnormal wall motion at follow-up in the non-Q than in the Q group. The mean endocardial surface area index was not significantly different between the 2 groups at entry or at follow-up. In conclusion, failure to develop Q waves after thrombolysis predicts a lower likelihood of developing regional left ventricular dysfunction and, when such dysfunction is present, predicts a greater degree of recovery.

Interstitial Collagen Metabolism Changes as Predictors of Rethrombosis

Collagen plays a specific role in the maintenance of vascular integrity and in the thrombosis and scar formation processes. Therefore, Peuhkurinen and associates[145] from Oulu, Finland, studied the changes in interstitial collagen metabolism during AMI treated with thrombolytic agents. Changes in collagen synthesis were evaluated by obtaining assays of the serum concentrations of the carboxyterminal propeptide of type I procollagen. Fibrin plasmin is capable of degrading extracellular matrix components, including collagen, and this capability was evaluated by monitoring the serum concentrations of the aminoterminal propeptide of type III procollagen. Twenty-four patients with suspected AMI and indications for thrombolytic therapy were randomized to receive either streptokinase (n = 11) or tPA (n = 13). The patient groups were identical in their clinical characteristics. Serum levels of the aminoterminal propeptide of type III collagen increased rapidly on infusion of the thrombolytic agents, with the maximal mean increases of 44% and 16% in the streptokinase and tPA-treated groups. Levels of the carboxyterminal propeptide of type I collagen did not change during the thrombolytic therapy. A transient decrease occurred in the type I propeptide concentration at postinfarction day 2, and this decrease was followed by a secondary increase at days 4 to 6 in both patient groups studied. It was concluded that thrombolytic agents stimulate the breakdown of interstitial collagen and that the collagen-degrading activity of tPA is lower than that of streptokinase. This factor may contribute to the relatively higher rethrombosis rate seen after tPA, because exposed collagen in the affected vascular wall stimulates thrombosis formation. On the other hand, increased collagen degradation followed by inhibition of collagen synthesis in the infarcted myocardium might increase the risk for cardiac rupture, especially after streptokinase treatment.

Myocardial Perfusion Scintigraphy as a Predictor of Coronary Events

Dakik and colleagues[146] determined whether myocardial perfusion scintigraphy is of prognostic value in patients undergoing thrombolytic therapy. Seventy-one patients who received thrombolytic therapy for AMI had exercise thallium-201 tomography and coronary angiography before hospital discharge. Eleven (15%) of 71 patients had ischemic ST segment depression during exercise, but 27 patients (38%) had scintigraphic evidence of ischemia. Twenty-five (37%) of 68 patients had a cardiac event, including either cardiac death (n = 2), recurrent AMI (n = 5), CHF (n = 7), or unstable angina (n = 11) during a follow-up of 26 ± 18 months. By multivariate analysis, the significant joint predictors of risk were LVEF, and ischemic perfusion defect size (Figure 2-74). The combination of LVEF and thallium tomography added significant incremental prognostic information to the clinical data, but angiography did not further improve a model that included clinical, LVEF, and tomographic variables. Thus, quantitative thallium-201 tomography provides important and incremental long-term prognostic information in patients receiving thrombolytic therapy for AMI.

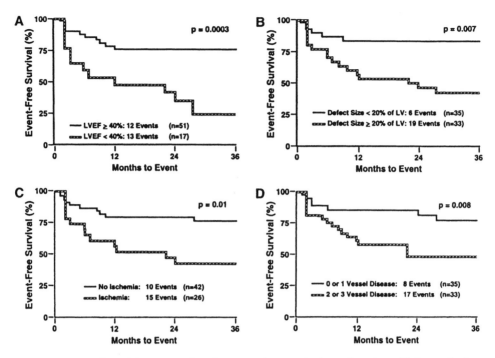

FIGURE 2-74. Kaplan-Meier curves showing event-free survival as a function of left ventricular ejection fraction (LVEF) **(A)**; perfusion defect size **(B)**; presence of myocardial ischemia **(C)**; and extent of coronary artery disease **(D)**. Events were defined as cardiac death, myocardial reinfarction, unstable angina, or CHF. LV indicates left ventricle. Reproduced with permission from Dakik et al.[146]

Predischarge Exercise Testing, Ejection Fraction, and Ventricular Ectopic Activity with Streptokinase

The relative importance of prognostic parameters that delineate left ventricular function, myocardial ischemia, and arrhythmogenic potential after thrombolytic therapy is not clear. Khattar and associates[147] from Harrow, United Kingdom, investigated 112 patients with AMI who were treated with thrombolysis to determine the relative prognostic value of predischarge treadmill exercise testing, radionuclide ventriculography, and ambulatory electrocardiographic monitoring for ventricular ectopic activity. During a mean follow-up period of 18 months (range 6 to 30), 42 first cardiac events were recorded, consisting of 3 deaths, 6 reinfarctions, 16 bouts of unstable angina, 16 episodes of CHF, and 1 arrhythmic event. Univariate analysis revealed EF, exercise time, and ventricular ectopic count of 10 per hour or greater to be predictive of future cardiac events. Subsequent multivariate analysis showed EF and exercise time to have independent prognostic value, but ventricular ectopic activity did not provide additional information. Ventricular ectopic count of 10 per hour or greater was additionally predictive only when combined with either EF (R2 = 5.4%) or exercise time (R2 = 2.9%). Event-free survival analysis revealed hazard ratios for EF less than 40% and exercise time less than 7 minutes of 3.63 and 2.16. Although EF and exercise time were able to predict future episodes of CHF, neither could adequately identify patients at risk of recurrent ischemic events.

Brouwer and Associates[148] for the Myocardial Infarction Triage and Intervention (MITI) project investigators earlier compared prehospital versus hospital administration of thrombolytic therapy. They found that the prehospitalization therapy markedly reduced hospital treatment times, but the 2 groups had similar outcomes. The patients, however, treated less than 70 minutes from symptom onset had better short-term outcomes. The present study was to determine the long-term influence of very early thrombolytic treatment for AMI. A total of 360 patients were followed for vital status and cardiac-related hospital admissions over a period of 34 ± 16 months. Patients enrolled in the trial had symptoms for a 6 hours or less ST segment elevation on the prehospital electrocardiogram, and no risk factors for serious bleeding. They received aspirin and recombinant tPA either before or after hospital arrival. Primary end points in this study included long-term survival and survival free of death, or readmission to the hospital for angina, AMI, CHF, or revascularization. Two-year survival was 89% for prehospital- and 91% for hospital-treated patients. Event-free survival at 2 years was 56% and 64% for prehospital- and hospital-treated patients. In patients treated within 70 minutes of symptom onset, 2-year survival was 98%, and it was 88% for those treated later. Two-year event-free survival was 65% for patients treated early and 59% for patients treated later. In this trial, poorer long-term survival was associated with advanced age, history of CHF, and CABG performed before the index hospitalization, but not with time to treatment.

Older Age and Increased Mortality with tPA

White and colleagues[149] in the Global Utilization of Streptokinase and Tissue Plasminogen Activator for Occluded Coronary Arteries (GUSTO-I) trial were able to evaluate outcomes according to age of patients receiving thrombolysis in patients after AMI. Patients were randomly assigned to streptokinase and subcutaneous heparin, streptokinase and intravenous heparin, accelerated tPA and intravenous heparin, or streptokinase and accelerated tPA plus intravenous heparin. Clinical outcomes at 30 days, including death; stroke; and nonfatal, disabling stroke; and 1-year mortality were summarized descriptively for patients aged younger than 65 (n = 24,708), 65 to 74 (n = 11,201), 75 to 85 (n = 4625), and older than 85 years (n = 412) and assessed as continuous functions of age. Older patients had a higher risk profile with regard to baseline clinical and angiographic characteristics. Mortality at 30 days increased markedly with age (3%, 9.5%, 19.6%, and 30% in the 4 groups, respectively) as did stroke, cardiogenic shock, bleeding, and reinfarction (Figures 2-75 and 2-76). Combined death or disabling stroke occurred less often with accelerated tPA in all but the oldest patients. Accelerated tPA treatment resulted in a lower 1-year mortality in all but the oldest patients (47% tPA vs. 40.3% streptokinase). Thus, lower mortality and greater net clinical benefit were seen with accelerated tPA in patients aged 85 years or younger.

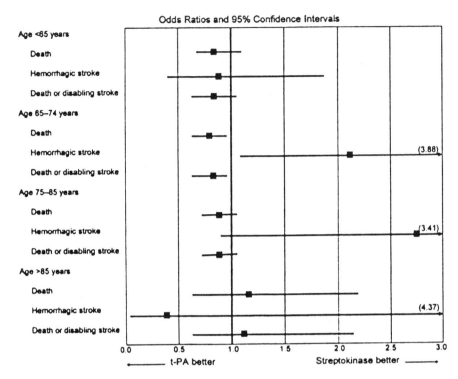

FIGURE 2-75. Odds ratios and 95% CIs for the risk of death, hemorrhagic stroke, and death or disabling stroke at 30 days with treatment with accelerated tPA and intravenous heparin vs. streptokinase and subcutaneous heparin. Reproduced with permission from White et al.[149]

Wall Motion Score to Predict Mortality

To recognize patients prone to subsequent left ventricular dilation after AMI treated by thrombolysis, Peels and associates,[150] on behalf of the CATS (Captopril and Thrombolysis Study) Investigators Group, studied 233 patients with a first anterior wall AMI treated with thrombolysis with 2-dimensional echocardiography within 12 hours after admission and then 3 months later. A wall motion score index and left ventricular volumes were assessed, and enzymatic infarct size was expressed as cumulative alphahydroxybutyrate dehydrogenate determined within the first 72 hours after infarction. Patients who died (17 of 233, 7%) after a mean follow-up of 517 days had a significantly higher acute wall motion score index (2.1 ± 0.3, mean ± SD) than did those who survived (1.9 ± 0.4). With use of this cutoff value of 2 for wall motion score index, ventricles with an acute wall motion score index of 2 or less (62%) showed no increase in end-diastolic volume index or end-systolic volume index, whereas ventricles with an acute wall motion score index greater than 2 (38%) showed a significant increase in end-systolic volume index (6.1 ± 12.2 mL/m^2) and in end-diastolic volume index (10.3 ± 16.6 mL/m^2) in the first 3 months. Using a cutoff value of 1,000 U/L for cumulative alphahydroxybutyrate dehydrogenase, only infarcts with a value of more than 1,000 U/L (52%) caused a

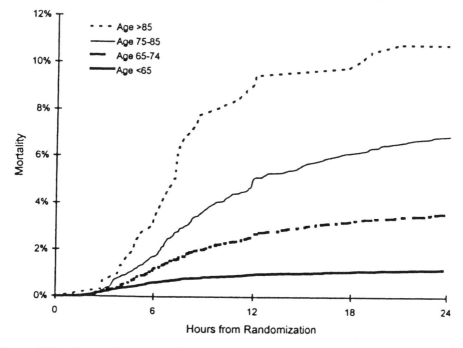

FIGURE 2-76. Twenty-four hour Kaplan-Meier mortality estimates by age group. Reproduced with permission from White et al.[149]

significant increase in end-systolic volume index (10.8 ± 14.3 mL/m^2) and end-diastolic volume index (6.5 ± 10.0 mL/m^2) in the first 3 months. Thus, acutely assessed wall motion score index of more than 2 is a predictor of subsequent dilation in patients with a first anterior infarction treated with streptokinase, and it is also a good predictor of mortality. Enzymatic infarct size also is a good predictor of dilation, although this measurement is not available until 3 days after infarction.

Heart Rate Variability and Mortality

Zuanetti and colleagues[151] in Milan, Italy, evaluated whether heart rate variability adds information relevant to risk stratification in post-MI patients treated with fibrinolytic therapy. From 24-hour electrocardiographic recordings, obtained at discharge in patients treated with recombinant tissue type plasminogen activator (rtPA) or streptokinase, Zuanetti et al.[151] measured several time-domain indexes of heart rate variability, including standard deviation, root-mean-square of successive differences, and number of RR interval increases greater than 50 msec. The prognostic value of heart rate variability for total and cardiovascular mortality was assessed. Among 567 patients with valid recordings, 52 (9%) died during the 1000 days of follow-up, 44 (7.8%) of cardiovascular causes. All indexes of low heart rate variability identified pa-

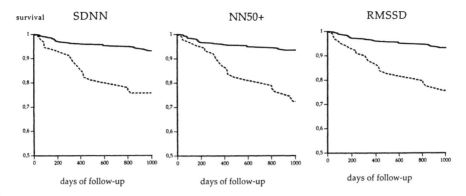

FIGURE 2-77. Survival curves for patients with low (dashed lines) and high (solid lines) HRV for the 3 indexes used. Cutoff values were SDNN, 70 ms; NN50+, 200 per 24 hours; and RMSSD, 17.5 msec. Reproduced with permission from Zuanetti et al.[151]

tients with a higher total mortality (Figure 2-77). The independent predictive value of low heart rate variability was confirmed by the adjusted analysis. Advanced age, previous MI, Killip class at entry, and use of digitalis were also predictors of higher mortality. Thus, in this study, time-domain indexes of heart rate variability retain their independent prognostic significance even in the post-MI patients treated with fibrinolytic therapy.

Ventricular Premature Complex Frequency for Risk Stratification

The independent predictive role of ventricular premature complex (VPC) frequency in the stratification of mortality risk after AMI was established in the prethrombolytic era by extensive multicenter trials. Thrombolysis has led to important changes in the natural history of patients after AMI, so that reassessment of established risk factors is now required. Statters and associates[152] from London, United Kingdom, assessed the prognostic significance of VPCs in 680 patients, of whom 379 received early thrombolytic therapy. All patients underwent 24-hour Holter monitoring in a drug-free state between 6 and 10 days after AMI. Patients were followed up for 1 to 8 years. During the first year of follow-up, cardiac death occurred in 33 patients, sudden death in 24, and sustained ventricular tachycardia in 20. Mean VPC frequency was significantly higher in patients who died of cardiac causes, in those who died suddenly, and in those with arrhythmic events during the first year of follow-up. This was also true when patients who did and did not undergo thrombolysis were considered separately. The positive predictive accuracy of VPC frequency in predicting adverse cardiac events was greater in patients who underwent thrombolysis than in those who did not. At a sensitivity level of 40%, the positive predictive accuracy for cardiac mortality and arrhythmic events for the group with thrombolysis was 19.4% and 25.8%, compared with 16% and 16% for those without thrombolysis. Moreover, the highest VPC frequency for the dichotomy of patients into high- and low-risk groups was 25 VPCs/hour after thrombolysis, but 10 VPCs per hour for patients without thrombolysis. VPC frequency appears to be more highly predictive of prognosis after AMI in patients who have undergone thrombolysis than in those who have not, but the optimal frequency for dichotomy is higher in the former.

Evolution of Early TIMI 2 Flow After Thrombolysis

Reiner and colleagues[153] for Investigators in the Global Utilization of Streptokinase and Tissue Plasminogen Activator for Occluded Arteries (GUSTO-1) trial evaluated the origin and evolution of early TIMI 2 flow by examining early and late angiograms and ventriculographic data from patients entered into this trial. Of 914 patients with both 90-minute and 5- to 7-day angiograms, 278 patients had TIMI grade 2 flow at 90 minutes. At follow-up, 188 (67%) had improved to TIMI grade 3 flow. At 90 minutes, patients with TIMI grade 2 flow had greater infarct vessel narrowing and a significantly greater incidence of thrombus than did patients with TIMI grade 3 flow. At the 5- to 7-day follow-up, patients whose flows had improved from TIMI grade 2 at 90 minutes to grade 3 flow at follow-up had larger caliber vessels and a lower incidence of visible thrombus (26% versus 38%) than did those with persistent TIMI grade 2 flow. These patients also had a higher mean LVEF and better infarct zone wall motion at the 5- to 7-day follow-up. Patients in whom flow improved from TIMI grade 2 at 90 minutes to TIMI grade 3 by 5 to 7 days had better LVEFs than did patients with persistent TIMI grade 0, 1, or 2 flow (Figure 2-78). Thus, these data suggest that incomplete clot lysis may play a role in the pathogenesis of TIMI grade 2 flow. Furthermore, early TIMI grade 2 flow may be sufficient to provide myocyte viability, which will further recover if flow normalizes.

Ito and colleagues[154] in Osaka, Japan, viewed the cineangiograms of 86 patients who had coronary revascularization within 12 hours of the onset of AMI and underwent myocardial contrast echocardiography before and soon after recanalization of the infarct-related artery with the intracoronary injection of sonicated microbubbles. Antegrade coronary flow after recanalization was graded by 2 observers and based on the TIMI trial flow grades. Left ventricular ejection fraction was measured on the day of infarction and 1 month later. TIMI grade 2 was observed in 18 patients (21%), and the other 68 patients manifested TIMI grade 3 after recanalization. All patients with TIMI 2 flow showed substantial myocardial contrast echocardiography no reflow, whereas only 11 patients (16%) with TIMI 3 showed myocardial contrast echocardiography no reflow. Functional improvement was worse in patients with TIMI 2 than in patients with TIMI 3 (Figure 2-79). Among patients with TIMI 3 flow, significant functional improvement was found only in patients with myocardial contrast echocardiography reflow. Thus, this study demonstrates the presence of TIMI 2 flow even in some post-AMI patients who have received recanalization therapy and have no obstructive lesion of the infarct-related artery. TIMI 2 flow appears to be caused by advanced microvascular damage and is a specific, although not very sensitive, predictor of poor functional outcome in patients with AMI. TIMI 3 flow does not necessarily indicate myocardial salvage, and

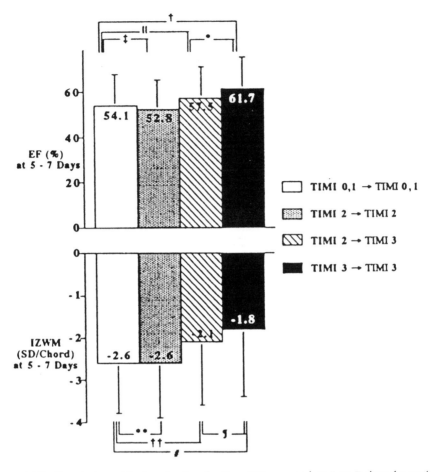

Figure 2-78. Top, Left ventricular ejection fraction (EF) assessed at 5 to 7 days for patients with specific early (90 minutes) and late (5 to 7 days) TIMI flow grade pairs. TIMI 0, 1→TIMI 0, 1 refers to the group of patients with closed arteries at both the 90-minute and follow-up angiographies; TIMI 2→TIMI 2, the group of patients with TIMI grade 2 flow at both the 90-minute and 5- to 7-day angiographies; TIMI 2→TIMI 3, the group of patients with TIMI grade 2 flow at the 90-minute angiography and improved (TIMI grade 3) flow at follow-up; and TIMI 3→TIMI 3, the group of patients with TIMI 3 flow at both the 90-minute and follow-up angiographies. Numbers within bars are means; vertical lines represent SD. Bottom, Regional wall motion in the infarct zone (IZWM) for the same groups of patients. *p = .002, †p = .0001, ‡p = .60, ‖p = .10, ¶p = .04, #p < .0001, **p = .95, ††p = .007. Reproduced with permission from Reiner et al.[153]

detection of myocardial contrast echocardiography no reflow in these patients is useful in predicting functional outcome (Figure 2-80).

Bundle Branch Block

Newby and colleagues[155] in Durham, North Carolina, examined the occurrence of new onset BBB, both transient and permanent, in 681 patients with

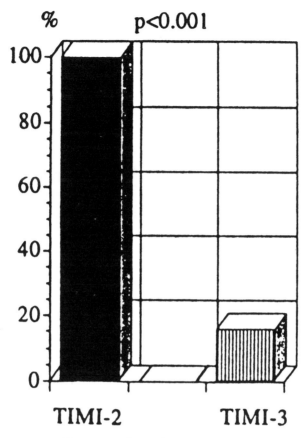

FIGURE 2-79. Comparison of frequency of no reflow phenomenon between patients with TIMI grades 2 and 3 reflow. Reproduced with permission from Ito et al.[154]

AMI enrolled in the Thrombolysis and Angioplasty in Myocardial Infarction (TAMI) 9 and GUSTO 1 protocols. Each patient underwent continuous 12-lead electrocardiographic monitoring for 36 to 72 hours. Bundle branch block was characterized as right, left, alternating, transient, or persistent. The overall incidence of bundle-branch block was 24%, with transient block in 18% and persistent block in 5%. Left bundle-branch block occurred in 7% (n = 48) and right bundle-branch block in 13% (n = 89) of the total population. Alternating bundle-branch block was seen in 4% (n = 24) of patients. Left anterior descending coronary artery MIs accounted for most bundle branch abnormalities (54%, n = 79). Patients with BBB had lower LVEFs, higher peak serum CK levels, and more diseased vessels. Mortality rates in patients with and without bundle-branch block were 9% and 4% (Figure 2-81). A higher mortality rate was observed in the presence of persistent (20%) versus transient (6%) or no (4%) bundle-branch block (Figure 2-82). Thus, thrombolytic therapy may reduce the overall mortality associated with persistent bundle-branch block. However, persistent bundle-branch block remains predictive of a higher mortality than either transient or no bundle-branch block. Continuous 12-lead electrocardio-

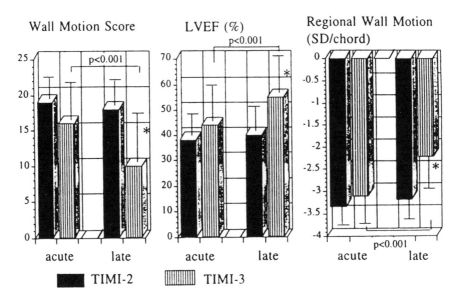

FIGURE 2-80. Comparison of left ventricular functional outcomes (wall motion score, left ventricular ejection fraction [LVEF], and regional wall motion) between patients with Thrombolysis in Myocardial Infarction (TIMI) grades 2 and 3 reflow. There are no differences in baseline left ventricular performance between the 2 subsets except that wall motion score is slightly greater in TIMI grade 2 reflow. Patients with TIMI grade 3 reflow showed substantial improvement in left ventricular performance in the late stage. Values are expressed as mean ± SD. *p<.001 vs. TIMI 2. Reproduced with permission from Ito et al.[154]

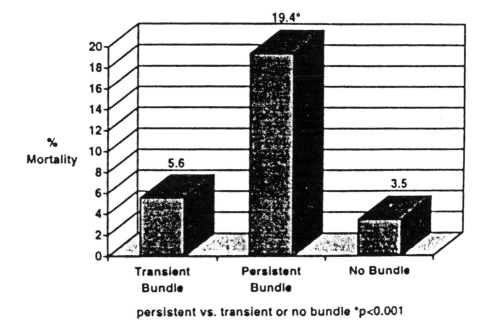

FIGURE 2-81. Incidence of 30-day mortality in the persistent, transient, and no bundle-branch block groups. Reproduced with permission from Newby et al.[155]

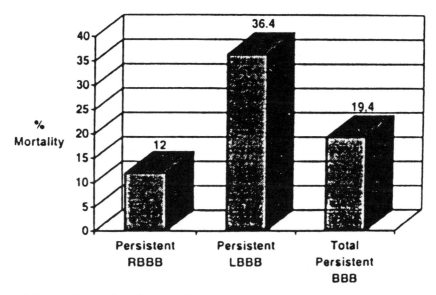

Figure 2-82. Incidence of 30-day mortality in the persistent right bundle-branch block (RBBB), persistent left bundle-branch block (LBBB), and total persistent bundle-branch block (BBB) groups. Reproduced with permission from Newby et al.[155]

graphic monitoring provides an accurate means for identifying conduction disturbances after AMI.

Acceleration of Early Cardiac Rupture

Several clinical trials have suggested the possibility that thrombolytic therapy may slightly increase early deaths from cardiac rupture. Becker and colleagues[156] reviewed the national registry of AMI participants to determine the incidence, timing, and prevalence of death from cardiac rupture in patients with AMI. Among 350,755 patients enrolled, 122,243 received thrombolytic therapy. The in-hospital mortality for those not treated with thrombolytics was 12.9%; for those treated with thrombolytics, it was 5.9%. Cardiogenic shock was the most common cause of death in each group. Although the incidence of cardiac rupture was less than 1%, it was responsible for 6.1% and 12.1%, respectively, of in-hospital deaths (Figure 2-83). Death from rupture occurred earlier in patients given thrombolytic therapy, with a clustering of events within the first day of drug administration. Multivariate analysis identified thrombolytics, prior AMI, advancing age, female gender, and intravenous beta blocker use as being independently associated with cardiac rupture. These authors concluded from this large registry experience that thrombolytic therapy accelerates cardiac rupture, typically to within 24 to 48 hours of treatment. This raises the possibility that rupture represents an early hemorrhagic complication of thrombolytic therapy.

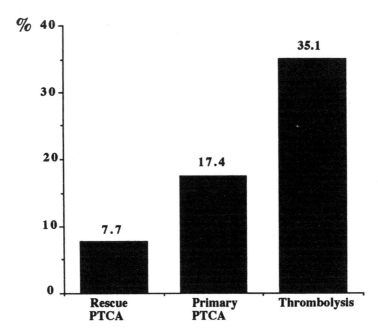

FIGURE 2-83. Prevalence of late potentials according to the reperfusion method after AMI. Reproduced with permission from Becker et al.[156]

Uncomplicated AMI and Early Hospital Discharge

In the past, hospital discharge has been accomplished by day 7 to 10 after AMI. Because of the potential for earlier discharge of patients with uncomplicated AMI after thrombolysis, Newby and colleagues[157] in the multicenter GUSTO trial re-addressed the definition of uncomplicated AMI as clinical criteria for early discharge of patients in the thrombolytic era. Uncomplicated AMI was defined as the absence of death, reinfarction, ischemia, stroke, shock, heart failure, bypass, surgery, balloon pumping, emergency catheterization, or cardioversion or defibrillation in the first 4 days. This definition was applied to 41,021 patients in the GUSTO-I trial. These criteria defined 57% of the patients as uncomplicated at day 4, with a very low risk of death and in-hospital complications: 30-day mortality, 1%; reinfarction, 1.7%; heart failure, 2.6%; recurrent ischemia, 6.7%; shock, 0.4%, and stroke, 0.2%. One-year mortality was 3.6%. The median hospital stay was 9 days, with a median cardiac care unit stay of 3 days. These authors concluded that simple clinical characteristics can identify a very low-risk post-AMI population by the 4th hospital day. They postulate that use of these criteria could substantially reduce the length of stay for patients with uncomplicated AMI.

(Thrombolysis) Compared with PTCA

After AMI, late potentials are associated with an increased risk of ventricular tachyarrhythmias and sudden death. In general, their prevalence is lower in patients with coronary reperfusion. Karam and colleagues[158] from Paris, France, retrospectively analyzed 109 patients with AMI who were treated within 6 hours of symptom onset and had angiographically proven early reperfusion. Reperfusion was achieved by intravenous thrombolysis in 34%, by rescue PTCA in 24%, and by primary percutaneous transluminal angioplasty (PTCA) in 42%. The prevalence of late potentials was similar in the 2 groups in which patency was achieved by primary and rescue PTCA (17.4% and 7.7%, respectively), but was higher in patients who had successful thrombolysis (35.1%). These authors concluded that after AMI, the prevalence of late potentials is lower when reperfusion is achieved by PTCA than by thrombolysis.

(Thrombolysis) After PTCA

Labinaz and associates[159] for the GUSTO-I investigators from multiple medical centers evaluated the outcomes of patients with prior coronary angioplasty who underwent thrombolysis for new AMI in the GUSTO-I trial. Baseline characteristics and clinical outcomes were compared between patients with and without previous angioplasty. The relations among prior angioplasty, clinical outcomes, and treatment effects were examined with logistic regression modeling. Patients with previous angioplasty tended to be younger and presented sooner after symptom onset, but had more multivessel CAD and lower EFs. Unadjusted mortality was significantly lower in the prior-angioplasty group at 24 hours (1.8% vs. 2.7%) and 30 days (5.6% vs. 7.0%). Although most of the survival advantages were due to low-risk characteristics in this group (lower age and heart rate and fewer anterior wall AMIs), prior angioplasty remained a weak but independent predictor of survival. Recurrent myocardial ischemia and reinfarction occurred more often in the prior-angioplasty group, as did CABG (12.2% vs. 8.5%). Treatment effects on 30-day mortality were similar among patients with prior infarction alone (6.3% vs. 12.6%). Treatment effects on 30-day mortality were similar among patients with prior angioplasty (odds ratio 1.2 for accelerated tPA vs. combined streptokinase arms). Patients with prior angioplasty who presented with AMI had fewer in-hospital adverse events and lower 30-day mortality than did those without such a history (Figures 2-84 and 2-85; Table 2-11).

Laster and associates[160] from Kansas City, Missouri, and Rochester, Minnesota, analyzed flow and myocardial salvage in 180 patients who underwent primary PTCA without antecedent thrombolytic therapy for AMI. TIMI flow grade was analyzed visually before and after PTCA. All patients underwent paired baseline (before angioplasty) and predischarge quantitative tomographic perfusion imaging with technetium-99m (Tc-^{99m}) sestamibi techniques for assessment of the initial area at risk and final infarct size. The myocardial salvage index was defined as the proportion of jeopardized myocardium that was salvaged. After primary PTCA, TIMI grade 3 flow was obtained in 163 patients (91%), TIMI grade 2 flow in 13 patients (7%), and TIMI grade 0 or 1 flow in 4 patients (2%). There was a significant association between TIMI flow and both infarct size and salvage index. Infarct size was significantly smaller in patients with TIMI grade 3 flow than in those with TIMI grade 2 flow (15%

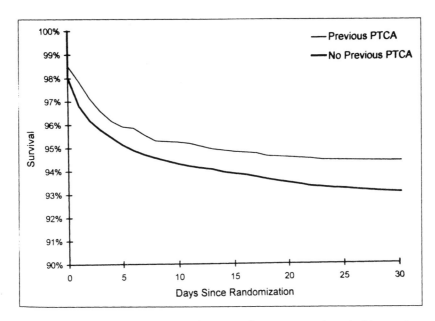

Figure 2-84. Kaplan-Meier curves for 30-day survival in patients with and without prior percutaneous transluminal coronary angioplasty (PTCA). Mortality was significantly lower in patients with prior PTCA (5.6% vs. 7.0%, p = .036). Reproduced with permission from Labinaz et al.[159]

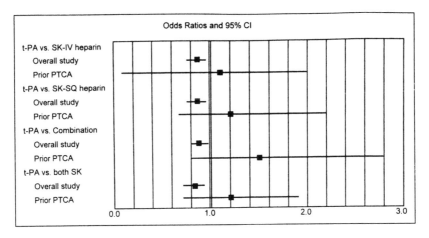

Figure 2-85. Odds ratios and 95% confidence intervals (CI) for survival with accelerated tPA treatment vs. other regimens, for the overall study population and for patients with prior PTCA. Values to the left of 1.0 indicate better survival with accelerated tPA treatment; values to the right of 1.0 indicate better survival with the other treatment strategy. Combination = tPA and streptokinase (SK) with intravenous (IV) heparin; SQ = subcutaneous. Reproduced with permission from Labinaz et al.[159]

TABLE 2-11
Major Clinical Outcomes

Outcome	Prior Angioplasty (n = 1,647)	No Prior Angioplasty (n = 39,260)
Unadjusted 24-hour mortality	30 (1.8%)	1,060 (2.7%)
Unadjusted in-hospital mortality	88 (5.4%)	2,584 (6.6%)
Unadjusted 30-day mortality	92 (5.6%)	2,715 (7.0%)
In-hospital reinfarction	75 (4.6%)	1,552 (4.0%)
Recurrent ischemia	392 (24.0%)	7,733 (20.0%)
Cardiogenic shock	86 (5.3%)	2,337 (6.0%)
Peak creatine kinase (IU)	1,105 (456, 2312)	1,433 (660, 2680)
Peak creatine kinase (IU)	102 (42, 205)	122 (57, 237)
CHF or pulmonary edema	233 (14.2%)	6,380 (16.3%)
In-hospital bypass surgery	200 (12.2%)	3,322 (8.5%)
Intra-aortic balloon pump	87 (5.3%)	1,392 (3.6%)
In-hospital angioplasty	564 (34.5%)	8,362 (21.4%)
Pacemaker insertion	139 (8.5%)	2,713 (6.9%)
Swan-Ganz catheter	291 (17.7%)	4,760 (12.2)
Sustained hypotension	184 (11.2%)	4,663 (11.9%)
Atrioventricular block	136 (8.3%)	3,234 (8.3%)
Sustained ventricular tachycardia	114 (7.0%)	2,399 (6.1%)
Ventricular fibrillation	134 (8.2%)	2,588 (6.6%)
Asystole	103 (6.3%)	2,218 (5.7%)
Atrial fibrillation/flutter	144 (8.8%)	3,678 (9.4%)
Acute MR	23 (1.4%)	549 (1.4%)
Ventricular septal defect	9 (0.6%)	185 (0.5%)
Cardiac tamponade	12 (0.7%)	299 (0.8%)
Stroke		
Hemorrhagic	9 (0.6%)	259 (0.7%)
Nonhemorrhagic	11 (0.7%)	236 (0.6%)
Bleeding		
Moderate or severe	211 (12.9%)	4,936 (12.6%)
Any blood transfusion	200 (12.2%)	4,385 (11.2%)

Values are medians with interquartile ranges in parentheses or number (%) of patients.

CHF = congestive heart failure.

Reproduced with permission from Labinaz et al.[159]

± 16% vs. 29% ± 21% of left ventricular mass). The salvage index was 55% ± 41% of the area at risk in the TIMI 3 group and 27% ± 38% of the area at risk in the TIMI 2 group. After primary PTCA, restoration of TIMI grade 3 flow was necessary for optimal myocardial salvage. TIMI grade 2 flow was associated with a larger final infarct size and a lower salvage index.

PTCA

Excessive Body Mass Index as a Risk Factor

Recognized risk factors account for only a small percent of the variant in the 4% to 10% incidence of major ischemic events associated with percutaneous coronary intervention. Body mass index (body weight in kg/{height in m}^{2})

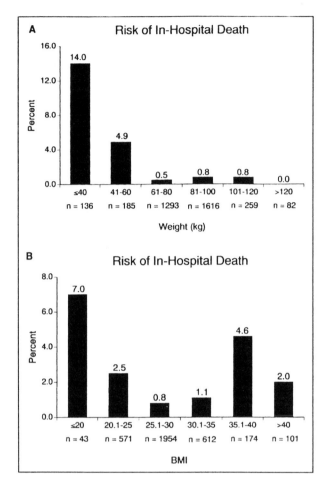

FIGURE 2-86. **A,** relation of in-hospital death to body weight in kilograms (kg). Lower weight individuals are identified to be at risk, but there is no apparent risk at higher body weights. **B,** relation of in-hospital death to body mass index (BMI) (see text for definition). Mortality is significantly higher at the extremes of this measure of body weight in relation to height. Reproduced with permission from Ellis et al.[161]

is a clinically useful estimate of body fat and has been shown to correlate with mortality from several causes. Ellis and associates[161] from Cleveland, Ohio, evaluated the effect of body mass index as a potential risk factor for the complications of percutaneous coronary intervention in 3571 consecutive percutaneous coronary intervention patients treated at a single referral center. Patients were prospectively divided into the nonobese (body mass index ≤25), mildly obese (body mass index 26–35), and very obese (body mass index >35), based on accepted definitions. Multiple logistic regression analyses were used to determine the correlates of major complications from 25 candidate variables, including body mass index of 25 or less (n = 614 patients) and body mass index greater than 35 (n = 275 patients), recorded prospectively in a relational database. Death occurred in 2.8% of the body mass index of 25 or less group, in 3.7% of the body mass index of greater than 35 group, and in 0.9% of the body mass index 26–34 group, but there was no difference in the incidence of other ischemic events. Blood product transfusion was required in 12% of the body mass index of 25 or less group, in 7% of the body mass index 25–34 group, and in 8% of the body mass index greater than 35 group. Multivariate analysis, after adjustment for other significant correlates, demonstrated that both body mass index of 25 or less (odds ratio = 27 and body mass index >35 odds ratio = 7.4) were independent correlates of death. Low normal or high BMI is a newly described and powerful risk factor for in-hospital death after percutaneous coronary intervention (Figure 2-86).

Coronary Thrombi as a Risk Factor

White and colleagues[162] evaluated the clinical importance of thrombi detectable by angioscopy but not by angiography in 122 patients undergoing PTCA at 6 medical centers. Unstable angina was present in 95 and stable angina in 27. Therapy was not guided by angioscopic findings, and no patient received thrombolytic therapy as an adjunct to angioplasty. Coronary thrombi were identified in 74 target lesions by angioscopy (61%), as compared with only 24 (20%) by angiography. Major in-hospital complications, including death, AMI, or emergency CABG occurred in 10 of 74 patients (14%) with angioscopic intracoronary thrombus, as compared with only 1 of 48 patients (2%) without thrombi (Figure 2-87). In-hospital recurrent ischemia occurred in 19 of 74 patients (26%) with angioscopic intracoronary thrombi compared to only 5 of 48 (10%) without thrombi. A relative risk analysis demonstrated that angioscopic thrombus was strongly associated with adverse outcomes (Figure 2-88) and that angiographic thrombi were not associated with these complications. Thus, the presence of intracoronary thrombus associated with coronary stenoses is significantly underestimated by angiography. Angioscopic intracor-

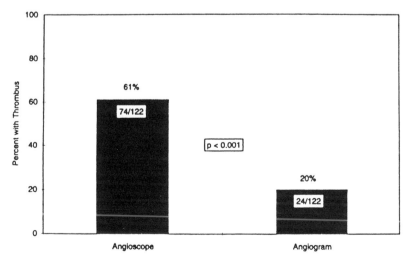

Figure 2-87. Bar graph showing incidence of angioscopic vs. angiographic thrombi. Reproduced with permission from White et al.[162]

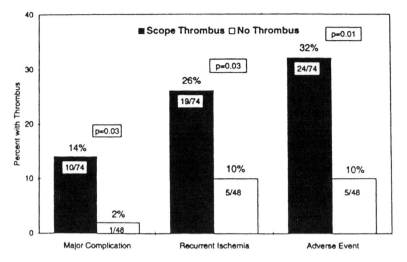

FIGURE 2-88. Bar graph showing relationship of angioscopic intracoronary thrombi to in-hospital adverse outcomes after angioplasty. Reproduced with permission from White et al.[162]

onary thrombi, many of which are not detected by angiography, are associated with an increased incidence of adverse outcomes after PTCA.

Heparin-Resistant Thrombin Activity

Oltrona and colleagues[163] in St. Louis, Missouri, conducted a study to detect the presence of heparin-resistant thrombin activity and define its relationship to acute ischemic complications during coronary interventions in 58 patients. Plasma levels of fibrinopeptide A, a marker of thrombin, and prothrombin fragment 1.2, a marker of factor Xa activity, were measured in the coronary sinus with heparin-bonded catheters. Activated coagulation times were maintained for more than 300 seconds by the Hemochron method. Mean fibrinopeptide A levels decreased significantly from 7.0 nmol/L before the procedure, to 5 ± 0.5 nmol/L after the heparin bolus, and to 2.9 nmol/L after the procedure (Figure 2-89). In 26 patients, fibrinopeptide A levels remained above the threshold for suppression of thrombin activity determined during PTCA in 7 patients without CAD (>3 nmol/L). Fibrinopeptide A concentrations after coronary interventions were increased in patients with intracoronary thrombus, abrupt coronary occlusion, postprocedural non-Q wave MI, and clinically unsuccessful procedures (Table 2-12). Prothrombin fragment 1.2 levels were low before the procedure and did not change significantly. Thus, heparin administration suppresses thrombin activity in most but not all patients undergoing coronary interventions. Heparin-resistant thrombin activity is associated with angiographic evidence of intracoronary thrombus and ischemic complications of coronary interventions.

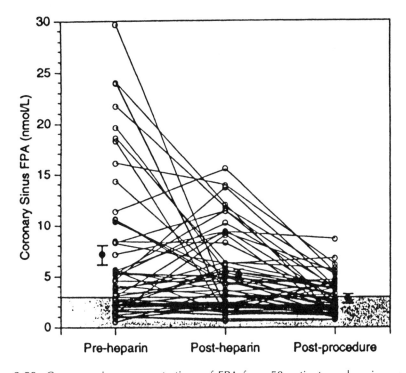

Figure 2-89. Coronary sinus concentrations of FPA from 58 patients undergoing coronary interventions. Lines connect individual patient FPA levels (○) before and after administration of the heparin bolus and after the coronary intervention. Mean concentrations of FPA (±SEM) (●) decreased from 7.0 ± 0.9 nmol/L before heparin, to 5.2 ± 0.5 nmol/L after heparin, and to 2.9 ± 0.2 nmol/L after the procedure (p = .0001). Transient increases in FPA concentrations in some patients after the heparin bolus are related to sampling soon after insertion of the arterial sheath. After the procedure, 45% of patients had FPA values above the threshold for suppression of thrombin activity as determined after low-dose heparin and angiography in 7 patients without coronary disease (3.0 nmol/L, shaded area). Reproduced with permission from Oltrona et al.[163]

Angioscopic Predictors of Early Adverse Outcome

Waxman and colleagues[164] from Boston, Massachusetts, investigated whether the use of angioscopy can improve prediction of early adverse outcome after PTCA in patients with unstable angina and non-Q wave MIs. Angioscopic characterization of the culprit lesion was performed before PTCA in 32 patients with unstable angina and 10 with non-Q wave MI. Seven patients (17%) had an adverse outcome, including MI, repeat PTCA, or need for CABG within 24 hours of PTCA. Six of 18 with a yellow culprit lesion had an adverse outcome compared with 1 of 24 in whom the culprit lesion was white. Six of 20 patients with plaque disruption suffered an adverse outcome compared with 1 of 22 with nondisrupted plaques (Figure 2-90). Six of 17 patients with intraluminal thrombus had an adverse outcome, whereas only 1 of 25 patients without thrombus had an adverse outcome (Figure 2-90). Yellow color, disruption, and thrombus at the culprit lesion site were associated with an 8-fold increase in

Table 2-12

Relationship of Postprocedural FPA and F1.2 Concentrations to Clinical Features, Angiographic Characteristics, and Complications of Interventional Patients

	Coronary Sinus FPA, nmol/L			Coronary Sinus F1.2, mol/L		
	Yes	No	p	Yes	No	p
Preprocedure heparin	3.1 ± 0.3	2.7 ± 0.3	*	0.19 ± 0.02	0.18 ± 0.02	*
Acute clinical presentation	3.0 ± 0.3	2.8 ± 0.4	*	0.18 ± 0.02	0.19 ± 0.02	*
Ambrose class (complex)	3.4 ± 0.4	2.7 ± 0.2	.14	0.20 ± 0.02	0.18 ± 0.02	*
Coronary thrombus	6.2 ± 1.6	2.8 ± 0.2	.01	0.19 ± 0.04	0.19 ± 0.01	*
Non-PTCA procedure	3.1 ± 0.3	2.7 ± 0.3	*	0.19 ± 0.02	0.19 ± 0.02	*
Angiographic success	2.9 ± 0.2	3.2 ± 0.6	*	0.18 ± 0.01	0.23 ± 0.03	.23
Minor dissection	2.8 ± 0.3	2.7 ± 0.3	*	0.20 ± 0.02	0.20 ± 0.02	*
Abrupt coronary occlusion	4.1 ± 0.8	2.8 ± 0.2	.06	0.22 ± 0.02	0.18 ± 0.01	.28
Clinical success	2.8 ± 0.2	3.9 ± 0.6	.04	0.18 ± 0.02	0.22 ± 0.02	.14
Postprocedure non-Q-wave MI	4.9 ± 1.2	2.8 ± 0.2	.04	0.21 ± 0.04	0.18 ± 0.01	*
Any major complication	3.8 ± 0.7	2.9 ± 0.2	.08	0.21 ± 0.02	0.18 ± 0.02	*

* $p \geq .40$.
Reproduced with permission from Oltrona et al.[163]

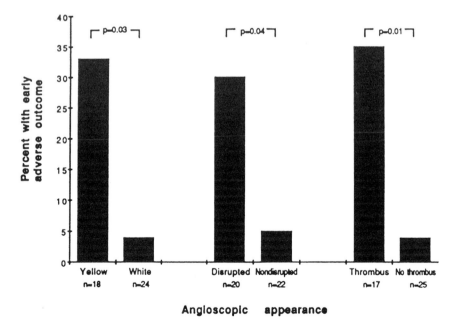

Figure 2-90. Relation between the angioscopic appearance of the culprit lesion and early adverse outcome after PTCA in 42 patients with unstable angina and non-Q wave myocardial infarction. n indicates the total number of patients in each group. Reproduced with permission from Waxman et al.[164]

risk of adverse outcome after PTCA. The prediction of PTCA outcome, based on characteristics of the plaque that were identifiable by angioscopy, was superior to that estimated from angiographic variables. Thus, in patients with unstable angina and non-Q wave MI, angioscopic features of disruption, yellow color, or thrombus at the culprit lesion identify patients at high risk of early adverse outcome after PTCA.

Diabetic Patients

Kip and colleagues[165] in Pittsburgh, Pennsylvania, obtained data on baseline clinical and angiographic characteristics and short- and long-term outcomes of 281 diabetic and 1833 nondiabetic PTCA patients in the multicenter National Heart, Lung, and Blood Institute 1985–1986 PTCA Registry. Diabetic patients were older, they were more likely to be female, and they had more comorbid baseline conditions, triple-vessel CAD, and atherosclerotic lesions. Angiographic success and completeness of revascularization did not differ significantly, yet diabetic patients experienced a higher incidence of in-hospital death (women) and nonfatal AMI. Nine-year mortality was twice as high in diabetic patients (35.9% vs. 17.9%) (Figure 2-91). Nine-year rates of nonfatal

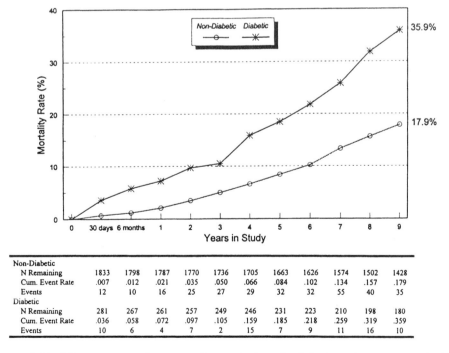

Non-Diabetic											
N Remaining	1833	1798	1787	1770	1736	1705	1663	1626	1574	1502	1428
Cum. Event Rate	.007	.012	.021	.035	.050	.066	.084	.102	.134	.157	.179
Events	12	10	16	25	27	29	32	32	55	40	35
Diabetic											
N Remaining	281	267	261	257	249	246	231	223	210	198	180
Cum. Event Rate	.036	.058	.072	.097	.105	.159	.185	.218	.259	.319	.359
Events	10	6	4	7	2	15	7	9	11	16	10

FIGURE 2-91. Nine-year mortality curve after angioplasty in diabetic patients compared with nondiabetics. Cum. indicates cumulative. Reproduced with permission from Kip et al.[165]

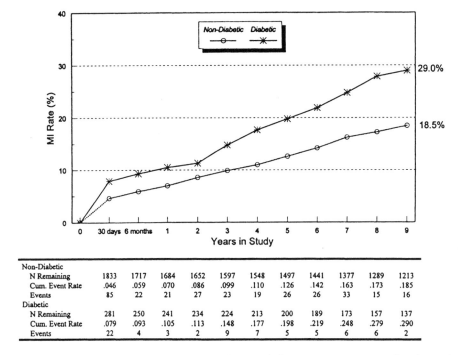

FIGURE 2-92. Nine-year rate of MI after angioplasty in diabetic patients compared with nondiabetics. Reproduced with permission from Kip et al.[165]

MI, CABG, and repeat PTCA were also higher in diabetics (Figures 2-92–2-94). In multivariate analysis, diabetes was a significant predictor of decreased 9-year survival and other untoward events. Thus, compared with nondiabetic patients receiving PTCA, diabetic patients have more extensive and diffuse atherosclerotic disease, and they are more likely to suffer in-hospital death and nonfatal MI. Long-term survival and freedom from MI and CABG are also reduced in diabetic patients.

Significance of Release of CK-MB Fraction

Abdelmeguid and colleagues[166] in Cleveland, Ohio, examined 4484 patients who underwent successful PTCA or directional coronary atherectomy and whose peak serum CK levels did not exceed twice the upper limit of laboratory normal. Group 1 (3776 patients) had no CK or MB elevation after the procedure. Group 2 (450 patients) had a peak CK level between 100 and 180 IU/L, with MB fraction greater than 4%, and group 3 (258 patients) had a peak serum CK level between 180 and 360 IU/L with MB fraction greater than 4%. The strongest correlation of postprocedure CK-MB elevation was with directional coronary atherectomy followed by the development of 1 or more in-lab minor procedural complications. Clinical follow-up was available in 4461 patients, (99.5%) with a mean duration of 36 ± 22 months. Survival analysis,

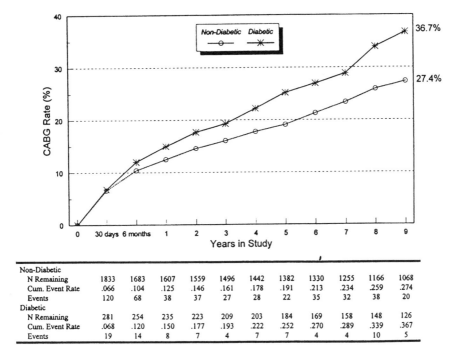

Non-Diabetic											
N Remaining	1833	1683	1607	1559	1496	1442	1382	1330	1255	1166	1068
Cum. Event Rate	.066	.104	.125	.146	.161	.178	.191	.213	.234	.259	.274
Events	120	68	38	37	27	28	22	35	32	38	20
Diabetic											
N Remaining	281	254	235	223	209	203	184	169	158	148	126
Cum. Event Rate	.068	.120	.150	.177	.193	.222	.252	.270	.289	.339	.367
Events	19	14	8	7	4	7	7	4	4	10	5

FIGURE 2-93. Nine-year rate of CABG after angioplasty in diabetic patients compared with nondiabetics. Reproduced with permission from Kip et al.[165]

after adjustment with the Cox proportional hazards regression model, demonstrated that the groups with elevated CK-MB had a significantly higher incidence of cardiac death and MI (Figure 2-95). Major ischemic complications, including death, MI, and coronary revascularization, occurred more frequently in the groups with increased CK-MB (Figure 2-96). Thus, this study demonstrates that relatively minor elevations of CK-MB after successful coronary intervention identifies a population with a poorer long-term prognosis compared with patients with no enzyme elevation.

Susceptibility to Pain During PTCA

Silent myocardial ischemia is frequently observed in patients with CAD. Higher pain thresholds have been documented in asymptomatic subjects, suggesting a generalized hyposensitivity to pain. Falcone and associates[167] from Pavia, Italy, studied patients with CAD to determine the dental pain threshold and reaction to tooth pulp stimulation and to correlate the clinical, ergometric, and angiographic features of patients with and without pain during PTCA to pulpal test response. Thus, they were trying to determine whether dental pulp stimulation could help identify patients particularly prone to silent ischemia. Eighty-six consecutive male patients with reproducible exercise-induced ischemia and CAD documented by angiography underwent PTCA. A pulpal test was performed in all patients by means of an electrical tooth pulp stimulator.

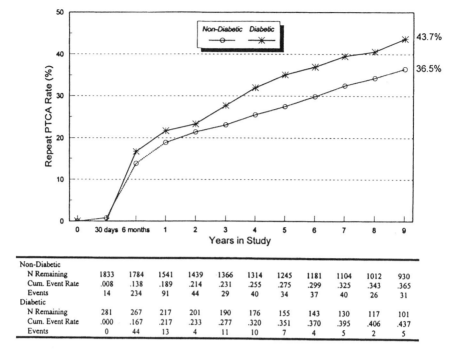

Non-Diabetic											
N Remaining	1833	1784	1541	1439	1366	1314	1245	1181	1104	1012	930
Cum. Event Rate	.008	.138	.189	.214	.231	.255	.275	.299	.325	.343	.365
Events	14	234	91	44	29	40	34	37	40	26	31
Diabetic											
N Remaining	281	267	217	201	190	176	155	143	130	117	101
Cum. Event Rate	.000	.167	.217	.233	.277	.320	.351	.370	.395	.406	.437
Events	0	44	13	4	11	10	7	4	5	2	5

FIGURE 2-94. Nine-year rate of repeat PTCA in diabetic patients compared with nondiabetics. Reproduced with permission from Kip et al.[165]

Seventy one patients with and 15 patients without angina during daily life were studied. During the pulpal test, 57 patients reported dental pain, whereas 29 were asymptomatic even at maximal stimulation. Patients were divided into group 1 (58 patients) or group 2 (28) who exhibited the presence or absence of angina during myocardial ischemia induced by PTCA. Dental pain was provoked by pulpal test in 81% of patients with and 36% of patients without symptoms during PTCA. The absence of dental pain even at maximal tooth pulp stimulation was observed in 11 patients in group 1 and 18 in group 2. Patients

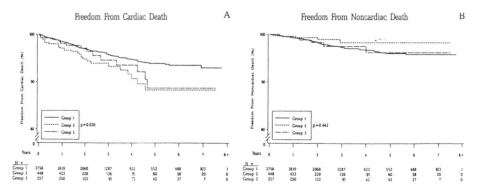

FIGURE 2-95. Plots showing freedom from cardiac (A) and noncardiac (B) death according to postprocedure cardiac enzyme level. Reproduced with permission from Abdelmeguid et al.[166]

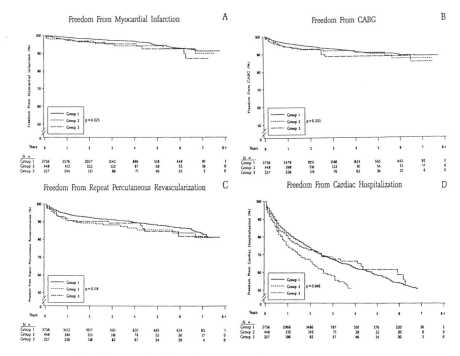

FIGURE 2-96. Plots showing freedom from myocardial infarction **(A)**, coronary artery bypass surgery (CABG) **(B)**, repeat percutaneous revascularization **(C)**, and cardiac hospitalization **(D)** for the three study groups. Reproduced with permission from Abdelmeguid et al.[166]

who were asymptomatic during PTCA had a higher mean dental pain threshold, lower mean threshold reaction, and lower mean maximal reaction than those who were symptomatic during both PTCA and the pulpal test. These authors concluded that a higher dental pain threshold and lower reactivity characterizes those subjects who are prone to silent ischemia both during daily life and during PTCA. Response to the pulpal test and the presence of symptoms during daily life were highly related to the presence of angina during PTCA.

Flexible Versus Nonflexible Sheaths and Patient Comfort

Patients who undergo PTCA by the femoral approach are usually required to lie flat in bed for 6 to 24 hours, which may result in significant discomfort. This study by Waksman and associates[168] from Atlanta, Georgia, was performed to evaluate the safety and benefit of a flexible sheath that enables patients to sit at a 60° angle while the sheath is in place in the femoral artery. Sixty patients were randomly assigned to receive either flexible or nonflexible sheaths before PTCA. Patients with flexible sheaths were allowed to sit an angle of 60° after the procedure. Heparin management was the same in both groups. Frequency of calls to nurses for back pain was recorded for both groups. For analgesia, nalbuphine was administered in 2-mg increments. All sheaths were removed the day after the procedure. Femoral ultrasound was used to detect groin complications (hematoma, pseudoaneurysm, or arteriovenous fistula) and was performed in all patients. Baseline characteristics were similar in both groups. There were no differences in ease of sheath insertion or guide catheter movement through the sheaths. The arterial pressure waveform was not dampened in any of the flexible sheath patients while in the sitting position. Patients with flexible sheaths had fewer calls for back pain and required less nalbuphine than did patients with nonflexible sheaths. Groin complications were similar in both groups. In conclusion, by allowing patients to sit up to an angle of 60°, flexible sheaths have a beneficial effect in reducing back pain and the need for analgesics after PTCA.

Delayed PTCA After AMI

A number of studies have shown that persistent coronary occlusion after anterior AMI will lead to ventricular dilation and CHF. One of the more important questions, therefore, is whether all patients with occlusion of the coronary artery should have it opened after AMI to prevent this subsequent remodeling and dilation. Pizzetti and colleagues[169] from Milan, Italy, studied 73 consecutive patients with anterior AMI as a first cardiac event; all had an isolated lesion or occlusion of the proximal LAD. Six patients died before hospital discharge. The 67 survivors were classified into 2 groups: group I (patent LAD and good distal flow, n = 40) and group II (LAD occlusion or subocclusion, n = 27). The 20 patients in group I who had significant residual restenosis and all patients in group II underwent elective PTCA within 18 days of AMI. The procedure was successful in 17 patients in group I and in 16 patients in group II; in the remaining 11 patients of group I, patency could not be re-established. Left ventricular volumes, EF, and a dysfunction score were measured echocardiographically on admission, before PTCA, at discharge, and after 3 and 6 months. Results showed that EF and dysfunction score were significantly worse in group II. However, ventricular function and volumes progressively improved in group IIA in the patients who had successful PTCA, whereas group IIB exhibited progressive deterioration of function. Ejection fraction decreased from 43% to 37%, and systolic volumes increased from 34 to 72 mL/min/m². Patients in group IIB also had worse effort tolerance, higher heart rate at rest, lower blood pressure, and significantly greater prevalence of CHF. These authors concluded that delayed PTCA of an occluded LAD can frequently restore vessel patency. Success appears to be associated with better ventricular function and a lack of chronic dilation. Large randomized studies are warranted to evaluate the effect of delayed PTCA on late mortality.

Whether angioplasty of occluded arteries after AMI may have beneficial effects on left ventricular function remains unknown. Garot and associates[170] from Crèteil, France, studied patients referred for coronary angioplasty that was performed between 3 and 4 weeks after onset of their first AMI. During that time, they received thrombolytic therapy and were found to have an occluded infarct-related artery at delayed coronary angiography. All patients underwent stress-redistribution-reinjection thallium-201 SPECT for myocardial viability assessment. Prior angioplasty, a quantitative evaluation of global and regional left ventricular function, was performed. The study group consisted of 38 patients (aged 57 ± 10 years): 18 had anterior wall infarctions, and 20 had inferior wall infarctions, but before angioplasty, 3 had a patent artery and were excluded. Angioplasty was successful in 30 patients. At follow-up, 13 patients (43%) had an occluded coronary artery. In contrast with patients with an occluded coronary artery at follow-up, those with a patent coronary artery had no left ventricular enlargement and had an improvement in both LVEF (from 48% ± 9% to 52% ± 9.8%) and regional wall motion index (Δ = +0.95 SD). In patients with a patent vessel at follow-up, there was a positive correlation between the number of myocardial viable segments and improvement of the infarct zone wall motion, and the number of necrotic segments at baseline was positively correlated to the 4-month changes in end-diastolic volume indexes. Thus, elective revascularization of occluded coronary arteries with viable myocardium after AMI improves left ventricular function and lessens remodeling if the artery remains patent during follow-up.

Complications of PTCA

Abrupt Closure

Narins and colleagues[171] in Durham, North Carolina, evaluated 62 patients undergoing PTCA with in- and out-of-cardiac catheterization laboratory abrupt closure and in whom intraprocedure activated clotting times had been measured among a population of 1290 consecutive patients undergoing nonemergency PTCA. These patients were compared with a matched control population of 124 patients who did not experience abrupt closure. Relative to the control population, patients who had abrupt closure had significantly lower initial and minimum activated clotting times (Figure 2-97). Higher activated clotting times were not associated with an increased likelihood of major bleeding complications. There was a strong inverse linear relationship between the activated clotting time and the probability of abrupt closure (Figure 2-97 and 2-98). Thus, the data in this study demonstrate a significant inverse relation between the degree of anticoagulation during PTCA and the risk of abrupt closure. The higher the intensity of anticoagulation, the lower the risk of abrupt closure after elective PTCA.

Elastic Recoil

Daniel and associates[172] from Dallas, Texas, assessed the incidence and magnitude of elastic recoil occurring within 15 minutes of successful coronary angioplasty and determined the effects of subsequent additional balloon inflations on coronary luminal diameter in patients displaying substantial recoil. The coronary angiograms of 50 consecutive patients who underwent a successful PTCA were analyzed using computer-assisted quantitative analysis. The patients were divided into 2 groups based on the magnitude of early elastic

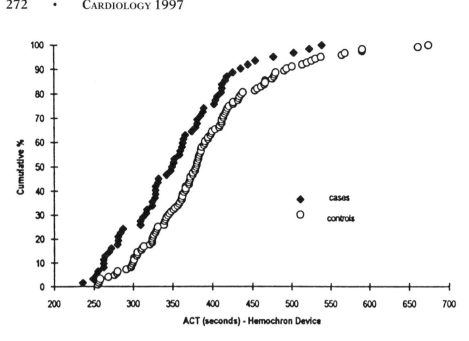

FIGURE 2-97. Cumulative distribution curves of initial activated clotting times for patients who experienced abrupt closure (n = 62) and a matched control group (n = 124). ACT indicates activated clotting time. Reproduced with permission from Narins et al.[171]

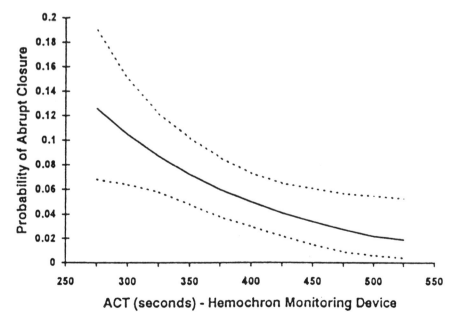

FIGURE 2-98. Graph showing probability of abrupt closure with upper and lower 95% confidence limits vs. the initial activated clotting time (seconds) measured with the Hemochron device. ACT indicates activated clotting time. Reproduced with permission from Narins et al.[171]

recoil following angioplasty: those with 10% or less loss of minimal lumen diameter (group 1, n = 30) and those with greater than 10% loss of minimal lumen diameter (group 2, n = 20). Lumen diameter was assessed by comparing the angiogram obtained immediately after successful angioplasty with that obtained 15 minutes later. The 2 groups were similar in clinical, angiographic, and procedural characteristics. Of the 20 group 2 subjects, 18 (90%) underwent repeat balloon dilatations, and 2 (10%) had no further intervention. After additional balloon inflations were performed in these 18 patients, 16 (90%) had a final result with less than 10% loss of minimal luminal diameter 15 minutes later. In conclusion, elastic recoil 15 minutes after apparently successful PTCA is frequent, occurring in approximately 40% of patients, and is attenuated in 90% of subjects with additional balloon inflations. The resultant larger lumen diameter may exert a salutary effect on long-term outcome.

AMI

PTCA has been associated with the procedural complication of AMI. Abrupt closure, distal coronary embolization, intimal dissection, coronary spasm, and acute thrombosis are the principal etiologies. New interventional devices (stent, laser, and atherectomy catheters) have been introduced as alternatives or as adjuncts to balloon angioplasty. With use of the New Approaches to Coronary Intervention Registry, Waksman and associates[173] for the NACI investigators from several medical centers studied the incidence, predictors, and outcome of AMI as a complication of using these devices as the primary mode of intervention. There were 3265 patients from 39 participating centers in the cohort treated with new devices. AMI was reported as an in-hospital complication of using new devices in 154 patients (4.7%), including Q wave AMI in 36 patients (1.1%), and non-Q wave AMI in 119 patients (3.6%). AMI rates were not significantly different among all patients with devices in the cohort treated with atherectomy (directional, extractional, rotational), laser (AUS, Spectranetics) or the Palmaz-Schatz stent. Multivariate logistic regression showed that postprocedure AMI was associated with multivessel CAD, high surgical risk, postinfarction, angina, and presence of a thrombus prior to the procedure. Prior PTCA was inversely related to the incidence of AMI. When a specific cause of AMI could be detected, the main etiologies were: coronary embolus 17%, and abrupt closure 27%. Other major in-hospital complications were higher in the AMI group than the non-AMI group: death, 7.8% versus 0.8%; and bypass surgery, 13.6% versus 1.7%. At 1 year, mortality rates remain higher at 12.9% in the AMI group versus 4.9% in the non-AMI group. Despite different indications for the use of new devices, they were not predictors for AMI with the exception of the rotablator. The incidence of AMI (1.1% Q wave, 3.6% non-Q wave) was comparable to previously reported rates from balloon angioplasty. The occurrence of AMI is associated with an increase in other in-hospital complications and a doubling of 1-year mortality.

PTCA: Follow-Up

Glycoprotein IIb/IIIa Effect on Outcome

Abrupt closure of a vessel occurs in 4% to 8% of PTCA procedures. Kereiakes and colleagues[174] in a multicenter study examined the safety and tolerability of a new nonpeptide platelet IIb/IIIa receptor antagonist given as an adjunct to heparin and aspirin therapy. Seventy three patients received this new agent tirofiban (MK-383) in 3 sequential dose panels, and 20 patients received placebo. Tirofiban was associated with a dose-dependent inhibition of ex vivo adenosine diphosphate-mediated platelet aggregation that was sustained during intravenous infusion and resolved rapidly after drug cessation. Adverse bleeding events, mainly at the vascular access site, were slightly increased at the higher dose. There were no differences in adverse clinical outcomes among the 2 groups. This study established a well-tolerated dosing regimen for administration of tirofiban as adjunctive therapy in high-risk PTCA patients. A larger trial will determine any impact on adverse clinical outcome.

PTCA for AMI is an attractive alternative to thrombolysis, but it is still limited by recurrent myocardial ischemia and coronary restenosis. Lefkovits and associates[175] for the EPIC Investigators determined whether adjunctive platelet glycoprotein IIb/IIIa receptor blockade improved outcomes in patients undergoing direct and rescue PTCA in the Evaluation of c7E3 for Prevention of Ischemic Complications (EPIC) trial. In the study, 2,099 patients undergoing percutaneous intervention were randomized to receive 1 of the following: chimeric 7E3 Fab (c7E3) as a bolus, a bolus and 12-hour infusion, or placebo. Forty-two patients underwent direct PTCA for AMI, and 22 patients had rescue PTCA after failed thrombolysis. The primary composite end points consisted of death, reinfarction, repeat intervention, or bypass surgery. Outcomes were assessed at 30 days and 6 months. Baseline characteristics were similar in direct and rescue PTCA patients. Pooling the 2 groups, c7E3 bolus and 12-hour infusion reduced the primary composite end points by 83% (26.1% placebo vs. 4.5% c7E3 bolus and infusion). No reinfarctions or repeat urgent interventions occurred in c7E3 bolus and infusion patients at 30 days, although there was a trend toward more deaths in c7E3-treated patients. Major bleeding was increased with c7E3 (24% vs. 13%). At 6 months, ischemic events were reduced from 47.8% with placebo to 4.5% with c7E3 bolus and infusion, particularly reinfarction and repeat revascularization. The authors concluded that adjunctive c7E3 therapy during direct and rescue PTCA decreased acute ischemic events and clinical restenosis in the EPIC trial. These data provide initial evidence of benefit for glycoprotein IIb/IIIa receptor blockade during PTCA for AMI (Figures 2-99 and 2-100).

Arterial Remodeling After

Mintz and colleagues[176] from Washington, D.C., obtained serial intravascular ultrasound images to study 212 native coronary lesions in 209 patients

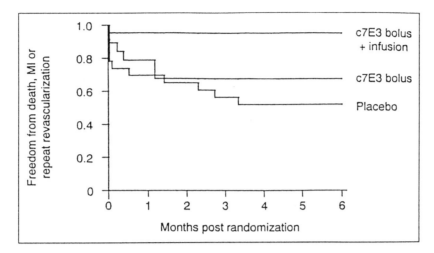

FIGURE 2-99. Kaplan-Meier plot of the composite clinical event rates up to 6 months for patients undergoing PTCA for AMI in the Evaluation of c7E3 for Prevention of Ischemic Complications trial. Adverse events were significantly reduced in the c7E3 bolus and infusion group compared with the placebo group (p = .002). Event rates in the c7E3 bolus group were not significantly different from the placebo group. Reproduced with permission from Lefkovits et al.[175]

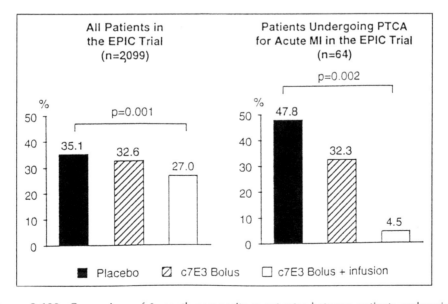

FIGURE 2-100. Comparison of 6-month composite event rates between patients undergoing PTCA for AMI in the Evaluation of c7E3 for Prevention of Ischemic Complications (EPIC) trial and the overall EPIC trial patient population. Reproduced with permission from Lefkovits et al.[175]

after PTCA, directional coronary atherectomy, rotational atherectomy, or excimer laser angioplasty. The external elastic membrane and lumen cross-sectional area were measured. Plaque plus media luminal cross-sectional area was calculated as the external elastic membrane minus lumen cross-sectional area. The anatomic slide selected for serial analysis had an axial location within the target lesion at the smallest follow-up lumen cross-sectional area. At follow-up, 73% of the decrease in lumen from 7 ± 2.5 to 4.0 ± 3.7 mm^2 was due to a decrease in external elastic membrane from 20 ± 6.4 to 18 ± 6.4 mm^2. Twenty-seven percent of the decrease was due to an increase in plaque plus media from 13.5 ± 5.5 to 14 ± 5.4 mm^2. The change in lumen cross-sectional area correlated more strongly with the change in external elastic membrane cross-sectional area than with a change in plaque plus media cross-sectional area. The change in external elastic membrane was bidirectional; 47 lesions showed an increase. Despite a greater increase in plaque plus media, lesions exhibiting an increase in external elastic membrane had (1) no change in lumen, (2) a reduced restenosis rate (26% versus 62%), and (3) a 49% frequency of late lumen gain compared with lesions with *no increase* in external elastic membrane. Thus, restenosis appears to be determined importantly by the direction and magnitude of vessel wall remodeling. An increase in external elastic membrane is adaptive to interventional therapy, whereas a decrease in external elastic membrane contributes to restenosis (Figure 2-101).

Glycoprotein IIb/IIIa Blockade in High-Risk Cases

Mark and colleagues[177] for the multicenter Evaluation of 7E3 for the Prevention of Ischemic Complications (EPIC) trial demonstrated that an antiplatelet monoclonal antibody to the platelet glycoprotein IIb/IIIa receptor reduced 30-day ischemic end points among high-risk patients undergoing PTCA by 35% and 6-month ischemic events by 23%, but increased in-hospital bleeding episodes. Among the 2099 patients randomized in EPIC, data were collected on 2038 (97%) to determine prospective hospital costs and major resources utilized. Physician fees were estimated from the Medicare Fee Schedule. Regression analysis was used to examine the economic trade-off between reduced ischemic events and increased major bleeding during the initial hospitalization. A potential cost savings of $622 per patient during the initial hospitalization from reduced ischemic events in patients receiving the monoclonal antibody was offset by an equivalent rise ($521) in cost as the result of an increase in bleeding episodes. Baseline medical costs for the bolus and infusion of the antibody arm averaged $13,577 exclusive of drug cost, compared with $13,434 for placebo. During the 6-month follow-up, patients treated with the antibody decreased repeat hospitalization rates by 23% (p = 0.004) and the need for repeat revascularization by 22% (p = 0.04), producing a mean $1270 savings per patient (exclusive of drug cost) (p = 0.018). With a cost of $1407 for the bolus and infusion antibody regimen, the cumulative net 6-month cost to switch from standard care to routine monoclonal antibody therapy averaged $293 per patient. Thus, in high-risk patients undergoing PTCA, aggressive platelet inhibition with the monoclonal antibody to the platelet glycoprotein IIb/IIIa

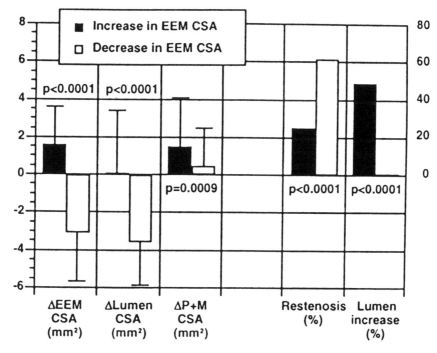

FIGURE 2-101. During the follow-up period, 47 lesions (22%) showed an increase in external elastic membrane (EEM) cross-sectional area (CSA) (3.1 $\pm$ 2.6 mm^2); 165 lesions had a decrease in EEM CSA (1.6 $\pm$ 2.0 mm^2). Lesions exhibiting an increase in EEM CSA had (1) no change in lumen CSA (Δlumen CSA $= -0.1 \pm 3.3$ mm^2 vs. 3.6 $\pm$ 2.3, p<.0001), (2) a greater increase in plaque (P)+ median (M) CSA (ΔP + M CSA $= 1.5 \pm 2.5$ mm^2 vs. 0.5 $\pm$ 2.0 mm^2, p = .0009), (3) a reduced restenosis rate (26% vs. 62% for lesions with a decrease in EEM CSA, p<.0001), and (4) a 49% frequency of late lumen gain (vs. 1% for lesions with a decrease in EEM CSA, p<.0001). Reproduced with permission from Mintz et al.[176]

receptor recoups most of the cost of therapy and has the potential to essentially pay for itself by significantly reducing ischemic events and repeat revascularization.

Quantitative Angiography After PTCA

Faxon and associates[178] for the NHLBI PTCA Registry Investigators examined the optimal angiographic definition for long-term success after coronary angioplasty and compared visual and quantitative angiographic measurements in assessing outcome. The National Heart, Lung, and Blood Institute's Percutaneous Transluminal Coronary Angioplasty Registry prospectively followed 1768 patients from 15 clinical centers. Symptom-free survival, which was defined as survival without angina, AMI, bypass surgery, or death, occurred in 59% of patients. In a subset of 393 patients, quantitative coronary angiography (QCA), done at a core angiographic laboratory, was compared with visual site readings. Although there was considerably more variability for visual readings, a site reading of a change in percent stenosis of greater than 20% correlated highly with symptom-free survival (64.6% for patients who had all lesions successfully dilated, 48% for patients with partial success, and only 21% for patients without angiographic success. Similar findings were seen for other angiographic definitions, but a change of more than 20% was most discriminatory. In contrast, QCA readings had little or no predictive value. This study confirms that visual assessment of the immediate change in percent stenosis is predictive of a successful 1-year outcome. A change of greater than 20% is most discriminatory and should still be used to define angiographic success. QCA does not appear to be superior to visual assessment in predicting 1-year outcome.

Angiography provides limited information on plaque morphology and composition before balloon angioplasty. Identification of plaques associated with reduced lumen gain or a high complication rate may provide the rationale for using alternative revascularization devices. Baptista and associates[179] from Rotterdam, The Netherlands, studied 60 patients with quantitative angiography and intracoronary ultrasound before and after balloon dilation. Angiography was used to measure transient wall stretch and elastic recoil. Intracoronary ultrasound was used to investigate the mechanisms of lumen enlargement among different plaque compositions and in the presence of a disease-free wall (minimal thickness ≤ 0.6 mm). Compared with ultrasound, angiography underestimated the presence of vessel calcification (13% vs. 78%), lumen eccentricity (35% vs. 62%), and wall dissection (32% vs. 57%). Intracoronary ultrasound measurements showed that balloon angioplasty increased lumen area from 1.82 ± 0.51 to 4.81 ± 1.43 mm^2. Lumen enlargement was the result of the combined effect of an increase in the total cross-sectional area of the vessel (wall stretching, 43%) and of a reduction in the area occupied by the plaque (plaque compression or redistribution, 57%). Vessels with a disease-free wall had smaller lumen gain than did other types of vessels ($2.13\% \pm 1.26$ vs. 3.59 ± 1.51 mm^2, respectively). Wall stretching was the most important mechanism of lumen enlargment in vessels with a disease-free wall (79% vs. 37% in the other vessels). Angiography revealed a direct correlation between temporary stretch and elastic recoil that was responsible for 26% of the loss of the potential lumen gain. Thus, lumen enlargement after balloon angioplasty is the combined result of wall stretch and plaque compression or redistribution. Intracoronary ultrasound indicates that vessels with a remnant arc of disease-free wall are dilated mainly by wall stretching compared with other types of vessels and are associated with a smaller lumen gain.

Effect of Late Recanalization of Total Occlusions

The clinical benefit of late recanalization of complete coronary occlusion is debated. Left ventricular function and volumes are major prognostic determinants in patients with CAD. Danchin and associates[180] from Van Doeuvreles-Nancy, France, sought to assess comprehensively the evolution of global and regional left ventricular function and left ventricular volumes after percutaneous recanalization of chronic complete coronary artery occlusions. The study group comprised a consecutive series of 55 patients who underwent successful percutaneous recanalization of a chronic (≥ 10 days), total occlusion (TIMI flow grade of 0) of the LAD or dominant right coronary arteries, and in whom a complete angiographic evaluation was available before angioplasty and at follow-up. At follow-up, 38 patients had a patent artery (group 1) and 17 had a reocclusion (group 2). Baseline parameters were similar in the 2 groups. In group 1, LVEF increased from 55% $\pm$ 14% to 62% $\pm$ 13%, with an increase in fractional shortening in the occluded artery territory (0.43 $\pm$ 0.30 to 0.71 $\pm$ 0.34), while left ventricular end-diastolic volume remained unchanged. In group 2, EF and regional wall motion were unchanged, while left ventricular end-diastolic volume index increased (86 $\pm$ 22 mL/m^2 to 99 $\pm$ 34 mL/m^2). The evolution in left ventricular global and regional function was similar in patients with or without previous AMI; however, prevention of left ventricular remodeling was observed only in patients with previous AMI. Maintained patency after successful recanalization of totally occluded coronary arteries improves global and regional left ventricular function and, in patients with previous AMI, avoids left ventricular remodeling.

Myocardial Velocity After PTCA

Doppler tissue imaging is a new noninvasive imaging modality that directly interrogates myocardial velocity with high temporal and spatial resolution. This study by Bach and associates[181] from Ann Arbor, Michigan, was designed to test the hypothesis that quantitative Doppler tissue imaging provides unique information regarding regional myocardial systolic and diastolic function during acute ischemic events. Myocardial velocities were quantified during the acute ischemic and reperfusion phases of 13 elective PTCA procedures in 12 patients. In myocardium subtended by angioplasty vessels, peak velocities decreased during occlusive balloon inflation (from 21 $\pm$ 9.8 to -0.6 ± 4.0 mm/sec in systole and from 22 $\pm$ 9.2 to -0.6 ± 3.9 mm/sec in diastole. During early reperfusion, velocities exceeded those observed at baseline. In regions remote from the treated artery, peak myocardial velocities increased in the absence of significant stenosis but remained unchanged or decreased in the presence of significant stenosis of the associated vessel. It was concluded that: 1) myocardial velocities rapidly decrease during acute ischemia and show a rebound increase after reperfusion; and 2) in regions remote from ischemia, velocities display distinct patterns on the basis of the presence or absence of obstructive coronary disease in the associated vessel. Quantitative Doppler tissue imaging is a useful tool for the assessment of myocardial velocity and may provide new insights into myocardial systolic and diastolic function.

Cyclic Flow Variations After PTCA

Experimental studies and studies in human beings have indicated that cyclic flow variation is a reliable marker of the formation of platelet aggregates and thus may be predictive of immediate complications after coronary angioplasty. In this study by Sunamura and associates[182] from Rotterdam, The Netherlands, the incidence and clinical relevance of cyclic flow variation in a large patient population after elective PTCA was assessed. One hundred and two patients with 1-vessel disease and no previous Q wave AMI underwent angiographically successful PTCA of a single lesion of a major coronary artery. A Doppler guidewire inserted distal to the stenosis was used to monitor flow velocity continuously after PTCA for 15 minutes. In 19 (92%) of 102 patients, a stable and reliable Doppler signal could be recorded for 15 minutes after the procedure. Cyclic flow variation, defined as gradual decline in flow over several minutes followed by a sudden restoration to higher values, was observed in 4 patients. In 3 of these patients, the occurrence of cyclic flow variation was predictive of immediate complications (2 intracoronary thrombosis and 1 acute closure), whereas none of the patients without cyclic flow variation (n = 90) showed acute closure during hospital stay. In conclusion, cyclic flow variations in patients after angiographically successful elective PTCA are rare (4.3%) but highly sensitive for the prediction of abrupt closure.

Leukocyte and Platelet Adhesion After PTCA

Increased expression of CD11b on monocytes and neutrophils promotes their adhesion to endothelial cells, extracellular matrix, and smooth muscle cells. Thrombin-activated platelets adhere to monocytes and neutrophils through P-selectin. Mickelson and colleagues[183] from Houston, Texas, evaluated whether leukocyte activation influences clinical outcome after PTCA. During this pilot trial in 11 men undergoing elective single-vessel PTCA, they measured flow cytometric detection of CD11b as well as the percentage of leukocytes with adherent platelets and the intensity of bound platelet fluorescence. After PTCA, there was an increase in CD11b and leukocytes with adherent platelets. Values for leukocyte CD11b expression, the percent of leukocytes with adherent platelets, and the intensity of bound platelet fluorescence were higher both before and after PTCA in the 6 patients experiencing clinical events. These authors concluded that despite standard aspirin and heparin therapy, leukocyte activation with platelet adherence occurs after PTCA and may be related to late clinical events.

Creatine Kinase Levels After PTCA

The threshold of creatine kinase elevation after coronary interventions has been set at levels ranging in different studies from 2 to greater than 5 times the laboratory's upper limit of normal. This high variability is caused by the absence of any systematic evaluation of the prognostic implications of cardiac-enzyme elevation in this setting. This study by Abdelmeguid and associates[184] from Cleveland, Ohio, was undertaken to evaluate the clinical, morphological, and procedural correlates, and the long-term follow-up of 2 commonly used thresholds of creatine kinase elevation after successful percutaneous coronary interventions. Their goal was to define the level of postprocedural cardiac enzymes that correlates with adverse clinical outcome. These investigators examined 4664 consecutive patients who underwent successful coronary angioplasty or directional atherectomy at the Cleveland Clinic. Group 1 (4480 patients) had creatine kinase ≤2 times control levels after the procedure (≤360 IU/L). Group II (123 patients) had a peak level between 361 and 900 IU/L, and group III (61 patients) had a peak level higher than 900 IU/L with positive myocardial isoenzymes (creatine kinase-MB>4%). Elevation of cardiac enzymes was associated with distinct clinical, morphologic, and procedural characteristics, including coronary embolism, recent infarction, transient in-laboratory closure, hemodynamic instability, vein graft procedure, and large dissections. Clinical follow-up was available in 4644 (99.6%) patients, with a mean follow-up of 36 ± 22 months. Kaplan-Meier survival analysis adjusted with Cox proportional hazards regression model showed that cardiac-enzyme elevation was an important correlate of cardiac death (risk ratio, 2.19). The groups with elevated cardiac enzymes had a higher incidence of cardiac death compared with group I. There was also a trend toward more cardiac hospitalizations in the same groups. The incidence of cardiac death and cardiac hospitalization on follow-up was not different between groups II and III. This study shows that creatine kinase elevations between 2 and 5 times control values after successful coronary interventions are associated with an adverse long-term outcome. The findings suggest that an appropriate creatine kinase threshold that has prognostic implications would be twice the upper limit of normal.

Determining Perfusion Defects After PTCA

In this investigation by Miller and associates[185] from St. Louis, Missouri, 34 consecutive patients had coronary flow velocity assessed under basal and hyperemic conditions in the proximal and distal coronary artery, followed by rest-stress technetium-99m sestamibi myocardial tomography within 3 months of successful coronary angioplasty. In spite of significant angiographic improvement, 29% of patients had a persistent reversible myocardial perfusion defect associated with a residual abnormality of the proximal-to-distal coronary average peak velocity ratio. Patients with an abnormal peak velocity ratio (>1.7) had more numerous angioplasty-zone perfusion defects (4.2 ± 3.3 vs. 0.8 ± 2.0). Multivariable analysis of clinical, angiographic, coronary flow, and scintigraphic data demonstrated that the relative risk of cardiac events (n = 11) was greatest in patients with a reversible angioplasty-zone perfusion defect (relative risk 5.5), post-stenotic coronary flow reserve less than 2.0 (relative risk 8.3) and peak velocity ratio greater than 1.7 (relative risk 6.2). Residual basal coronary flow-velocity abnormalities are significant physiologic correlates of stress-induced myocardial perfusion defects and are a prognostic covariable associated with future ischemic cardiac events.

In Octogenarians

Direct PTCA has emerged as effective reperfusion therapy for AMI. Few data exist on its use in octogenarians. Thrombolytic therapy in this age group has reduced early mortality from approximately 30% to 20%, but it is associated with an increased risk of stroke and major hemorrhage. Laster and associates[186] from Kansas City, Missouri, analyzed the acute and long-term results of direct PTCA performed on patients aged 80 years or older between 1980 and 1993. The study group consisted of 55 patients (mean patient age, 83.3 ± 2.3 years). Infarcts were anterior in 27 patients (49%). Cardiogenic shock was present in 6 patients (11%). The mean time to reperfusion was 4.3 ± 2.8 hours. Direct PTCA was successful in 53 patients (96%). There were no emergent bypass operations. In-hospital death occurred in 9 patients (16%), including 4 of 6 (67%) presenting in cardiogenic shock. There were no strokes during hospitalization. Bleeding complications requiring blood transfusion were present in 4 patients (7%). Thirty-day mortality was 16%, and 1-year actuarial survival was 67%. Direct PTCA in patients older than 80 years of age can be performed safely with a high procedural success rate. The clinical outcome with PTCA in this high-risk subset of patients compares favorably with that reported previously for both thrombolytic and medical therapy.

Long-Term Follow-Up of PTCA

Clinical Outcome at Ten Years

PTCA was first performed in 1977. There are only a few reports on the clinical outcome 10 or more years after PTCA. Ruygrok and colleagues[187] from Rotterdam, The Netherlands, evaluated the 10-year outcome of 856 patients who underwent PTCA during the years 1980 to 1985. The procedural clinical success rate was 82%. At 10 years, 77% were alive, of whom 53% were symptom free and 40% were taking no antianginal medications. Factors that were found to adversely influence 10-year survival were age older than 60, multivessel disease, impaired LVEF, and a history of previous MI. These authors concluded that the long-term prognosis of patients after PTCA is good, particularly in those who are younger than 60 with single-vessel disease and normal left ventricular function. Most patients, however, are likely to experience a further cardiac event in the 10 years after their first PTCA (Figure 2-102).

Outcome in Patients Older Than 75 Years of Age

No prospective studies have been undertaken to compare the long-term results of PTCA in patients over 75 years of age with those in a younger patient group. Berg and associates[188] from Nieuwegein, The Netherlands, matched a total of 192 consecutive PTCA patients, aged 75 years or older (group I), with 192 control patients, aged 40 to 65 years (group II). The groups were matched for gender, angina pectoris class, left ventricular function, 1-, 2-, and 3-vessel CAD, and previous AMI. The mean follow-up was 40.4 months (range 0–110 months). Actuarial analysis (freedom from events) after 5 years yielded the following results for group I versus group II: freedom from death remained

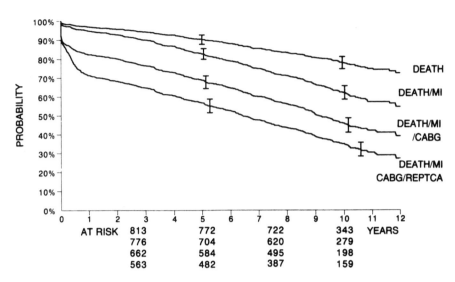

FIGURE 2-102. Ten year cumulative survival and event-free survival rate in 856 patients who underwent coronary angioplasty during the years 1980 to 1985. Reproduced with permission from Ruygrok et al.[187]

77.1% versus 97.9%, from cardiac death 92.4% versus 97.9%, and from angina pectoris 54.6% versus 75.1%. The differences were not significant for those remaining free from myocardial infarction, repeat balloon angioplasty, or coronary artery bypass grafting. (When elderly patients with complete revascularization (n = 127) were compared with a matched control group of 127 patients aged 40 to 65 years who underwent complete revascularization, a significant difference was found only in noncardiac death rates). We conclude that patients older than 75 years of age have a significantly higher cardiac and noncardiac death rate and a higher incidence of angina pectoris after successful balloon angioplasty. However, the incidence of reintervention and myocardial infarction is lower in the elderly. If complete revascularization is achieved in the elderly, then freedom from cardiac death and recurrence of angina pectoris would be comparable to that in younger patients (Tables 2-13 and 2-14).

Patent Infarct-Related Artery and Mortality

Welty and colleagues[189] in Boston, Massachusetts, compared long-term outcome, studying reinfarction and death in patients with open versus closed coronary arteries after PTCA. All patients had experienced MI complicated by persistent ischemia. Between 1981 and 1989, 505 patients underwent PTCA for post-MI ischemia at the Deaconess Hospital in Boston, Massachusetts. Long-term incidence of death, nonfatal reinfarction, repeat PTCA, and CABG were determined for 479 patients and compared on the basis of the status of the artery, open versus closed, at the end of PTCA. The 5-year Kaplan-Meier actuarial mortality rate was 5% for 456 patients with open infarct-related arteries and 19% for 23 patients with closed infarct-related arteries (Figure 2-103).

TABLE 2-13
Actuarial Freedom from Events (%) at Five Years in 192 Patients Aged ≥ 75 Years (group I) Versus 192 Patients Aged 40 to 65 Years (group II)

	Group I (n = 192)	Group II (n = 192)	p Value
All death	77.1% (0.05)	97.9% (0.01)	0.0001
Cardiac death	92.4% (0.03)	97.9% (0.01)	0.049
Noncardiac death	83.4% (0.05)	100% (0.00)	0.0001
Myocardial infarction	96.7% (0.02)	96.0% (0.02)	0.55
Reintervention	86.6% (0.03)	79.9% (0.03)	0.16
Repeat balloon angioplasty	89.9% (0.02)	86.2% (0.03)	0.51
Related repeat balloon angioplasty	94.1% (0.02)	89.5% (0.02)	0.18
Bypass surgery	95.9% (0.02)	93.1% (0.02)	0.25
Major events	80.3% (0.03)	74.6% (0.03)	0.44
Angina pectoris	54.6% (0.09)	75.1% (0.03)	0.03

Numbers in parentheses are SEM.

Reintervention = repeat balloon angioplasty or bypass surgery; Major events = cardiac death, repeat balloon angioplasty, bypass surgery, myocardial infarction.

Reproduced with permission from Berg et al.[188]

Multivariate Cox proportional hazards analysis controlling for age, sex, number of diseased vessels, type and location of MI, and year of PTCA revealed a hazard ratio for death for closed compared with open arteries of 6. Among patients with LVEFs lower than 50%, a closed artery was associated with a higher mortality compared with patients with open arteries. However, the status of the artery was not associated with a difference in mortality in patients with LVEFs of 50% or higher (Figure 2-104). Thus, an open artery after PTCA for post MI ischemia is associated with significantly lower long-term mortality, especially in patients with LVEFs of less than 50%.

Comparison of Costs for Low- and High-Volume Operators

Whether higher operator case volume is associated with improved PTCA clinical and cost outcomes was studied by Shook and associates[190] from Los

TABLE 2-14
Actuarial Freedom from Events (%) at Five Years in 127 Patients Aged ≥ 75 Years (group III) Versus 127 Patients Aged 40 to 65 Years (group IV) With Complete Revascularization

	Group III (n = 127)	Group IV (n = 127)	p Value
All death	86.4% (0.05)	97.6% (0.01)	0.02
Cardiac death	96.1% (0.03)	97.6% (0.01)	0.9
Noncardiac death	89.9% (0.04)	100% (0.00)	0.0007
Myocardial infarction	97.1% (0.02)	96.2% (0.02)	0.78
Reintervention	84.8% (0.04)	80.0% (0.04)	0.31
Related repeat balloon angioplasty	94.6% (0.02)	89.7% (0.03)	0.2
Repeat balloon angioplasty	94.6% (0.02)	89.7% (0.03)	0.2
Bypass surgery	95.7% (0.04)	92.0% (0.02)	0.16
Major events	82.0% (0.04)	74.2% (0.04)	0.21
Angina pectoris	59.8% (0.12)	75.0% (0.04)	0.34

Numbers in parentheses are SEM.

Reproduced with permission from Berg et al.[188]

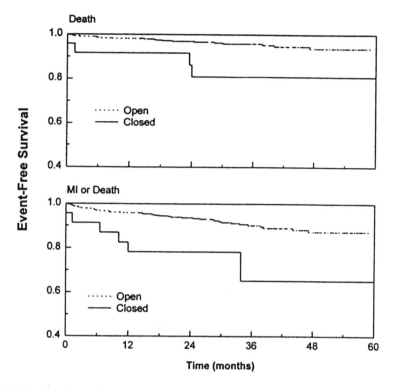

FIGURE 2-103. The 5-year Kaplan-Meier actuarial event-free survival curves for 456 patients with open arteries and 23 patients with closed arteries after coronary angioplasty for post-myocardial infarction (MI) ischemia. **Top,** freedom from death; **bottom,** freedom from reinfarction or death. Dashed line indicates open artery; solid lines, closed artery. Reproduced with permission from Welty et al.[189]

Angeles, California. Hospital volume-related improvement in clinical outcomes has been shown for CABG and PTCA. Physician case volume-related differences in clinical outcomes have not been clearly demonstrated, and differences in hospital costs have not been examined. For clinical and cost outcomes, risk-adjusted analysis of differences in PTCA outcomes has not been reported. In addition, controversy exists about the appropriate annual case volume considered adequate to maintain skills and achieve optimal clinical outcomes in performing PTCA procedures. Shook's group studied 2350 PTCAs performed between March 1, 1991, and February 28, 1994. Physicians were divided into 2 volume groups: high ($\geq$50 cases/year) and low (<50 cases/year). The rate of emergency CABG after PTCA was 2.1% for high- and 3.9% for low-volume operators. Hospital morbidity associated with PTCA was lower in high- than in low-volume operators (6.46% vs. 10.73%). The risk-adjusted ratios for emergency CABG and morbidity were 2.05 and 1.79, respectively. The length of stay averaged 4.07 ± 4.54 days for high- and 4.49 ± 4.33 days for low-volume operators. Hospital costs averaged $7,977 ± $7,269 for high- and $8,278 ± $6,289 for low-volume operators. The risk-adjusted ratio was 1.091 for length of stay and 1.050 for cost. Thus, PTCA performed by high-volume operators is significantly less likely to require emergency CABG and is also significantly associated with lower hospital morbidity, shorter hospital length of stay, and lower hospital costs (Figure 2-105).

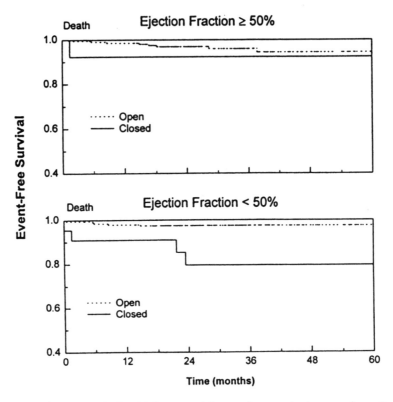

FIGURE 2-104. The 5-year Kaplan-Meier actuarial event-free survival curves for patients with open vs closed arteries stratified by ejection fraction after coronary angioplasty for post-myocardial infarction ischemia. **Top,** freedom from death in patients with ejection fractions ≥50%; bottom, freedom from death in patients with ejection fractions <50%. Dashed line indicates open artery; solid lines, closed artery. Reproduced with permission from Welty et al.[189]

Impact of Operator on Cost

Heidenreich and associates[191] from San Francisco, California, reviewed the hospital charts and billing records of 250 consecutive admissions for PTCA at a university hospital. Clinical characteristics, performing physician, angiographic features of the dilated lesion, procedural outcome, length of stay, and total and departmental hospital costs were recorded for each patient. The authors identified several independent predictors of hospital cost, including the physician ($4,400 increase from highest- to lowest-cost physician), age ($790 increase per 10-year increase in age), urgency of the procedure ($4,100 increase for urgent vs elective), and combined angiography and PTCA ($850 increase vs separate angiography). Independent predictors of catheterization laboratory cost included the physician ($1,280 increase from highest- to lowest-cost physician), American College of Cardiology/American Heart Association lesion type B2 or C ($320 increase), and combined angiography and PTCA ($430 increase). Expensive operators used more catheterization laboratory resources than did inexpensive operators; however, there were no significant differences in suc-

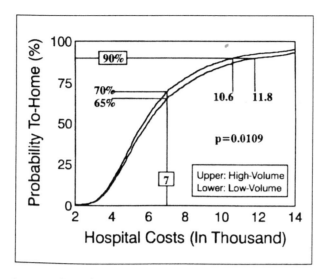

FIGURE 2-105. The Cox adjusted estimates of discharge (To-Home) distributions among 2,204 consecutive patients who underwent PTCA patients: high-volume operators (**top curve**), and low-volume operators (**bottom curve**). Variables adjusted include patient age, gender, race, body surface area, procedural priority, procedural complexity, preprocedural heart rate, and preprocedural blood pressure. Reproduced with permission from Shook et al.[190]

cess rate or need for emergent bypass surgery between physicians. PTCA cost is determined by both patient characteristics and the performing physician. The increase in cost due to the physician was not explained by patient variables, lesion characteristics, success rate, or complications (Table 2-15).

Restenosis

Time Course by Angiographic Follow-Up

Nakagawa and associates[192] from Kitakyushu, Japan, designed a serial follow-up study to identify the time course of reocclusion and/or restenosis after direct angioplasty for AMI. Direct angioplasty for AMI was attempted in 160 patients. Of the 141 who underwent successful reperfusion and were discharged, 137 (97%) were enrolled in this study. At the 3-week follow-up study (100% eligible), angiographic restenosis of the infarct-related artery was documented in 21 patients (16%), 9 (43%) of whom had reocclusions. At 4 months in 100 patients (92% of those eligible), restenosis was newly documented in 28 infarct-related arteries (28%), 3 of which had reocclusion (11%). At 1 year in 64 patients (89% of those eligible), restenosis was newly documented in 5-infarct-related arteries (7.8%), with no reocclusions. The cumulative restenosis rate was 20% at 3 weeks, 43% at 4 months, and 47% at 1 year; when divided into occlusive and nonocclusive types, restenosis rates were 12%

Table 2-15
Distribution of Hospital Costs by Department for the 10 Departments With Highest Costs

Department	Mean Cost (95% CI)	Percentage of Total Cost*
Catheterization laboratory	$4,020 ($4,300-$3,800)	47%
Coronary care unit	$1,690 ($1,900-$3,400)	20%
Pharmacy	$550 ($480-$620)	6%
General hospital ward	$470 ($370-$570)	6%
Material services	$300 ($260-$340)	4%
Laboratory	$230 ($200-$260)	3%
Operating room	$210 ($100-$320)	2%
Respiratory therapy	$200 ($140-$260)	2%
Radiology	$130 ($100-$160)	2%
Blood bank	$110 ($60-$160)	1%

* Accounted for 92% of all hospital costs.
CI = confidence interval.
Reproduced with permission from Heidenreich et al.[191]

and 8.8% at 3 weeks and 14% and 29% at 4 months, respectively. Restenosis was most prevalent within the first 4 months and rarely occurred after that. When restenosis is manifested as reocclusion, it occurs earlier than in nonocclusive restenosis, often within 3 weeks (Figure 2-106).

Role of Thrombus in Restenosis

Violaris and colleagues[193] in Rotterdam, The Netherlands, examined the role of angiographically identifiable thrombus in the clinical situation to deter-

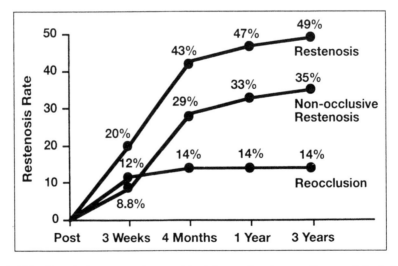

Figure 2-106. Cumulative restenosis rate of the infarct-related artery. Restenosis included both nonocclusive restenosis and reocclusion. The timing of reocclusion was earlier than the timing of nonocclusive restenosis. Reproduced with permission from Nakagawa et al.[192]

mine its role in postangioplasty restenosis. The study population consisted of 2950 patients with 3583 lesions. The presence of angiographically identifiable thrombus either before or after the procedure was defined as the presence of a generalized haziness or filling defect within the arterial lumen. Restenosis was assessed by both a categorical (>50% diameter stenosis at follow-up) or a continuous approach (absolute and relative losses). The study population included 160 lesions with and 3423 lesions without angiographically identifiable thrombus. The categorical restenosis rate was significantly higher in lesions containing angiographically identifiable thrombus: 43% versus 34% (Figure 2-107). The absolute and relative losses were also higher in lesions containing angiographically identifiable thrombus with an absolute loss of 0.43 versus 0.32 and the relative loss of 0.16 versus 0.13. The higher restenosis rate in these lesions was due primarily to the increased incidence of occlusion at follow-up angiography in this group: 14% versus 6%. When lesions proceeding to occlu-

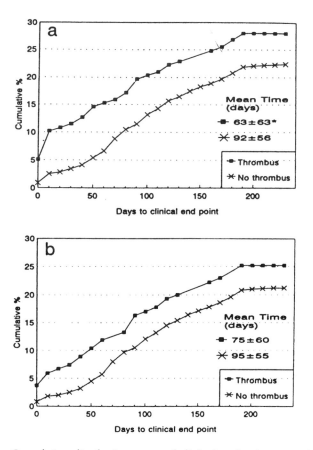

FIGURE 2-107. **a,** Cumulative distribution curve of clinical end points over time for patients with and without the presence of thrombus at the time of angioplasty. **b,** Cumulative distribution curve of clinical end points over time for patients with and without the presence of thrombus at the time of angioplasty (excluding lesions that went on to occlude at the time of follow-up angiography). Numbers given are mean ± SD. * + t.05. Reproduced with permission from Violaris et al.[193]

sion by the time of follow-up angiography were excluded from analysis, the categorical versus relative risk and continuous versus relative loss were not significant. The results of this study indicate that the presence of an angiographically identifiable thrombus at the time of the angioplasty procedure is associated with a higher restenosis rate.

Association with Fibrinolysis

This study by Sakata and associates[194] from Shizuoka, Japan, examined the role of fibrinolytic components in the process of restenosis after PTCA. Seventy-two patients with single-vessel disease who underwent successful PTCA were prospectively selected. tPA, free plasminogen activator inhibitor-1, and total free plasminogen activator inhibitor-1 antigen levels were measured before, at 1 week after, and at 3 months after PTCA. Six months after PTCA, the study patients were divided into 2 groups: 41 patients without restenosis and 31 patients with restenosis. There were no significant differences with regard to sex, age, coronary risk factors, or morphological changes in the target lesions between the 2 groups. There were no significant differences in plasma tPA, or total plasminogen activator inhibitor-1 levels at each sampling period, or in the time courses between the 2 groups except for total plasminogen activator inhibitor-1 levels at 1 week after PTCA. Although no significant differences in free plasminogen activator inhibitor-1 levels after PTCA were observed, free plasminogen activator inhibitor-1 levels after PTCA in the patients with restenosis were significantly higher than those in the patients without restenosis. In addition, each group had a significant change in the time course of free plasminogen activator inhibitor-1 levels. The results suggest that impaired fibrinolysis early after PTCA might affect the repair process of vascular injury, which leads to restenosis, and also that serial determination of free plasminogen activator inhibitor-1 levels could help predict restenosis.

Lipoprotein(a) as a Risk Factor

To determine the relation between the concentration of lipoprotein(a) and restenosis after PTCA in Japan, Miyata and associates[195] from Kagoshima, Japan, studied 80 consecutive patients with single-vessel disease who successfully underwent PTCA. All were evaluated by follow-up angiography a mean of 6.9 months after PTCA and were divided into the restenosis (30 patients) and the nonrestenosis (50 patients) groups. The serum lipoprotein(a) concentration of 29 ± 17 mg/dL in the restenosis group was significantly higher than that of 17 ± 14 mg/dL in the nonrestenosis group. Multiple logistic regression analysis for risk factors revealed a significant correlation between restenosis and lipoprotein(a). The serum lipoprotein(a) concentration was positively correlated with the coronary artery percent stenosis at the time of follow-up angiography. High serum concentration of lipoprotein(a) is therefore a risk factor for restenosis after PTCA in Japan.

Transforming βig-H3 as a Risk Factor

Transforming growth factor-β plays an important role in vascular lesion formation and, possibly, in the renarrowing process (restenosis) that occurs after balloon angioplasty. Secreted in a latent form by most cells, transforming growth factor-β requires enzymatic conversion before it is biologically active. Transforming growth factor-β-inducible gene h3 (βig-h3) is a novel molecule that is induced when cells are treated with transforming growth factor-β1. A study by O'Brien and coworkers[196] in Seattle, Washington, examined the expression of βig-h3 in normal and diseased human vascular tissue. To determine the expression pattern of βig-h3 in human arteries, immunochemistry was performed on tissue sections from: 1) normal internal mammary arteries; 2) the proximal left anterior descending coronary artery (with minimal intimal) thickening of 15 patients aged 18–40 years; 3) primary and restenotic coronary lesions from 7 patients; and 4) fresh directional atherectomy tissue from 11 patients. A polyclonal antibody consistently immunodetected βig-h3 protein in endothelial cells of all vascular tissue. In normal coronary arteries of young individuals, βig-h3 protein was absent from the intima and media but was found in the subendothelial smooth muscle cells of some arteries with modest intimal thickening. In diseased arteries, βig-h3 protein was more abundant in the intima than in the media. Restenotic coronary lesions tended to show higher levels of immunodetectable βig-h3 protein, especially in areas of dense fibrous connective tissue. βig-h3 protein was immunodetected in the cytoplasm of plaque macrophages as well as smooth muscle and endothelial cells. By using in situ hybridization on fresh directional atherectomy specimens, the investigators found βig-h3 mRNA to be overexpressed by plaque macrophages and smooth muscle cells. Nondiseased human internal mammary arteries also expressed βig-h3 mRNA in endothelial cells but not in the smooth muscle cells of the normal intima and media. The results documented the expression of βig-h3 in diseased human arterial tissue and support the hypothesis that active transforming growth factor-β plays a role in atherogenesis and restenosis.

Influence of Vessel Dilatation

The aim of the study by Schmitz and associates[197] from Bergisch Gladbach, Germany, and Aachen, Germany, was to evaluate the influence of vessel dilatation on restenosis after successful PTCA on the basis of quantitative angiographic analysis. To have the best comparison possible, these investigators retrospectively studied a homogenous series of patients from the early 1980s treated according to a standardized PTCA procedure. The study group consisted of 86 patients with stable angina pectoris and single-vessel disease, all of whom underwent successful PTCA for a short concentric lesion in proximal vessel parts. The overall restenosis rate was 27%. Angiographically measured balloon size remained below specifications. The size of the inflated balloon at the site of minimal lumen diameter averaged 2.6 ± 0.5 mm, and nominal balloon size was 3.3 ± 0.4 mm. In 22 patients with an oversized balloon (mean balloon/artery ratio, 1.1 ± 0.16) the restenosis rate was 5% compared with 34% in the corresponding group. Minimal lumen diameters that were similar after the procedure (2.4 ± 0.3 vs. 2.3 ± 0.4) were 2.3 ± 0.4 mm and 1.8 ± 0.7 mm, respectively, at follow-up. Multivariate analysis revealed balloon/vessel size ratio, postprocedure diameter stenosis, and percentage diameter increase produced by PTCA as independent correlates of the late outcome. Postangioplasty minimal lumen diameter was not related to restenosis. The strongest and most significant predictor of late PTCA outcome both by univariate and multivariate analysis was balloon/vessel size ratio, especially when balloon expansion at the site of minimal lumen diameter was regarded. In patients with continued success at follow-up, the ratio was 0.81 ± 0.15 compared with 0.60 ± 0.11 in patients with restenosis. These results suggest that the late angiographic outcome of PTCA is strongly influenced by procedural factors. It appears that in a selected group of patients, an increased balloon/artery ratio, supposedly associated with increased vessel wall stretch, favorably affects the restenosis process.

Circumferential Coronary Constriction

Therapies that inhibit intimal hyperplasia do not prevent restenosis after coronary artery balloon angioplasty, suggesting that additional mechanisms may be responsible for restenosis in humans. Using an intravascular ultrasound monorail imaging catheter, Luo and colleagues[198] in Los Angeles, California, studied 17 patients with clinical and angiographic restenosis at an average of 7 months after balloon angioplasty (12 LAD arteries, 4 right coronary arteries, and 1 left coronary artery). The lumen area, vessel wall area, and total cross-sectional area within the external elastic lamina were measured at the restenosis site and at proximal and distal reference sites which were defined as adjacent segments with the least amount of plaque. Consistent with coronary angiography findings, decreased lumen area at the restenotic site was detected in all 17 patients. The unique finding was that total cross-sectional area at the restenotic site was significantly decreased compared with both proximal and distal reference sites, whereas vessel wall area was slightly increased at the angioplasty site compared with both proximal and distal reference sites. Eighty-three percent of the loss in lumen area at the restenotic site was due to constriction of the total cross-sectional area, whereas the increase in vessel wall area at the restenotic site accounted for only a 17% loss in lumen area. The investigators then compared these results with the morphology of coronary artery segments in 14 patients without restenosis. These coronary artery segments had been previously treated with balloon angioplasty. Unlike that in restenotic lesions, the total cross-sectional area within the external elastic lamina at the sites of previous angioplasty was similar to that in distal and proximal reference sites. Significant and consistent reduction in arterial cross-sectional area with a minor increase in vessel wall area, characterizes human coronary lesions that cause angiographic restenosis. These data suggested that in humans "recoil" and/or vascular contraction with healing in response to balloon injury is a major contributor to restenosis after balloon angioplasty.

REDUCE Trial: Role of Low Molecular Weight Heparin

Unfractionated heparin and its low molecular weight fragments possess antiproliferative effects and have been shown to reduce neointimal smooth muscle cell migration and proliferation in response to vascular injury in experimental studies. Karsch and colleagues[199] in a multicenter trial (REDUCE)* evaluated the effect of low molecular weight heparin on the incidence and occurrence of restenosis in patients undergoing PTCA. Twenty-six centers in Europe and Canada enrolled 625 patients with single-lesion coronary artery obstruction suitable for PTCA. Three hundred six patients received reviparin as a 7000-U bolus before PTCA followed by 10,500 U as an infusion over 24 hours, then twice daily 3500 U subcutaneous application for 28 days. The 306 patients in the control group received a bolus of 10,000 U of unfractionated heparin followed by an infusion of 24,000 U over 24 hours. These patients then underwent 28 days of subcutaneous placebo injections. The primary end points were efficacy defined as a reduction in the incidence of major adverse events (death, myocardial infarction, need for reintervention or bypass surgery), absolute loss of minimum lumen diameter and incidence of restenosis during the observation period of 30 weeks after PTCA. Using the intention to treat analysis for all patients, 33.3% in the reviparin group and 32% in the control group reached a primary clinical end point. Likewise, no difference in late loss of minimum lumen diameter was evident for either group. Acute events within 24 hours occurred in 3.9% in the reviparin group and 8.2% in the control group during or immediately after the initial procedure. In the control group, 8 major bleeding complications were observed, and in the reviparin group 7 were observed within 35 days after PTCA. In the REDUCE trial, reviparin use during and after PTCA did not reduce the recurrence of major clinical events or the incidence of angiographic restenosis over 30 weeks.

Preventive Effects of Probucol

This protocol by Watanabe and associates[200] from Ehime, Japan, was performed to elucidate the preventive effects of probucol on restenosis after PTCA. A total of 118 patients with 134 vessels undergoing successful PTCA were randomly and prospectively assigned to the probucol group (group P) or the control group (group C). The groups comprised 91 men and 27 women, with a mean age of 63.4 ± 2.3 years. Sixty-six vessels of 59 patients in group P and 68 vessels of 59 patients in group C were evaluated by coronary angiography at 3 months after PTCA. Probucol (0.5 mg/day) was administered between at least 7 days before PTCA and 3 months after PTCA. Serum total cholesterol level and LDL cholesterol in group P decreased from 204 ± 43 to 170 ± 39 mg/dl and from 131 ± 0.7 to 109 ± 2.5 mg/dL; in group C; however, the levels decreased from 202 ± 32 to 194 ± 30 mg/dL and from 129 ± 38 to 124 ± 32 mg/dL. The restenosis rate was significantly lower in group P (20%, 13 of 66 vessels) than in group C (40%; 27 of 68 vessels). In the probucol group, the probucol blood concentration was significantly higher in the individuals without restenosis (31 ± 9 μg/mL) than in those with restenosis (18 ± 8 μg/mL), but the serum total cholesterol and LDL cholesterol levels were not significantly different between these 2 groups. In summary, long-term administration of probucol significantly reduced the incidence of restenosis after PTCA. It is suggested that the mechanism of this preventive effect was not reducing the serum total cholesterol or LDL cholesterol levels, but rather an inhibitory action on smooth muscle cell proliferation.

Estrogen Replacement Therapy in Reduction of Restenosis

Although estrogen replacement therapy has been associated with a reduction in cardiovascular events and improvement in endothelial function, no study has examined whether estrogen reduces restenosis rates after percutaneous coronary interventions. O'Brian and colleagues[201] from the Coronary Angioplasty Versus Excisional Atherectomy Trial (CAVEAT) contacted 204 women during follow-up and determined their estrogen replacement status. Late loss in minimal lumen diameter, late loss index, minimal lumen diameter, rate of restenosis greater than 50%, and actual percentage of stenosis were compared in estrogen users and nonusers by quantitative coronary angiography at 6-month follow-up. Late loss in minimal lumen diameter was significantly less in women using estrogen than in nonusers who underwent atherectomy. A regression analysis of the determinants of late loss in minimal lumen diameter revealed that estrogen use was the single most important predictor of subsequent late loss. In contrast, estrogen had minimal effects on restenosis end points after angioplasty. These authors concluded that there is a potential for estrogen replacement therapy to reduce angiographic measures in postmenopausal women after coronary intervention, particularly in those undergoing atherectomy.

Directional Coronary Atherectomy

Cytomegalovirus Infection as a Risk Factor for Restenosis after Coronary Atherectomy

Zhou and colleagues[202] at the National Institutes of Health in Bethesda, Maryland, prospectively studied 75 consecutive patients undergoing directional coronary atherectomy for symptomatic CAD. Before atherectomy was performed, they measured blood levels of anti-CMV IgG (anti-cytomegalovirus) antibodies to determine whether previous exposure to CMV increased the risk of restenosis as determined by coronary angiography performed 6 months after atherectomy. After atherectomy, the mean luminal diameter of the target vessel was greater in the 49 patients who were seropositive for CMV than in the 26 patients who were seronegative (3.2 mm vs. 3.0 mm, p = 0.01). After 6 months, however, the seropositive patients had a greater reduction in the luminal diameter (1.2 mm vs. 0.68 mm, p = 0.003) resulting in a significantly higher rate of restenosis in the seropositive patients (43% vs. 8%, p = 0.002). In a multivariable logistic-regression model, CMV seropositivity and the CMV titer were independently predictive of restenosis (odds ratios, 12.9 and 8.1, respectively). There was no evidence of acute infection since the titer of anti-CMV IgG antibodies did not increase over time, and tests for anti-CMV IgM antibodies were negative in all patients. Prior infection with CMV is a strong independent risk factor for restenosis after coronary atherectomy. The authors suggest that these findings may help identify patients at high risk for restenosis.

Atherectomy in Patients with AMI

Although PTCA has been an effective treatment for primary reperfusion in AMI, patients with thrombolytic ineligibility, thrombolytic failure, cardiogenic shock, and vein graft occlusion remain at high risk for complications with PTCA treatment. The transluminal extraction catheter may be useful for treatment of such patients owing to its ability to aspirate thrombus. Kaplan and associates[203] from 2 medical centers (1 in Royal Oak, Michigan, and the other in Chicago, Illinois) prospectively evaluated extraction atherectomy in 100 patients, age 62 ± 10 years. High-risk features included thrombolytic failure in 40%, postinfarct angina in 28%, presence of angiographic thrombus in 66%, presence of cardiogenic shock in 11%, and a saphenous vein graft occlusion in 29%. Procedural success, defined as a final residual stenosis <50% and TIMI 2 or 3 grade flow, was seen in 94%. Events during the hospitalization included death in 5%, bypass surgery in 4%, and blood transfusion in 18%. In a substudy, patients enrolled at William Beaumont Hospital (n = 65) underwent elective predischarge angiography, which revealed a patent infarct-related vessel in 95%. These patients were also followed for 6 months, with angiographic follow-up in 60%. Target vessel revascularization was necessary in 38%, and 6-month mortality was 10%. Although long-term vessel patency was 90%, angiographic restenosis occurred in 68%. AMI patients can be treated with extraction atherectomy with a high technical success rate and a low incidence of complications. Infarct artery patency at 1 week and 6 months was excellent; however, angiographic restenosis remains a problem. Extraction of thrombus in this high-risk group of patients is associated with low in-hospital mortality and a high rate of vessel patency at 6 months.

With Adjunctive Balloon PTCA

The purpose of this study by Khoury and associates[204] from St. Louis, Missouri, was to examine the influence of sequential percutaneous transluminal coronary rotational atherectomy and PTCA on coronary blood flow and flow reserve in patients. Rotational coronary atherectomy restores lumen patency by partially ablating fibrocalcific plaque, which releases microparticulate debris into the distal coronary circulation. Adjunctive balloon PTCA is usually performed to optimize the angiographic luminal dimensions. Serial alterations in coronary physiology have not been reported. Fourteen lesions in 13 patients were treated by sequential rotational atherectomy followed by adjunctive balloon angioplasty. Poststenotic baseline coronary blood flow velocity was measured by using a Doppler flow wire, and coronary blood flow was calculated by using the distal vessel cross-sectional area obtained by quantitative coronary angiography. Data were acquired at baseline and during hyperemia (12 to 18 μg of intracoronary adenosine), before and after percutaneous transluminal coronary rotational atherectomy, and again after balloon angioplasty. The mean stenosis decreased from 76% $\pm$ 12% at baseline to 21% $\pm$ 11% at the completion of the procedure. The minimal luminal diameter (by quantitative coronary angiography), which was 0.7 $\pm$ 0.4 mm at baseline, increased to 1.9 $\pm$ 0.4 mm after rotational atherectomy, and to 2.4 $\pm$ 0.5 mm after balloon angioplasty. Distal (poststenotic) coronary blood flow at baseline was 47 $\pm$ 23 mL/min and 57 $\pm$ 38 mL/min during hyperemia. After percutaneous transluminal coronary rotational atherectomy, coronary blood flow increased to 104 $\pm$ 59 mL/min and to 132 $\pm$ 73 mL/min with hyperemia. After adjunctive angioplasty, coronary blood flow was 84 $\pm$ 40 mL/min and increased to 143 $\pm$ 81 mL/min with hyperemia. The poststenotic coronary flow reserve increased from an initial value of 1.1 $\pm$ 0.2 mL/min to 1.3 $\pm$ 0.3 mL/min after percutaneous transluminal coronary rotational atherectomy and to 1.6 $\pm$ 0.3 mL/min after adjunctive balloon angioplasty. Percutaneous transluminal coronary rotational atherectomy significantly increased resting coronary blood flow. Adjunctive balloon angioplasty did not significantly augment resting or hyperemic coronary blood flow more than that achieved by rotational atherectomy alone. These data demonstrate that percutaneous transluminal coronary rotational atherectomy alone improves baseline coronary blood flow with minimal additional physiological change after adjunctive balloon angioplasty.

Effect of Glycoprotein IIb/IIIa Receptor Blockade on Adverse Outcomes

Randomized trials comparing directional atherectomy with PTCA have demonstrated modest benefits favoring atherectomy but at a cost of increased acute ischemic complications, notably non-Q wave AMI. Lefkovits and colleagues[205] evaluated data from the EPIC trial to determine the effects of platelet glycoprotein IIb/IIIa receptor blockade on adverse outcomes, especially non-Q wave AMI in patients undergoing directional atherectomy in the EPIC trial. Of 2038 high-risk patients undergoing coronary intervention in the EPIC trial, directional atherectomy was performed in 10%. Patients randomly received the glycoprotein IIb/IIIa antibody as a bolus, or a bolus and 12-hour infusion, or placebo. Patients undergoing directional atherectomy had a lower baseline risk for acute complications, but had a higher incidence of any AMI (10.7% vs. 6.3%) and non-Q wave myocardial infarction (9.6% vs. 4.9%). Bolus and infusion of IIb/IIIa antibody reduced non-Q wave myocardial infarctions by 71% after atherectomy (15.4% for placebo vs. 4.5%). Non-Q wave AMI rates after PTCA were not affected by the antibody, although Q wave infarcts were reduced from 2.6% to 0.8%. The EPIC trial had confirmed the increased risk of non-Q wave myocardial infarction with directional atherectomy as compared with PTCA. A bolus and 12-hour infusion of the glycoprotein IIb/IIIa receptor inhibitor abolished this excess risk. Thus, directional atherectomy-related non-Q wave myocardial infarction appears to be platelet-aggregation dependent.

Coronary Stenting

In AMI

Data on the feasibility, safety, and clinical outcome of intracoronary stenting in AMI are limited. Le May and associates[206] from Ottawa, Canada, examined the immediate angiographic results and the early and late outcomes in 32 patients who had coronary stenting during AMI. Coronary angiograms recorded at the time of stenting were reviewed with quantitative measurements obtained on the "target" coronary lesion before and after stenting. Immediate angiographic success was achieved in 30 patients (94%). The minimal luminal diameter increased from 0.36 ± 0.37 to 2.58 ± 0.41 mm. Two patients died in the hospital. Of the remainder, none had reinfarction or required CABG, whereas 2 required repeat PTCA for recurrent ischemia. Although thrombus at the infarct-related coronary lesion was initially detected in 41% of the patients, its presence was not associated with adverse procedural stenting, which resolved with intracoronary urokinase. At a mean follow-up of 6.1 ± 4.1 months, there was 1 additional cardiac death, and no patient had AMI or required repeat PTCA or bypass; among the 29 survivors, 86% were free of angina. Thus, intracoronary stenting of the infarct-related artery in the setting of AMI is associated with excellent immediate angiographic success and a favorable clinical outcome and remains an option even in the presence of thrombus.

Stent implantation in patients with coronary disease appears to provide better short- and long-term outcomes than PTCA. Saito and colleagues[207] from Kamakura, Japan, evaluated the feasibility and efficacy of primary stent implantation without coumadin in 74 patients within 8 hours of the onset of AMI. Stent implantation was successful in 72 patients, and stent thrombosis was noted in only 1 patient, who was not given ticlopidine, aspirin, or coumadin. The rates of restenosis and frequency of major clinical events during the hospital period were less in the patients undergoing stenting as compared with angioplasty. These authors concluded that primary stent implantation can improve clinical outcomes of patients with AMI when the stent is dilated adequately and antiplatelet drugs are used.

Although coronary stenting has been useful in conjunction with PTCA for patients with suboptimal results, abrupt closure, and threatening occlusion, its use in patients with AMI is controversial because of the presence of intracoronary thrombus. Rodriguez and associates[208] from Boston, Massachusetts, used intracoronary stenting to treat suboptimal results and complications in 30 patients (35 narrowings) undergoing PTCA during AMI. There were 28 men and 2 women, mean age 58 ± 12 years. Thirteen patients (43%) had undergone rescue PTCA because of unsuccessful thrombolysis. Four patients had Killip's grade IV, 5 Killip's grade III, and 21 Killip's grade II (or under) heart failure. Stents were placed in the 35 lesions because of suboptimal results (n = 19), early loss (n = 9), abrupt closure (n = 2), and coronary dissection with threatening occlusion (n = 5). All stents were deployed successfully. In-hospital complications included 1 in-hospital death (3.0%); no patient required emergency CABG. One patient (3.0%) developed abrupt closure and was successfully treated with PTCA and intracoronary thrombolysis. Vascular complications requiring blood transfusion developed in 3 of 30 patients (10%). At 11.8 months (range 4 to 24) follow-up, there were no deaths or myocardial infarction. One patient underwent coronary artery bypass grafting. The remaining patients were free of angina at follow-up. Thus, intracoronary stents can be used successfully to treat both suboptimal results and complications occurring in patients undergoing PTCA during AMI.

Garcia-Cantu and associates[209] from Paris, France, and Le Chesnay, France, studied 35 patients who had coronary stent implantation among 138 patients treated with coronary angioplasty during AMI. The mean age was 56 years, and 83% were men. Mean time from onset of chest pain was 6.0 ± 5.3 hours, and previous thrombolytic therapy had been given to 10 patients (29%). Infarct location was anterior in 19 (54%), inferior in 14 (40%), and lateral in 2 patients (6%). TIMI grade flows 0, 1, and 2 were seen in 24 (69%), 6 (17%), and 5 patients (14%), respectively. The culprit vessel was the left anterior descending artery in 18 patients (51%), right coronary artery in 14 patients (40%), left circumflex in 2 patients (6%), and left main coronary artery in 1 patient (3%). Mean vessel diameter was 3.3 ± 0.3 mm. Indications were: primary in 5 (14%), suboptimal result in 8 (23%), nonocclusive dissection in 14 (40%), and occlusive dissection in 8 patients (23%). Angiographic thrombus after initial angioplasty was present in 12 patients (34%). A total of 46 stents were implanted; mean balloon diameter and pressure were 3.4 ± 0.4 mm and 15.5 ± 2.2 atm, respectively. Residual diameter stenosis was 4 ± 7%. There were 2 deaths: sudden in 1, and postelective CABG in the other; 2 patients (6%) had groin hematomas. Mean hospitalization was 9.9 ± 5.0 days. Repeat angiography revealed no stent occlusion. With initial intravenous heparin for 3 to 7 days, all patients received aspirin and ticlopidine for 1 month. Thus, AMI is not a contraindication for stent implantation. The benefits of stenting are a high success rate, low residual diameter stenosis, and low incidence of in-hospital recurrent ischemia. Reduction in restenosis rate in this setting is likely but remains to be determined.

For Chronic Coronary Occlusions

Restenosis is common after PTCA. Stenting has the potential for improving results. Sirnes and colleagues[210] from Feiring, Norway, and Oslo, Norway and Göteborg, Sweden investigated in the SICCO trial whether stenting improved long-term results after PTCA of chronic coronary occlusions. One hundred nineteen patients with satisfactory results after successful recanalization by PTCA of a chronic coronary occlusion were randomly assigned to: 1) a control group with no other intervention or 2) a group in which PTCA was followed by implantation of Palmaz-Schatz stents with full anticoagulation. Coronary angiography was performed before randomization, after stenting, and at 6-month follow-up. There were no deaths, but inguinal bleeding was more frequent in the stent group. One patient with stenting had an AMI. Subacute occlusion within 2 weeks occurred in 4 patients in the stent group and in 3 in the PTCA group. At follow-up, 57% of patients with stenting were free from angina compared with 24% of patients with PTCA only. Angiographic follow-up data were available in 114 patients. Restenosis developed in 32% of patients with stenting and in 74% of patients with PTCA only. Reocclusion occurred in 12% and 26%, respectively. Minimum lumen diameter at follow-up was 1.92 mm and 1.11 mm, respectively. Target lesion revascularization within 300 days was less frequent in patients with stenting than in patients with PTCA only. Although the incidence of reocclusion was quite high in the control group, these authors concluded that stent implantation improved long-term angiographic and clinical results after PTCA of chronic coronary occlusions.

For Right Coronary Artery Lesions

This study by Eeckhout and associates[211] from Lausanne, Switzerland, compared the clinical and angiographic outcome during a 6-month follow-up period, of 84 patients with new-onset lesions of the right coronary artery randomly assigned to either Wiktor stent implantation (42 patients) or conventional balloon angioplasty (42 patients). At hospital discharge, 3 patients in each group (7%) reached a clinical end point. At 6 months, these proportions were 24% (10 patients with stents) and 29% (12 patients with angioplasty). There were no incidents of death or myocardial infarction. Despite a larger minimal luminal diameter after stenting (2.87 mm vs. 2.37 mm), no difference was observed at 6 months of follow-up (1.75 mm vs. 1.74 mm, respectively). Accordingly, angiographic restenosis rates were 48% (19 of 40 patients with stents) and 35% (14 of 40 patients with angioplasty). Elective stenting with the Wiktor stent and conventional balloon angioplasty are safe and immediately effective therapeutic options for symptomatic, obstructive right coronary artery disease. At 6 months of follow-up, clinical and angiographic outcome did not differ. The role of Wiktor stent placement in primary restenosis prevention remains to be determined for lesions of the right coronary artery.

After Unsuccessful Emergency Angioplasty

In a report by Steffenino and colleagues[212] from Cuneo, Italy, 19 consecutive procedures of coronary stenting were attempted in 70 consecutive patients (27%) with evolving AMI due to threatened vessel reocclusion after primary (16 cases) or rescue (3 cases) angioplasty. Two patients were in cardiogenic shock. Stent delivery was successful in 18 patients with a TIMI flow grade 3; residual diameter stenosis was 19% ± 11%, and minimum luminal diameter was 2.98 ± 0.62 mm. After the procedure, heparin was continued for 4 days, and 250 mg ticlopidine was given twice a day for 1 month. Acute stent occlusion occurred in 1 patient 1 hour after the procedure and was successfully treated with emergency repeat angioplasty. Subacute stent occlusion occurred 6 days after the procedure in 1 patient, with multivessel CAD and a suboptimal stent result. He had been referred for surgery, and emergent CABG was performed. CABG was performed in another patient before discharge because of severe multivessel disease. Persistent cardiogenic shock and new myocardial infarction in another location were the causes of death in 2 patients, 3 and 10 days after the procedure. Fifteen patients were discharged with a patent infarct vessel and without reinfarction or the need for coronary bypass surgery. One patient had repeat angioplasty for intrastent restenosis at 3 months. The remaining 14 patients were free from new coronary events 4 ± 2 months after the procedure. Although AMI is generally considered a contraindication to the use of coronary stents, stents may play a role in increasing the rates of successful infarct artery reperfusion.

Versus Balloon Angioplasty (Palmaz-Schatz)

Mori and associates[213] from Himeji, Japan, and Kobe, Japan, compared angiographic and clinical outcomes after successful revascularization of chronic total coronary occlusion with the placement of the Palmaz-Schatz stent (43 patients) and conventional balloon angioplasty (53 patients). After the procedure, the coronary stent led to a greater minimal lumen diameter than did conventional balloon angioplasty (2.6 vs. 1.7 mm), resulting in a smaller residual stenosis (6.5% vs. 36.7%). At 6-month follow-up, there was no significant difference in late loss between the groups, resulting in a larger minimal lumen diameter at follow-up in the stent group (1.8 vs. 1.1 mm). The incidence of restenosis was lower in the stent group (27.9% vs. 56.6%). The frequency of the combination of AMI and CABG surgery tended to be less in the stent group (2.3% vs. 11.3%). Placement of the Palmaz-Schatz stent improved LVEF by 26% in patients who had reduced LVEF, but conventional balloon angioplasty did not. Thus, placement of the Palmaz-Schatz stent provided a wider lumen than did conventional balloon angioplasty and therefore reduced the incidence of restenosis in chronic total coronary arterial occlusion. The lower restenosis rate of coronary stenting would be beneficial for long-term clinical outcome in patients with chronic total occlusion.

Antiplatelet Versus Anticoagulant Therapy

Schömig and colleagues[214] in Munich, Germany, compared antiplatelet therapy with conventional anticoagulant therapy with respect to clinical outcome 30 days after coronary artery stenting by randomly assigning 257 patients after successful placement of Palmaz-Schatz coronary artery stents to receive antiplatelet therapy, including ticlopidine and aspirin (n = 257), and to receive anticoagulant therapy, with intravenous heparin, phenprocoumon, and aspirin (n = 260). The primary cardiac end point was a composite measure reflecting death from cardiac causes or the occurrence of myocardial infarction, CABG, or repeated PTCA. The primary noncardiac end point comprised death from noncardiac causes, cerebrovascular accident, severe hemorrhage, and peripheral vascular events. Among the patients assigned to antiplatelet therapy, 1.6% reached a primary cardiac end point, as did 6.2% of those assigned to anticoagulant therapy for a relative risk of 0.25, 95% confidence interval, 0.06 to 0.77. With antiplatelet therapy, there was an 82% lower risk of AMI than in the anticoagulant therapy group, and a 78% reduced need for repeated interventions. Occlusion of the stented vessel occurred in 0.8% of the antiplatelet therapy group and in 5.4% of the anticoagulant group. A primary noncardiac end point was reached by 1.2% of the antiplatelet-therapy group and 12% of the anticoagulant group. Hemorrhagic complications occurred only in the anticoagulant therapy group in 6.5% of patients. There was an 87% reduction in the risk of peripheral vascular events in patients treated with antiplatelet therapy. Thus, as compared with conventional anticoagulant therapy, combined antiplatelet therapy after the placement of coronary artery stents reduces the incidence of both cardiac events and hemorrhagic and vascular complications.

Without Anticoagulant Therapy (French Multicenter Registry)

Karrillon and colleagues[215] in Antony, France, evaluated the 1-month outcome of a prospective registry of 2900 patients in whom successful coronary artery stenting was performed without coumadin anticoagulation. Patients received 100 mg/day of aspirin and 250 mg/day ticlopidine for 1 month. Low molecular weight heparin treatment was progressively reduced in 4 consecutive stages, from 1 month treatment to none. Event-free outcome at 1 month was achieved in 2816 patients (97%). Major stent-related cardiac events were subacute closure in 51 patients (1.8%), including death in 12 (0.5%); acute MI in 17 (0.6%); and CABG in 9 (0.3%). Stent thrombosis was more frequent with balloon size of less than 3.0 mm, bail-out situations, and in patients with unstable angina or AMI (Table 2-16). Bleeding complications that required transfusion, surgical repair, or both occurred in 55 patients (1.9%). Bleeding complications were related to female gender (4% vs. 1.5%), duration of low molecular weight heparin treatment, sheath size, bail-out situations, and saphenous vein graft stenting (Table 2-17). Thus, these data suggest that treatment by ticlopidine/aspirin after stent placement is an effective alternative to coumadin anticoagulation, achieving a low rate of subacute closure and bleeding complications. Low molecular weight heparin treatment did not appear to improve subacute reocclusion rates but did increase bleeding complications.

Without Anticoagulant Therapy

Goods and colleagues[216] in Birmingham, Alabama, determined whether anticoagulation may be removed from the treatment of patients after coronary artery stent placement, thereby reducing comorbidity without increasing stent thrombosis. Between September 1994 and May 1995, 369 patients received balloon-expandable coil stents in native coronary arteries. Among these pa-

TABLE 2-16
Clinical and Procedural Univariate and Multivariate Predictors of Subacute Stented Artery Occlusion at 1 Month Follow-up

	Subacute Closure		Univariate Analysis		Multivariate Analysis	
	Percentage of Patients (n = 2900)	Complication Rate, %	Univariate P	Odds Ratio (CI)	Multivariate P	Adjusted Odds Ratio (CI)
Participating centers						
Nonexperiment	11.0	3.13	.07	2.01 (0.99–4.04)	.04	1.46 (1.03–2.08)
Experiment	89.0	1.59				
Age, Y						
>75	7.1	3.38	.10	2.11 (0.94–4.74)	.14	1.36 (0.90–2.06)
≤75	92.9	1.63				
Sex						
Female	15.5	2.22	.43	1.33 (0.32–1.59)		
Male	64.5	1.67				
Type of stent						
Palmaz-Schatz	81.9	1.81	.40	1.40 (0.63–3.12)		
Other	18.1	1.34				
Balloon size, mm						
≤2.5	3.5	10.0	<.001	10.30 (4.67–22.73)	<.001‡	
3.0	34.9	2.3		2.16 (1.17–4.00)	<.01§	3.22 (1.92–5.26)
≥3.5	61.6	1.0			f§.32§	1.22 (0.83–1.01)
No. of stents/patient*						
One	82.1	1.72	.85	0.89 (0.44–1.79)		
Multiple	17.9	1.93				
Sheath size†						
6F	43.3	1.48	.49	0.77 (0.38–1.56)		
7F	29.0	2.21		1.16 (0.57–2.38)		
≥8F	25.2	1.99				
Maximal final inflation pressure, atm						
≤8	4	4.92	.23		.42	
8–15	70.6	2.03				
>15	25.2	1.30				
Clinical presentation						
Unstable angina/acute MI	57.0	2.24	.02	2.02 (1.09–3.75)	.04	1.39 (1.02–1.90)
Stable angina/ elective/restenosis	43.0	1.12				
Reason for stenting						
Occlusive dissection	7.2	6.67	<.001	5.12 (2.72–9.63)	<.001	1.82 (1.02–2.54)
Other	92.0	1.38				
Vessel type						
Native artery	94.5	1.79	.60	1.4 (0.35–5.97)		
Graft	5.5	1.25				
Duration of LMWH therapy (phase)						
II-III	26.1	1.32	.27	0.68 (0.34–1.37)		
IV-V	73.9	1.91				

Factors not included in the multivariate model analysis ($p > .15$).

* For methodological reasons, patients with multiple various stent implantation procedures were excluded from this analysis.

† Data were not available for phase II.

‡ Compared with the third level.

§ Overall comparison.

Reproduced with permission from Karillon et al.[215]

TABLE 2-17
Clinical and Procedural Univariate and Multivariate Predictors of Local Bleeding Complications at 1-Month Follow-up

	Local Bleeding Complications		Univariate Analysis		Multivariate Analysis	
	Percentage of Patients (n = 2900)	Complication Rate, %	Univariate P	Odds Ratio (CI)	Multivariate P	Adjusted Odds Ratio (CI)
Participating centers						
Experiment	89.0	2.01	.15	2.17 (0.67–7.14)		
Nonexperiment	11.0	0.94				
Age, y						
>75	7.1	2.90	.31	1.61 (0.66–3.81)		
≤75	92.9	1.62				
Sex						
Female	15.5	4.00	.001	2.70 (1.53–4.76)	<.001	1.95 (1.40–2.72)
Male	84.5	1.51				
Type of stent						
Palmaz-Schatz	81.9	1.95	.52	1.28 (0.6–2.72)	.15	1.39 (0.89–2.18)
Other	16.1	1.53				
No. of stents/patient						
One	82.1	1.81	.46	0.78 (0.41–1.47)	.12	1.33 (0.92–1.94)
Multiple*	17.9	2.31				
Sheath size†						
≥6F	27.7	4.23	<.001	8.45 (3.49–20.26)	<.001‡	
7F	29.0	1.04		2.00 (0.69–5.80)	<.01§	3.13 (1.61–6.09)
8F	43.3	0.52			.90§	1.03 (0.58–1.87)
Clinical presentation						
Stable angina/elective/ restenosis	43.0	1.92	.93	1.02 (0.60–1.75)		
Unstable angina/acute MI	57.0	1.58				
Reason for stenting						
Occlusive dissection	7.2	4.76	.002	2.94 (1.46–5.92)	<.01	1.72 (1.18–2.49)
Other	92.6	1.67				
Vessel type						
Graft	5.5	4.38	.04	2.56 (1.14–5.88)		
Native artery	94.5	1.75				
Duration of LMWH therapy (phase)						
II-III	26.1	3.83	<.001	5.08 (2.39–10.75)	.12‡	
IV	34.0	1.72		2.23 (1.00–5.05)	.06§	1.55 (0.97–2.50)
V	39.9	0.69			.62§	1.12 (0.71–1.75)

Factors not included in the multivariate model analysis (P>.15).

* For methodological reasons, patients with multiple various stent implantation were excluded from this analysis.

† Data were not available for phase II.

‡ Overall comparison.

§ Compared with the third level.

Reproduced with permission from Karillon et al.[215]

tients, 216 were selected for a protocol of aspirin and ticlopidine for 1 month without anticoagulation. Eligibility for the protocol followed satisfaction of certain procedural and angiographic criteria, including adequate coverage of the intimal dissections, absence of residual filling defects, and normal TIMI grade 3 flow in the stented vessel after high-pressure balloon inflations. Intravascular ultrasound was not used to guide stent deployment. The stenting procedure was planned in 37% of patients and unplanned in 63% of them, including 25 (12%) for acute or threatened closure. During the 30-day follow-up period, 2 patients had stent thrombosis (0.9%), 1 patient died (0.5%), and 2 patients (0.9%) had CABG. Four patients had vascular access-site complications (2%), and 4 had bleeding that required blood transfusion (2%). These data suggest that patients who receive a coronary balloon expandable coil stent with optimal angiographic results without intravascular ultrasound guidance may be managed safely with a combination of aspirin and ticlopidine without anticoagulation.

Effect of Antithrombotic Therapy on Platelet Activation

Gawaz and colleagues[217] in München, Germany, evaluated the effects of 2 different antithrombotic regimens on platelet function after coronary Palmaz-Schatz stent implantation. The study group consisted of 46 low-risk patients who were treated with ticlopidine (250 mg twice a day) and aspirin (100 mg twice a day) after stenting. The control group was derived from a group of 151 patients receiving conventional anticoagulation therapy, including phenprocoumon, heparin, and aspirin after stenting. The following were criteria for matching: indication for stenting, target vessel, balloon size, inflation pressure, and number of inserted stents. Matches were obtained for 38 patients. Platelet function was evaluated before stenting and daily for 12 days after stenting in venous blood samples with immunologic activation markers. Those patients receiving anticoagulation therapy showed a significantly increased surface exposure of activated fibrinogen receptors and of P-selectin. In contrast, in patients receiving ticlopidine, expression of the activated fibrinogen receptor decreased and expression of P-selectin remained basically unchanged after stenting (Figure 2-108). Platelet count significantly decreased after stenting in patients treated by anticoagulation, but no significant changes were found in the ticlopidine group. Thus, significant platelet activation occurs in patients receiving anticoagulation therapy after stenting, while platelet deactivation is found in patients treated with combined antiplatelet therapy. Such therapy may lead to a reduction in the incidence of subacute stent thrombosis.

Aspirin Versus Aspirin and Ticlopidine

Hall and colleagues[218] in Milan, Italy, and Tokyo, Japan, evaluated the importance of specific antiplatelet agents when stenting is performed without any coagulation. After successful intravascular ultrasound guided stenting, 226 patients were randomly assigned to receive either aspirin therapy alone (n = 103) or a combination of ticlopidine and short-term aspirin therapy (n = 123). Primary angiographic and clinical end points were stent thrombosis, death, myocardial infarction, the need for postprocedure CABG or repeat PTCA and significant medication side effects requiring termination of the medication within the first month of a successful procedure. The data demonstrate that at 1 month, the rate of stent thrombosis was 2.9% in the aspirin-only group and

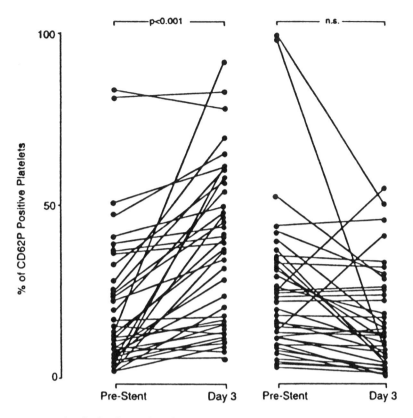

FIGURE 2-108. Individual values of surface expression of P-selectin (CD62P) before and day 3 after implantation of coronary stents. Left, patients receiving heparin, phenprocoumon, and aspirin; right, patients receiving ticlopidine and aspirin as antithrombotic therapy. Reproduced with permission from Gawaz et al.[217]

0.8% in the ticlopidine-aspirin group; these differences were not statistically different. Major clinical events after successful stenting occurred in 3.9% of the patients in the aspirin group and 0.8% in the ticlopidine-aspirin group. There were no medication side effects in the aspirin group. In the combined ticlopidine-aspirin group, medication side effects occurred in 3 patients. Therefore, there were no differences in the incidence of stent thrombosis or other clinical end points between the 2 post-stent antiplatelet regimens of aspirin alone as compared with aspirin and ticlopidine. The relatively small size of the study, however, and the low incidence of thrombotic events may have contributed to the failure to detect differences in end points between the groups.

Recent studies have demonstrated that antiplatelet therapy using a combination of aspirin and ticlopidine without anticoagulation after native coronary artery stenting is associated with a low incidence of stent thrombosis (<1%), as well as a low incidence of bleeding and vascular access complications. The use of this antiplatelet regimen is rapidly becoming standard practice. Ticlopidine, however, may cause significant adverse reactions, in particular, neutropenia. This makes extra physician and laboratory monitoring necessary and increases the cost of the procedure. Currently, it is not known whether anti-

TABLE 2-18
Patient Characteristics

	Aspirin + Ticlopidine (n = 338)	Aspirin (n = 46)	p Value
Age (yrs)	60 ± 11	63 ± 11	0.08
Male	246 (73)	27 (59)	0.07
Previous balloon angioplasty	128 (38)	16 (35)	0.8
Previous coronary bypass	56 (17)	7 (15)	0.9
Number narrowed coronary arteries			
1	108 (32)	19 (41)	
2	134 (40)	14 (31)	0.4
3	96 (28)	13 (28)	
Indication for coronary angioplasty			
Unstable angina	143 (42)	16 (35)	
Recent myocardial infarction	43 (13)	0 (0)	0.003
Stable angina	119 (35)	28 (61)	
Other	33 (10)	2 (4)	
Indication for Stenting			
Suboptimal result	156 (46)	8 (17)	
De novo	100 (30)	27 (59)	
Acute or threatened closure	33 (10)	1 (2)	<0.001
Restenosis	36 (10)	9 (20)	
Ostial lesion	12 (4)	1 (2)	

Reproduced with permission from Goods et al.[219]

platelet therapy with aspirin alone would be as effective as the combination of aspirin and ticlopidine in preventing stent thrombosis. Goods and associates[219] from Birmingham, Alabama, performed a prospective comparative study to determine whether aspirin alone would be as effective as aspirin and ticlopidine in preventing stent thrombosis after the stenting of native coronary arteries. The patients studied, the coronary anatomy, and the clinical outcome at 1-month clinical follow-up are shown in Tables 2-18–2-20. In this study the pa-

TABLE 2-19
Quantitative Data

	Aspirin + Ticlopidine	Aspirin	p Value
Number of coronary arteries	367	48	
Reference vessel size (mm)	2.9 ± 0.5	2.9 ± 0.5	1.0
Narrowing length (mm)	12 ± 7.3	10 ± 5.4	0.07
Diameter stenosis: Pre %	77 ± 13	72 ± 10	0.01
Post %	5 ± 11	7 ± 10	0.2
Lesion type*			
A	18 (5)	4 (8)	
B1	91 (25)	16 (33)	0.3
B2	198 (54)	23 (48)	
C	60 (16)	5 (11)	
Stents per vessel	1.4 ± 0.7	1.4 ± 0.8	1.0
Stent-to-vessel ratio	1.17 ± 0.17	1.17 ± 0.15	1.0
Maximum pressure, ATM	15 ± 2	15 ± 2	1.0

* Modified American Heart Association-American College of Cardiology criteria. ATM indicates atmospheres.
Data presented are mean ± SD or number (%) of lesions.
Reproduced with permission from Goods et al.[219]

TABLE 2-20
Clinical Outcome at 1-Month Clinical Follow-up

	Aspirin + Ticlopidine n = 338	Aspirin n = 46	p Value
Stent thrombosis	3 (0.9%)	3 (6.5%)	0.02
Deaths	1 (0.3%)	2 (4.4%)	0.04
Q-wave myocardial infarction	0 (0%)	3 (6.5%)	0.002
Non-Q-wave myocardial infarction	14 (4.1%)	0 (0%)	0.2
Vascular access complications	6 (1.8%)	0 (0%)	0.5
Hemorrhage	4 (1.2%)	1 (2.2%)	0.4

Reproduced with permission from Goods et al.[219]

tients treated with aspirin alone had a significantly worse outcome than those treated with a combination of aspirin and ticlopidine. This difference was evident despite the finding that the aspirin group was at a lower risk for stent thrombosis than was the group on combination therapy. The aspirin group was less likely to have an unstable ischemic syndrome as an indication for coronary balloon angioplasty and less likely to have acute or threatened closure as an indication for stenting. In summary, this prospective non-randomized study demonstrated an increased incidence of stents, thrombosis, Q-wave AMI, and cardiac death in a group of patients managed with aspirin alone compared with a group of patients managed with a combination of aspirin and ticlopidine following native coronary artery stenting.

For Ostial Lesions

De Cesare and associates[220] from Milan, Italy, evaluated acute and long-term clinical and angiographic results of elective Palmaz-Schatz coronary stent implantation for LAD coronary artery ostial stenosis in 23 consecutive patients. Eight patients had stable angina, 14 had unstable angina, and 1 had recent myocardial infarction. Sixteen patients had single-vessel, 5 had double-vessel, and 2 had triple-vessel disease. Clinical success without major complications (death, AMI, emergency CABG) was obtained in all cases, and technical success was obtained in 20 cases (87%). After stenting, minimal lumen diameter increased from 1.05 ± 0.45 mm to 2.89 ± 0.52 mm and percent diameter stenosis decreased from $65\% \pm 13\%$ to $2.94\% \pm 20\%$. There was 1 case of subacute thrombosis, and there were no major bleeding complications. Twenty patients were followed for 6 months, during which no acute cardiac event (death, AMI) was observed. Eighteen patients were eligible for follow-up coronary angiography; restenosis ($\geq 50\%$ diameter stenosis) was observed in 4 (11%). Minimal lumen diameter was 1.77 ± 0.55 mm, percent diameter stenosis was $40\% \pm 18\%$, late loss was 1.01 ± 0.69 mm, net gain was 0.79 ± 0.55 mm, and loss index (late loss/acute gain) was 0.53 ± 0.37. This study suggests that elective Palmaz-Schatz stent implantation may be a safe and successful treatment of LAD ostial lesions and provides a large increase in lumen diameter.

Heparin-Coated Stents

Serruys and investigators[221] in the BENESTENT-II Pilot Study evaluated the safety of delaying or eliminating anticoagulant therapy in patients receiving a heparin-coated stent in association with antiplatelet drugs (Figure 2-109). The study consisted of 3 initial phases (I, II, III) during which resumption of heparin therapy after sheath removal was deferred progressively by 6, 12, and 36 hours. In phase IV, coumadin and heparin were replaced by 250 mg ticlopidine and 100 mg aspirin. Of the 207 patients with stable angina and a de novo lesion in whom heparin-coated stent implantation was attempted, implantation was successful in 202 patients. Stent thrombosis did not occur during all 4 phases, and overall clinical success rate at discharge was 99%. Bleeding complications requiring blood transfusion or surgery fell from 7.9% in phase I to 5.9%, 4%, and 0% in the 3 following phases. Hospital stay was 7.4, 6.1, 7.2 and 3.1 days for the consecutive phases. The restenosis rate for the combined 4 phases was 13%, with 15% in phase I, 20% in phase II, 11% in phase III, and 6% in phase IV. The need for reintervention for the 4 phases was 8.9%. After 6 months, 84%, 75%, 94%, and 92% of the patients in phase I to IV were event free. Among the 4 phases, the event-free rate was 86%, which compares favorably with the rate of 80% observed in the earlier BENESTENT-I study. These data indicate that the implantation of stents coated with polyamine and

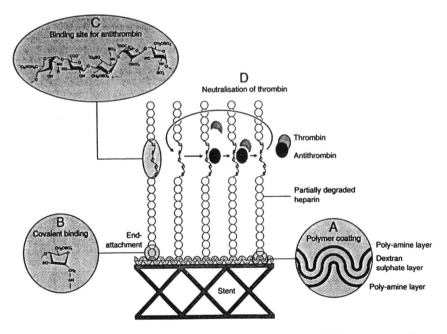

FIGURE 2-109. Schematic illustrations of the prominent features of a heparin-coated stent. **A,** The stent is coated with a polymer made of multiple layers of polyamine and dextran sulphate; **B,** deploymerized molecules of heparin are covalently bound to this polymer and the nature of the covalent binding is described; **C,** pentasaccharide constituting the binding site for antithrombin of each heparin molecule is depicted; and **D,** continuous neutralization cycle of thrombin is illustrated. Reproduced with permission from Serruys et al.[221]

end-point-attached heparin in stable patients with 1 significant de novo coronary lesion is well tolerated and is associated with no acute stent thrombosis and a favorable event-free survival after 6 months.

Nonheparin-Coated Stents

Intracoronary stenting has been shown to have better immediate and long-term clinical outcomes and less restenosis than standard balloon angioplasty. However, the benefit has been achieved at the cost of higher rates of coronary thrombosis, bleeding complications, the need for anticoagulation, and longer hospital stay. For the latter reasons, there is a tendency to replace the anticoagulants by antiplatelet agents alone after stenting. However, Lee and associates[222] from Hong Kong and Beijing, China, prospectively monitored 150 consecutive patients (133 men, 17 women; mean age 59 years) from 2 centers beginning in February 1993. They all had CAD and underwent percutaneous implantation of nonheparin-coated Palmaz-Schatz coronary stents under a full but lower dose of anticoagulation. The femoral approach was used in all patients except 1. In the 150 patients, 200 stents were implanted in 165 target arteries with 172 lesions. Stenting was performed without the guidance of intravascular ultrasonography; high-pressure poststenting inflation was used in only 17% of patients with less than optimal angiographic results. Coronary angiography was performed at baseline, immediately after the procedure, and after 6 months (mean 207 ± 54 days) of stenting. The mean coronary minimum luminal diameter increased from 0.52 mm to 3.13 ± 0.42 mm immediately after stenting was performed and was 2.12 ± 0.91 mm at 6 months. There was a 0% subacute thrombosis rate and a 0% femoral bleeding complication rate in the whole series. Only 3 (2%) major events occurred: 1 Q-wave AMI from closure of an angioplasty site distal to the stent on a very long lesion, 1 cerebrovascular accident, and 1 noncoronary-related death. The only patient who underwent the brachial approach had hematoma; otherwise, no other minor event occurred. The mean hospital stay was 4.5 days in 1 of the 2 study centers. The long-term clinical follow-up rate was 97%. The mean clinical follow-up period was 589 ± 363 days. Clinical symptoms improved; the percentage of patients who had angina according to the Canadian Cardiovascular society functional class II, III, and IV was 31%, 45%, and 4%, respectively, before stenting was performed and was reduced to 4.7%, 3.7%, and 0%, respectively, at 6-month follow-up after stenting. The 6-month angiographic restudy rate was 91%, and the restenosis rate was 18%. In contrast to other reported series, these results support the idea that with careful puncture technique and meticulous postoperative wound care, intracoronary stenting can be successfully performed with the patient under full anticoagulation without major risks of bleeding and femoral vascular complications. Furthermore with a full but comparatively lower dose of anticoagulation, subacute thrombotic complications can be reduced to 0% even with non-heparin-coated stents without the use of intravascular ultrasound guidance and without the use of adjunctive high-pressure poststenting inflation in most patients. The restenosis rate and long-term clinical outcomes remained very favorable.

Long-Term Outcome (In Vein Grafts)

Patients with stenosis of coronary artery bypass grafts pose a particular problem in the management of angina. de Jaegere and colleagues[223] from Rotterdam, The Netherlands, sought to determine the role of stent implantation in vein grafts by evaluating the long-term clinical outcome at 5 years in 62 patients and comparing this data with other treatment modalities. A total of 93 stents were implanted in 62 patients. During the in-hospital period, 11% sustained a major cardiac event with 3% deaths, 3% AMI, and 5% urgent CABG. The clinical success rate was 89%. During a median follow-up period of 2.5 years, 8% of patients died and 23% sustained an AMI. Twenty percent underwent CABG, and 23% underwent PTCA. The estimated 5-year survival and event-free survival rates were 83% and 30%. These authors observed an acceptable in-hospital outcome of patients who underwent stent implantation in a vein graft, but their long-term clinical outcome was poor. They concluded that it was unlikely that mechanical intervention alone would provide a satisfactory or definitive answer for patients with graft sclerosis over the long term.

Saphenous vein graft (SVG) disease remains a therapeutic conundrum. The use of stents after excluding the presence of thrombus has proved highly successful at short- and long-term follow-up. Ceceña and Hoelzinger[224] reported 60 severely symptomatic patients with multiple subtotal and total thrombotic SVG occlusions who were treated with a combination of intragraft urokinase-verapamil infusion and insertion of multiple biliary stents. The success rate for stent deployment was 100%. No case of clinical subacute thrombosis was registered, and major in-hospital complications were uncommon (<1%). The clinical outcome was encouraging, with a 12-month event-free survival rate of 87% in the 57 evaluable patients. This method of therapy appears to be highly successful in the treatment of thrombus-containing occlusive SVG disease, in preventing the "no-reflow" phenomenon, and in lessening the incidence of periprocedural non-Q-wave myocardial infarction.

Complications

Thrombosis remains a feared complication of stent procedures. Hasdai and colleagues[225] from Rochester, Minnesota, evaluated treatment of early intracoronary stent thrombosis. Twenty-nine patients with early (<30 days) coronary stent thrombosis over a 5-year period were identified, 23 patients were treated with catheter-based therapies, including PTCA alone and/or intracoronary urokinase. Of the 23 patients, 2 died despite restoration of anterograde flow, and 9 were referred for emergent or urgent CABG. Of the remaining 6 patients, 5 were treated medically and 1 with CABG; 3 died. Thus, severe adverse outcomes are associated with stent thrombosis. Although catheter-based therapies are effective in restoring patency in a majority of patients, patients are referred frequently for CABG. This emphasizes the need for alternative or adjunctive therapies for stent thrombosis.

In a study by Pan and associates[226] from Córdoba, Spain, and Las Palmas de Gran Canaria, Spain, 2 consecutive antithrombotic strategies after Palmaz-Schatz stent implantation were compared in 918 patients. Patients treated between May 1991 and May 1994 (group 1; n = 379) received aspirin, dipyridamole, and intravenous unfractionated heparin until oral anticoagulation was effective. Between June 1994 and August 1995, 539 patients (group 2) were treated for 1 month with subcutaneous low molecular weight heparin (Fragmin), ticlopidine, and aspirin. There were no differences between the groups in terms of sex, clinical condition, vessel diameter, and severity and location of stenosis. Patients in group 1 were younger than those in group 2. Group 1 patients had more frequent unplanned stenting (48% vs. 18%, respectively) and fewer endoprostheses in the same artery than did group 2 patients (1.1 ± 0.5 vs. 1.2 ± 0.5, respectively). Among group 2 patients, there was a significant reduction in thrombotic and hemorrhagic complications compared with group 1 patients. No subacute thrombosis occurred in patients in group 2 in contrast with a 5.8% incidence in patients in group 1. In addition, a lower incidence of groin and systemic bleeding was observed in patients in group 2 compared with patients in group 1 (2.6% vs. 15%). The association of low molecular weight heparin and antiplatelets provides a simpler antithrombotic strategy in patients treated with intracoronary stents and reduces the incidence of stent thrombosis and hemorrhagic complications. These findings suggest that this antithrombotic regimen may prevent or completely avoid stent thrombosis.

Restenosis within tubular slotted stents is secondary to intimal hyperplasia and is usually treated with PTCA. Mehran and associates[227] from Washington, D.C., used sequential intravascular ultrasound to assess the mechanisms and results of PTCA for in-stent stenosis. Sixty-four restenotic Palmaz-Schatz stents were studied by IVUS imaging before and after PTCA. Intravascular ultrasound measurements of stent and lumen cross-sectional areas at 5 segments (proximal and distal stent edges, proximal and distal stent bodies, and the central articulation) were used to calculate intimal hyperplasia cross-sectional area (stent-lumen cross-sectional area) The results of 5 segments were then averaged. Mean and minimum cross-sectional areas were compared before and after PTCA. Quantitative angiographic measurements showed a minimal lumen diameter increase from 1.05 ± 0.63 mm (mean ± 1 SD) before intervention to 2.77 ± 0.51 mm after PTCA. Conversely, the diameter stenosis decreased from 63% ± 19% to 18 ± 12%. IVUS measurements showed a minimum lumen CSA increase from 2.3 ± 1.3 mm^2 to 6.1 ± 2.2 mm^2 as a result of an increased minimum stent CSA (7.2 ± 2.4 mm^2 to 8.7 ± 2.6 mm^2) and a decreased intimal hyperplasia CSA within the stent (4.9 ± 2.2 mm^2 to 2.7 ± 2.0 mm^2). Of the total mean lumen enlargement, 56% ± 28% was the result of additional stent expansion and 44% ± 28% was the result of a decrease in neointimal tissue. The minimum lumen CSA after PTCA was significantly smaller than the minimum stent CSA before PTCA (presumably an accurate reflection of lumen dimensions immediately after stent implantation). The mechanism of PTCA for restenosis is a combination of additional stent expansion and tissue extrusion out of the stent; there is a relatively high residual stenosis (angiographic diameter stenosis of 18% ± 12%) (Figure 2-110).

Hoffmann and colleagues[228] used serial intravascular ultrasound after intervention and at follow-up in 142 stents in 115 lesions to evaluate restenosis within Palmaz-Schatz stents and to determine its mechanism. Intravascular

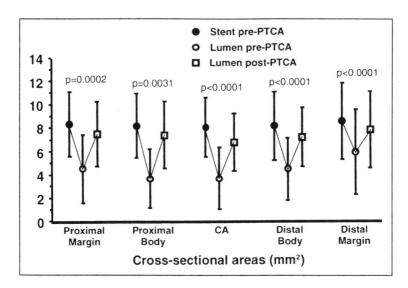

FIGURE 2-110. Because stent dimensions do not change over time, stent dimensions before (Pre) PTCA should reflect lumen dimensions at the time of stent implantation. The stent cross-sectional areas (CSAs, *solid circles*) before PTCA, the lumen CSAs (*open circles*) before PTCA, and the lumen CSAs (*open squares*) after (Post) PTCA are shown for each stent segment analyzed. This sequence is representative of the changes in lumen dimensions from immediately after the acute stent implantation procedure to the time of instent restenosis to after PTCA for the in-stent restenosis process. Within each of the 5 stent segments analyzed, lumen dimensions after PTCA were smaller than stent dimensions before PTCA. The p values compare the stent CSAs before PTCA with the lumen CSAs after PTCA. CA = central articulation. Reproduced with permission from Mehran et al.[227]

ultrasound measurements, stent, and luminal cross-sectional areas and diameters were measured, and plaque cross-sectional surface area, late lumen loss, remodeling, and tissue growth were calculated. After intervention, the lumen tended to be smallest at the articulation because of tissue prolapse. At follow-up, tissue growth was uniformly distributed throughout the stent. The tendency for greater neointimal tissue accumulation at the central articulation reached statistical significance only when normalized for the smaller postintervention lumen cross-sectional area. In stented segments, late lumen loss correlated strongly with tissue growth, but only weakly with remodeling. Stents affected adjacent vessel segments and remodeling progressively increased whereas tissue growth progressively decreased at distances from the edge of the stent. These findings were similar in native arteries and saphenous vein grafts and in lesions treated with 1 or 2 stents. There was no difference in the post-intervention or follow-up lumen when overlapped stents were compared with non-overlapped stents. Thus, these data suggest that late lumen loss and in-stent restenosis were the result of neointimal tissue proliferation that tended to be uniformly distributed over the length of the stent.

The introduction of coronary stents for the treatment of acute vessel closure has probably improved the safety of angioplasty, but little data are available regarding angioplasty complication rates when bailout stenting is available. Therefore, in a study conducted by Altmann and associates[229] from New

York, New York, baseline and patient outcome data for 2242 consecutive patients treated at a single tertiary referral center were compared before and after bailout coronary stenting was introduced. Patients treated after stents became available were more likely to have diabetes (16% pre-stent availability vs. 19% post-stent), unstable angina (61% pre-stent vs. 70% post-stent), and treatment with intravenous nitroglycerin before the procedure (22% pre-stent vs. 28% post-stent). Major complications occurred in 4.1% of patients before stent availability and in 2.0% afterwards. These complications included in hospital death (1.1% pre-stent vs. 0.7% post-stent), Q wave myocardial infarction (0.5% prestent vs. 0.3% post-stent), and emergency CABG (2.9% prestent vs. 1.1% post-stent). The introduction of coronary stents was associated with a more than 50% reduction in major complications despite greater patient acuity. The traditionally reported complication rates for angioplasty appear not to apply when bailout stenting is available.

Follow-Up

Kimura and colleagues[230] in Japan evaluated clinical and angiographic follow-up information for up to 3 years after the implantation of Palmaz-Schatz metallic coronary artery stents in 143 patients with 147 lesions of native coronary arteries. The rate of survival free of AMI, CABG, and repeat PTCA for stented lesions was 74.6% at 3 years. After 14 months, revascularization of the stented lesion was necessary in only 3 patients (2%). In contrast, PTCA for a new lesion was required in 11 patients (7.7%). Follow-up coronary angiography of 137 lesions at 6 months, 114 lesions at 1 year, and 72 lesions at 3 years revealed a decrease in minimal luminal diameter from 2.54 ± 0.44 mm immediately after stent implantation to 1.87 ± 0.56 mm at 6 months, but no further decrease in diameter at 1 year. Significant late improvement in luminal diameter was observed at 3 years in patients with paired angiograms: 1.94 ± 0.48 mm at 6 months, and 2.09 ± 0.48 mm at 3 years, p<0.001. Thus, these data suggest that coronary artery stenting is followed by favorable outcomes, with a low rate of revascularization of the stented lesions during a 3-year period of follow-up. Late improvement in luminal diameter appears to occur between 6 months and 3 years in at least some patients.

Using stents is an effective strategy in the treatment of native CAD and saphenous vein bypass graft disease. The STRESS and BENESTENT trials have demonstrated a decrease in both angiographic restenosis and the need for repeat revascularization in the first year for vessels treated by stenting rather than balloon angioplasty. Laham and colleagues[231] from Boston, Massachusetts, evaluated the longer-term outcome of stent placement by following 175 consecutive patients who underwent elective placement of 194 Palmaz-Schatz stents in 185 vessels. Clinical events (death, myocardial infarction, recurrent angina, or any revascularization) were assessed at 6 weeks; 2, 4, and 6 months; 1 year and yearly thereafter. Clinical follow-up was available on all patients for a mean of 54 months. Initial angiographic success was achieved in 98.9%, angiographic restenosis was observed at 6 months in 26.1% of target sites. The survival rate was 86.7% at 5 years with a 5-year event-free survival rate decreasing progressively to 50.7%, reflecting primarily repeat revascularization procedures (41.2% at 5 years). However, the rate of repeat revascularization of the treatment site was 14.4%, 17.7%, and 19.8% at 1, 3 and 5 years, respectively. For patients who underwent saphenous vein graft stenting vs. those with native coronary artery stenting, rates of both 5-year survival (70.5% vs. 93.4%) and event-free survival (21% vs. 63%) were lower. These authors concluded that the long-term outcome of stenting, shows stability of the treated lesion, with only a slight increase in treatment site revascularization between 2 and 5 years (17.1% to 19.8%). The progressive increase in repeat revascularization over that period (24% to 41%) and most ongoing late events can be attributed to the progression of coronary disease at other sites, rather than to late deterioration of the stent result itself. These data provide continuing assurance that the good short-term results of the stents will, in fact, be repeated in the long term.

Reperfusion Outcomes/Injury

Outcome in Nonsmokers Versus Smokers

Bowers and associates[232] for the TAMI Investigators analyzed 399 patients randomized into the primary angioplasty in myocardial infarction PAMI trial to receive tPA or to undergo primary PTCA for AMI. Of these, 168 were current smokers, and 128 had never smoked. Univariate analyses of baseline characteristics and outcome, including death, recurrent AMI, and recurrent ischemia, were done by chi-square analysis. Multivariate stratified analysis was then performed controlling for age and gender, which were found to be confounders of outcome. The combined in-hospital outcomes of death, recurrent AMI, and recurrent ischemia were similar for smokers and nonsmokers. When stratified according to treatment modality, nonsmokers treated with PTCA had a lower frequency of death and nonfatal recurrent AMI (7% vs. 18%), in-hospital ischemia (11% vs. 33%), or the combined event (13% vs. 40%). At 6 months, nonsmokers treated with PTCA continued to have a lower incidence of death or nonfatal recurrent AMI (11% vs. 24%) compared with those receiving tPA. Conversely, in smokers, the treatment strategy did not significantly affect hospital outcomes: recurrent ischemia (12% vs. 23%), death and recurrent AMI (6% vs. 8%), or the combined event (15% vs. 25%). The statistical significance of these associations was maintained when multivariate analysis controlling for age and gender was used. Thus, nonsmokers presenting with AMI had a significantly better outcome when treated with primary angioplasty; these differences were not seen in smokers (Figures 2-111–2-113).

Free Radical Scavengers

Early reperfusion after myocardial infarction improves survival rate and is thought to preserve myocardial function, but the reperfusion of ischemic

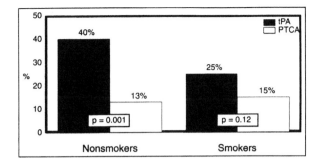

FIGURE 2-111. In-hospital clinical outcomes (death, recurrent myocardial infarction, or recurrent ischemia) stratified according to treatment status in the nonsmokers and smokers. Reproduced with permission from Bowers et al.[232]

tissue may release oxygen free radicals, which could adversely affect left ventricular function and diminish the beneficial effects of reperfusion. Measurements related to free radical scavenging (plasma and erythrocyte enzyme systems, which are involved in free radical control, α-tocopherol, selenium, and manganese superoxide dismutase) may be indirect markers of free radical production. Lafont and colleagues[233] from Paris, France; Cleveland, Ohio; and Sioux Falls, South Dakota, evaluated 10 patients undergoing PTCA within 4 hours of AMI to measure the impact of abrupt reperfusion on free radical

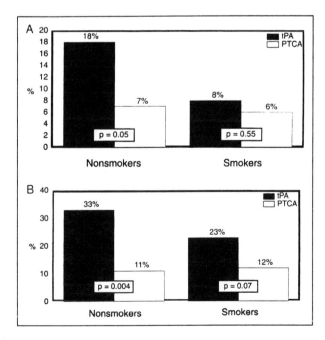

FIGURE 2-112. In-hospital clinical outcomes divided into subgroups of death and recurrent acute myocardial infarction (the 2 primary end points of the Primary Angioplasty in Myocardial Infarction trial) **(A)** and recurrent ischemia **(B)** stratified according to treatment status in nonsmokers and smokers. Reproduced with permission from Bowers et al.[232]

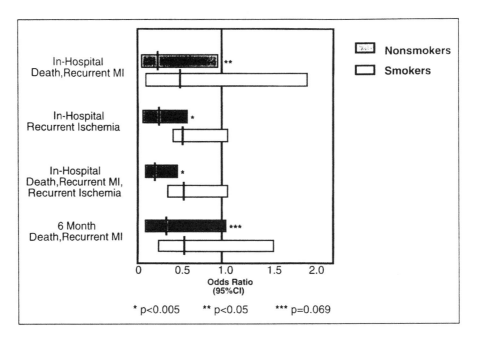

FIGURE 2-113. Effect of the reperfusion modality (PTCA vs. tPA) on outcome after controlling for age and gender, found to be confounders of outcome. *Vertical lines* represent the odds ratio; *horizontal bars* depict 95% confidence intervals (CI). Angioplasty resulted in a significant decrease in events in nonsmokers, but did not affect the outcome in smokers. MI = myocardial infarction. Reproduced with permission from Bowers et al.[232]

scavenger-related indexes. Pulmonary artery samples were taken before, immediately after, and 3 hours after PTCA. During reperfusion, significant reductions occurred in α-tocopherol (1.1 $\pm$ 0.3 mg/dL before, 0.9 $\pm$ 0.2 mg/dL immediately after, and 0.8 $\pm$ 0.2 mg/dL 3 hours after PTCA, and selenium levels (14 $\pm$ 2.4 μg/dL before, 13 $\pm$ 2.4 μg/dL $\pm$ 2.4 μg/dL immediately after, and 10 $\pm$ 3.0 μg/dL 3 hours after PTCA). Erythrocyte markers (glutathione peroxidase and superoxide dismutase) were not altered by reperfusion, possibly reflecting the relatively long half-life of the erythrocyte. The erythrocyte glutathione peroxidase value before reperfusion in patients (31 $\pm$ 5.1 IU/gm of hemoglobin) was lower than in a control group (36 $\pm$ 6.5 IU/gm of hemoglobin). Thus, the decrease in plasma α-tocopherol and selenium after reperfusion in this group of patients may reflect a general alteration in plasma free radical scavenger levels, suggesting consumption of plasma free radical scavengers with reperfusion after AMI.

In nonhuman animals, oxygen-derived free radicals have been found to be important mediators of reperfusion injury to ischemic but viable myocardium. In humans, there is no direct evidence of free radical production after the restoration of coronary artery patency in AMI. Grech and associates[234] from Manchester, United Kingdom, quantitated and assessed the time course of free radical production in coronary venous outflow in patients with AMI undergoing successful recanalization of the infarct-related artery by primary PTCA. Primary PTCA was performed in 17 patients with AMI of less than 6 hours duration. Direct free radical production was assessed by coronary venous effluent blood sampling before PTCA and at timed intervals up to 24 hours (or 48 hours in 6 patients) after recanalization. All samples were added to the spin trapping agent α-phenyl N-tert butyl nitrone and analyzed by electron paramagnetic resonance spectroscopy. Vessel patency resulted in a sharp increase in free radical signal. Relative to the level before PTCA, the changes reached statistical significance after only 15 minutes. Peak signals were observed between 1½ and 3½ hours, then declined up to 5 hours. A second increase in signal level was detected between 18 and 24 hours despite no angiographic evidence of reocclusion. A gradual decline was observed after 24 hours. These findings provide the first direct and quantitative evidence of free radical production in the immediate postrecanalization phase after thrombotic occlusion of a major coronary artery in humans.

Temporal Changes in Regional End-Diastolic Wall Thickness

Oh and associates[235] from Osaka, Japan, investigated early temporal changes in end-diastolic wall thickness of the infarcted myocardium in relation to myocardial viability in 46 patients with reperfused anterior AMI. Two-dimensional echocardiography was performed on days 1 and 2 of AMI, and the end-diastolic wall thickness of the anterior segment was measured in the short-axis view. Patients were divided into 3 groups on the basis of day 1 to day 2 ratio of end-diastolic wall thickness: the ratio ≤0.85 as group A (n = 13), greater than 0.85 but 1.15 or less as group B (n = 23), and greater than 1.15 as group C (n = 10). LV functional improvement was significantly better in group B than in groups A and C. Substantial size of "no reflow" phenomenon was observed only in groups A (n = 9, 69%) and C (n = 6, 60%). The frequency of transient ST re-elevation after reperfusion was the highest in group C (70%), and left ventricular expansion was observed at day 2 only in group A. It was concluded that changes in the end-diastolic wall thickness of the infarct segment early after reperfusion, either decreases or increases, are related to irreversibly damaged myocardium. A decrease in end-diastolic wall thickness and concomitant ventricular expansion may be related to impaired myocardial perfusion. An increase in end-diastolic wall thickness after reperfusion may be caused by accelerated myocardial and microvascular damage after reperfusion.

No-Reflow Phenomenon

The no-reflow phenomenon is observed as reduction of coronary blood flow on angiograms (angiographic no-reflow) after immediate PTCA in patients with AMI. To assess whether a potent coronary microvascular dilator—papaverine—could attenuate the no-reflow phenomenon, 9 patients with AMI who were found to have angiographic no-reflow after PTCA were studied by Ishihara and associates[136] from Hiroshima, Japan. Angiographic no-reflow was defined as TIMI flow grade 1 or 2 without any mechanical obstructions in the epicardial artery. A bolus dose of 10 mg of intracoronary papaverine was administered, and the flow grade was again evaluated. Intracoronary papaverine caused a significant improvement of the flow grade. The number of cineframes that were required for the contrast medium to pass 2 selected landmarks on the angiograms also significantly decreased (41 $\pm$ 17 frames to 18 $\pm$ 8 frames). Thus, intracoronary papaverine attenuated angiographic no-reflow that occurred after PTCA for AMI.

Low-Osmolar Ionic Contrast Media to Reduce Ischemic Complications

Retrospective observations have suggested an increased risk of thrombosis with the use of nonionic contrast media. Grines and colleagues[237] from Royal Oak, Michigan, sought to prospectively determine whether angiographic or clinical outcomes in patients with unstable ischemic syndromes undergoing PTCA are altered by these differences in anticoagulant and antiplatelet effects of ionic and nonionic contrast media. A total of 211 patients with AMI or unstable angina undergoing PTCA were randomized to receive nonionic or ionic low osmolar contrast media. Patients receiving ionic media were significantly less likely to experience decreased blood flow during the procedure (8.1% vs. 17.8%). After PTCA, residual stenosis, vessel patency, the incidence of moderate-to-large thrombi and use of adjunctive thrombolytic therapy were similar between the 2 groups. However, patients receiving ionic media had fewer recurrent ischemic events requiring repeat catheterization (3% vs. 11.4%) and repeat PTCA during the initial hospital stay (1% vs. 5.8%). These authors concluded that in patients with unstable ischemic syndromes undergoing PTCA, the use of ionic low osmolar contrast media reduces the risk of ischemic complications acutely (1 month) after the procedure.

Platelet Function in AMI Treated with Direct Angioplasty

Gawaz and colleagues[238] München, Germany, evaluated platelet function in 15 patients with anterior AMI who were treated by direct PTCA. Peripheral venous blood samples were obtained before and 4, 8, 24, and 48 hours after recanalization of the occluded artery by PTCA. Fifteen patients who had stable CAD and were undergoing elective PTCA served as controls. Fibrinogen receptor function and surface expression of P-selectin on platelets were determined by flow cytometry. The authors evaluated the generation of platelet-derived microparticles and the effect of systemic plasma from patients with AMI on normal platelet function and on platelet adhesion to human endothelial cells in culture. Fibrinogen receptor activity and P-selectin expression on circulating platelets 8 hours after direct PTCA were decreased (Figure 2-114). This coincided with a decrease in peripheral platelet count and an increase in the generation of microparticles. Twenty-four to 48 hours after PTCA, fibrinogen receptor activity and P-selectin expression increased. Systemic plasma obtained before and after direct PTCA sensitized normal platelets to hyperaggregate *in vitro*

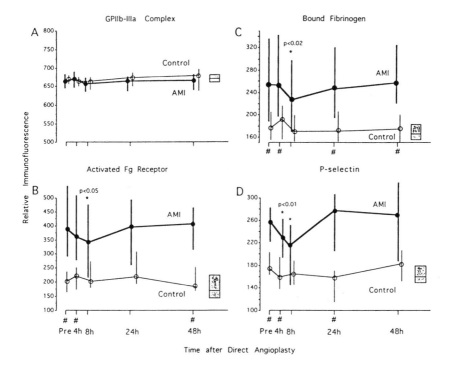

FIGURE 2-114. Plots of time course of platelet surface markers after direct angioplasty showing surface expression of GPIIb-IIIa **(A)** P-selectin **(B)** bound fibrinogen **(C)** and activated fibrinogen receptor **(D)** on circulating platelets in AMI patients (n = 15) before and after (4,8,24, and 48 hours) successful recanalization of the infarct-related vessel (●). Patients undergoing elective angioplasty (n = 15) served as controls (○). * and # indicate significance compared with time before angioplasty (*) and compared with control group (#). Shaded boxes indicate median (quartiles) of relative immunofluorescence of normal individuals (n = 20). Circles indicate median values; horizontal lines, quartiles. Reproduced with permission from Gawaz et al.[238]

and stimulated platelet adhesion to endothelial cells in culture. None of the changes found in patients with AMI were obvious in the control individuals. Thus, after transient deactivation of circulating platelets, possibly caused by sequestration of hyperactive platelets, platelet activation increased in patients with AMI treated by PTCA. These data emphasize the need for effective antiplatelet strategies in patients with AMI.

Influence of Infarct-Related Artery Patency on Survival

Infarct-related artery patency improves late survival, perhaps by its effects on LV function in reducing remodeling. Brodie and colleagues[239] from Greensboro, North Carolina, evaluated the importance of late infarct-related artery patency for recovery of left ventricular function and late survival after primary angioplasty for acute myocardial infarction. They followed 576 hospital survivors of AMI treated with PTCA for 5.3 years. Patients with patent arteries had more improvement and a better late EF than did patients with occluded arteries

(56.3% vs. 47.9%). In patients with acute EF less than 45%, late survival was better than in those with patent vs. occluded arteries (89% vs. 44%). These authors concluded that infarct-related artery patency is important for recovery of left ventricular function and in patients with an acute EF less than 45% is important for late survival.

Early Coronary Patency Grades: Relation to Mortality

Coronary patency has been used as a measure of thrombolysis success after AMI. The TIMI study grading scale for coronary perfusion has gained wide acceptance, but the significance of individual grades on clinical outcome has not been adequately tested. Anderson and associates[240] hypothesized that optimal outcomes would be achieved only with early (and maintained) TIMI grade 3 (complete) perfusion compared with TIMI grade 2 (partial perfusion, previously classified as a reperfusion success) or grades 0 or 1 (occluded arteries). Five recent, angiographically controlled, prospectively performed studies of thrombolysis in AMI were identified, representing 3969 patients. Odds ratios for mortality by early perfusion grades were calculated, using the Mantel-Haenszel test, and combined in a weighted fashion. Results for selected clinical and laboratory outcomes by patency grade were also assessed. Overall, mortality averaged 8.8% for TIMI grade 0/1; 7.0% for grade 2; and 3.7% for grade 3 perfusion. The odds ratio for early mortality was substantially reduced for grade 3 vs. <3 perfusion (odds ratio = 0.45). In pairwise comparisons, grade 3 was clearly superior to grade 2 (odds ratio = 0.54) as well as grades 0/1 (odds ratio = 0.41). Acute and convalescent ejection fraction, regional wall motion, time to enzyme peaks (creatine kinase [CK], creatine kinase myocardial bond [CK-MB], peak enzyme levels (CK, lactate dehydrogenase [LDH], LDH-1), and risk of heart failure were each significantly less in patients achieving grade 3 than grade 2 (or lower grades) perfusion. Results were observed despite the frequent use of interventions after angiography. This meta-analysis demonstrates that early and complete (grade 3) flow is associated with superior survival and clinical outcome; grade 2 perfusion results in an inferior outcome, closer to that of an occluded than an open artery. The goal of reperfusion strategies should be early and maintained TIMI grade 3 perfusion (Figures 2-115–117).

Influence of AMI Location on Outcome

In the Primary Angioplasty in Myocardial Infarction (PAMI) trial, 395 patients with AMI were prospectively randomized by Stone and associates[241] from Royal Oak, Michigan, to tPA or primary PTCA. In 138 patients with anterior wall AMI, in-hospital mortality was significantly reduced by treatment with PTCA compared with tPA (1.4% vs. 11.9%). PTCA also resulted in lower rates of death or reinfarction (1.4% vs. 18.0%), recurrent myocardial ischemia (11.3% vs. 28.4%), and stroke (0.0% vs. 6.0%) in anterior wall AMI. The independent beneficial effect of treatment with primary PTCA rather than tPA in

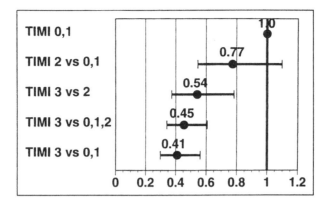

FIGURE 2-115. Odds ratios by meta-analysis (Mantel-Haenszel) for short-term mortality (<30 days) by early angiographic perfusion grade for the meta-analysis of 5 studies, expressed as point estimate of risk together with 95% confidence intervals. TIMI = Thrombolysis in Myocardial Infarction trial. Reproduced with permission from Anderson et al.[240]

anterior wall AMI was confirmed by multivariate analysis and interaction testing. The in-hospital mortality of 257 patients with nonanterior wall AMI was similar after PTCA and tPA (3.2% vs. 3.8%). Compared with tPA, however, primary PTCA resulted in a markedly lower rate of recurrent myocardial ischemia (9.7% vs. 27.8%), fewer unscheduled catheterization and revascularization procedures, and a shorter hospital stay (7.0 vs. 8.6 days) in nonanterior wall AMI. Thus, compared with tPA, primary PTCA in patients with anterior

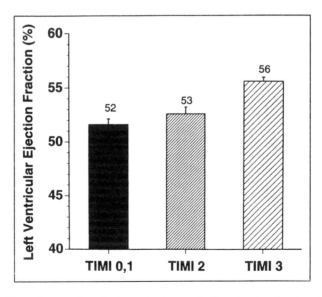

FIGURE 2-116. Convalescent (predischarge) left ventricular ejection fraction by early angiographic perfusion grade: overview of 3 studies. Results shown as approximate overall mean ejection fraction in percentage points ± SEM. TIMI = Thrombolysis in Myocardial Infarction trial. Reproduced with permission from Anderson et al.[240]

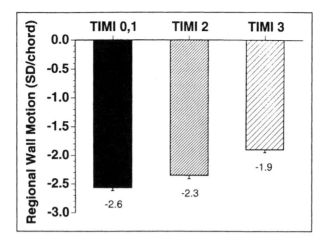

FIGURE 2-117. Convalescent (predischarge) regional wall motion by early angiographic perfusion grade: overview of 2 studies. Results given as approximate overall mean SD (from normal) per chord ± SEM. TIMI = Thrombolysis in Myocardial Infarction trial. Reproduced with permission from Anderson et al.[240]

wall AMI results in significantly improved survival with lower rates of stroke, reinfarction, and recurrent myocardial ischemia. In nonanterior wall AMI, treatment with PTCA and tPA results in similar early mortality, although PTCA-treated patients have a more stable hospital course characterized by reduced recurrent ischemia, fewer subsequent invasive procedures, and earlier discharge (Figures 2-118–2-120).

Superoxide Dismutase as a Predictor of Reperfusion

Tomoda and associates[242] from Kanagawa, Japan, attempted to predict successful myocardial reperfusion and salvage in AMI by using measurements of plasma superoxide dismutase, a plasma free-radical scavenger. Forty-nine patients with AMI were studied within 6 hours of symptoms onset. In group 1 (n = 26), primary PTCA was undertaken, and plasma superoxide dismutase activity was measured for 8 hours by the nitrite method. Left ventricular angiography was assessed before and 3 months after PTCA by computer left ventricular contraction analysis. In group 2 (n = 23), tissue-type plasminogen activator was infused intravenously over a 60-minute period, and plasma superoxide dismutase activity was measured before and after tissue-type plasminogen activator infusion. In group 1, occluded coronary arteries were successfully dilated in 24 of 26 patients, and plasma superoxide dismutase activity increased from 3.20 ± 0.17 UL/mL to 4.66 ± 0.29 UL/mL at 1 hour after PTCA, returning to the basal level by 8 hours after PTCA. Plasma superoxide dismutase activity did not significantly change in patients with unsuccessful PTCA or in those with the no-reflow phenomenon. The maximal increase in plasma superoxide dismutase activity was significantly correlated with the grade of improvement

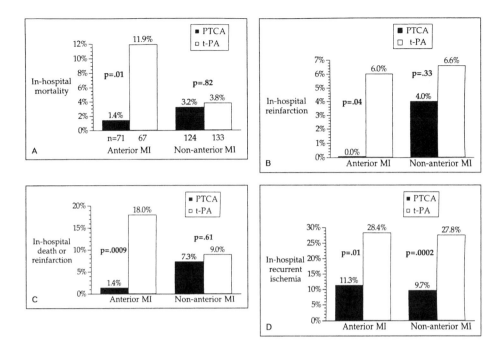

FIGURE 2-118. Effect of reperfusion modality on in-hospital outcome stratified by infarct location. **(A)** Mortality. **(B)** Nonfatal reinfarction. **(C)** Death or reinfarction. **(D)** Recurrent ischemia. MI = myocardial infarction; PTCA = percutaneous transluminal coronary angioplasty. Reproduced with permission from Stone et al.[241]

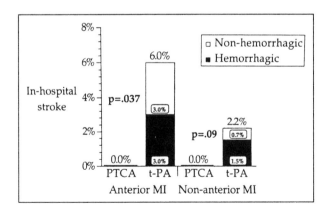

FIGURE 2-119. Effect of reperfusion modality on in-hospital stroke stratified by infarct location. Reproduced with permission from Stone et al.[241]

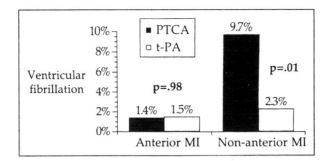

FIGURE 2-120. Effect of reperfusion modality on the development of ventricular fibrillation after study entry stratified by infarct location. Reproduced with permission from Stone et al.[241]

in left ventricular contraction. In group 2, the sensitivity and specificity of predicting coronary recanalization was 86% and 89%. In conclusion, myocardial reperfusion and salvage in AMI can be predicted by changes in plasma superoxide dismutase activity.

Correlation of Regional Wall Motion Abnormalities and Perfusion Defects

In this study by Oh and associates[243] from Rochester, Minnesota, 20 patients (13 men and 7 women; mean age 61 ± 12 years) with more than 30 minutes of chest pain and new ST-segment elevation who were treated with reperfusion therapy underwent technetium-99m sestamibi imaging and 2-dimensional echocardiography simultaneously before and within 2 hours of each test after acute reperfusion therapy. Nine patients had anterior wall myocardial infarction. Fifteen patients were initially treated with intravenous thrombolytic agents, and 5 patients underwent urgent PTCA. Both myocardial perfusion defect and wall motion score index improved after reperfusion therapy (perfusion defect from 28% to 15%, wall motion score index from 1.68 to 1.45, respectively). The overall correlation between wall motion score index and perfusion defect as a measure of myocardium at risk was significant during the acute phase and at hospital dismissal. Thus myocardial perfusion defect and wall motion abnormalities correlated fairly well in patients with AMI during the acute phase and a predismissal study.

Coronary Angioplasty Versus Coronary Artery Bypass

Several trials have compared the revascularization techniques of PTCA and CABG. One of the important questions that has arisen from these trials is whether the results can be generalized to the population of patients at large in the United States: that is, are patients who are routinely undergoing these procedures similar to patients who have been entered into large trials? The

BARI trial is a multicenter investigation comparing initial revascularization with PTCA and CABG in patients with symptomatic multivessel CAD. Detre and colleagues[244] from Pittsburgh, Pennsylvania; Boston, Massachusetts; and Rochester, Minnesota, assessed the potential of the BARI trial by surveying 75 United States hospitals offering PTCA and CABG as compared with all BARI hospitals. At both United States and BARI hospitals, 57% of all revascularization procedures were PTCA and 43% were CABG. The United States hospitals had more patients with single-vessel disease, AMI, and primary procedures. Older patients were more likely and younger patients less likely to undergo CABG in BARI vs. United States hospitals. The majority of revascularization procedures were PTCA for single-vessel disease (United States 32% vs. BARI 25%) and CABG for triple-vessel disease (United States 31% vs. BARI 31%). Overall, the choice between CABG and PTCA was similar in BARI and United States hospitals. The BARI protocol would have excluded 65% of all candidates for revascularization, for whom indications already exist for PTCA or CABG and another 23% for whom PTCA would be contraindicated for individual lesions. These authors concluded that patients undergoing coronary revascularization in BARI and United States hospitals were generally similar as was the choice between types of revascularization.

The BARI Investigation randomly assigned 1829 patients to PTCA or CABG. Clinical site angiographers categorized lesions of 50% or greater diameter stenosis (n=4977) as clinically significant (86.4%) or nonsignificant (13.6%), and as favorable or nonfavorable for PTCA or CABG. The results of this analysis were described by Botas and colleagues[245] for the BARI Investigators. More narrowings were considered favorable for revascularization by CABG than by PTCA (91.5% vs. 78.5%), particularly in the subgroup of 99% to 100% lesions (77.6% for CABG vs. 21.9% for PTCA). Lesion features, characterized by the BARI core laboratory, were correlated with clinical site angiographers' assessment of clinical importance and suitability for PTCA or CABG. By multivariate analysis, positive predictors of clinical importance for 50% to 95% stenoses were greater stenosis severity, more jeopardized myocardium, larger reference diameter, and proximal vessel location. For 99% to 100% occlusions, predictors were shorter duration of occlusion and more jeopardized myocardium. PTCA suitability for 50% to 95% stenoses was inversely related to lesion length, ostial location, locations on a bend, difficult access, and age, and was directly associated with greater TIMI flow rate and more jeopardized myocardium. Predictors of PTCA suitability for 99% to 100% lesions were a lower American College of Cardiology/American Heart Association class and higher TIMI grade. Predictors for 50% to 95% stenoses were more jeopardized myocardium, larger reference diameter, and more proximal vessel location, and for 99% to 100% occlusions, more jeopardized myocardium and shorter duration of occlusion. Suitability for PTCA depended on lesion patency (<99%) and multiple morphologic characteristics that contrasted with the few angiographic features that adversely affect CABG suitability.

Zhao and colleagues[246] from Seattle, Washington, and Atlanta, Georgia, for the Emory Angioplasty Versus Surgery Trial (EAST) investigators determined whether PTCA is as effective as CABG in restoring arterial perfusion capacity in eligible patients with multivessel CAD. Among 392 patients in the EAST study, 198 were randomly assigned to PTCA and 194 to CABG. Index lesions were those with 50% or greater stenosis judged treatable by both PTCA and CABG. Coronary segments jeopardized by these lesions were designated as index segments, and there were 4 ± 1.4 per patient. Percent stenosis was measured by quantitative angiography at the point of greatest obstruction in the main perfusion path of each index segment. The EAST primary arteriographic end point was the percent of the patient's index segments with less than 50% stenosis in the main perfusion pathways at 1 and 3 years. At baseline, the percent of index segments for which revascularization was attempted was 85% for PTCA and 98% for CABG. At 1 year, PTCA patients had a smaller percentage of successfully revascularized index segments than did CABG patients (59% vs. 88%) (Figure 2-121). At 3 years, the findings were similar, but less striking (70% vs. 87%). When only high-priority index segments were considered, baseline attempts were comparable, but CABG remained more successful at 1 and 3 years. However, the mean percent of index segments free of severe stenosis of 70% or greater did not differ between PTCA and CABG at 3 years (93% vs. 95%). In addition, the frequency of patients with all index seg-

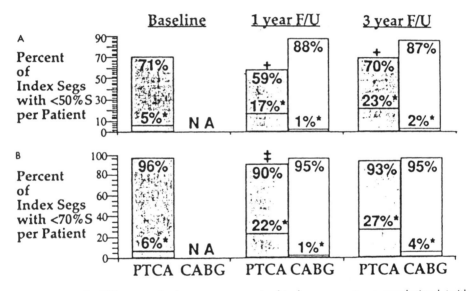

FIGURE 2-121. **A,** Differences in the mean percent of index segments revascularized (with percent stenosis [S] <50%) between PTCA and CABG at the protocol time points. The mean percentage of index segments revascularized with QCA measurements was 71% for PTCA (the previously published 75% was determined with digital caliper measurements performed at Emory University Hospital) for PTCA and not assessed (NA) for CABG at baseline after the procedure. From operative reports, 99% of index segments were initially bypassed. Revascularization averaged 59% for PTCA vs. 88% for CABG at 1 year (p<.001), and 70% for PTCA vs. 87% for CABG at 3 years (p<.001). *Mean percent of index segments successfully revascularized through additional procedures. **B,** Differences in the mean percent of index segments free of severe stenosis (≥70%) between PTCA and CABG at the protocol time points. At baseline after the procedure, the mean percent of index segments free of severe stenosis was 96% for PTCA and not assessed (NA) for CABG. It was 90% for PTCA vs. 95% for CABG at 1 year (p<.05) and 93% for PTCA vs. 95% for CABG at 3 years (p=NS). *Mean percent of index segments free of severe stenosis as a result of additional procedures. F/U indicates follow-up. †p<.001, ‡p<.05 vs. CABG group by t test. Reproduced with permission from Zhao et al.[246]

ments free of severe stenosis did not differ between the 2 groups at 1 (76% vs. 83%) or 3 (82% for both PTCA and CABG) years. Thus, in the EAST study, in patients with multivessel CAD, index segment revascularization was more complete with CABG than with PTCA at both 1 and 3 years. However, when physiological priority of the target lesion and the measured severity of the residual stenosis are taken into account, the advantage of CABG becomes less significant. These same investigators had reported earlier that PTCA and CABG-treated patients did not differ with regard to the EAST primary clinical end points over 3 years.

The BARI[247] Investigators tested the hypothesis that in selected patients with multivessel CAD suitable for treatment with either procedure, an initial strategy of PTCA does not result in a poorer 5-year clinical outcome than CABG. Patients with multivessel CAD were randomly assigned to an initial treatment strategy of CABG (n = 914) or PTCA (n = 915) and were followed for an average of 5.4 years. Analysis of outcome events was performed according to the intention to treat. The respective in-hospital event rates for CABG and PTCA were 1.3% and 1.1% for mortality, 4.6% and 2.1% for Q-wave AMI (p<.01), and 0.8% and 0.2% for stroke. The 5-year survival rate was 89% for those assigned to CABG and 86% for those assigned to PTCA (p = NS). The respective 5-year survival rates free from Q-wave AMI were 80% and 79%. By 5 years after study entry, 8% of the patients assigned to CABG had undergone additional revascularization procedures, as compared with 54% of those assigned to PTCA. Sixty-nine percent of those assigned to PTCA originally did not subsequently undergo CABG. Among diabetic patients who were being treated with insulin or oral hypoglycemic agents at baseline, a subgroup not specified by the protocol, 5-year survival was 81% for the CABG group as compared with 66% for the PTCA group (p = .003). These data indicate that as compared with CABG, an initial strategy of PTCA did not significantly compromise 5-year survival in patients with multivessel CAD, although subsequent revascularization was more often necessary with this strategy. In treated diabetics, 5-year survival was significantly better after CABG than after PTCA.

Pocock and colleagues[248] in London, United Kingdom, for the Randomized Intervention of Treatment (RITA) trial investigators assessed the impact of PTCA and CABG in 1011 patients with angina with regard to the impact of these revascularization procedures on angina frequency, quality of life, and employment during 3 years of follow-up. Both interventions produced marked improvement in all quality-of-life dimensions, including energy, pain, emotional reactions, sleep, social isolation, and mobility, and 7 aspects of daily living (Figure 2-122). Patients with angina at 2 years had more quality-of-life impairment than did angina-free patients. There was a close correlation at baseline between angina grade and quality of life. There was slightly greater impairment of quality of life in the PTCA-treated patients compared with the CABG-treated patients as a result of their significantly higher likelihood of having angina, especially after 6 months. Employment status was investigated mainly for men 60 years of age or younger. The patients receiving PTCA returned to work sooner (40% at 2 months, compared with 10% of CABG patients), but patients treated with CABG caught up by 5 months. After 2 years, 22% of CABG and 26% of PTCA patients were not working for cardiac reasons. Patients with angina at 2 years were more likely to be unemployed than were those without. Thus, the impact of angina on quality of life and unemployment

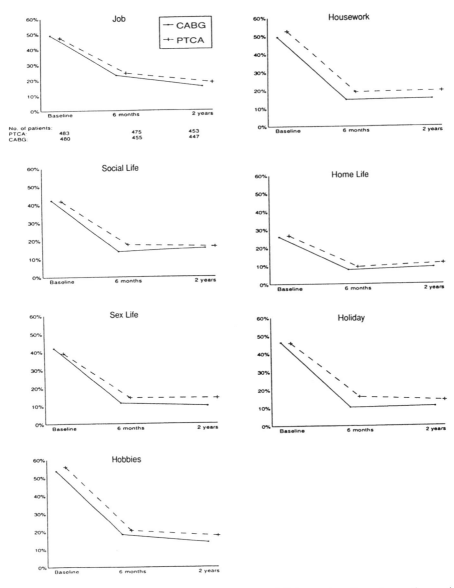

FIGURE 2-122. Effect of patient's health on 7 aspects of living at baseline, 6 months, and 2 years from part 2 of the NHP (self reported % affected plotted by life aspect, time, and treatment group). Reproduced with permission from Pocock et al.[248]

is alleviated by PTCA and CABG. Angina is avoided more successfully with CABG, but PTCA offers a more rapid return to work.

The relative value of PTCA and CABG is emerging in several trials. Rodriguez and colleagues[249] from Buenos Aires, Argentina, and Boston, Massachusetts, reported the 3-year follow-up results of the Argentine randomized trial of PTCA vs. CABG in multivessel disease (ERACI). One hundred twenty seven patients with multivessel disease who were candidates for revascularization were randomized to undergo PTCA (63) or CABG (64). Freedom from combined cardiac events of death, Q-wave infarction, angina, and repeat revascularization procedures was significantly greater for the CABG group than for the PTCA group (77% vs. 47%). There were no differences in overall cardiac mortality (4.7% for both) or in the frequency of acute myocardial infarction (7.8% for both). Patients who had CABG, however, had more freedom from angina (79% vs. 57%) and required fewer additional re-interventions (6.3% vs. 37%). These authors concluded that in this 3-year follow-up, freedom from combined cardiac events was greater with CABG than with PTCA, although the accumulative mortality was the same.

CABG

In Unstable Angina and Non-Q Wave MI

Kleiman and associates[250] for the TIMI IIIR investigators performed a study to characterize patients with and without prior CABG among a prospectively identified cohort of patients presenting with unstable angina or non-Q wave AMI. Patients in the Thrombolysis in Myocardial Infarction Phase III Registry prospective study presented within 96 hours of an episode of unstable angina or non-Q wave AMI. Of 2048 patients, 336 (16.4%) had prior CABG. Compared with those without prior CABG, patients were the same age, but were more likely to be men, white, diabetic, have a history of angina or myocardial infarction, to have received anti-ischemic medications in the prior week, and to receive intravenous heparin or nitroglycerin, or both, during hospitalization. They were equally likely to undergo coronary angioplasty or CABG. Death or nonfatal AMI occurred by day 10 in 4.5% of patients with prior CABG and in 2.8% of patients without prior CABG; and by day 42 in 7.7% and 5.1%, respectively. The composite of death, AMI, or recurrent ischemia at 1 year was more common among patients with prior CABG (39.3% vs. 30.2%). By multiple logistic regression, prior CABG was not independently associated with the occurrence of death or AMI, or the composite of death, AMI, or recurrent ischemia either at 6 weeks or at 1 year. The likelihood of recurrent ischemic events is greater among patients with than without prior CABG, but is most likely explained by differences in baseline or treatment characteristics which reflect the degree of underlying cardiac disease (Table 2-21).

Managed Delay of CABG

Universal access to medical services in Canada comes at the expense of waiting lists of which the impact has been incompletely assessed. Cox and colleagues[251] from Halifax, Nova Scotia, sought to determine the impact to delaying CABG at 1 Canadian academic referral center. A prospective, observational study was carried out on all residents of Nova Scotia and Prince Edward Island who were accepted for CABG between April 1, 1992, and October 31, 1992. Of 423 patients referred, 35% were triaged as urgent, 9.7% as semiurgent

TABLE 2-21
Outcome at 10 and 42 Days, and at One Year

	Prior CABG (n = 335)	No Prior CABG (n = 1712)	p Value
	Outcome at 10 Days		
Death	6 (1.8)	14 (1.0)	0.09
MI	10 (3.1)	37 (2.2)	0.35
Death or MI	15 (4.5)	48 (2.8)	0.11
Stroke	0 (0)	6 (0.4)	0.28
Recurrent ischemia			
with ECG changes	39 (11.6)	191 (11.1)	0.97
without ECG changes	112 (33.3)	636 (39.1)	0.08
	Outcome at 42 Days		
Death	16 (4.8)	44 (2.6)	0.03
MI	16 (4.8)	58 (3.4)	0.21
Death or MI	27 (7.7)	87 (5.1)	0.03
Stroke	0 (0)	11 (6.4)	0.14
Death, MI, or recurrent ischemia	68 (20.2)	280 (16.4)	0.10
	Outcome at One Year		
Death	40 (11.9)	158 (9.2)	0.12
MI	27 (8.0)	91 (5.3)	0.04
Death or MI	58 (17.3)	213 (12.4)	0.02
Death, MI, or recurrent ischemia	132 (39.3)	516 (30.2)	0.002

Values are expressed as number (%).

ECG = electrocardiographic; MI = myocardial infarction.

Reproduced with permission from Kleiman et al.[250]

A, 39% as semiurgent B, and 16.3% as elective. Operation occurred at less than 1 week in 25%, less than 1 month in 47%, and more than 6 months in 1.4%. There were no nonfatal AMIs, but 5 cardiac deaths occurred (1.2%). Of 275 patients not initially classified as urgent, 12.4% required reclassification to higher priorities because of worsening symptoms. These authors concluded that the triage system equitably stratified patients in a queue. Deaths were rare and could not be attributed to the triage process. Thus, patients with worsening clinical status were safely accommodated with earlier waiting times, but concerns remain regarding excessive waiting times and patient anxiety.

Influence of Graft Selection on Survival

Cameron and colleagues[252] in New York, New York, and Rochester, Minnesota, identified all the patients in the registry of the Coronary Artery Surgery Study who had undergone first-time CABG. Those with internal-thoracic-artery bypass grafts (n = 749) were compared with those with saphenous-vein bypass grafts (4888 patients) only with respect to survival over a 15-year follow-up period. Using multivariate analysis to account for differences between the 2 groups, the presence of an internal-thoracic-artery graft was an independent predictor of improved survival and was associated with a relative risk of dying of 0.73. This improved survival was also observed in subgroups, including patients 65 years of age or older, both men and women, and patients with reduced ventricular function. The survival curves of the 2 groups showed further separation over the years of follow-up with a more marked downsloping after 8 years in the curve for the group with saphenous-vein grafts only than for the group with internal thoracic artery grafts. As compared with saphenous vein coronary bypass grafts, internal thoracic artery grafts conferred a survival advantage throughout a 15-year follow-up period. The survival advantage increased with time, suggesting that the initial selection of the conduit was a more important factor in survival than problems appearing long after surgery, including the progression of CAD.

A New Anastomosis Site Restraining Device

Borst and colleagues[253] from Utrecht, The Netherlands, and Amsterdam, The Netherlands, evaluated the feasibility of CABG on the beating heart without interruption of native coronary blood flow using a novel anastomosis site restraining device. This suction device (Octopus) was evaluated in 31 pigs. These authors found that coronary bypass on the beating heart was feasible without interruption of coronary flow. This was done in both open and in closed chest procedures. Further evaluation is warranted with this device in patients.

Use of Unilateral and Biradial Arteries

A number of previous surgical studies have noted that internal mammary artery patency is much greater than saphenous vein graft patency after CABG. Brodman and colleagues[254] from the Bronx, New York, evaluated the routine use of radial artery grafts in patients undergoing CABG. They reviewed 175 of 249 consecutive patients. In 54 patients, bilateral radial arteries were harvested. The operative mortality was 1.6%. No deaths were related to the grafts, and there were no harvest site hematomas or infections. Transient dysesthesia 1 day to 4 weeks in duration occurred in the distribution of the lateral antebrachial cutaneous nerve in 2.6% of patients. Elective catheterization in 60 patients at 12 weeks postoperatively demonstrated a 95.7% patency rate. These authors concluded that there is the potential benefit of long-term patency associated with arterial grafts, in terms of minimal morbidity and mortality associated with the use of the radial artery and excellent short-term patency rates. They believe that use of 1 or both radial arteries as additional conduits will be helpful in surgical revascularization procedures.

Intravascular Imaging of Grafts

In this investigation by Komlyama and associates[255] from Tokyo, Japan, to clarify the structural changes of saphenous vein grafts after CABG, intravascular ultrasound and angioscopic images were obtained from 23 grafts *in vivo* and 5 grafts and 3 new veins *in vitro*; the images were compared with histologic findings. Intravascular ultrasound demonstrated a single-layered appearance of new veins and all of the angiographically normal grafts within 6 months after surgery. A triple-layered appearance that might be related to the remarkably proliferative and degenerated intima was revealed histologically in 73% of the normal sites of grafts between 5 and 10 years after operation. In 83% of the stenoses at several years after operation, angioscopy showed yellow atheromatous plaques, often with a friable surface; a heterogeneous, lucent echo pattern was revealed on intravascular ultrasound. Thus, intravascular ultrasound and angioscopy may be used to identify more precisely than conventional angiography the morphological changes of grafts at different time points after implantation.

Nishioka and colleagues[256] from Cedars-Sinai Medical Center in Los Angeles, California, used intravascular ultrasound to determine whether lumen reduction in human coronary saphenous vein bypass grafts is accompanied by vessel wall thickening and arterial wall constriction. Forty-three saphenous vein bypass grafts from 42 patients (32 men, 10 women, with a mean age of 72 years) were examined 8 to 23 years after bypass graft procedures. Intravascular ultrasound images were obtained with a 3.5F ultrasound catheter with a 30-MHz frequency and were analyzed at the lesion site, the reference site, and an intermediate site. The lumen area was significantly decreased in these vein bypass grafts. The vessel wall area and the plaque area were significantly increased from the reference site through the lesion site. However, the saphenous vein bypass graft cross-sectional area was the same at these 3 sites, and the external elastic lamina area was also constant (Figure 2-123). Thus, intravascular ultrasound data from human coronary saphenous vein bypass grafts demonstrate that there is no focal compensatory enlargement or vessel constriction occurring in stenotic segments compared with the reference segments. The absence of focal compensatory enlargement appears to be a potentially important factor in the progression of stenoses in the coronary saphenous vein bypass grafts.

MRI of Grafts

Galjee and colleagues[257] from Amsterdam, The Netherlands, investigated whether magnetic resonance cine gradient-echo images performed in addition to standard spin-echo have additional value in the assessment of graft patency. They also assessed graft functioning by measuring the flow pattern and flow rate with magnetic resonance phase velocity imaging in 47 patients with CAD who had previous CABG. These patients had angiography and magnetic resonance spin-echo and gradient-echo phase velocity imaging. The magnetic resonance images were evaluated by 3 independent observers blinded to the angiographic results. The spatial mean velocity and volume flow were measured and repeated of each image at consecutive 50-msec intervals throughout the cardiac cycle. Forty-seven patients had 98 proximal aortotomies, of which 60 were single and 38 were sequential grafts. Seventy-three grafts were patent; 25 were occluded. Eighty-four grafts (86%) were eligible for comparison of the results

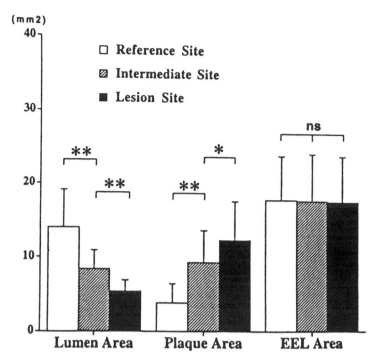

FIGURE 2-123. Bar graph shows comparison of lumen area, plaque area, and external elastic lamina area in saphenous vein bypass grafts at the reference site, intermediate site, and lesion site. In saphenous vein bypass grafts, lumen area gradually decreased and plaque area increased as the lumen area became smaller. However, saphenous vein bypass graft external elastic lamina; area was similar at the lesion site, intermediate site, and reference site. *$p<.01$, **$p<.001$. Reproduced with permission from Nishioka et al.[256]

of spin-echo and gradient-echo images. The assessment of patency was inconclusive in spin-echo images in 7 grafts (5 occluded by angiography) and on gradient-echo images in 7 grafts (2 occluded). A comparison of the results of contrast angiography and spin-echo and gradient-echo MRI techniques demonstrated that both techniques had a high sensitivity (98%) and lower specificity (85% and 88%, respectively) for graft patency. Combined analysis of the spin-echo and gradient-echo images did not improve the accuracy. The strength of the interobserver agreement on gradient-echo images was good, but on spin-echo images the agreement was only moderate. Adequate magnetic resonance phase velocity profiles were obtained in 62 of 73 angiographically patent grafts. Graft flow was characterized by a balanced biphasic forward flow pattern. The volume flow of sequential grafts to 3 regions was significantly higher than in single grafts. These data suggest that gradient-echo phase MRI with velocity mapping is a promising clinical tool in the noninvasive assessment of coronary artery graft patency and function.

Complications of Bypass Surgery

Arrhythmias are common after coronary surgery and are associated with hemodynamic compromise, stroke, and prolonged hospitalization. β-Blockers prevent atrial fibrillation postoperatively, but there are few data regarding the prophylactic use of type I antiarrhythmia agents or of the prevention of ventricular arrhythmias. Gold and associates[258] from Boston, Massachusetts, performed a randomized, double-blind, placebo-controlled study of the effects of oral procainamide on 100 patients undergoing elective CABG. Procainamide was received for 4 days; the dosage was adjusted for body weight. Patients receiving procainamide had a significant reduction in AF (16 vs. 29 patient-days) and VT (2% vs. 20%). However, the incidence of atrial fibrillation was not significantly reduced (38% vs. 26%). In the group achieving therapeutic serum procainamide levels, there was a reduction in all measured postoperative arrhythmias. No serious cardiac or noncardiac adverse events were noted during procainamide therapy, although there was a significant increase in the incidence of nausea. The authors concluded that procainamide reduces arrhythmias in the early postoperative period after CABG, most prominently in patients who achieve therapeutic serum levels. This was associated with no serious cardiac adverse reactions (Table 2-22).

Increasingly, patients undergoing CABG are elderly, have had previous CABG, and have poor left ventricular function. To evaluate determinants of perioperative myocardial infarction after isolated CABG, 499 consecutive patients were reviewed by Greaves and associates[259] from Boston, Massachusetts. Definite perioperative myocardial infarction (total peak creatine kinase>700 U/L, creatine kinase-MB>30 ng/mL, and new pathological electrocardiographic Q-waves) occurred in 25 patients (5.0%), and probable perioperative myocardial infarction (total peak creatine kinase>700 U/L, creatine-kinase-MB>30 ng/mL, and a new wall motion abnormality) occurred in 10 (2.0%) patients. According to multivariate logistic regression analysis, independent risk factors for definite or probable perioperative myocardial infarction were emergency surgery, aortic cross-clamp time shorter than 100 minutes, myocardial infarction in the preceding week, and previous revascularization. In conclusion, both preoperative and intraoperative factors influence the risk of perioperative myocardial infarction after CABG. Despite changes in the profile of patients undergoing CABG, the incidence of perioperative myocardial infarction in this tertiary center is comparable with that found in earlier series, probably because of improvements in surgical techniques and postoperative care.

There is an expanding population of patients with surgically treated CAD, a number of whom require repeat revascularization procedures. Although there are randomized comparative data for CABG vs. medical therapy and more

TABLE 2-22
Subgroup Analysis of Arrhythmias

Characteristic	Therapeutic	Subtherapeutic	Placebo
Number	30	20	50
Atrial fibrillation	13%*	45%	38%
Ventricular tachycardia	0%*	5%	20%
Premature ventricular complexes/hr	5±2*	36±16	21±7
Atrial premature complexes/hr	5±3*	54±28	22±7

* $p<0.05$ versus placebo.
Reproduced with permission from Greaves et al.[259]

TABLE 2-23
Troponin T for Diagnosis of Acute Myocardial Infarction

Parameter	TnT>0.1 ng/mL	TnT>0.2 ng/mL
First sample only		
Sensitivity	8/17 (47%)	4/17 (24%)
Specificity	1,093/1,158 (94%)	1,126/1,158 (97%)
Positive predictive value	8/73 (11%)	4/36 (11%)
Negative predictive value	1,093/1,102 (99%)	1,126/1,139 (99%)
Relative risk	13.4	9.7
Peak troponin value:*		
Sensitivity	13/15 (87%)	12/15 (80%)
Specificity	860/1,018 (84%)	914/1,018 (90%)
Positive predictive value	13/171 (8%)	12/116 (10%)
Negative predictive value	860/862 (99%)	914/917 (99%)
Relative risk	32.8	31.6

* Among 1033 patients with more than one troponin value.
TnT = troponin T.

recently versus PTCA, these studies have generally excluded patients with previous CABG. Stephan and colleagues[260] from Kansas City, Missouri, attempted to determine the relative risks and benefits of PTCA and repeat CABG in patients with previous CABG. They retrospectively analyzed data from 632 patients with previous CABG who required either elective repeat CABG (n = 164) or PTCA (n = 468) at a single center during 1987 through 1988. Both groups were similar with respect to gender, age greater than 70 years, mean left ventricular ejection fraction, presence of class III or IV angina, and 3-vessel CAD. Complete revascularization was achieved in 38% of patients with PTCA and in 92% of those with repeat CABG. The in-hospital complication rates were significantly lower in the PTCA group (death 0.3% vs. 7.3%, and Q-wave myocardial infarction 0.9% vs. 6.1%). Actuarial survival was equivalent at 1 year and 6 years. However, the need for repeat PTCA or surgical revascularization or both was significantly higher in the PTCA group by 6 years (PTCA 64% vs. repeat CABG 8%). Multivariate analysis identified age greater than 70 years, left ventricular ejection fraction less than 40%, unstable angina, number of diseased vessels, and diabetes mellitus as independent correlates of mortality for the entire group. These authors concluded that in this nonrandomized series of patients with previous CABG requiring revascularization, an initial strategy of either PTCA or repeat CABG resulted in equivalent overall survival, event-free survival, and relief of angina. PTCA offers lower procedural morbidity and mortality risks, although it is associated with less complete revascularization and a greater need for subsequent revascularization procedures.

Bypass Graft Patency in the Long Term

There are considerable data available about bypass graft patency in the long term. However, there are less data on the precise relation between fate of grafts and patient outcome. Fitzgibbon and colleagues[261] from Ottawa, On-

TABLE 2-24
Troponin T and Major Cardiac Complications Among Patients
Without AMI

Parameter	TnT>0.1 ng/mL	TnT>0.2 ng/mL
First sample only:		
Sensitivity	7/17 (41%)	4/17 (24%)
Specificity	1,091/1,141 (96%)	1,113/1,141 (98%)
Positive predictive value	7/57 (12%)	4/32 (12.5%)
Negative predictive value	1,091/1,110 (99%)	1,113/1,126 (99%)
Relative risk	13.5	10.8
*Peak troponin value**		
Sensitivity	10/16 (62%)	8/16 (50%)
Specificity	854/1,002 (85%)	906/1,002 (90%)
Positive predictive value	10/158 (6%)	8/104 (8%)
Negative predictive value	854/860 (99%)	906/914 (99%)
Relative risk	9.1	8.8

* Among patients with more than one troponin T sample.
TnT = troponin T.

tario, Canada, evaluated the long-term fate of a large number of patients undergoing CABG to correlate graft patency and disease with patient survival and reoperation. A total of 1388 patients underwent a first CABG procedure at a mean age of 49 years. Of those, 234 had a second bypass procedure at a mean age of 53, and 15 had a third bypass procedure at a mean age of 58 during the 25-year period from 1969 to 1994. Most were male military personnel or veterans. Of 5284 grafts placed, 91% were venous and 9%, arterial. Angiograms were performed on 5065 (98% of surviving) grafts early: on 3,993 grafts at 1 year, and on 1,978 grafts at 5 years after operation. The perioperative mortality was 1.4% for an isolated first CABG, and 6.6% for reoperation. Vein graft patency was 88% early, 81% at 1 year, 75% at 5 years, and 50% at greater than 15 years. After the early study, the vein graft occlusion rate was 2.1% per year. Internal mammary artery graft patency was significantly better but decreased with time. Survival of all patients was 93.6% at 5 years, 81% at 10 years, 61.1% at 15 years, and 46.7% at 20 years. Survival decreased as age increased, but curves approximated normal life expectancy for older patients. Survival curves at all ages showed a steeper decline after 7 years. The rate of reoperation increased significantly 5 years after the first coronary bypass procedure; plateaued at 10 to 14 years; and then decreased to a lower, but steady level. Vein graft patency and disease were temporally and closely related to reoperation and survival. These authors concluded that coronary bypass graft disease and occlusion are common after CABG and increase with time. They are the major determinants of clinical prognosis as measured by reoperation rate and survival. Intraoperative graft atheroembolism was a major reoperation hazard. Reoperation is worthwhile but entails identifiable risks that must be considered.

Effect of Smoking on Bypass Surgery

Voors and colleagues[262] in The Netherlands determined the long-term clinical effects of smoking and smoking cessation after venous CABG by studying

415 patients who underwent CABG with the use of venous bypass grafts between April 1976 and April 1977. These patients were followed prospectively for 15 years. Survival analysis evaluations revealed that patients who smoked at the time of surgery had no elevated risks for clinical events compared with nonsmokers. However, smoking behavior at 1 and 5 years after surgery appeared to be an important predictor of clinical events during the subsequent follow-up period, as compared with cessation of smoking at the time of surgery. Smokers at 1 year after CABG had more than twice the risk for AMI and reoperation (Figure 2-124). Patients who were still smoking at 5 years after CABG had even more elevated risks for AMI and reoperation and a significantly increased risk for angina pectoris compared with patients who stopped smoking at the time of surgery and those who never smoked (Figure 2-124). In those patients who started to smoke again within 5 years of CABG, there were increased risks for reoperation and angina pectoris. No differences in outcome were found between patients who stopped smoking at the time of surgery and nonsmokers. These data indicate that smoking cessation after CABG may have important beneficial effects in the reduction of clinical events during subsequent follow-up.

Effect of Thrombolysis

Patients with chronically occluded aortocoronary vein grafts and uncontrolled angina have limited therapeutic options. Based on previous work that had shown that chronically occluded vein grafts can be recanalized by thrombolysis, a multicenter study ROBUST, Recanalization of Chronically Occluded Aortocoronary Saphenous Vein Bypass Grafts with Long-Term, Low-Dose Direct Infusion of Urokinase. (ROBUST)[263] was organized to evaluate the effect of low-dose direct urokinase infusion in recanalizing chronically occluded saphenous vein bypass grafts. Urokinase 100,000 U/h was infused directly into occluded vein grafts in 107 patients, followed by PTCA. Patients were discharged on warfarin and aspirin therapy. Initial patency was achieved in 69% of patients after a mean infusion duration of 25.4 hours and a mean urokinase dose of 3.7 million U. AMI occurred in 5% of patients, enzyme level elevation in 17%, emergency CABG in 4%, stroke in 3%, and death in 6.5%. Recanalization was unsuccessful in all 7 patients who died. At 6-month follow-up, patent grafts were noted in 40% of the patients who were restudied. These authors concluded that chronically occluded bypass grafts can be recanalized in about 70% of appropriately selected patients. There was an improvement in angina during follow-up. They believe that this therapy should only be used in patients with 1 occluded vein graft.

Effect of Diet

Epidemiological and experimental data suggest that a high dietary intake of long-chain polyunsaturated n-3 fatty acids may reduce the risk of atherothrombotic disease. In a randomized, controlled study, Eritsland and associates[264] from Oslo, Norway, assigned 610 patients undergoing CABG either to

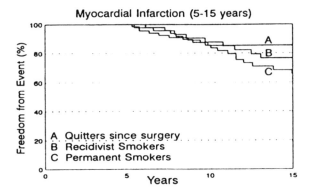

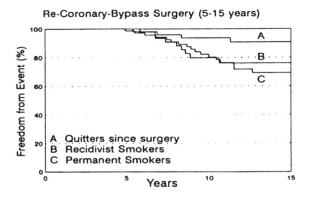

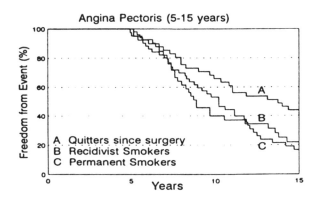

FIGURE 2-124. Kaplan-Meier survival curves representing freedom from clinical events for those who discontinued smoking after surgery, those who resumed smoking, ie, recidivist smokers, and permanent smokers, from 5 to 15 years after coronary bypass surgery. Reproduced with permission from Voors et al.[262]

a fish oil group, receiving 4 g/day of fish oil concentrate, or to a control group. All patients received antithrombotic treatment, either aspirin or warfarin. Their diet and serum phospholipid fatty acid profiles were monitored. The primary end point was 1-year graft patency, which was assessed by angiography in 95% of patients. Vein graft occlusion rates per distal anastomoses were 27% in the fish oil group and 33% in the control group (odds ratio 0.77). In the fish oil group, 43% of the patients had 1 or more occluded vein graft(s) compared with 51% in the control group (odds ratio, 0.72). Moreover, in the entire patient group, there was a significant trend to fewer patients with vein graft occlusions with increasing relative change in serum phospholipid n-3 fatty acids during the study period. Thus, in patients undergoing CABG, dietary supplementation with n-3 fatty acids reduced the incidence of vein graft occlusion, and an inverse relation between relative change in serum phospholipid n-3 fatty acids and vein graft occlusions was observed.

Cardiac Rehabilitation

Participation in a standard-length outpatient cardiac rehabilitation program for 3 months is known to result in positive changes in body composition, functional capacity, and blood lipids in patients with CAD. There has been little attempt, however, to compare patients who remain active in a formal cardiac rehabilitation program for a length greater than 1 year with patients who exit after the standard length of 3 months. Consequently, Brubaker and associates[265] from Winston-Salem, North Carolina, performed a series of tests in 50 patients, including a maximal graded exercise treadmill test, assessment of body composition, and fasting blood lipid analysis, at entry to cardiac rehabilitation program and after a follow-up period that ranged from 1 to 5 years. All patients participated in a standard multidisciplinary cardiac rehabilitation program for 3 months. Twenty-five patients discontinued participation after 3 months and received no other contact from the program staff until follow-up, whereas 25 patients remained active in the program until follow-up. After statistically adjusting baseline differences between the groups, significant differences were observed between the extended- and standard-length groups at follow-up for body weight (177 vs. 183 lbs), percent fat (22% vs. 24%), METS (10.5 vs. 8.4), HDL level cholesterol (44 vs. 39) mg/dL, total cholesterol/HDL ratio (5.2 vs. 6.1), and triglycerides (134 vs. 204 mg/dL), respectively. No significant differences in the adjusted means were observed between the groups at follow-up for total cholesterol (209 vs. 219 mg/dL) and LDL cholesterol (136 vs. 138 mg/dL). Data from this study demonstrate the efficacy of extended participation in CRP on body composition, functional capacity, and blood lipids.

The purpose of this study by Gagliardi and associates[266] from Buenos Aires, Argentina, was to evaluate whether combined treatment with a cardiovascular exercise rehabilitation program and low doses of heparin can induce changes in ergometric parameters of ischemia in patients with CAD. Heparin may potentiate the development of new vessels promoted by ischemia and therefore may produce important clinical improvement. Thirty-six patients with stable CAD and evidence of myocardial ischemia on exercise testing were randomized into 3 groups: a control group (n = 11) received the usual medical treatment; another group (n = 11) underwent 3 exercise sessions per week during 12 weeks; and a third group (n = 14) undertook this exercise program and also received calcium heparin 12,500 IU subcutaneously 20 to 30 minutes before each exercise session. Pretreatment and posttreatment exercise tests were compared. Patients who underwent the rehabilitation program had an increase in exercise duration and workload at the onset of 1-mm ST-segment depression, but only patients who received calcium heparin showed a significant increase in rate-pressure product at the ST-segment ischemic threshold. This result suggests that higher levels of myocardial oxygen consumption were now tolerated, a change that may be related to an improvement in myocardial perfusion.

Milani and associates[267] from New Orleans, Louisiana, evaluated the effect of cardiac rehabilitation and exercise training on depression after major cardiac events. They studied 338 consecutive patients in whom a major cardiac event had occurred 4 to 6 weeks previously and who were participating in phase II cardiac rehabilitation, consisting of 36 sessions over a 3-month period. Depressive symptoms and other behavioral characteristics and quality-of-life parameters were analyzed by validated questionnaire. Depression was prevalent in patients with CAD, occurring in 20% of the patients evaluated. At baseline, depressed patients had lower exercise capacity, reduced HDL cholesterol level, and higher triglyceride levels; had lower scores for mental health, energy or fatigue, general health, pain, overall function, well-being, and total quality of life; and had greater scores for somatization, anxiety, and hostility than those of nondepressed patients. After cardiac rehabilitation, depressed patients had marked improvements in depression scores and other behavioral parameters (anxiety, somatization, and hostility) and quality of life. Depressed patients also showed improved exercise capacity, percentage of body fat, and levels of triglycerides and HDL cholesterol. Depressed patients exhibited statistically greater improvements in certain behavioral and quality-of-life parameters than did nondepressed patients. Two-thirds of the patients who were initially depressed resolved their symptoms by study completion. In conclusion, depression is reduced in patients with symptomatic CAD enrolled in cardiac rehabilitation. Greater emphasis is needed to ensure that depressed patients are referred to and attend formal cardiac rehabilitation programs after major cardiac events.

Ades and colleagues[268] in Burlington, Vermont, studied the effects of a 3-month and a 1-year program of intense aerobic exercise in 60 CAD patients with a mean age of 68 ± 5 years beginning 8 ± 5 weeks after AMI or CABG, Outcome measures included peak aerobic capacity, cardiac output, arterial venous oxygen difference, hyperemic calf blood flow, and skeletal muscle fiber morphometry, oxidative enzyme activity, and capillarity. Training results were compared with a sedentary, age-, and diagnosis-matched control groups (n = 10). Peak aerobic capacity increased in the intervention group at 3 months, and at 1 year by 16% and 20%, respectively. Peak exercise, cardiac output, hyperemic calf blood flow, and vascular conductance were unaffected by the conditioning protocol. At 3 and 12 months, arteriovenous oxygen difference at peak exercise was increased in the exercise group, but not in the control group. Histochemical analysis of skeletal muscle documented a 34% increase in capillary density and a 23% increase in succinate dehydrogenase activity after 3 months of conditioning. At 12 months, individual fiber area increased by 29%, compared with baseline. Thus, in older patients with CAD, exercise rehabilitation successfully improves peak aerobic capacity after 3 and 12 months.

Surgery for Left Ventricular Aneurysm

Rastegar and colleagues[269] undertook reconstruction of the left ventricle with a pericardial patch or endoaneurysmorrhaphy performed with mapping-guided subendocardial resection for recurrent VT in 25 patients over a 5-year period. Postoperatively, electrophysiological studies were conducted to assess the results of surgery, which were further evaluated during long-term follow-up with survival analyses. The study included 25 patients (mean age, 60 years) with CAD, discrete left ventricular aneurysms, and malignant VT. LVEF was 24% preoperatively. Left ventricular endocardial mapping, endocardial resection, and endoaneurysmorrhaphy were performed in all patients. There was no operative or perioperative (30 day) mortality. Postoperative VT was induced in 2 of the 25 patients (8%). Left ventricular function increased to 32% postoperatively. At a mean follow-up period of 37 months (range, 6 to 65 months), there had been 6 deaths, including 1 sudden death, 2 CHF deaths, and 3 noncardiac deaths. Analysis of multiple variables failed to identify predictors of postoperative inducibility, sudden cardiac death, cardiac death, or total mortality. Thus, endoaneurysmorrhaphy with a pericardial patch combined with mapping-guided subendocardial resection frequently cures recurrent VT with low operative mortality and some improvement in LVEF (Figures 2-125 and 2-126).

Cardiac Risk in Noncardiac Procedures

The value of dipyridamole technetium-99m sestamibi tomography for preoperative cardiac risk stratification was assessed in 285 consecutive patients being considered for nonvascular surgery in this study performed by Stratmann and colleagues[270] from St. Louis, Missouri. A major (n = 140) or minor (n = 89) nonvascular procedure was later done in 229 of these patients within 4 months after dipyridamole testing. Perioperative cardiac events (unstable angina, acute ischemic pulmonary edema, nonfatal myocardial infarction, or cardiac death) occurred in 11 (8%) patients undergoing major nonvascular surgery and 1 (1%) undergoing a minor procedure. The only clinical or scintigraphic variables associated with significantly increased perioperative cardiac risk in patients having major surgery were Goldman class II or higher, an abnormal dipyridamole technetium-99m sestamibi tomography scan, and a fixed perfusion defect. In these patients, cardiac events occurred in 1% of those who had a normal dipyridamole technetium-99m sestamibi tomography study, 14% of those with an abnormal scan, 12% with a reversible defect, and 17%

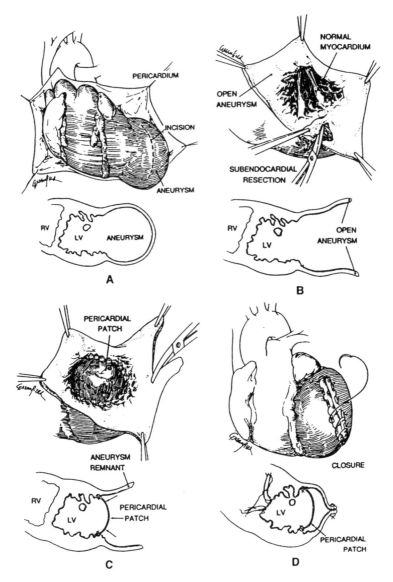

FIGURE 2-125. Left ventricular (LV) endoaneurysmorrhaphy for an anterior LV aneurysm. After completion of epicardial mapping by use of normothermic cardiopulmonary bypass, ventriculotomy was performed with a longitudinal incision parallel to the intraventricular septum at the apex of the aneurysm **(A).** Subsequently, endocardial mapping was performed, and after completion of mapping-guided subendocardial resection **(B)** and cryoablation, ventricular endoaneurysmorrhaphy was undertaken with an elliptical pericardial patch pretreated with glutaraldehyde. The patch was attached to the edge of the healthy myocardium with a continuous suture **(C).** The ventriculotomy was then repaired using either felt buttresses or direct suture **(D).** RV, right ventricle. Reproduced with permission from Rastegar et al.[269]

Survival

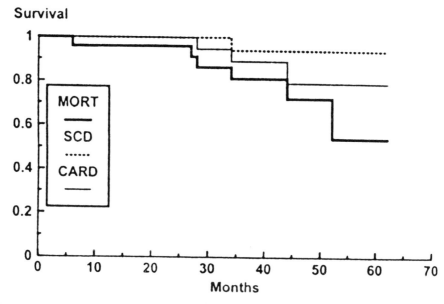

FIGURE 2-126. Survival analysis indicating 94% freedom from sudden cardiac death (SCD), during 3 to 65 months of follow-up, and showing increased total mortality (MORT) and cardiac mortality (CARD) after 30 months of follow-up. Reproduced with permission from Rastegar et al.[269]

with a fixed dipyridamole technetium-99m sestamibi tomography defect. In the 60 patients whose Goldman class was II or higher, only an abnormal dipyridamole technetium-99m sestamibi study and a fixed perfusion defect were associated with incremental risk of a perioperative cardiac event. The incidence of perioperative cardiac events in these patients was 4% with a normal dipyridamole technetium-99m sestamibi tomography scan, 27% with an abnormal study, 24% with a reversible defect, and 37% with a fixed defect. Event rates were low in patients having minor nonvascular surgery; none of the 25 with a normal study and only 1 of the 64 with an abnormal scan had a perioperative cardiac event. It was concluded that dipyridamole technetium-99m sestamibi tomography can provide important prognostic information in patients having major nonvascular surgery. A normal study indicates a low risk of perioperative cardiac events, whereas an abnormal study in patients with Goldman class II or higher undergoing major surgery is associated with significantly increased risk. The prognostic value of dipyridamole technetium-99m sestamibi tomography in patients at low clinical risk undergoing minor surgery is limited.

To assess the diagnostic performance of cardiac troponin T as a marker for myocardial injury in patients undergoing major noncardiac surgery, Lee and associates[271] from Boston, Massachusetts, prospectively collected preoperative and postoperative clinical data, including measurements for creatine kinase (CK), CK-MB, and troponin T for 1,175 patients undergoing major noncardiac surgery. AMI was diagnosed in 17 patients (1.4%) by a reviewer who was blinded to troponin T data and used CK-MB and electrocardiographic criteria to define AMI. Other predischarge major cardiac complications were detected for another 17 patients. Troponin T elevations (>0.1 ng/mL) occurred in 87%

of patients with and in 16% of patients without AMI. Among patients without AMI, troponin T was elevated in 62% of patients with and in 15% of patients without major cardiac complications. Receiver-operating characteristic analysis indicated that for the diagnosis of AMI, troponin T performed similarly to CK-MB, and had a significantly better correlation with other major cardiac complications in patients without definitive infarction. Future research should help to determine the significance of troponin T elevations in patients without complications.

Although perfusion imaging studies are used extensively as a preoperative screening test for risk stratification of patients undergoing noncardiac surgery, no single cardiac noninvasive test has been shown to be ideal for risk stratification. Kontos and associates[272] from Richmond, Virginia, investigated the relative impact of transthoracic 2-dimensional echocardiography compared with dipyridamole thallium scintigraphy in predicting major cardiac complications in patients undergoing noncardiac surgery. Eighty-seven consecutive patients undergoing 96 procedures (56 vascular, 40 general) underwent preoperative evaluation: first with dipyridamole thallium scintigraphy and then with 2-dimensional echocardiography before surgery. Complications were prospectively defined as AMI, cardiac death (AMI, CHF, or arrhythmia), or need for revascularization before surgery. Dipyridamole thallium scintigraphy showed 1 or more reversible defects in 44 (51%) patients, whereas 2-dimensional echocardiography demonstrated a reduced LVEF in 25 (29%) patients. Major postoperative cardiac complications occurred in 10 patients: 5 deaths (2 VF, 3 fatal AMIs) and 5 nonfatal AMIs. Four additional patients required urgent revascularization (CABG in 3 and PTCA in 1). Of the 20 patients with both abnormal dipyridamole thallium scintigraphy and 2-dimensional echocardiography, 11 (55%) had major complications, compared with 1 of the 26 with an abnormal dipyridamole thallium scintigraphy but normal LVEF. The sensitivity of dipyridamole thallium scintigraphy and 2-dimensional echocardiography were not significantly different (79% vs. 86%, respectively), although the specificity of dipyridamole thallium scintigraphy was lower (51% vs 81%). The positive predictive value of dipyridamole thallium scintigraphy was significantly improved from 22% (12% to 35%) to 52% (32% to 72%) when both dipyridamole thallium scintigraphy and 2-dimensional echocardiography were abnormal. The results were not significantly different when the 4 patients who underwent revascularization were excluded. In conclusion, 1) in spite of similar sensitivity of 2-dimensional echocardiography and dipyridamole thallium scintigraphy, 2-dimensional echocardiography appears to be relatively more specific in predicting major cardiac complications, and 2) when 2-dimensional echocardiography and dipyridamole thallium scintigraphy are both abnormal, the risk of cardiac complications related to noncardiac surgery is significantly increased. Use of the combination of dipyridamole thallium scintigraphy and 2-dimensional echocardiography before major noncardiac surgery can improve the identification of patients at risk for complications.

1. Tosteson ANA, Goldman L, Udvarhelyi IS, Lee TH: Cost-effectiveness of a coronary care unit versus an intermediate care unit for emergency department patient with chest pain. Circulation 1996 (July 15);94:143–150.

2. Oopik AJ, Dorogy M, Devereux RB, Yeh J-L, Okin PM, Lee ET, Cowan L, Fabsitz RR, Howard BV, Welty TK: Major electrocardiographic abnormalities among American Indians aged 45 to 74 years. (The Strong Heart Study). Am J Cardiol 1996 (December 15);78:1400–1405.

3. Sigurdsson E, Sigfusson N, Sigvaldason H, Thorgeirsson G: Silent ST-T changes in an epidemiologic cohort study—a marker of hypertension or coronary heart disease, or both: The Reykjavik Study. J Am Coll Cardiol 1996 (April);27:1140–1147.

4. Moursi MH, Bhatnagar SK, Vilacosta I, San Roman JA, Espinal MA, Nanda NC: Transesophageal echocardiographic assessment of papillary muscle rupture. Circulation 1996 (September 1);94:1003–1009.

5. Pizzulli L, Hagendorff A, Zirbes M, Fehske W, Ewig S, Jung W, Luderitz B: Influence of captopril on nitroglycerin-mediated vasodilation and development of nitrate tolerance in arterial and venous circulation. Am Heart J 1996 (February);131:342–349.

6. Chauhan A, Mullins PA, Taylor G, Petch MC, Schofield PM: Cardioesophageal reflex: A mechanism for "linked angina" in patients with angiographically proven coronary artery disease. J Am Coll Cardiol 1996 (June);27:1621–1628.

7. Hachamovitch R, Berman DS, Kiat H, Cohen I, Cabico JA, Friedman J, Diamond GA: Exercise myocardial perfusion SPECT in patients without known coronary artery disease. Incremental prognostic value and use in risk stratification. Circulation 1996 (March 1);93:905–914.

8. Perrone-Filardi P, Pace L, Prastaro M, Squame F, Betocchi S, Soricelli A, Piscione F, Indolfi C, Crisci T, Salvatore M, Chiariello M: Assessment of myocardial viability in patients with chronic coronary artery disease. Rest-4-hour-24-hour ^{201}Tl tomography versus dobutamine echocardiography. Circulation 1996 (December 1);94:2712–2719.

9. Matsunari I, Fujino S, Taki J, Senma J, Aoyama T, Wakasugi T, Hirai J, Saga T, Ichiyanagi K, Hisada K: Impaired fatty acid uptake in ischemic but viable myocardium identified by thallium-201 reinjection. Am Heart J 1996 (March);131:458–465.

10. Schulman SP, Fleg JL, Goldberg AP, Busby-Whitehead J, Hagberg JM, O'Connor FC, Gerstenblith G, Becker LC, Katzel LI, Lakatta LE, Lakatta EG: Continuum of cardiovascular performance across a broad range of fitness levels in healthy older men. Circulation 1996 (August 1);94:359–367.

11. Blumenthal RS, Becker DM, Moy TF, Coresh J, Wilder LB, Becker LC: Exercise thallium tomography predicts future clinically manifest coronary heart disease in a high-risk asymptomatic population. Circulation 1996 (March 1);93:915–923.

12. Varga A, Picano E, Cortigiani L, Petix N, Margaria F, Magaia O, Heyman J, Bigi R, Mathias W, Gigli G, Landi P, Raciti M, Pingitore A, Sicari R: Does stress echocardiography predict the site of future myocardial infarction? A large-scale multicenter study. J Am Coll Cardiol 1996 (July);28:45–51.

13. Weiss EJ, Bray PF, Tayback M, Schulman SP, Kickler TS, Becker LC, Weiss JL, Gerstenblith G, Goldschmidt-Clermont PJ: A polymorphism of a platelet glycoprotein receptor as an inherited risk factor for coronary thrombosis. N Engl J Med 1996 (April 25);334:1090–1094.

14. Wang XL, McCredie RM, Wilcken DEL: Genotype distribution of angiotensin-converting enzyme polymorphism in Australian healthy and coronary populations in relevance to myocardial infarction and coronary disease. Atheroscl Thromb Vasc Biol 1996 (January);16:115–119.

15. Pingitore A, Picano E, Colosso MQ, Reisenhofer B, Gigli G, Lucarini AR, Petix N, Previtali M, Bigi R, Chiaranda G, Minardi G, de Alcantara M, Lowenstein J, Sclavo MG, Palmieri C, Galati A, Seveso G, Heyman J, Mathias W Jr, Casazza F, Sicari R, Raciti M: The atropine factor in pharmacologic stress echocardiography. J Am Coll Cardiol 1996 (April);27:1164–1170.

16. Senior R, Raval U, Lahiri A: Prognostic value of stress dobutamine technetium-99m sestamibi single-photon emission computed tomography (SPECT) in patients with suspected coronary artery disease. Am J Cardiol (November 15) 1996;78:1092–1096.

17. He ZX, Dakik HA, Vaduganathan P, Qureshi U, Mahmarian JJ, Verani MS: Clinical and angiographic significance of a normal thallium-201 tomographic study in patients with a strongly positive exercise electrocardiogram. Am J Cardiol 1996 (September) 150;78:638–641.

18. Meza MF, Mobarek S, Sonnemaker R, Shuler S, Ramee SR, Collins TJ, White CJ, Aristizabal D, Murgo JP, Cheirif J: Myocardial contrast echocardiography in human beings: Correlation of resting perfusion defects to sestamibi single photon emission computed tomography. Am Heart J 1996 (September);132:528–535.

19. Ginzton LE, Rodrigues D, Shapiro SM, Laks MM, Conant R, Lobodzinski SM: Estimation of regional end-systolic wall stress during exercise in coronary artery disease. Am Heart J 1996 (October);132:733–746.

20. Lauer MS, Okin PM, Larson MG, Evans JC, Levy D: Impaired heart rate response to graded exercise. Prognostic implications of chronotropic incompetence in the Framingham Heart Study. Circulation 1996 (April 15);93:1520–1526.

21. Barthélémy J-C, Roche F, Gaspoz J-M, Geyssant A, Minini P, Antoniadis A, Page É, Wolf J-É, Wilner C, Isaaz K, Cavallaro C, Lacour J-R: Maximal blood lactate level acts as a major discriminant variable in exercise testing for coronary artery disease detection in men. Circulation 1996 (January);93:246–252.

22. Krittayaphong R, Biles PL, Christy CG, Sheps DS: Association between angina pectoris and ischemic indexes during exercise testing and ambulatory monitoring. Am J Cardiol 1996 (August 1);78:266–270.

23. Ambrosio G, Betocchi S, Pace L, Losi MA, Perrone-Filardi P, Soricelli A, Piscione F, Taube J, Squame F, Salvatore M, Weiss JL, Chiariello M: Prolonged impairment of regional contractile function after resolution of exercise-induced angina. Evidence of myocardial stunning in patients with coronary artery disease. Circulation 1996 (November 15);94:2455–2464.

24. Maybaum S, Ilan M, Mogilevsky J, Tzivoni D: Improvement in ischemic parameters during repeated exercise testing: a possible model for myocardial preconditioning. Am J Cardiol (November 15) 1996;78:1087–1091.

25. Marcovitz PA, Shayna V, Horn RA, Hepner A, Armstrong WF: Value of dobutamine stress echocardiography in determining the prognosis of patients with known or suspected coronary artery disease. Am J Cardiol 1996 (August 15);78:404–408.

26. Merz CNB, Moriel M, Rozanski A, Klein J, Berman DS: Gender-related differences in exercise ventricular function among healthy subjects and patients. Am Heart J 1996 (April);131:704–709.

27. Bax JJ, Cornel JH, Visser FC, Fioretti PM, van Lingen A, Reijs AEM, Boersma E, Teule GJJ, Visser CA: Prediction of recovery of myocardial dysfunction after revascularization comparison of fluorine-18 fluorodexoyglucose/thallium-201 SPECT, thallium-201 stress-reinjection SPECT and dobutamine echocardiography. J Am Coll Cardiol 1996 (September);28:558–564.

28. vom Dahl J, Muzik O, Wolfe ER Jr, Allman C, Hutchins G, Schwaiger M: Myocardial rubidium-82 tissue kinetics assessed by dynamic positron emission tomography as a marker of myocardial cell membrane integrity and viability. Circulation 1996 (January);93:238–245.

29. Mäki M, Luotolahti M, Nuutila P, Iida H, Voipio-Pulkki L-M, Ruotsalainen U, Haaparanta M, Solin O, Hartiala J, Härkönen R, Knuuti J: Glucose uptake in the chronically dysfunctional but viable myocardium. Circulation 1996 (May 1);93:1658–1666.

30. Schwarz ER, Schaper J, vom Dahl J, Altehoefer C, Grohmann B, Schoendube F, Sheehan FH, Uebis R, Buell U, Messmer BJ, Schaper W, Hanrath P: Myocyte degeneration and cell death in hibernating human myocardium. J Am Coll Cardiol 1996(June);27:1577–1585.

31. Indolfi C, Piscione F, Perrone-Filardi P, Prastaro M, Di Lorenzo E, Sacca L, Salvatore M, Condorelli M, Chiariello M: Inotropic stimulation by dobutamine increases left ventricular regional function at the expense of metabolism in hibernating myocardium. Am Heart J 1996 (September);132:542–549.

32. Conversano A, Walsh JF, Geltman EM, Perez JE, Bergmann SR, Gropler RJ: Delineation of myocardial stunning and hibernation by positron emission tomography in advanced coronary artery disease. Am Heart J 1996 (March);131:440–450.

33. Gerber BL, Vanoverschelde J-LJ, Bol A, Michel C, Labar D, Wijns W, Melin JA: Myocardial blood flow, glucose uptake, and recruitment of inotropic reserve in chronic left ventricular ischemic dysfunction. Implications for the pathophysiology of chronic myocardial hibernation. Circulation 1996 (August 15);94:651–659.

34. Gibson CM, Cannon CP, Daley WL, Dodge JT Jr, Alexander B, Marble SJ, McCabe CH, Raymond L, Fortin T, Poole WK, Braunwald E, for the TIMI 4 Study Group. TIMI frame count: a quantitative method of assessing coronary artery flow. Circulation 1996 (March 1);93:879–888.

35. Hundley WG, Lange RA, Clarke GD, Meshack BM, Payne J, Landau C, McColl R, Sayad DE, Willett DL, Willard JE, Hillis LD, Peshock RM: Assessment of coronary arterial flow and flow reserve in humans with MRI. Circulation 1996 (April 15); 93:1502–1508.

36. Nakamura M, Tsunoda T, Wakatsuki T, Ui K, Degawa T, Yabuki S, Yamaguchi T: Distal coronary flow velocity immediately after direct angioplasty for acute myocardial infarction. Am Heart J 1996 (August);132:251–257.

37. Nakamura M, Tsunoda T, Wakatsuki T, Ui K, Degawa T, Yabuki S, Yamaguchi T: Safety and feasibility of continuous monitoring of coronary flow velocity in acute myocardial infarction by Doppler guide wire. Am Heart J 1996 (September); 132:567–571.

38. Tron C, Donohue TJ, Bach RG, Wolford T, Caracciolo EA, Aguirre FV, Khoury A, Kern MJ: Differential characterization of human coronary collateral blood flow velocity. Am Heart J 1996 (September);132:508–515.

39. Nitzsche EU, Choi Y, Czernin J, Hoh CK, Huang S-C, Schelbert HR: Noninvasive quantification of myocardial blood flow in humans. A direct comparison of the [^{13}N]ammonia and the [^{15}O]water techniques. Circulation 1996 (June 1);93: 2000–2006.

40. Thieme T, Wernecke KD, Meyer R, Brandenstein E, Habedank D, Hinz A, Felix SB, Baumann G, Kleber FX: Angioscopic evaluation of atherosclerotic plaques: Validation by histomorphologic analysis and association with stable and unstable coronary syndromes. J Am Coll Cardiol 1996(July);28:1–6.

41. Juhan-Vague I, Pyke SDM, Alessi MC, Jespersen J, Haverkate F, Thompson SG, on behalf of the ECAT Study Group. Fibrinolytic factors and the risk of myocardial infarction or sudden death in patients with angina pectoris. Circulation 1996 (November 1);94:2057–2063.

42. de Maat MPM, de Bart ACW, Hennis BC, Meijer P, Havelaar AC, Mulder PGH, Kluft C: Interindividual and intraindividual variability in plasma fibrinogen, tPA antigen, PAI activity, and CRP in healthy, young volunteers and patients with angina pectoris. Arterioscl Thromb Vasc Biol 1996 (September);16:1156–1162.

43. Savonitto S, Ardissino D, Egstrup K, Rasmussen K, Bae EA, Omland T, Schjelderup-Mathiesen PM, Marraccini P, Wahlqvist I, Merlini PA, Rehnqvist N: Combination therapy with metoprolol and nifedipine versus monotherapy in patients with stable angina pectoris: results of the International Multicenter Angina Exercise (IMAGE) Study. J Am Coll Cardiol 1996 (February);27:311–316.

44. von Arnim T: Prognostic significance of transient ischemic episodes: Response to treatment shows improved prognosis—Results of the Total Ischemic Burden Bisoprolol Study (TIBBS) follow-up. J Am Coll Cardiol 1996 (July);28:20–24.

45. Gomez MA, Anderson JL, Karagounis LA, Muhlestein JB, Mooers FB: An emergency department-based protocol for rapidly ruling out myocardial ischemia reduces hospital time and expense: Results of a randomized study (ROMIO). J Am Coll Cardiol 1996 (July);28:25–33.

46. Krantz DS, Kop WJ, Gabbay FH, Rozanski A, Barnard M, Klein J, Pardo Y, Gottdiener JS: Circadian variation of ambulatory myocardial ischemia. Triggering by daily activities and evidence for an endogenous circadian component. Circulation 1996 (April 1);93:1364–1371.

47. Pepine CJ, Andrews T, Deanfield JE, Forman S, Geller N, Hill JA, Pratt C, Rogers WJ, Sopko G, Steingart R, Stone PH, Conti CR, for the ACIP Study Group: Relation of patient characteristics to cardiac ischemia during daily life activity (an asymptomatic cardiac ischemia pilot data bank study). Am J Cardiol 1996 (June 15);77: 1267–1272.

48. Stone PH, Chaitman BR, McMahon RP, Andrews TC, MacCallum G, Sharaf B, Frishman W, Deanfield JE, Sopko G, Pratt C, Goldberg AD, Rogers WJ, Hill J, Proschan M, Pepine CJ, Bourassa MG, Conti CR, for the ACIP Investigators. Asymptomatic cardiac ischemia pilot (ACIP) study: Relationship between exercise-induced and ambulatory ischemia in patients with stable coronary disease. Circulation 1996 (October 1);94:1537–1544.

49. Pratt CM, McMahon RP, Goldstein S, Pepine CJ, Andrews TC, Dyrda I, Frishman WH, Geller NL, Hill JA, Morgan NA, Stone PH, Knatterud GL, Sopko G, Conti CR, for the ACIP Investigators: Comparison of subgroups assigned to medical regimens used to suppress cardiac ischemia (The Asymptomatic Cardiac Ischemia Pilot (ACIP) Study). Am J Cardiol 1996 (June 15);77:1302–1309.

50. Després J-P, Lamarche B, Mauriège P, Cantin B, Dagenais GR, Moorjani S, Lupien P-J: Hyperinsulinemia as an independent risk factor for ischemic heart disease. N Engl J Med 1996 (April 11);334:952–957.

51. Madjlessi-Simon T, Mary-Krause M, Fillette F, Lechat P, Jaillon P: Persistent transient myocardial ischemia despite beta-adrenergic blockade predicts a higher risk of adverse cardiac events in patients with coronary artery disease. J Am Coll Cardiol 1996 (June);27:1586–1591.

52. Mulcahy D, Dakak N, Zalos G, Andrews NP, Proschan M, Waclawiw MA, Schenke WH, Quyyumi AA: Patterns and behavior of transient myocardial ischemia in stable coronary disease are the same in both men and women: A comparative study. J Am Coll Cardiol 1996 (June);27:1629–1636.

53. Harpaz D, Benderly M, Goldbourt U, Kishon Y, Behar S, for the Israeli BIP Study Group. Effect of aspirin on mortality in women with symptomatic or silent myocardial ischemia. Am J Cardiol 1996 (December 1);78:1215–1219.

54. van Boven AJ, Jukema JW, Zwinderman AH, Crijns HJGM, Lie KI, Bruschke AVG, on behalf of the REGRESS Study Group. Reduction of transient myocardial ischemia with pravastatin in addition to the conventional treatment in patients with angina pectoris. Circulation 1996 (October 1);94:1503–1505.

55. Ylitalo K, Jama L, Raatikainen P, Peuhkurinen K: Adaptation to myocardial ischemia during repeated dynamic exercise in relation to findings at cardiac catheterization. Am Heart J 1996 (April);131:689–697.

56. Onaka H, Hirota Y, Shimada S, Kita Y, Sakai Y, Kawakami Y, Suzuki S, Kawamura K: Clinical observation of spontaneous anginal attacks and multivessel spasm in variant angina pectoris with normal coronary arteries: Evaluation by 24-hour 12-lead electrocardiography with computer analysis. J Am Coll Cardiol 1996 (January);27:38–44.

57. Bøtker HE, Sonne HS, Sørensen KE: Frequency of systemic microvascular dysfunction in syndrome X and in variant angina. Am J Cardiol 1996 (July 15);78:182–186.

58. Miwa K, Miyagi Y, Igawa A, Nakagawa K, Inoue H: Vitamin E deficiency in variant angina. Circulation 1996 (July 1);94:14–18.

59. Kugiyama K, Yasue H, Okumura K, Ogawa H, Fujimoto K, Nakao K, Yoshimura M, Motoyama T, Inobe Y, Kawano H: Nitric oxide activity is deficient in spasm arteries of patients with coronary spastic angina. Circulation 1996 (August 1);94:266–272.

60. De Servi S, Arbustini E, Marsico F, Bramucci E, Angoli L, Porcu E, Costante AM, Kubica J, Boschetti E, Valentini P, Specchia G: Correlation between clinical and morphologic findings in unstable angina. Am J Cardiol 1996 (January 15);77:128–132.

61. Lindahl B, Venge P, Wallentin L, for the FRISC Study Group. Relation between troponin T and the risk of subsequent coronary events in unstable coronary artery disease. Circulation 1996 (May 1);93:1651–1657.

62. Biasucci LM, Liuzzo G, Caligiuri G, Quaranta G, Andreotti F, Sperti G, van de Greef W, Rebuzzi AG, Kluft C, Maseri A: Temporal relation between ischemic episodes and activation of the coagulation system in unstable angina. Circulation 1996 (June 15);93:2121–2127.

63. Kikuta K, Yasue H, Yoshimura M, Morita E, Sumida H, Kato H, Kugiyama K,

Ogawa H, Okumura K, Ogawa Y, Nakao K: Increased plasma levels of B-type natriuretic peptide in patients with unstable angina. Am Heart J 1996 (July);132: 101–107.

64. Liuzzo G, Biasucci LM, Rebuzzi AG, Gallimore JR, Caligiuri G, Lanza GA, Quaranta G, Monaco C, Pepys MB, Maseri A: Plasma protein acute-phase response in unstable angina is not induced by ischemic injury. Circulation 1996 (November 15);94:2373–2380.

65. Fujita M, Ikemoto M, Kishishita M, Otani H, Nohara R, Tanaka T, Tamaki S, Yamazato A, Sasayama S: Elevated basic fibroblast growth factor in pericardial fluid of patients with unstable angina. Circulation 1996 (August 15);94:610–613.

66. Moreno PR, Bernardi VH, López-Cuéllar J, Murcia AM, Palacios IF, Gold HK, Mehran R, Sharma SK, Nemerson Y, Fuster V, Fallon JT: Macrophages, smooth muscle cells, and tissue factor in unstable angina. Implications for cell-mediated thrombogenicity in acute coronary syndromes. Circulation 1996 (December 15); 94:3090–3097.

67. Ott I, Neumann F-J, Gawaz M, Schmitt M, Schömig A: Increased neutrophil-platelet adhesion in patients with unstable angina. Circulation 1996 (September 15);94:1239–1246.

68. Théroux P, Kouz S, Roy L, Knudtson ML, Diodati JG, Marquis J-F, Nasmith J, Fung AY, Boudreault J-R, Delage F, Dupuis R, Kells C, Bokslag M, Steiner B, Rapold HJ, on Behalf of the Investigators. Platelet membrane receptor glycoprotein IIb/IIIa antagonism in unstable angina. The Canadian Lamifiban study. Circulation 1996 (September 1);94:899–905.

69. Schulman SP, Goldschmidt-Clermont PJ, Topol EJ, Califf RM, Navetta FI, Willerson JT, Chandra NC, Guerci AD, Ferguson JJ, Harrington RA, Lincoff AM, Yakubov SJ, Bray PF, Bahr RD, Wolfe CL, Yock PG, Anderson HV, Nygaard TW, Mason SJ, Effron MB, Fatterpacker A, Raskin S, Smith J, Brashears L, Gottdiener P, du Mee C, Kitt MM, Gerstenblith G: Effects of integrelin, a platelet glycoprotein IIb/IIIa receptor antagonist, in unstable angina. A randomized multicenter trial. Circulation 1996 (November 1);94:2083–2089.

70. Moreno PR, Bernardi VH, López-Cuéllar J, Newell JB, McMellon C, Gold HK, Palacios IF, Fuster V, Fallon JT: Macrophage infiltration predicts restenosis after coronary intervention in patients with unstable angina. Circulation 1996 (December 15);94:3098–3102.

71. Biasucci LM, Vitelli A, Liuzzo G, Altamura S, Caligiuri G, Monaco C, Rebuzzi AG, Ciliberto G, Maseri A: Elevated levels of interleukin-6 in unstable angina. Circulation 1996 (September 1);94:874–877.

72. Ardissino D, Merlini PA, Gamba G, Barberis P, Demicheli G, Testa S, Colombi E. Poli A, Fetiveau R, Montemartini C: Thrombin activity and early outcome in unstable angina pectoris. Circulation 1996 (May 1);93:1634–1639.

73. Langford EJ, Wainwright RJ, Martin JF: Platelet activation in acute myocardial infarction and unstable angina is inhibited by nitric-oxide donors. Atheroscl Thromb Vasc Biol 1996 (January);16:51–55.

74. Peters RW, Brooks MM, Zoble RG, Liebson PR, Seals AA, for the CAST Investigators. Chronobiology of acute myocardial infarction: Cardiac Arrhythmia Suppression Trial (CAST) experience. Am J Cardiol 1996 (December 1);78:1198–1201.

75. Ornato JP, Peberdy MA, Chandra NC, Bush DE: Seasonal Pattern of Acute Myocardial Infarction in the National Registry of Myocardial Infarction. J Am Coll Cardiol 1996 (December);28:1684–1688.

76. Lee RT, Schoen FJ, Loree HM, Lark MW, Libby P: Circumferential stress and matrix metalloproteinase 1 in human coronary atherosclerosis: implications for plaque rupture. Arterioscl Thromb Vasc Biol. 1996 (August);16:1070–1073.

77. Kern MJ, Moore JA, Aguirre FV, Bach RG, Caracciolo EA, Wolford T, Khoury AF, Mechem C, Donohue TJ: Determination of angiographic (TIMI grade) blood flow by intracoronary Doppler flow velocity during acute myocardial infarction. Circulation 1996 (October 1);94:1545–1552.

78. Every NR, Spertus J, Fihn SD, Hlatky M, Martin JS, Weaver WD: Length of hospital stay after acute myocardial infarction in the myocardial infarction triage and intervention (MITI) project registry. J Am Coll Cardiol 1996(August);28:287–293.

79. Barefoot JC, Schroll M: Symptoms of depression, acute myocardial infarction, and total mortality in a community sample. Circulation 1996 (June 1);93:1976–1980.

80. Leor J, Kloner RA, for the Investigators: The Northridge earthquake as a trigger for acute myocardial infarction. Am J Cardiol 1996 (June 1);77:1230–1232.

81. Muller JE, Mittleman MA, Maclure M, Sherwood JB, Tofler GH, for the Determinants of Myocardial Infarction Onset Study Investigators. Triggering myocardial infarction by sexual activity: Low absolute risk and prevention by regular physical exertion. JAMA 1996 (May 8);275:1405–1409.

82. Müllner M, Sterz F, Binder M, Brunner M, Hirschl MM, Mustafa G, Schreiber W, Kürkciyan I, Domanovits H, Laggner AN: Creatine kinase and creatine kinase-MB release after nontraumatic cardiac arrest. Am J Cardiol 1996 (March 15);77: 581–585.

83. Midgette AS, Griffith JL, Califf RM, Laks MM, Dietz SB, Beshansky JR, Selker HP: Prediction of the infarct-related artery in acute myocardial infarction by a scoring system using summary ST-segment and T-wave changes. Am J Cardiol 1996 (August 15);78:389–395.

84. Birnbaum Y, Kloner RA, Sclarovsky S, Cannon CP, McCabe CH, Davis VG, Zaret BL, Wackers FJT, Braunwald E, for the TIMI 4 Investigators: Distortion of the terminal portion of the QRS on the admission electrocardiogram in acute myocardial infarction and correlation with infarct size and long-term prognosis (Thrombolysis in Myocardial Infarction 4 Trial). Am J Cardiol 1996 (August 15);78: 396–403.

85. Peterson ED, Hathaway WR, Zabel M, Pieper KS, Granger CB, Wagner GS, Topol EJ, Bates ER, Simoons ML, Califf RM: Prognostic significance of precordial ST segment depression during inferior myocardial infarction in the thrombolytic era: Results in 16,521 patients. J Am Coll Cardiol 1996 (August);28:305–312.

86. Schröder K, Völler H, Dingerkus H, Münzberg H, Dissman R, Linderer T, Schultheiss HP: Comparison of the diagnostic potential of four echocardiographic stress tests shortly after acute myocardial infarction: Submaximal exercise, transesophageal atrial pacing, dipyridamole, and dobutamine-atropine. Am J Cardiol 1996 (May 1);77:909–914.

87. Elhendy A, Trocino G, Salustri A, Cornel JH, Roelandt JRTC, Boersma E, van Domburg RT, Krenning EP, El-Said GM, Fioretti PM. Low-dose dobutamine echocardiography and rest-redistribution thallium-201 tomography in the assessment of spontaneous recovery of left ventricular function after recent myocardial infarction. Am Heart J 1996 (June);131:1088–1096.

88. Naito J, Masuyama T, Yamamoto K, Mano T, Kondo H, Nagano R, Doi Y, Morozumi T, Ito H, Fujii K, Hori M, Kamada T. Myocardial integrated ultrasonic backscatter in patients with old myocardial infarction: Comparison with radionuclide evaluation. Am Heart J 1996 (July);132:54–60.

89. Kuntz KM, Tsevat J, Goldman L, Weinstein MC. Cost-effectiveness of routine coronary angiography after acute myocardial infarction. Circulation 1996 (September 1);94:957–965.

90. Køber L, Torp-Pedersen C, Ottesen M, Burchardt H, Korup E, Lyngborg K, on behalf of the TRACE Study Group: Influence of age on the prognostic importance of left ventricular dysfunction and congestive heart failure on long-term survival after acute myocardial infarction. Am J Cardiol 1996 (July 15);78:158–162.

91. Njølstad I, Arnesen E, Lund-Larsen PG. Smoking, serum lipids, blood pressure, and sex differences in myocardial infarction. A 12-year follow-up of the Finnmark study. Circulation 1996 (February);93:450–456.

92. Moriel M, Benhorin J, Brown MW, Raubertas RF, Severski PK, Van Voorhees L, Bodenheimer MM, Tzivoni D, Wackers FJT, Moss AJ, The Multicenter Myocardial Ischemia Research Group: Detection and significance of myocardial ischemia in women versus men within six months of acute myocardial infarction or unstable angina. Am J Cardiol 1996 (April 15);77:798–804.

93. Phillips GB, Pinkernell BH, Jing T-Y: The association of hyperestrogenemia with coronary thrombosis in men. Arterioscl Thromb Vasc Biol 1996 (November);16: 1383–1387.

94. Singh N, Mironov D, Armstrong PW, Ross AM, Langer A, for the GUSTO ECG Substudy Investigators. Heart rate variability assessment early after acute myocardial infarction: pathophysiological and prognostic correlates. Circulation 1996 (April 1);93:1388–1395.

95. Ito H, Maruyama A, Iwakura K, Takiuchi S, Masuyama T, Hori M, Higashino Y, Fujii K, Minamino T. Clinical implications of the 'no reflow' phenomenon. A predictor of complications and left ventricular remodeling in reperfused anterior wall myocardial infarction. Circulation 1996 (January);93:223–228.

96. Becker RC, Cannon CP, Bovill EG, Tracy RP, Thompson B, Knatterud GL, Randall A, Braunwald E, for the TIMI III Investigators: Prognostic value of plasma fibrinogen concentration in patients with unstable angina and non-Q-wave myocardial infarction (TIMI IIIB Trial). Am J Cardiol 1996 (July 15);78:142–147.

97. Behague I, Poirier O, Nicaud V, Evans A, Arveiler D, Luc G, Cambou J-P, Scarabin P-Y, Bara L, Green F, Cambien F. β fibrinogen gene polymorphisms are associated with plasma fibrinogen and coronary artery disease in patients with myocardial infarction. The ECTIM study. Circulation 1996 (February);93:440–449.

98. Kobayashi K, Kitamura K, Hirayama N, Date H, Kashiwagi T, Ikushima I, Hanada Y, Nagatomo Y, Takenaga M, Ishikawa T, Imamura T, Koiwaya, Eto T. Increased plasma adrenomedullin in acute myocardial infarction. Am Heart J 1996 (April); 131:676–680.

99. Haider AW, Andreotti F, Thompson GR, Kluft C, Maseri A, Davies GJ. Serum lipoprotein(a) level is related to thrombin generation and spontaneous intermittent coronary occlusion in patients with acute myocardial infarction. Circulation 1996 (November 1);94:2072–2076.

100. Stampfer MJ, Krauss RM, Ma J, Blanche PJ, Holl LG, Sacks FM, Hennekens CH. A prospective study of triglyceride level, low-density lipoprotein particle diameter, and risk of myocardial infarction. JAMA 1996 (September 18);276:882–888.

101. Stubbs P, Collinson P, Moseley D, Greenwood T, Noble M. Prognostic significance of admission troponin T concentrations in patients with myocardial infarction. Circulation 1996 (September 15);94:1291–1297.

102. Arakawa N, Nakamura M, Aoki H, Hiramori K: Plasma brain natriuretic peptide concentrations predict survival after acute myocardial infarction. J Am Coll Cardiol 1996 (June);27:1656–1661.

103. Omland T, Aakvaag A, Bonarjee VVS, Caidahl K, Lie RT, Nilsen DWT, Sundsfjord JA, Dickstein K. Plasma brain natriuretic peptide as an indicator of left ventricular systolic function and long-term survival after acute myocardial infarction. Comparison with plasma atrial natriuretic peptide and N-terminal proatrial natriuretic peptide. Circulation 1996 (June 1);93:1963–1969.

104. Zoni-Berisso M, Molini D, Mela GS, Vecchio C: Value of programmed ventricular stimulation in predicting sudden death and sustained ventricular tachycardia in survivors of acute myocardial infarction. Am J Cardiol 1996 (April 1);77:673–680.

105. Brand FN, Larson M, Friedman LM, Kannel WB, Castelli WP. Epidemiologic assessment of angina before and after myocardial infarction. The Framingham Study. Am Heart J 1996 (July);132:174–178.

106. Ueda S, Ikeda U, Yamamoto K, Takahashi M, Nishinaga M, Nago N, Shimada K. C-reactive protein as a predictor of cardiac rupture after acute myocardial infarction. Am Heart J 1996 (May);131:857–860.

107. Figueras J, Curos A, Cortadellas J, Soler-Soler J. Reliability of electromechanical dissociation in the diagnosis of left ventricular free wall rupture in acute myocardial infarction. Am Heart J 1996 (May);131:861–864.

108. Huikuri HV, Seppänen T, Koistinen MJ, Airaksinen KEJ, Ikäheimo MJ, Castellanos A, Myerburg RJ. Abnormalities in beat-to-beat dynamics of heart rate before the spontaneous onset of life-threatening ventricular tachyarrhythmias in patients with prior myocardial infarction. Circulation 1996 (May 15);93:1836–1844.

109. Van Dantzig JM, Delemarre BJ, Koster RW, Bot H, Visser CA. Pathogenesis of MR in acute myocardial infarction: Importance of changes in left ventricular shape and regional function. Am Heart J 1996 (May);131:865–871.

110. Irimpen AM, Tenaglia AN, Shin DJ, Buda AJ. Lack of ventricular remodeling in non-Q-wave myocardial infarction. Am Heart J 1996 (March);131:466–471.

111. Mortara A, Specchia G, La Rovere MT, Bigger JT Jr., Marcus FI, Camm JA, Hohn-loser SH, Nohara R, Schwartz PJ, on behalf of the ATRAMI Investigators. Patency of infarct-related artery: effect of restoration of anterograde flow on vagal reflexes. Circulation 1996 (March 15);93:1114–1122.

112. LeFeuvre CA, Connolly SJ, Cairns JA, Gent M, Roberts RS: Comparison of mortality from acute myocardial infarction between 1979 and 1992 in a geographically defined stable population. Am J Cardiol 1996 (December 15);78:1345–1349.

113. Rouleau JL, Talajic M, Sussex B, Potvin L, Warnica W, Davies RF, Gardner M, Stewart D, Plante S, Dupuis R, Lauzon C, Ferguson J, Mikes E, Balnozan V, Savard P: Myocardial infarction patients in the 1990s—their risk factors, stratification and survival in Canada: The Canadian Assessment of Myocardial Infarction (CAMI) study. J Am Coll Cardiol 1996 (April);27:1119–1127.

114. Gheorghiade M, Ruzumna P, Borzak S, Havstad S, Ali A, Goldstein S. Decline in the rate of hospital mortality from acute myocardial infarction: Impact of changing management strategies. Am Heart J 1996 (February);131:250–256.

115. Misao J, Hayakawa Y, Ohno M, Kato S, Fujiwara T, Fujiwara H. Expression of bcl-2 protein, an inhibitor of apoptosis, and Bax, an accelerator of apoptosis, in ventricular myocytes of human hearts with myocardial infarction. Circulation 1996 (October 1);94:1506–1512.

116. Hattori T, Sumimoto T, Yuasa F, Kaida M, Jikuhara T, Hikosaka M, Sugiura T, Iwasaka T. Influence of intrinsic limb vasodilator capacity on exercise tolerance in patients with recent myocardial infarction. Am Heart J 1996 (September);132: 593–598.

117. Oka RK, Fortmann SP, Varady AN: Differences in treatment of acute myocardial infarction by sex, age, and other factors (The Stanford Five-City Project). Am J Cardiol (October 15) 1996;78:861–865.

118. Kudenchuk PJ, Maynard C, Martin JS, Wirkus M, Weaver WD, for the MITI Project Investigators: Comparison of presentation, treatment, and outcome of acute myocardial infarction in men versus women (The Myocardial Infarction Triage and Intervention Registry). Am J Cardiol 1996 (July 1);78:9–14.

119. Azar AJ, Cannegieter SC, Deckers JW, Briët E, van Bergen PMM, Jonker JJC, Rosendaal FR: Optimal intensity of oral anticoagulant therapy after myocardial infarction. J Am Coll Cardiol 1996 (May);27:1349–1355.

120. Singh RB, Niaz MA, Rastogi SS, Rastogi S: Usefulness of antioxidant vitamins in suspected acute myocardial infarction (The Indian Experiment of Infarct Survival-3). Am J Cardiol 1996 (February 1);77:232–236.

121. Rengo F, Carbonin P, Pahor M, DeCaprio L, Bernabei R, Ferrara N, Carosella L, Acanfora D, Parlati S, Vitale D, CRIS Investigators: A controlled trial of verapamil in patients after acute myocardial infarction: Results of the calcium antagonist reinfarction Italian study (CRIS). Am J Cardiol 1996 (February 15);77:365–369.

122. Zuanetti G, Latini R, Avanzini F, Franzosi MG, Maggioni AP, Colombo F, Nicolis E, Mauri F, on behalf of the GISSI Investigators: Trends and determinants of calcium antagonist usage after acute myocardial infarction (The GISSI Experience). Am J Cardiol 1996 (July 15);78:153–157.

123. Waldo AL, Camm AJ, deRuyter H, Friedman PL, MacNeil DJ, Pauls JF, Pitt B, Pratt CM, Schwartz PJ, Veltri EP, for the SWORD Investigators. Effect of d-sotalol on mortality in patients with left ventricular dysfunction after recent and remote myocardial infarction. Lancet 1996 (July 6);348:7–12.

124. Bonarjee VVS, Carstensen S, Caidahl K, Nilsen DWT, Edner M, Lindvall K, Snapinn SM, Berning J. Benefit of converting enzyme inhibition on left ventricular volumes and ejection fraction in patients receiving β-blockade after myocardial infarction. Am Heart J 1996 (July);132:71–77.

125. Gruppo Italiano per Lo Studio Della Sopravvivenza Nell'Infarto Miocardico: Six-month effects of early treatment with isinopril and transdermal glyceryl trinitrate singly and together withdrawn six weeks after acute myocardial infarction: The GISSI-3 trial. J Am Coll Cardiol 1996 (February);27:337–344.

126. Boersma E, Maas ACP, Deckers JW, Simoons ML. Early thrombolytic treatment in acute myocardial infarction: reappraisal of the golden hour. Lancet 1996 (September 21);348:771–775.

127. O'Connor CM, Meese RB, McNulty S, Lucas KD, Carney RJ, LeBoeuf RM, Maddox W, Bethea CF, Shadoff N, Trahey TF, Heinsimer JA, Burks JM, O'Donnell G, Krucoff MW, Califf RM, DUCCS-II Investigators: A randomized factorial trial of reperfusion strategies and aspirin dosing in acute myocardial infarction. Am J Cardiol 1996 (April 15);77:791–797.

128. Glick A, Kornowski R, Michowich Y, Koifman B, Roth A, Laniado S, Keren G: Reduction of reinfarction and angina with use of low-molecular-weight heparin therapy after streptokinase (and heparin) in acute myocardial infarction. Am J Cardiol 1996 (June 1);77:1145–1148.

129. Mahaffey KW, Granger CB, Collins R, O'Connor CM, Ohman EM, Bleich SD, Col JJ, Califf RM: Overview of randomized trials of intravenous heparin in patients with acute myocardial infarction treated with thrombolytic therapy. Am J Cardiol 1996 (March 15);77:551–556.

130. Califf RM, White HD, Van de Werf F, Sadowski Z, Armstrong PW, Vahanian A, Simoons ML, Simes RJ, Lee KL, Topol EJ, for the GUSTO-I Investigators. One-year results from the Global Utilization of Streptokinase and tPA for Occluded Coronary Arteries (GUSTO-I) trial. Circulation 1996 (September 15);94:1233–1238.

131. The Global Use of Strategies to Open Occluded Coronary Arteries (GUSTO) IIb Investigators. A comparison of recombinant hirudin with heparin for the treatment of acute coronary syndromes. N Engl J Med 1996 (September 12);335:775–82.

132. Antman EM, for the TIMI 9B Investigators. Hirudin in acute myocardial infarction: Thrombolysis and thrombin inhibition in myocardial infarction (TIMI) 9B trial. Circulation 1996 (September 1);94:911–921.

133. Leschke M, Schoebel FC, Mecklenbeck W, Stein D, Jax TW, Muller-Gartner HW, Strauer BE: Long-term intermittent urokinase therapy in patients with end-stage coronary artery disease and refractory angina pectoris: A randomized dose-response trial. J Am Coll Cardiol 1996 (March 1);27:575–584.

134. Bode C, Smalling RW, Berg G, Burnett C, Lorch G, Kalbfleisch JM, Chernoff R, Christie LG, Feldman RL, Seals AA, Weaver WD, for the RAPID II Investigators. Randomized comparison of coronary thrombolysis achieved with double-bolus reteplase (recombinant plasminogen activator) and front-loaded, accelerated alteplase (recombinant tPA) in patients with acute myocardial infarction. Circulation 1996 (September 1);94:891–898.

135. Kono T, Morita H, Nishina T, Fujita M, Hirota Y, Kawamura K, Fujiwara: Circadian variations of onset of acute myocardial infarction and efficacy of thrombolytic therapy. J Am Coll Cardiol 1996 (March 15);27:774–778.

136. Newby LK, Rutsch WR, Califf RM, Simoons ML, Aylward PE, Armstrong PW, Woodlief LH, Lee KL, Topol EJ, van de Werf F: Time from symptom onset to treatment and outcomes after thrombolytic therapy. J Am Coll Cardiol 1996 (June);27:1646–1655.

137. Raitt MH, Maynard C, Wagner GS, Cerqueira MD, Selvester RH, Weaver WD. Relation between symptom duration before thrombolytic therapy and final myocardial infarct size. Circulation 1996 (January);93:48–53.

138. Langer A, Goodman SAG, Topol EJ, Charlesworth A, Skene AM, Wilcox RG, Armstrong PW: Late Assessment of Thrombolytic Efficacy (LATE) Study: Prognosis in patients with non-Q wave myocardial infarction. J Am Coll Cardiol 1996 (May);27:1327–1332.

139. Granger CB, Hirsh J, Califf RM, Col J, White HD, Betriu A, Woodlief LH, Lee KL, Bovill EG, Simes J, Topol EJ, for the GUSTO-I Investigators. Activated partial thromboplastin time and outcome after thrombolytic therapy for acute myocardial infarction. Results from the GUSTO-I trial. Circulation 1996 (March 1);93:870–878.

140. Becker RC, Cannon CP, Tracy RP, Thompson B, Bovill EG, Desvigne-Nickens P, Randall AMY, Knatternud G, Braunwald E. Relation between systemic anticoagulation as determined by aPTT and heparin measurements and in-hospital clinical events in unstable angina and non-Q wave myocardial infarction. Am Heart J 1996 (March);131:421–433.

141. Scharfstein JS, Abendschein DR, Eisenberg PR, George D, Cannon CP, Becker RC, Sobel B, Cupples LA, Braunwald E, Loscalzo J, for the TIMI-5 Investigators: Usefulness of fibrinogenolytic and procoagulant markers during thrombolytic therapy in predicting clinical outcomes in acute myocardial infarction. Am J Cardiol 1996 (September 1);78:503–510.

142. Popović AD, Nešković AN, Marinković J, Thomas JD: Acute and long-term effects of thrombolysis after anterior wall acute myocardial infarction with serial assessment of infarct expansion and late ventricular remodeling. Am J Cardiol 1996 (March 1);77:446–450.

143. Bär FW, Volders PGA, Höppener P, Vermeer F, Meyer J, Wellens HJJ: Development of ST-segment elevation and Q- and R-wave changes in acute myocardial infarction and the influence of thrombolytic therapy. Am J Cardiol 1996 (February 15); 77:337–343.

144. Isselbacher EM, Siu SC, Weyman AE, Picard MH. Absence of Q waves after thrombolysis predicts more rapid improvement of regional left ventricular dysfunction. Am Heart J 1996 (April);131:649–654.

145. Peuhkurinen K, Risteli L, Jounela A, Risteli J. Changes in interstitial collagen metabolism during acute myocardial infarction treated with streptokinase or tPA. Am Heart J 1996 (January);131:7–13.

146. Dakik HA, Mahmarian JJ, Kimball KT, Koutelou MG, Medrano R, Verani MS. Prognostic value of exercise ^{201}T1 tomography in patients treated with thrombolytic therapy during acute myocardial infarction. Circulation 1996 (December 1); 94:2735–2742.

147. Khattar RS, Basu SK, Raval U, Senior R, Lahiri A: Prognostic value of predischarge exercise testing, ejection fraction, and ventricular ectopic activity in acute myocardial infarction treated with streptokinase. Am J Cardiol 1996 (July 15);78:136–141.

148. Brouwer MA, Martin JS, Maynard C, Wirkus M, Litwin PE, Verheught WAF, Weaver WD for the MITI Project Investigators: Influence of early prehospital thrombolysis on mortality and event-free survival (The Myocardial Infarction Triage and Intervention (MITI) randomized trial). Am J Cardiol 1996 (September 1); 78:497–502.

149. White HD, Barbash GI, Califf RM, Simes RJ, Granger CB, Weaver WD, Kleiman NS, Aylward PE, Gore JM, Vahanian A, Lee KL, Ross AM, Topol EJ, for the GUnited StatesTO-I Investigators. Age and outcome with contemporary thrombolytic therapy: Results from the GUSTO-I trial. Circulation 1996 (October 15);94: 1826–1833.

150. Peels KH, Visser CA, Dambrink JHE, Jaarsma W, Wielenga RP, Kamp O, Kingma JH, van Gilst WH, on behalf of the CATS Investigators Group: Left ventricular wall motion score as an early predictor of left ventricular dilation and mortality after first anterior infarction treated with thrombolysis. Am J Cardiol 1996 (June 1);77:1149–1154.

151. Zuanetti G, Neilson JMM, Latini R, Santoro E, Maggioni AP, Ewing DJ, on behalf of GISSI-2 Investigators. Prognostic significance of heart rate variability in post-myocardial infarction patients in the fibrinolytic era. The GISSI-2 Results. Circulation 1996 (August 1);94:432–436.

152. Statters DJ, Malik M, Redwood S, Hnatkova K, Staunton A, Camm AJ: Use of ventricular premature complexes for risk stratification after acute myocardial infarction in the thrombolytic era. Am J Cardiol 1996 (January 15);77:133–138.

153. Reiner JS, Lundergan CF, Fung A, Coyne K, Cho S, Israel N, Kazmierski J, Pilcher G, Smith J, Rohrbeck S, Thompson M, Van de Werf F, Ross AM, for the GUSTO-1 Angiographic Investigators. Evolution of early TIMI 2 flow after thrombolysis for acute myocardial infarction. Circulation 1996 (November 15);94:2441–2446.

154. Ito H, Okamura A, Iwakura K, Masuyama T, Hori M, Takiuchi S, Negoro S, Nakatsuchi Y, Taniyama Y, Higashino Y, Fujii K, Minamino T. Myocardial perfusion patterns related to thrombolysis in myocardial infarction perfusion grades after coronary angioplasty in patients with acute anterior wall myocardial infarction. Circulation 1996 (June 1);93:1993–1999.

155. Newby KH, Pisanó E, Krucoff MW, Green C, Natale A. Incidence and clinical relevance of the occurrence of bundle-branch block in patients treated with thrombolytic therapy. Circulation 1996 (November 15);94:2424–2428.

156. Becker RC, Gore JM, Lambrew C, Weaver WD, Rubison RM, French WJ, Tiefenbrunn AJ, Bowlby L, Rogers WJ: A composite view of cardiac rupture in the United States national registry of myocardial infarction. J Am Coll Cardiol 1996 (May); 27:1321–1326.

157. Newby LK, Califf RM, Guerci A, Weaver WD, Col J, Horgan JH, Mark DB, Stebbins A, Van de Werf F, Gore JM, Topol EJ: Early Discharge in the Thrombolytic Era: An Analysis of Criteria for Uncomplicated Infarction From the Global Utilization of Streptokinase and t-PA for Occluded Coronary Arteries (GUSTO) Trial. J Am Coll Cardiol 1996 (March 1);27:625–632.

158. Karam C, Golmard JL, Steg PG: Decreased prevalence of late potentials with mechanical versus thrombolysis-induced reperfusion in acute myocardial infarction. J Am Coll Cardiol 1996 (May);27:1343–1348.

159. Labinaz M, Sketch MH Jr, Stebbins AL, DeFranco AC, Holmes DR Jr, Kleiman NS, Betriu A, Rutsch WR, Vahanian A, Topol EJ, Califf RM, for the GUSTO-I Investigators: Thrombolytic therapy for patients with prior percutaneous transluminal coronary angioplasty and subsequent acute myocardial infarction. Am J Cardiol 1996 (December 15);78:1338–1344.

160. Laster SB, O'Keefe JH Jr, Gibbons RJ: Incidence and importance of thrombolysis in myocardial infarction grade 3 flow after primary percutaneous transluminal coronary angioplasty for acute myocardial infarction. Am J Cardiol 1996 (September 15);78:623–626.

161. Ellis SG, Elliott J, Horrigan M, Raymond RE, Howell G: Low-normal or excessive body mass index: newly identified and powerful risk factors for death and other complications with percutaneous coronary intervention. Am J Cardiol 1996 (September 15);78:642–646.

162. White CJ, Ramee SR, Collins TJ, Escobar AE, Karsan A, Shaw D, Jain SP, Bass TA, Heuser RR, Teirstein PS, Bonan R, Walter PD, Smalling RW. Coronary thrombi increase PTCA risk. Angioscopy as a clinical tool. Circulation 1996 (January);93:253–258.

163. Oltrona L, Eisenberg PR, Lasala JM, Sewall DJ, Shelton ME, Winters KJ. Association of heparin-resistant thrombin activity with acute ischemic complications of coronary interventions. Circulation 1996 (November 1);94:2064–2071.

164. Waxman S, Sassower MA, Mittleman MA, Zarich S, Miyamoto A, Manzo KS, Muller JE, Abela GS, Nesto RW. Angioscopic predictors of early adverse outcome after coronary angioplasty in patients with unstable angina and non-Q-wave myocardial infarction. Circulation 1996 (June 15);93:2106–2113.

165. Kip KE, Faxon DP, Detre KM, Yeh W, Kelsey SF, Currier JW, for the Investigators of the NHLBI PTCA Registry. Coronary angioplasty in diabetic patients: The National Heart, Lung, and Blood Institute Percutaneous Transluminal Coronary Angioplasty Registry. Circulation 1996 (October 15);94:1818–1825.

166. Abdelmeguid AE, Topol EJ, Whitlow PL, Sapp SK, Ellis SG. Significance of mild transient release of creatine kinase-MB fraction after percutaneous coronary interventions. Circulation 1996 (October 1);94:1528–1536.

167. Falcone C, Auguadro C, Sconocchia R, Catalano O, Ochan M, Angoli L. Montemartini C: Susceptibility to Pain During Coronary Angioplasty: Usefulness of Pulpal Test. J Am Coll Cardiol 1996 (October);28:903–909.

168. Waksman R, Scott NA, Ghazzal ZMB, Mays R, Frerichs FA, Petersen JY, King SB III. Randomized comparison of flexible versus nonflexible femoral sheaths on patient comfort after angioplasty. Am Heart J 1996 (June);131:1076–1078.

169. Pizzetti G, Belotti G, Margonato A, Cappelletti A, Chierchia SL: Coronary recanalization by elective angioplasty prevents ventricular dilation after anterior myocardial infarction. J Am Coll Cardiol 1996 (October);28:837–845.

170. Garot J, Scherrer-Crosbie M, Monin JL, DuPouy P, Bourachot ML, Teiger E, Rosso J, Castaigne A, Gueret P, Dubois-Randé JL: Effect of delayed percutaneous transluminal coronary angioplasty of occluded coronary arteries after acute myocardial infarction. Am J Cardiol 1996 (May 1);77:915–921.

171. Narins CR, Hillegass WB Jr., Nelson CL, Tcheng JE, Harrington RA, Phillips HR, Stack RS, Califf RM. Relation between activated clotting time during angioplasty and abrupt closure. Circulation 1996 (February);93:667–671.

172. Daniel WC, Pirwitz MJ, Willard JE, Lange RA, Hillis LD, Landau C: Incidence and treatment of elastic recoil occurring in the 15 minutes following successful percutaneous transluminal coronary angioplasty. Am J Cardiol 1996 (August 1); 78:253–259.

173. Waksman R, Ghazzal ZMB, Baim DS, Steenkiste AR, Yeh W, Ketre KM, King SB III, for the NACI Investigators. Myocardial infarction as a complication of new interventional devices. Am J Cardiol 1996 (October 1);78:751–756.

174. Kereiakes DJ, Kleiman NS, Ambrose J, Cohen M, Rodriguez S, Palabrica T, Herrmann HC, Sutton JM, Weaver WD, McKee DB, Fitzpatrick V, Sax FL: Randomized, double-blind, placebo-controlled dose-ranging study of tirofiban (MK-383) platelet IIb/IIIa blockade in high-risk patients undergoing coronary angioplasty. J Am Coll Cardiol 1996 (March 1);27:536–542.

175. Lefkovits J, Ivanhoe RJ, Califf RM, Bergelson BA, Anderson KM, Stoner GL, Weisman HF, Topol EJ for the EPIC Investigators: Effects of platelet glycoprotein IIb/IIIa receptor blockade by a chimeric monoclonal antibody (abciximab) on acute and six-month outcomes after percutaneous transluminal coronary angioplasty for acute myocardial infarction. Am J Cardiol 1996 (May 15);77:1045–1051.

176. Mintz GS, Popma JJ, Pichard AD, Kent KM, Satler LF, Wong SC, Hong MK, Kovach JA, Leon MB. Arterial remodeling after coronary angioplasty. A serial intravascular ultrasound study. Circulation 1996 (July 1);94:35–43.

177. Mark DB, Talley JD, Topol EJ, Bowman L, Lam LC, Anderson KM, Jollis JG, Cleman MW, Lee KL, Aversano T, Untereker WJ, Davidson-Ray L, Califf RM, for the EPIC Investigators. Economic assessment of platelet glycoprotein IIb/IIIa inhibition for prevention of ischemic complications of high-risk coronary angioplasty. Circulation 1996 (August 15);94:629–635.

178. Faxon DP, Vogel R, Yeh W, Holmes DR Jr., Detre K, NHLBI PTCA Registry Investigators: Value of visual versus central quantitative measurements of angiographic success after percutaneous transluminal coronary angioplasty. Am J Cardiol (May 15);77:1067–1072.

179. Baptista J, di Mario C, Ozaki Y, Escaned J, Gil R, de Feyter P, Roelandt JRTC, Serruys PW: Impact of plaque morphology and composition on the mechanisms of lumen enlargement using intracoronary ultrasound and quantitative angiography after balloon angioplasty. Am J Cardiol 1996 (January 15);77:115–121.

180. Danchin N, Angioï M, Cador R, Tricoche O, Dibon O, Jullière Y, Cuillière M, Cherrier F: Effect of late percutaneous angioplastic recanalization of total coronary artery occlusion on left ventricular remodeling, ejection fraction, and regional wall motion. Am J Cardiol 1996 (October 1);78:729–735.

181. Bach DS, Armstrong WF, Donovan CL, Muller DWM. Quantitative Doppler tissue imaging for assessment of regional myocardial velocities during transient ischemia and reperfusion. Am Heart J 1996 (October);132:721–725.

182. Sunamura M, di Mario C, Piek JJ, Schroeder E, Vrints C, Probst P, Heyndrickx GR, Fleck E, Serruys PW. Cyclic flow variations after angioplasty: A rare phenomenon predictive of immediate complications. Am Heart J 1996 (May);131:843–848.

183. Mickelson JK, Lakkis NM, Villarreal-Levy G, Hughes BJ, Smith CW: Leukocyte activation with platelet adhesion after coronary angioplasty: A mechanism for recurrent disease? J Am Coll Cardiol (August);28:345–353.

184. Abdelmeguid AE, Ellis SG, Sapp SK, Whitlow PL, Topol EJ. Defining the appropriate threshold of creatine kinase elevation after percutaneous coronary interventions. Am Heart J 1996 (June);131:1097–1105.

185. Miller DD, Esparza-Negrete J, Donohue TJ, Mechem C, Shaw LJ, Byers S, Kern MJ. Periprocedural Doppler coronary blood flow predictors of myocardial perfusion abnormalities and cardiac events after successful coronary interventions. Am Heart J 1996 (June);131:1058–1066.

186. Laster SB, Rutherford BD, Giorgi LV, Shimshak TM, McConahay DR, Johnson WL Jr, Huber KC, Ligon RW, Hartzler GO: Results of direct percutaneous transluminal coronary angioplasty in octogenarians. Am J Cardiol 1996 (January 1);77:10–13.

187. Ruygrok PN, de Jaegere PPT, van Domburg RT, van den Brand MJ, Serruys PW, de Feyter PJ: Clinical outcome 10 years after attempted percutaneous transluminal coronary angioplasty in 856 patients. J Am Coll Cardiol 1996 (June);27:1669–1677.

188. ten Berg JM, Voors AA, Suttorp MJ, Ernst SMPG, Mast EG, Bal E, Plokker HWT: Long-term results after successful percutaneous transluminal coronary angioplasty in patients over 75 years of age. Am J Cardiol 1996 (April 1);77:690–695.

189. Welty FK, Mittleman MA, Lewis SM, Kowalker WL, Healy RW, Shubrooks SJ, Muller JE. A patent infarct-related artery is associated with reduced long-term mortality after percutaneous transluminal coronary angioplasty for postinfarction ischemia and an ejection fraction <50%. Circulation 1996 (April 15);93: 1496–1501.

190. Shook TL, Sun GW, Burstein S, Eisenhauer AC, Matthews RV: Comparison of percutaneous transluminal coronary angioplasty outcome and hospital costs for low-volume and high-volume operators. Am J Cardiol 1996 (February 15);77: 331–336.

191. Heidenreich PA, Chou TM, Amidon TM, Ports TA, Browner WS: Impact of the operating physician on costs of percutaneous transluminal coronary angioplasty. Am J Cardiol 1996 (June 1);77:1169–1173.

192. Nakagawa Y, Iwasaki Y, Kimura T, Tamura T, Yokoi H, Yokoi H, Hamasaki N, Nosaka H, Nobuyoshi M: Serial angiographic follow-up after successful direct angioplasty for acute myocardial infarction. Am J Cardiol (November 1) 1996;78: 980–984.

193. Violaris AG, Melkert R, Herrman J-PR, Serruys PW. Role of angiographically identifiable thrombus on long-term luminal renarrowing after coronary angioplasty. A quantitative angiographic analysis. Circulation 1996 (March 1);93:889–897.

194. Sakata K, Miura F, Sugino H, Shinobe M, Shirotani M, Yoshida H, Mori N, Hoshino T, Takada A. Impaired fibrinolysis early after percutaneous transluminal coronary angioplasty is associated with restenosis. Am Heart J 1996 (January); 131:1–6.

195. Miyata M, Biro S, Arima S, Hamasaki S, Kaieda H, Nakao S, Kawataki M, Nomoto K, Tanaka H. High serum concentration of lipoprotein(a) is a risk factor for restenosis after percutaneous transluminal coronary angioplasty in Japanese patients with single-vessel disease. Am Heart J 1996 (August);132:269–273.

196. O'Brien ER, Bennett KL, Garvin MR, Zderic TW, Hinohara T, Simpson JB, Kimura T, Nobuyoshi M, Mizgala H, Purchio A, Schwartz SM: βig-h3, a transforming growth factor-β-inducible gene, is overexpressed in atherosclerotic and restenotic human vascular lesions. Arterioscl Thromb Vasc Biol 1996 (April);16:576–584.

197. Schmitz HJ, Erbel R, Meyer J, von Essen R. Influence of vessel dilatation on restenosis after successful percutaneous transluminal coronary angioplasty. Am Heart J 1996 (May);131:884–891.

198. Luo H, Nishioka T, Eigler NL, Forrester JS, Fishbein MC, Berglund H, Siegel RJ: Coronary artery restenosis after balloon angioplasty in humans is associated with circumferential coronary constriction. Arterioscl Thromb Vasc Biol 1996 (November);16:1393–1398.

199. Karsch KR, Preisack MB, Baildon R, Eschenfelder V, Foley D, Garcia E, Kaltenbach M, Meisner C, Selbmann HK, Serruys PW, Shiu MF, Sujatta M, Bonan R: Low molecular weight heparin (reviparin) in percutaneous transluminal coronary angioplasty: Results of a randomized, double-blind, unfractionated heparin and placebo-controlled, multicenter trial (REDUCE Trial). J Am Coll Cardiol 1996 (November 15);28:1437–1443.

200. Watanabe K. Sekiya M, Ikeda S, Miyagawa M, Hashida K: Preventive effects of probucol on restenosis after percutaneous transluminal coronary angioplasty. Am Heart J 1996 (July);132:23–29.

201. O'Brien JE, Peterson ED, Keeler GP, Berdan LG, Ohman EM, Faxon DP, Jacobs AK, Topol EJ, Califf RM: Relation between estrogen replacement therapy and restenosis after percutaneous coronary interventions. J Am Coll Cardiol 1996 (November 1);28:1111–1118.

202. Zhou YF, Leon MB, Waclawiw MA, Popma JJ, Yu ZX, Finkel T, Epstein SE: Association between prior cytomegalovirus infection and the risk of restenosis after coronary atherectomy. N Engl J Med 1996 (August 29);335:624–630.

203. Kaplan BM, Larkin T, Safian RD, O'Neill WW, Kramer B, Hoffman M, Schreiber

T, Grines CL: Prospective study of extraction atherectomy in patients with acute myocardial infarction. Am J Cardiol 1996 (August 15);78:383–388.

204. Khoury AF, Aguirre FV, Bach RG, Carracciolo EA, Donohue TJ, Wolford T, Mechem C, Herrmann SC, Kern MJ: Influence of percutaneous transluminal coronary rotational atherectomy with adjunctive percutaneous transluminal coronary angioplasty on coronary blood flow. Am Heart J 1996 (April);131:631–638.

205. Lefkovits J, Blankenship JC, Anderson KM, Stoner GL, Talley JD, Worley SJ, Weisman HF, Califf RM, Topol EF: Increased risk of non-Q wave myocardial infarction after directional atherectomy is platelet dependent: Evidence from the EPIC Trial. J Am Coll Cardiol 1996 (October);28:849–855.

206. LeMay MR, Labinaz M, Beanlands RSB, Laramée LA, O'Brien ER, Marquis J-F, Williams WL, Al-Sadoon K, Davies RF, Kearns SA, Johansen HL, Higginson LA: Usefulness of intracoronary stenting in acute myocardial infarction. Am J Cardiol 1996 (July 15);78:148–152.

207. Saito S, Hosokawa G, Kim K, Tanaka S, Miyake S: Primary stent implantation without coumadin in acute myocardial infarction. J Am Coll Cardiol 1996 (July); 28:74–81.

208. Rodriguez AE, Fernandez M, Santaera O, Larribau M, Bernardi V, Castaño H, Palacios IF: Coronary stenting in patients undergoing percutaneous transluminal coronary angioplasty during acute myocardial infarction. Am J Cardiol 1996 (April 1);77:685–689.

209. Garcia-Cantu E, Spaulding C, Corcos T, Hamda KB, Roussel L, Favereau X, Guérin Y, Chalet Y, Souffrant G, Guérin F: Stent implantation in acute myocardial infarction. Am J Cardiol 1996 (March 1);77:451–454.

210. Sirnes PA, Golf S, Myreng Y, Molstad P, Emanuelsson H, Albertsson P, Brekke M, Mangschau A, Endresen K, Kjekshus J: Stenting in chronic coronary occlusion (SICCO): A randomized, controlled trial of adding stent implantation after successful angioplasty. J Am Coll Cardiol 1996 (November 15);28:1444–1451.

211. Eeckhout E, Stauffer J-C, Vogt P, Debbas N, Kappenberger L, Goy J-J. Comparison of elective Wiktor stent placement with conventional balloon angioplasty for newonset lesions of the right coronary artery. Am Heart J 1996 (August);132:263–268.

212. Steffenino G, Dellavalle A, Ribichini F, Uslenghi E: Coronary stenting after unsuccessful emergency angioplasty in acute myocardial infarction: Results in a series of consecutive patients. Am Heart J 1996 (December);132:1115–1118.

213. Mori M, Kurogane H, Hayashi T, Yasaka Y, Ohta S, Kajiya T, Takarada A, Yoshida A, Matsuda Y, Nakagawa K, Murata T, Yoshida Y, Yokoyama M: Comparison of results of intra-coronary implantation of the Palmaz-Schatz stent with conventional balloon angioplasty in chronic total coronary arterial occlusion. Am J Cardiol 1996 (November 1);78:985–989.

214. Schömig A, Neumann F-J, Kastrati A, Schühlen H, Blasini R, Hadamitzky M, Walter H, Zitzmann-Roth E-M, Richardt G, Alt E, Schmitt C, Ulm K: A randomized comparison of antiplatelet and anticoagulant therapy after the placement of coronary-artery stents. N Engl J Med 1996 (April 25);334:1084–1089.

215. Karrillon GJ, Morice MC, Benveniste E, Bunouf P, Aubry P, Cattan S, Chevalier B, Commeau P, Cribier A, Eiferman C, Grollier G, Guerin Y, Henry M, Lefevre T, Livarek B, Louvard Y, Marco J, Makowski S, Monassier JP, Pernes JM, Rioux P, Spaulding C, Zemour G: Intracoronary stent implantation without ultrasound guidance and with replacement of conventional anticoagulation by antiplatelet therapy. 30-Day clinical outcome of the French multicenter registry. Circulation 1996 (October 1);94:1519–1527.

216. Goods CM, Al-Shaibi KF, Yadav SS, Liu MW, Negus BH, Iyer SS, Dean LS, Jain SP, Baxley WA, Parks JM, Sutor RJ, Roubin GS: Utilization of the coronary balloonexpandable coil stent without anticoagulation or intravascular ultrasound. Circulation 1996 (May 15);93:1803–1808.

217. Gawaz M, Neumann F-J, Ott I, May A, Schömig A: Platelet activation and coronary stent implantation. Effect of antithrombotic therapy. Circulation 1996 (August 1); 94:279–285.

218. Hall P, Nakamura S, Maiello L, Itoh A, Blengino S, Martini G, Ferraro M, Colombo

A: A randomized comparison of combined ticlopidine and aspirin therapy versus aspirin therapy alone after successful intravascular ultrasound-guided stent implantation. Circulation 1996 (January);93:215–222.

219. Goods CM, Al-Shaibi KF, Liu MW, Yadav JS, Mathur A, Jain SP, Dean LS, Iyer SS, Parks JM, Roubin GS: Comparison of *aspirin* alone versus aspirin plus triclopidine after coronary artery stenting. Am J Cardiol 1996 (November 1);78:1042–1044.

220. De Cesare NB, Bartorelli AL, Galli S, Loaldi A, Fabbiocchi F, Sganzerla P, Montorsi P, Guazzi MD. Treatment of ostial lesions of the left anterior descending coronary artery with Palmaz-Schatz coronary stent. Am Heart J 1996 (October);132:716–720.

221. Serruys PW, Emanuelsson H, van der Giessen W, Lunn AC, Kiemeney F, Macaya C, Rutsch W, Heyndrickx G, Suryapranata H, Legrand V, Goy JJ, Materne P, Bonnier H, Morice M-C, Fajadet J, Belardi J, Colombo A, Garcia E, Ruygrok P, de Jaegere P, Morel M-A, on behalf of the BENESTENT-II Study Group: Heparincoated Palmaz-Schatz stents in human coronary arteries. Early outcome of the BENESTENT-II pilot study. Circulation 1996 (February);93:412–422.

222. Lee SW, Chen M, Chan H, Lam L, Guo J, Mao J, Lam KKH, Guo L, Li H, Chan K: No subacute thrombosis and femoral bleeding complications under full anticoagulation in 150 consecutive patients receiving non-heparin-coated intracoronary Palmaz-Schatz stents. Am Heart J 1996 (December);132:1135–1146.

223. de Jaegere PP, van Domburg RT, de Feyter PJ, Ruygrok PN, van der Giessen WJ, van den Brand MJ, Serruys PW: Long-term clinical outcome after stent implantation in saphenous vein grafts. J Am Coll Cardiol 1996 (July);28:89–96.

224. Cecēna FA, Hoelzinger DH: Transcatheter therapy of thrombotic-occlusive lesions in saphenous vein grafts. Am J Cardiol 1996 (July 1);78:31–36.

225. Hasdai D, Garrat KN, Holmes DR Jr, Berger PB, Schwartz RS, Bell MR: Coronary angioplasty and intracoronary thrombolysis are of limited efficacy in resolving early intracoronary stent thrombosis. J Am Coll Cardiol 1996 (August);28:361–367.

226. Pan M, Suarez de Lezo J, Velasco F, Romero M, Medina A, Segura J, Hernandez E, Pavlovic D, Melian F, Gallardo A, Zayas R, Ruiz M, Torres A: Reduction of thrombotic and hemorrhagic complications after stent implantation. Am Heart J 1996 (December);132:1119–1126.

227. Mehran R, Mintz GS, Popma JJ, Pichard AD, Satler LF, Kent KM, Griffin J, Leon MB: Mechanisms and results of balloon angioplasty for the treatment of in-stent restenosis. Am J Cardiol 1996 (September 15);78:618–622.

228. Hoffmann R, Mintz GS, Dussaillant GR, Popma JJ, Pichard AD, Satler LF, Kent KM, Griffin J, Leon MB: Patterns and mechanisms of in-stent restenosis: a serial intravascular ultrasound study. Circulation 1996 (September 15);94:1247–1254.

229. Altmann DB, Racz M, Battleman DS, Bergman G, Spokojny A, Hannan EL, Sanborn TA: Reduction in angioplasty complications after the introduction of coronary stents: Results from a consecutive series of 2242 patients. Am Heart J 1996 (September);132:503–507.

230. Kimura T, Yokoi H, Nakagawa Y, Tamura T, Kaburagi S, Sawada Y, Sato Y, Yokoi H, Hamasaki N, Nosaka H, Nobuyoshi M: Three-year follow-up after implantation of metallic coronary-artery stents. N Engl J Med 1996 (February 29);334:561–6.

231. Laham RJ, Carrozza JP, Berger C, Cohen DJ, Kuntz RE, Baim DS: Long-term (4- to 6-Year) outcome of Palmaz-Schatz stenting: Paucity of late clinical stent-related problems. J Am Coll Cardiol 1996 (October);28:820–826.

232. Bowers TR, Terrien EF, O'Neill NW, Sachs D, Grines CL for the PAMI Investigators: Effect of reperfusion modality on outcome in nonsmokers and smokers with acute myocardial infarction (A Primary Angioplasty in Myocardial Infarction [PAMI] Study). Am J Cardiol 1996 (September 1);78:511–515.

233. Lafont A, Marwick TH, Chisolm GM, Van Lente F, Vaska KJ, Whitlow PL: Decreased free radical scavengers with reperfusion after coronary angioplasty in patients with acute myocardial infarction. Am Heart J 1996 (February);131:219–223.

234. Grech ED, Dodd NJF, Jackson MJ, Morrison WL, Faragher EB, Ramsdale DR:

Evidence for free radical generation after primary percutaneous transluminal coronary angioplasty recanalization in acute myocardial infarction. Am J Cardiol 1996 (January 15);77:122–127.

235. Oh H, Ito H, Iwakura K, Masuyama T, Takiuchi S, Maruyama A, Higashino Y, Fujii K, Azuma J, Minamino T: Temporal changes in regional end-diastolic wall thickness early after reperfusion in acute anterior myocardial infarction: Relation to myocardial viability and vascular damage. Am Heart J 1996 (June);131: 1113–1120.

236. Ishihara M, Sato H, Tateishi H, Kawagoe T, Shimatani Y, Kurisu S, Sakai K: Attenuation of the no-reflow phenomenon after coronary angioplasty for acute myocardial infarction with intracoronary papaverine. Am Heart J 1996 (November);132:959–963.

237. Grines CL, Schreiber TL, Savas V, Jones DE, Zidar FJ, Gangadharan V, Brodsky M, Levin R, Safian R, Puchrowicz-Ochocki S, Castellani MD, O'Neil WW: A randomized trial of low osmolar ionic versus nonionic contrast media in patients with myocardial infarction or unstable angina undergoing percutaneous transluminal coronary angioplasty. J Am Coll Cardiol 1996 (May);27:1381–1386.

238. Gawaz M, Neumann F-J, Ott I, Schiessler A, Schömig A: Platelet function in acute myocardial infarction treated with direct angioplasty. Circulation 1996 (January); 93:229–237.

239. Brodie BR, Stuckey TD, Kissling G, Hansen CJ, Weintraub RA, Kelly TA: Importance of infarct-related artery patency for recovery of left ventricular function and late survival after primary angioplasty for acute myocardial infarction. J Am Coll Cardiol 1996 (August);28:319–325.

240. Anderson JL, Karagounis LA, Califf RM: Metaanalysis of five reported studies on the relation of early coronary patency grades with mortality and outcomes after acute myocardial infarction. Am J Cardiol 1996 (July 1);78:1–8.

241. Stone GW, Grines CL, Browne KF, Marco J, Rothbaum D, O'Keefe J, Hartzler GO, Overlie P, Donohue B, Chelliah N, Vlietstra R, Puchrowicz-Ochocki S, O'Neill WW: Influence of acute myocardial infarction location on in-hospital and late outcome after primary percutaneous transluminal coronary angioplasty versus tPA therapy. Am J Cardiol 1996 (July 1);78:19–25.

242. Tomoda H, Morimoto K, Aoki N. Superoxide dismutase activity as a predictor of myocardial reperfusion and salvage in acute myocardial infarction. Am Heart J 1996 (May);131:849–856.

243. Oh JK, Gibbons RJ, Christian TF, Gerah BJ, Click RL, Sitthisook S, Tajik AJ, Seward JB. Correlation of regional wall motion abnormalities detected by two-dimensional echocardiography with perfusion defect determined by technetium 99m sestamibi imaging in patients treated with reperfusion therapy during acute myocardial infarction. Am Heart J 1996 (January);131:32–37.

244. Detre KM, Rosen AD, Bost JE, Cooper ME, Sutton-Tyrrell K, Holubkov R, Shemin RJ, Frye RL: Contemporary practice of coronary revascularization in U.S. hospitals and hospitals participating in the Bypass Angioplasty Revascularization Investigation (BARI). J Am Coll Cardiol 1996 (September);28:609–615.

245. Botas J, Stadius ML, Bourassa MG, Rosen AD, Schaff HV, Sopko G, Williams DO, McMillan A, Alderman EL, and the BARI Investigators: Angiographic correlates of lesion relevance and suitability for percutaneous transluminal coronary angioplasty and coronary artery bypass grafting in the Bypass Angioplasty Revascularization Investigation Study (BARI). Am J Cardiol 1996 (April 15);77:805–814.

246. Zhao X-Q, Brown BG, Stewart DK, Hillger LA, Barnhart HX, Kosinski AS, Weintraub WS, King SB III. Effectiveness of revascularization in the Emory Angioplasty versus Surgery Trial. A randomized comparison of coronary angioplasty with bypass surgery. Circulation 1996 (June 1);93:1954–1962.

247. The Bypass Angioplasty Revascularization Investigation (BARI) Investigators. Comparison of coronary bypass surgery with angioplasty in patients with multivessel disease. N Engl J Med 1996 (July 25);335:217–25.

248. Pocock SJ, Henderson RA, Seed P, Treasure T, Hampton JR, for the RITA Trial Participants. Quality of life, employment status, and anginal symptoms after coro-

nary angioplasty or bypass surgery. 3-year follow-up in the Randomized Intervention Treatment of Angina (RITA) trial. Circulation 1996 (July 15);94:135–142.

249. Rodriguez A, Mele E, Peyregne E, Bullon F, Perez-Baliño N, Liprandi MIS, Palacios IF: Three-year follow-up of the Argentine randomized trial of percutaneous transluminal coronary angioplasty versus coronary artery bypass surgery in multivessel disease (ERACI). JACC 1996 (April);27:1178–1184.

250. Kleiman NS, Anderson HV, Rogers WJ, Theroux P, Thompson B, Stone P: Comparison of outcome of patients with unstable angina and non-Q-wave acute myocardial infarction with and without prior coronary artery bypass grafting (Thrombolysis in Myocardial Ischemia III registry). Am J Cardiol 1996 (February 1);77: 227–231.

251. Cox JL, Petrie JF, Pollak PT, Johnstone DE: Managed delay for coronary artery bypass graft surgery: The experience at one Canadian center. J Am Coll Cardiol 1996 (May);27:1365–1373.

252. Cameron A, Davis KB, Green G, Schaff HV. Coronary bypass surgery with internal-thoracic-artery grafts-effects on survival over a 15-year period. N Engl J Med 1996 (January 25);334:216–219.

253. Borst C, Jansen EWL, Tulleken CAF, Gründeman PF, Beck HJM, van Dongen JWF, Hodde KC, Bredée JJ: Coronary artery bypass grafting without cardiopulmonary bypass anastomosis site restraining device ("Octopus"). J Am Coll Cardiol 1996 (May);27:1356–1364.

254. Brodman RF, Frame R, Camacho M, Hu E, Chen A, Hollinger I: Routine Use of Unilateral and Bilateral Radial Arteries for Coronary Artery Bypass Graft Surgery. J Am Coll Cardiol 1996 (October);28:959–963.

255. Komiyama N, Nakanishi S, Nishiyama S, Seki A. Intravascular imaging of serial changes of disease in saphenous vein grafts after coronary artery bypass grafting. Am Heart J 1996 (July);132:30–40.

256. Nishioka T, Luo H, Berglund H, Eigler NL, Kim C-J, Tabak SW, Siegel RJ. Absence of focal compensatory enlargement or constriction in diseased human coronary saphenous vein bypass grafts. An intravascular ultrasound study. Circulation 1996 (February);93:683–690.

257. Galjee MA, van Rossum AC, Doesburg T, van Eenige MJ, Visser CA. Value of MRI in assessing patency and function of coronary artery bypass grafts: an angiographically controlled study. Circulation 1996 (February);93:660–666.

258. Gold MR, O'Gara PT, Buckley MJ, DeSanctis RW: Efficacy and safety of *procainamide* in preventing arrhythmias after coronary artery bypass surgery. Am J Cardiol (November 1) 1996;78:975–979.

259. Greaves SC, Rutherford JD, Aranki SF, Cohn LH, Couper GS, Adams DH, Rizzo RJ, Collins JJ Jr, Antman EM. Current incidence and determinants of perioperative myocardial infarction in coronary artery surgery. Am Heart J 1996 (September); 132:572–578.

260. Stephan WJ, O'Keefe JH Jr, Piehler JM, McCallister BD, Dahiya RS, Shimshak TM, Ligon RW, Hartzler GO: Coronary angioplasty versus repeat coronary artery bypass grafting for patients with previous bypass surgery. J Am Coll Cardiol 1996 (November 1);28:1140–1146.

261. Fitzgibbon GM, Kafka HP, Leach AJ, Keon WJ, Hooper GD, Burton JR: Coronary bypass graft fate and patient outcome: Angiographic follow-up of 5,065 grafts related to survival and reoperation in 1,388 patients during 25 years. J Am Coll Cardiol 1996 (September);28:616–626.

262. Voors AA, van Brussel BL, Plokker HWT, Ernst SMPG, Ernst NM, Koomen EM, Tijssen JGP, Vermeulen FEE. Smoking and cardiac events after venous coronary bypass surgery. A 15-year follow-up study. Circulation 1996 (January);93:42–47.

263. Hartmann JR, McKeever LS, O'Neill WW, White CJ, Whitlow PL, Gilmore PS, Doorey AJ, Galichia JP, Enger EL: Recanalization of Chronically Occluded Aorto-coronary Saphenous Vein Bypass Grafts with Long-Term, Low Dose Direct Infusion of Urokinase (ROBUST): A serial trial. J Am Coll Cardiol 1996 (January);27: 60–66.

264. Eritsland J, Arnesen H, Grønseth K, Fjeld NB, Abdelnoor M: Effect of dietary supplementation with n-3 fatty acids on coronary artery bypass graft patency. Am J Cardiol 1996 (January 1);77:31–36.

265. Brubaker PH, Warner JG Jr, Rejeski WJ, Edwards DG, Matrazzo BA, Ribisl PM, Miller HS Jr, Herrington DM: Comparison of standard- and extended-length participation in cardiac rehabilitation on body composition, functional capacity, and blood lipids. Am J Cardiol 1996 (October 1);78:769–773.

266. Gagliardi JA, Prado NG, Marino JC, Lederer S, Ramos AO, Bertolasi CA. Exercise training and heparin pretreatment in patients with coronary artery disease. Am Heart J 1996 (November);132:946–951.

267. Milani RV, Lvie CJ, Cassidy MM. Effects of cardiac rehabilitation and exercise training programs on depression in patients after major coronary events. Am Heart J 1996 (October);132:726–732.

268. Ades PA, Waldmann ML, Meyer WL, Brown KA, Poehlman ET, Pendlebury WW, Leslie KO, Gray PR, Lew RR, LeWinter MM. Skeletal muscle and cardiovascular adaptations to exercise conditioning in older coronary patients. Circulation 1996 (August 1);94:323–330.

269. Rastegar H, Link MS, Foote CB, Wang PJ, Manolis AS, Estes NAM III. Perioperative and long-term results with mapping-guided subendocardial resection and left ventricular endoaneurysmorrhaphy. Circulation 1996 (September 1);94:1041–1048.

270. Stratmann HG, Younis LT, Wittry MD, Amato M, Mark AL, Miller DD. Dipyridamole technetium 99m sestamibi myocardial tomography for preoperative cardiac risk stratification before major or minor nonvascular surgery. Am Heart J 1996 (September);132:536–541.

271. Lee TH, Thomas EJ, Ludwig LE, Sacks DB, Johnson PA, Donaldson MC, Cook EF, Pedan A, Kuntz KM, Goldman L: Troponin T as a marker for myocardial ischemia in patients undergoing major noncardiac surgery. Am J Cardiol 1996 (May 15);77:1031–1036.

272. Kontos MC, Brath LK, Akosah KW, Mohanty PK. Cardiac implications in noncardiac surgery: Relative value of resting two-dimensional echocardiography and dipyridamole thallium imaging. Am Heart J 1996 (September);132:559–566.

3

Congestive Heart Failure

Congestive Heart Failure (General Topics)

Baseline Quality of Life as a Predictor of Mortality and Hospitalization

Konstam and associates[1] from multiple medical centers for the Studies of Left Ventricular Dysfunction (SOLVD) Investigators examined the independent relation of health-related quality of life to mortality and congestive heart failure (CHF) related hospitalizations in patients with ejection fractions (EFs) less than 35% followed for a mean of 36.5 months. A brief health-related quality of life questionnaire was administered at baseline to patients randomly assigned to placebo or enalapril in the SOLVD trial. Participants had EF less than 35% and either symptomatic CHF (treatment trial, n = 2465) or asymptomatic CHF (prevention trial, n = 2560). Baseline assessment of health-related quality of life predicted mortality and CHF-related hospitalizations in symptomatic and asymptomatic patients randomized to enalapril and placebo treatment. Domains that were the stronger univariate predictors of mortality and CHF-related hospitalizations were activities of daily living (relative risk [RR] for mortality, 1.163; for hospitalization, 1.215), general health (RR for mortality, 1.205; for hospitalization, 1.188), and social functioning (RR for mortality, 1.098; for hospitalization, 1.156). In the multivariate model, activities of daily living (RR for mortality, 1.41; for hospitalization, 1.43), general health (RR for mortality, 1.21; for hospitalization, 1.16) and heart failure symptoms (RR for mortality, 1.02; for hospitalization, 1.03) were found to be independent risk factors. Health-related quality of life independently predicted mortality and CHF-related hospitalizations after adjustment for EF, age, treatment, and New York Heart Association functional classification in patients with an EF less than 35% randomized to enalapril and placebo treatment. Health-related quality of life provides additional clinical information regarding disease course and outcome that is not captured by traditional indexes of clinical status.

Proinflammatory Cytokine Levels in Patients with Depressed Left Ventricular Ejection Fraction

Elevations of tumor necrosis factor-α have been found in patients with heart failure. Torre-Amione and colleagues[2] from Houston, Texas, evaluated

363

tumor necrosis factor-α and interleukin-6 levels in patients in the SOLVD study. Plasma levels of tumor necrosis factor-α were elevated in patients in functional classes I through III (1.95, 2.63, and 6.4 pg/mL, respectively) compared with age-matched control subjects (0.75 pg/mL). Plasma levels of interleukin-6 were elevated in patients in functional classes I through III (3.3, 6.2, and 5.22 pg/mL, respectively) compared with age-matched control subjects (1.8 pg/mL). These authors concluded that circulating levels of proinflammatory cytokines increase in patients as their functional heart failure classification deteriorates. Activation of the neurohumoral axis is unlikely to completely explain this increase since there was no significant correlation between neurohumoral and proinflammatory cytokine levels.

Nitric Oxide Synthase in Heart Failure

Haywood and colleagues[3] in Stanford, California, and St. George's Hospital in London, United Kingdom, analyzed inducible nitric oxide synthase (iNOS) expression in ventricular myocardium taken from 72 hearts: 11 hearts of control subjects who had died suddenly from noncardiac cause; 10 donor hearts before implantation; and 51 hearts of patients with heart failure, including 24 with dilated cardiomyopathy, 17 with coronary artery disease (CAD) heart disease, and 10 with valvular heart disease. Reverse transcription-polymerase chain reaction (RT-PCR) was used to confirm the presence of intact mRNA and to detect expression of iNOS and atrial natriuretic peptide (ANP). ANP was used as a molecular phenotypic marker of CHF. iNOS was expressed in 36 of 51 biopsies (71%) from patients with CHF and in none of the control individuals. iNOS expression could also be detected in 50% of the donor hearts. All samples that expressed iNOS also expressed ANP. iNOS gene expression occurred in 67% of patients with dilated cardiomyopathy, 59% of patients with coronary artery disease (CAD) heart failure, and 100% of patients with valvular heart disease (Figure 3-1). Immunohistochemistry was performed on 3 donor and 9 failing hearts. iNOS mRNA expression demonstrated that all failing hearts showed diffuse cytoplasmic staining in cardiac myocytes, but this was not found in donor myocardium and in control sections. Expression of iNOS was found in all 4 chambers. Western blot analysis with the same primary antibody showed a specific positive band for iNOS protein in the CHF specimens and minimal iNOS protein expression in donor heart samples. Thus, iNOS expression occurs in human cardiac myocytes in patients with CHF, and it may be involved in the heart failure of these patients.

Dobutamine Echocardiography for Predicting Severity

Functional status in chronic heart failure is evaluated in general by subjective means, such as the New York Heart Association class, or by invasive techniques difficult to use routinely. The aim of this study by Marmor and associates[4] from Haifa, Israel, was to evaluate noninvasively the contractile reserve in cases of heart failure as a means to define the functional status of the patients.

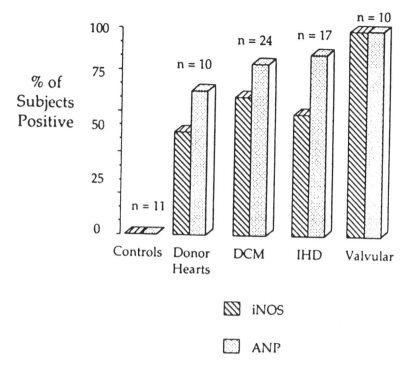

Figure 3-1. Frequency of iNOS and ANP mRNA expression in ventricular myocardium detected by RT-PCR. DCM indicates idiopathic dilated cardiomyopathy; IHD, ischemic heart disease; and Valvular, valvular heart disease. Reproduced with permission from Haywood et al.[3]

Cardiac peak power, a new noninvasively obtained afterload-independent index of contractility, was calculated from online Doppler and central arterial blood pressure estimated noninvasively in 35 patients with heart failure and in 10 healthy individuals during dobutamine infusion. Cardiac output increased in all patients to the same extent, without differentiation among the functional classes. Contractile reserve, as assessed by peak power, was found to be a good marker of functional class: it was significantly higher in functional class I than in functional classes II through IV. A correlation of r = 0.99 and probability of p < .001 was found with the functional status. This new, noninvasive contractility index, peak power, allows an objective evaluation of the severity of heart failure.

Cheyne-Stokes Respiration and Prognosis

Patients with CHF frequently demonstrate Cheyne-Stokes respiration (CSR) with repetitive arousals and oxygen desaturations during sleep. Although it is evident from early publications that CSR during the daytime is a poor prognostic indicator in patients with CHF, Andreas and associates[5] from Göttingen, Germany, speculated that CSR during sleep could impede left ventricular function and even survival. The authors therefore followed 36 patients with CHF and a left ventricular ejection fraction (LVEF) of 40% or less who underwent a sleep study at their institution. The patients had a reduced EF (20% ± 8%) and CSR with a median of 19% of total sleep time (lower and upper quartiles 9% and 56%). In 12% ± 9% of their time in bed, the arterial oxygen saturation was less than 90%. No patient was lost to follow-up, which lasted for 32 ± 15 months (range, 11 to 53). One-year survival was 86% ± 6%, and 2-year survival was 66% ± 8%. Univariate comparisons for survival between groups stratified by the amount of CSR revealed no significant difference. However, the 20 patients with LVEF less than 20% had a shorter mean survival time than did patients with an EF of 20% or more (9.5 vs. 28.3 months). Two patients with CSR during the daytime died within 1 month. No other patient had CSR during the daytime, and only 1 patient without daytime CSR died within 1 month. Higher age, reduced carbon dioxide end-tidal partial pressure, and increased transit time were found to be significantly related to the amount of nocturnal CSR. In conclusion, CSR occurring during sleep has no important prognostic impact in patients with CHF, but CSR present during the daytime suggests a high likelihood of dying within a few months.

Right Ventricular Diastolic Function

Yu and colleagues[6] in Hong Kong compared right ventricular diastolic function between 2 groups in a large cohort of patients with CHF: patients with pulmonary hypertension and normal left ventricular function and normal subjects. Transtricuspid and pulmonary artery flow were assessed by 2-dimensional echocardiography at maximum inspiration and expiration in 185 patients, including 114 symptomatic patients with CHF and right ventricular ejection fractions (RVEFs) less than 50%, 31 patients with pulmonary hypertension, and 40 normal subjects. The patients with pulmonary artery hypertension had pulmonary artery systolic pressures greater than 40 mm Hg. A subset was matched for age and heart rate. The results showed a high prevalence of right ventricular diastolic abnormalities. CHF patients had lower tricuspid E-A ratios, lower peak E-wave velocity, and prolonged right ventricular isovolumic relaxation time. Tricuspid E-wave deceleration time was shorter only in those who had a left ventricular restrictive filling pattern. The patients with pulmonary hypertension had similar findings. Compared with a normal range, more than half of the patients had lower tricuspid E-A ratios, and 61% of heart failure and 58% of patients with pulmonary hypertension had prolonged right ventricular isovolumic relaxation time. In the pulmonary hypertension group, right ventricular diastolic variables, including E-wave deceleration time, E-A ratio, and isovolumic relaxation time, correlated significantly with pulmonary artery systolic pressure. However, in the heart failure patients, only tricuspid E-wave deceleration time correlated significantly with pulmonary artery systolic pressure, and heart failure patients with normal pulmonary artery systolic pressures had lower tricuspid E-A ratios and prolonged right ventricular isovolumic relaxation times than did normal subjects. A close correlation existed between individual right ventricular and left ventricular diastolic variables, suggesting that left ventricular diastolic dysfunction may directly affect right ventricular function, but there was no relationship between left ventricular size or systolic function and right ventricular diastolic dysfunction. Thus, right ventricular diastolic function is frequently abnormal in heart failure patients. This is not related to elevated pulmonary artery (PA) systolic pressure alone, but high PA pressure by itself is associated with impaired right ventricular diastolic function. It may be important to assess right ventricular diastolic function in determining the symptoms and prognosis of patients with CHF.

Relation of Ventricular Size and Function to Heart Failure Status

Patients with severe left ventricular dysfunction may or may not have overt CHF and ventricular dysrhythmia. To study factors behind this variability, Koilpillai and associates[7] for the SOLVD Investigators examined a subset of 311 patients from the SOLVD study: 95 with a history of moderate CHF (treatment trial), and 216 with no CHF (prevention trial), all with an EF of less than 35%. Echocardiographic variables were compared between trials and also correlated with dysrhythmia in 258 patients and with neurohormones in 199 patients. Compared with prevention patients, treatment patients had larger left ventricular end-diastolic diameter, end-systolic volume, sphericity index, and ratio of early-to-late diastolic filling velocity by Doppler (E-A ratio); lower left ventricular ejection fraction and atrial contribution to ventricular filling; and similar LV mass, end-diastolic volume, and estimates of systolic wall stress. With prevention and treatment patients combined, the prevalence of abnormally elevated atrial natriuretic peptide was 92% in the highest tertile of E-A ratio, compared with 55% in the lower tertiles. Across tertiles of left ventricular end-diastolic volume, there was an increase in the prevalence of nonsustained ventricular tachycardia (24%, 45%, and 45%) and premature ventricular complexes greater than 10/hour (48%, 62%, and 80%). Thus, in severe left ventricular dysfunction, ventricular filling indexes suggestive of high filling pressures, along with larger and more spherical ventricles, are particularly common in patients with overt heart failure, thus suggesting that diastolic properties and the degree of ventricular remodeling affect clinical status. Once ejection fraction is significantly reduced, the prevalence of ventricular dysrhythmia correlates with left ventricular size rather than systolic function. This observation lends support to previous experimental findings on the role of myocardial stretch and scar in the genesis of dysrhythmia (Figure 3-2).

Left ventricular systolic function and CHF are important predictors of long-term mortality after acute myocardial infarction (AMI). The importance of transient CHF and the interaction of CHF and left ventricular function on prognosis has received little attention. Using data from the TRAndolopril Cardiac Evaluation (TRACE) Study, Kober and associates[8] on behalf of the TRACE Study Group quantified wall motion index by echocardiogram in 6676 consecutive patients who had experienced AMI 1 to 6 days earlier. To study the interaction of CHF and wall motion index on long-term mortality, separate analyses were performed in patients with different levels of left ventricular function.

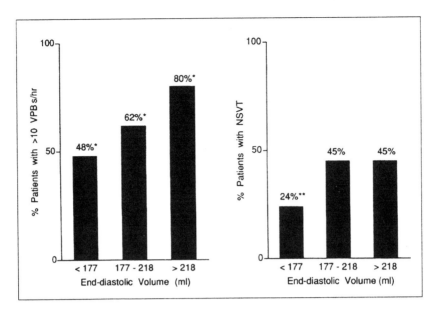

FIGURE 3-2. Prevalence of ventricular premature beat (VPB) frequency greater than 10/hour and nonsustained ventricular tachycardia (NSVT) across fertiles of left ventricular end-diastolic volume. Each tertile includes approximately one-third of patients who had both echocardiographic and ambulatory electrocardiographic studies. *p <.001 versus other 2 tertiles; **p =.007 versus the 2 highest tertiles. Reproduced with permission from Koilpillai et al.[7]

Risk ratios were determined from proportional hazard models subgrouped by wall motion index or CHF adjusted for age and gender. Heart failure was separated into transient or persistent. Wall motion index and CHF are correlated. Furthermore, there is an interaction between wall motion index and CHF. The prognostic importance of wall motion index depends on whether patients have CHF: the risk ratio associated with decreasing 1 wall motion index unit is 3.0 in patients with CHF, and 2.2 in patients without CHF when adjusted for age and gender. Similarly, the prognostic importance of CHF depends on the level of wall motion index: the risk ratio associated with CHF is 3.9 when the wall motion index is less than 0.8 and 1.9 when the wall motion index is greater than 1.6. Transient CHF is an independent risk factor (risk ratio 1.5) although it is milder than persistent CHF (risk ratio 2.8).

Response to Exercise Training/Exercise Capacity

Wilson and colleagues[9] in Nashville, Tennessee, postulated that patients with CHF with preserved cardiac output responses to exercise were limited by deconditioning and may respond to exercise training, whereas patients with CHF with reduced cardiac output responses to exercise are limited by skeletal muscle underperfusion and do not improve with exercise training. Thirty-two patients with CHF were evaluated. Hemodynamic responses to maximal treadmill exercise were measured, and patients were enrolled in a standard 3-month cardiac rehabilitation program. Peak exercise myocardial oxygen consumption, lactate threshold, and quality-of-life questionnaires were assessed at 1, 2, and 3 months. Twenty-one patients had normal cardiac output responses to exercise. Each of these 21 patients participated in the rehabilitation program without difficulty, and 9 (43%) responded to rehabilitation, defined as a greater than 10% increase in both peak exercise myocardial oxygen consumption and anaerobic threshold. Among the 11 patients with reduced cardiac output responses to exercise, 3 discontinued rehabilitation because of severe exhaustion and only 1 qualified as a responder. Thus, in patients with CHF and normal cardiac output responses to exercise, one may expect frequent improvement with exercise training. However, in patients with severe hemodynamic dysfunction during exercise, there is usually no improvement with training (Figure 3-3).

Previous exercise training studies in patients with chronic CHF were performed for periods lasting longer than 2 months, and effects of activity restriction on exercise-induced benefit were not systematically assessed. With the exception of 1 study, patients were not reported to be transplant candidates. Meyer and associates[10] from Bad Krozingen, Germany, examined in a random-order crossover study the effects of 3 weeks of exercise training and 3 weeks of exercise restriction on functional capacity in 18 hospitalized patients with

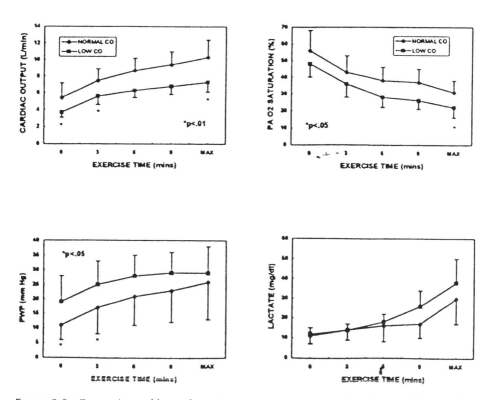

FIGURE 3-3. Comparison of hemodynamic responses to exercise in patients with normal vs. reduced cardiac output (CO) responses to exercise. Statistical comparisons were not performed at 6 and 9 minutes because many patients terminated exercise at 4 to 9 minutes. PWP indicates pulmonary wedge pressure. Reproduced with permission from Wilson et al.[9]

severe CHF (mean age 52 ± 2 years; EF 21% ± 1%); half were on a transplant waiting list. The training program consisted of interval exercise with bicycle ergometer (15 minutes, 5 times weekly), interval treadmill walking (10 minutes 3 times weekly) and exercises (20 minutes, 3 times weekly). With training, the onset of ventilatory threshold was delayed with increased work rate by 57% and oxygen uptake by 23.7%. On average, there was a 14.6% decrease in slope of ventilation/carbon dioxide production before the onset of ventilatory threshold and ventilatory equivalent of carbon dioxide production by 10.3%. At the highest comparable work rate (56 ± 5 W), the following variables were decreased: heart rate (7.3%), lactate (26.6%), and ratings of perceived leg fatigue and dyspnea (14.5% and 16.5%). At peak exercise, oxygen uptake was increased by 19.7% and oxygen pulse by 14.2%. There was a correlation of baseline peak oxygen uptake and increase of peak oxygen uptake due to training. Independently of the random order, data after activity restriction did not differ significantly from data measured at baseline. Patients with stable, severe CHF can achieve significant improvements in aerobic and ventilatory capacity and symptomology by short-term exercise training using interval exercise methods. Impairments due to activity restriction suggest the need for long-term exercise training.

Abnormalities of skeletal muscle appear to play a role in the limitation of exercise capacity in CHF. Massie and colleagues[11] from San Francisco, California, and Athens, Georgia, further characterized the skeletal muscle morphology and histochemistry in 18 men with mild-to-moderate CHF, as compared with 8 age- and gender-matched sedentary control subjects. Studies included measurements of peak systemic oxygen consumption during cycle ergometry, resistance to fatigue of the quadriceps femoris muscle group, and biopsy of the vastus lateralis muscle. Peak oxygen consumption and resistance to fatigue were lower in the patients with heart failure than in control subjects. Heart failure patients also had a lower proportion of slow-twitch, type I fibers (36% vs. 46%), and a higher proportion of fast-twitch, type IIab fibers (18% vs 17%). Cross-sectional area was smaller, and a mitochondrial oxidative marker was lower in patients. Peak oxygen consumption and resistance to fatigue correlated significantly with several measures of fiber size, especially of fast-twitch fibers in patients. These authors concluded that CHF is associated with changes in the characteristics of skeletal muscle and local, as well as systemic, exercise performance. There are fewer slow-twitch fibers, smaller fast-twitch fibers, and lower succinate dehydrogenase activity. The latter suggests that the mitochondrial content of muscle is reduced in heart failure and may play a role in the limitation of exercise capacity.

The aim of this study by Chati and associates[12] from Nancy, France, was to investigate the contribution of physical deconditioning in skeletal muscle metabolic abnormalities in patients with chronic CHF. Phosphate metabolism was studied in the leg muscle at rest and during exercise by using phosphate-31 nuclear magnetic resonance spectroscopy in a group of 14 patients with New York Heart Association class II and III CHF and LVEF less than 40%, and in 2 groups of age-matched healthy volunteers: 1 group of 7 sedentary and another group of 7 physically fit individuals. Phosphocreatine depletion rate, intracellular pH, and adenosine diphosphate levels in the muscle during exercise were not statistically different in the CHF patients and in the sedentary healthy individuals, but both groups were statistically different from the physically fit healthy individuals who had slower phosphocreatine depletion rates, as well as less intracellular acidosis and lower adenosine diphosphate levels during exercise. These results suggest that metabolic changes occurring in the skeletal muscle of patients with CHF contribute to the limitation of exercise capacity and are most likely a consequence of physical deconditioning because they are very similar to what is observed in sedentary and otherwise healthy individuals as compared with physically fit individuals.

Cardiac Sympathetic Nerve Function

In this study, Eisenhofer and colleagues[13] used a comprehensive neurochemical approach to examine the mechanisms responsible for increased availability of norepinephrine and depletion of myocardial norepinephrine stores in patients with heart failure. Fifty-four patients with CHF, including 42 men and 12 women, (mean age, 52 years), and 57 control subjects (mean age, 50 years) were evaluated. All patients with CHF had LVEFs of less than 35%. Most were in New York Heart Association functional class III, 6 were in class II, and 3 were in class IV. Ischemic cardiomyopathy was demonstrated in 25 patients by coronary angiography, one patient had CHF secondary to valvular heart disease, and the remainder had idiopathic dilated cardiomyopathy. Subjects with and without CHF received intravenous infusions of [^{3}H] norepinephrine. Cardiac spillover, reuptake, vesicular-axoplasmic exchange, and tissue stores of norepinephrine were assessed from arterial and coronary venous plasma concentrations of endogenous and [^{3}H]-labeled norepinephrine and dihydroxyphenylglycol. Tyrosine hydroxylase activity was assessed from plasma dopamine, and norepinephrine turnover was assessed from measurements of norepinephrine metabolites. Norepinephrine release and reuptake were both increased in the failing heart. However, the efficiency of norepinephrine uptake was reduced such that cardiac spillover of norepinephrine was increased disproportionately more than neuronal release of norepinephrine. Cardiac norepinephrine stores were 47% lower, and the rate of vesicular leakage of norepinephrine was 42% lower in the failing than in the normal heart. Cardiac spillover of dopamine and norepinephrine turnover were increased similarly in patients with congestive heart failure. These data indicate that increased neuronal release of norepinephrine and decreased efficiency of norepinephrine uptake both contribute to increased cardiac adrenergic drive in patients with CHF. Decreased vesicular leakage of norepinephrine, as a result of decreased myocardial stores of norepinephrine, limits the increase in cardiac norepinephrine turnover in patients with CHF. Decreased norepinephrine store size in the failing heart appears to result not from insufficient tyrosine hydroxylation, but from chronically increased norepinephrine turnover and reduced efficiency of norepinephrine uptake and storage (Figure 3-4).

Prognosis

There are conflicting data regarding the relation between gender, clinical characteristics, and survival in patients with CHF. Adams and colleagues[14]

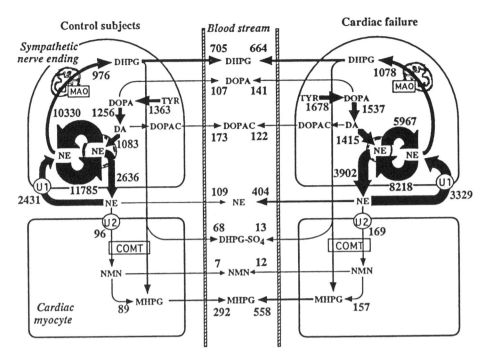

FIGURE 3-4. The processes of synthesis, vesicular-axoplasmic exchange, metabolism, release, neuronal and extraneuronal uptakes, spillover, and turnover of NE for sympathetic nerves of the normal (left) and failing (right) human heart at rest. U1 indicates neuronal uptake; U2, extraneuronal uptake; TYR, tyrosine; DHPG-SO$_4$, DHPG sulfate; MAO, monoamine oxidase; COMT, catechol-*O*-methyltransferase. Numbers with each arrow represent the rates of each process in picomoles per minute. Reproduced with permission from Eisenhofer et al.[13]

from Chapel Hill, North Carolina, examined the relation of these factors in 557 patients (380 men, 177 women) who had symptomatic heart failure predominantly ischemic in origin (68%) and typically associated with severe left ventricular dysfunction. Follow-up data were available in 99% of patients over an average of 2.4 years. By life-table analysis, women were significantly less likely to reach the endpoint of mortality. A significant association was found between female gender and better survival, which depended on the primary etiology of the heart failure but not on baseline ventricular function. Women survived longer than did men when heart failure was due to nonischemic causes. In contrast, outcome appeared similar when heart failure was due to ischemic heart disease. These authors concluded that women with heart failure due to nonischemic causes had significantly better survival than did men.

The DD genotype is a linkage marker for a mutation at or near the angiotensin-converting enzyme (ACE) gene and has been associated with increased risk for the development of CAD, left ventricular hypertrophy, and left ventricular dilation after acute myocardial infarction (AMI). Andersson and Sylvén[15] from Göteborg, Sweden, and Stockholm, Sweden, investigated the association between the DD genotype of the ACE gene and survival and cardiac function in patients with idiopathic heart failure. The genotype was determined in 193 patients recruited from a large, unselected population of patients with CHF and was compared with a control group from the general population. The frequency of the D allele was not significantly different in the study and control groups (0.57 vs. 0.56). Long-term survival was significantly worse in the patients with the DD genotype than in the remaining patients (5-year survival rate: 49% vs. 72%). The independent importance of the DD genotype for prognosis was verified by a multivariate Cox proportional hazards analysis. The odds ratio for mortality with the DD genotype was 1.69. These authors concluded that ACE gene DD polymorphism was associated with poorer survival and an increase in left ventricular mass in patients with idiopathic heart failure.

Survival with Advanced CHF and Atrial Fibrillation

Atrial fibrillation (AF) occurs in 15% to 30% of patients with heart failure. Despite the recognized potential for adverse effects, the impact of AF on prognosis is controversial. Stevenson and colleagues[16] from Boston, Massachusetts, and Los Angeles, California, evaluated whether changes in heart failure therapy since 1989 have altered the prognostic significance of AF. Two-year survival for 750 consecutive patients discharged from a single hospital after evaluation for heart transplantation from 1985 to 1989 (group I, n = 3359) and from 1990 to 1993 (group II, n = 391) was analyzed in relation to AF. In group I, class I antiarrhythmic drugs and hydralazine vasodilator drugs were routinely allowed. In group II, amiodarone and ACE-inhibitors were first line antiarrhythmic and vasodilating drugs. A history of AF was present in 20% of patients in group I and 24% of those in group II. Among patients with AF, those in group II had a markedly better 2-year survival (.66 vs. 39) and sudden death-free survival (.84 vs. 70) than those in group I. In each time period, survival was worse for patients with than without AF in group I (0.39 vs. 0.55) but not in group II (0.66 vs. 0.75). These authors concluded that the prognosis of patients with advanced heart failure and AF is improving. These findings also lend support to the practice of avoiding class I antiarrhythmic drugs in this group and may also reflect recent beneficial changes in heart failure therapy.

Oxidative Stress

In this study by Díaz-Vélez and associates[17] from San Juan, Puerto Rico, malondialdehyde, a marker of lipid peroxidation, was measured in the plasma of patients with CHF having varying degrees of clinical symptoms and in control individuals. The 53 patients studied were divided into 2 groups based on their LVEF. Group A consisted of 30 symptomatic patients with chronic CHF and LVEF less than 40%. Group B consisted of 23 asymptomatic patients with LVEF greater than 40%. Patients in group A (mean LVEF = 28) had a significantly greater history of myocardial infarction (88% vs. 48%) than did those in group B. Group B patients and the controls had similar LVEFs (58 vs. 62). Neither patients in group A nor those in group B showed correlation between malondialdehyde values and LVEF, unless controls were included. Mean malondialdehyde concentrations in groups A (2.65 ± 1.03 μmol/L) and B (2.1 ±

0.7 μmol/L) were significantly higher than those in the control group (1.45 ± 0.77 μmol/L), supporting the hypothesis that the CHF state and underlying risk conditions appear to be associated with abnormal oxidative stress. Moreover, a significant correlation was found in group A patients between the malondialdehyde values and the duration in years (chronicity) of the CHF state.

Treatment

Enalapril versus Hydralazine Isosorbide Dinitrate

Heart failure with mild systolic dysfunction occurs commonly but is generally understudied because clinical trials often exclude patients with an EF greater than 35%. Carson and colleagues[18] from Washington, D.C., evaluated such patients in the Vasodilator in Heart Failure (V-HEFT) I and II trials. In both studies, patients with an LVEF greater than 35% had higher functional capacity and lower cardiac dimensions than did patients with a lower EF. There was a lower cumulative mortality and less frequent hospital admissions for heart failure. Cumulative mortality and morbidity did not differ between treatment groups in V-HeFT-I, whereas enalapril versus hydralazine isosorbide dinitrate decreased overall mortality in V-HeFT-II. Enalapril also decreased VT at follow-up in this group. These authors concluded that in the 2 V-HeFT trials, CHF with mild systolic dysfunction had a more favorable prognosis and that enalapril decreased overall mortality and sudden death in this group compared with hydralazine isosorbide dinitrate. Prospective trials, however, are needed to address potential therapeutic differences in this group of patients.

Carvedilol

Packer and colleagues[19] in the Prospective Randomized Evaluation of Carvedilol in Symptoms and Exercise (PRECISE) trial enrolled 278 patients with moderate-to-severe heart failure and an LVEF of 35% or less at 31 centers. After an open-label, run-in period, each patient was randomly assigned to either placebo (n = 145) or carvedilol (n = 133, with a target dose of 25 to 50 mg twice a day) for 6 months. Additional therapy with digoxin, diuretics, and an angiotensin-converting enzyme ACE inhibitor remained constant. Compared with placebo, patients in the carvedilol group had a greater frequency of symptomatic improvement and lower risk of clinical deterioration as evaluated by changes in their New York Heart Association functional class and by global assessment of progress judged either by the patient or by the physician. In addition, treatment with carvedilol was associated with a significant increase in LVEF and a significant decrease in the combined risk of morbidity and mortality. Therapy with this drug was accompanied by an increase in LVEF of 0.08 on carvedilol versus 0.03 on placebo, p<.001. Twenty-four percent of the placebo group, but only 14.5% of the carvedilol group required hospitalization for cardiovascular reasons (p = .029). When death and cardiovascular hospitalizations were combined in a time-to-first-event analysis, the probability of a major fatal or nonfatal event was reduced by carvedilol from 31% to 19.6%

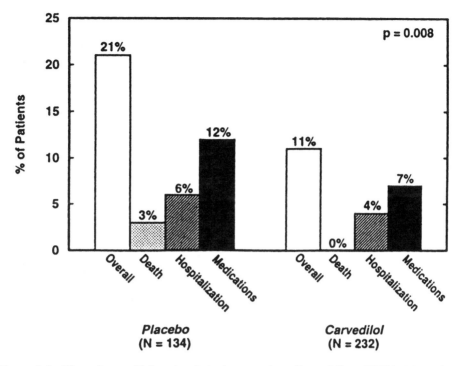

Figure 3-5. Effect of carvedilol on the clinical progression of heart failure (CHF) in 366 patients randomly assigned to carvedilol (n = 232) or placebo (n = 134). The progression of heart failure was defined as death due to heart failure, hospitalization for heart failure, or the need to increase heart failure medications. Reproduced with permission from Colucci et al.[20]

(p = 0.029). However, carvedilol therapy had little effect on indirect measures of patient benefit, including change in exercise tolerance or quality of life scores. The effects of the drug were similar in patients with CAD or idiopathic dilated cardiomyopathy as a cause of CHF. Thus, these findings indicate that in addition to its favorable effects on survival, carvedilol produces important clinical benefits in patients with moderate-to-severe CHF also treated with digoxin, diuretics, and an ACE inhibitor.

Colucci and colleagues[20] in the PRECISE trial tested the hypothesis that carvedilol inhibits clinical progression in patients with mildly symptomatic CHF due to left ventricular systolic dysfunction. Patients (n = 366) with mildly symptomatic CHF and with an LVEF of 0.35 or less and minimal functional impairment who were receiving optimized standard therapy, including ACE inhibitors, were double-blind randomly assigned to carvedilol (n = 232) or placebo (n = 134) and followed for 12 months. The primary end point was clinical progression, defined as death due to CHF, hospitalization for CHF, or a sustained increase in CHF medications. Clinical progression of CHF occurred in 21% of placebo patients and in 11% of carvedilol patients, reflecting a 48% reduction in the primary endpoint of CHF progression (Figures 3-5 and 3-6). This effect of carvedilol was not influenced by sex, age, race, etiology of CHF, or baseline LVEF. Carvedilol therapy also significantly improved several secondary endpoints, including LVEF, CHF score, New York Heart Association

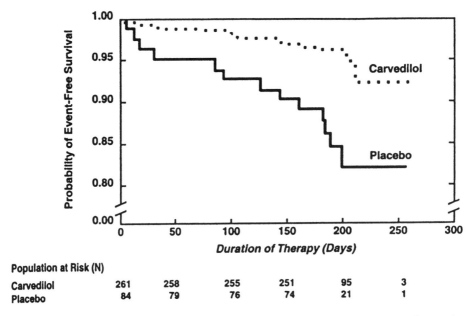

Figure 3-6. Kaplan-Meier plot of the progression of heart failure in patients randomized to carvedilol or placebo, as described in Fig 3-5. Carvedilol reduced the occurrence of heart failure progression by 48% (p = .007). The relative risk of heart failure was 0.52 (CI, 0.32 to 0.85). Reproduced with permission from Colucci et al.[20]

functional class, and the physician and patient global assessments. Carvedilol reduced all-cause mortality, but had no effects on the Minnesota Living With Heart Failure scale, the distance walked in 9 minutes on a self-powered treadmill, or cardiothoracic index. The drug was well tolerated. Thus, these data indicate that when carvedilol is added to standard therapy, including an ACE inhibitor, there is a reduction in the clinical progression to CHF in patients who are only mildly symptomatic and initially have well-compensated CHF.

Bristow and colleagues[21] conducted a multicenter, placebo-controlled trial designed to establish the efficacy and safety of carvedilol, a third-generation β-blocking agent with vasodilator properties in patients with CHF. Three hundred forty-five subjects with mild-to-moderate, stable but chronic CHF were randomly assigned to receive treatment with placebo, 6.25 mg twice daily of carvedilol (low-dose group), 12.5 mg twice daily carvedilol (medium-dose group), or 25 mg twice daily carvedilol (high-dose group). After a 2- to 4-week up-titration period, subjects remained on study medication for a period of 6 months. The primary efficacy variable was submaximal exercise measured by 2 different techniques: the 6-minute corridor walk and 9-minute self-powered treadmill test. Carvedilol had no detectable effect on submaximal exercise measured by either method. However, therapy with carvedilol was associated with a dose-related improvement in LV function by 5, 6, and 8 ejection fraction units in the low-, medium-, and high-dose carvedilol groups, compared with 2 ejection fraction units with placebo (p<0.001) for linear dose response. Survival was enhanced with increasing doses of carvedilol, with mortality rates of 6%, 6.7%, and 1% compared with 15.5% in the placebo group (p<.001) (Figures 3-7 and 3-8). When the 3 carvedilol groups were combined, the all-

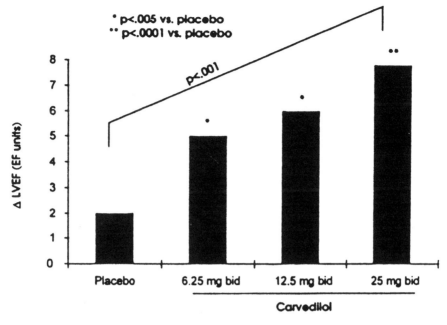

FIGURE 3-7. LVEF data at end of 6-month maintenance period as change (Δ) from baseline values. Reproduced with permission from Bristow et al.[21]

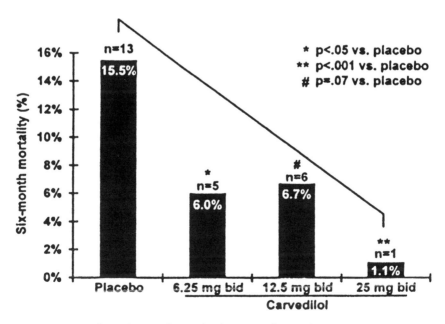

FIGURE 3-8. Six-month crude mortality as deaths per randomized patients × 100. Reproduced with permission from Bristow et al.[21]

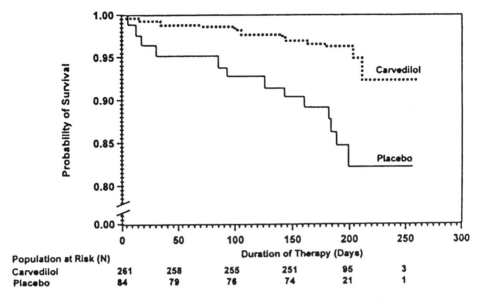

FIGURE 3-9. Actuarial survival curves for placebo group vs all carvedilol treatment groups combined. Reproduced with permission from Bristow et al.[21]

cause mortality risk was lowered by 73% in the carvedilol-treated subjects (Figure 3-9). Carvedilol also lowered the hospitalization rate by 58% to 64%, and was usually well tolerated. Thus, in subjects with mild-to-moderate CHF from systolic dysfunction, carvedilol produced dose-related improvements in left ventricular function and in mortality and hospitalization rates.

Packer and colleagues[22] in the U.S. Carvedilol Heart Failure Study Group enrolled 1094 patients with chronic heart failure in a double-blind, placebo-controlled, stratified program in which patients were assigned to 1 of 4 treatment protocols on the basis of their exercise capacity. Within each of the 4 protocols, patients with mild, moderate, or severe heart failure with LVEFs of 35% or less were randomly assigned to receive either placebo (n = 398) or the β-blocker carvedilol (n = 696). Patients were continued on digoxin, diuretics, and an angiotensin converting enzyme inhibitor. Patients were followed to determine the occurrence of death or hospitalization for cardiovascular reasons during the following 6 months (12 months for the group with mild heart failure). The overall mortality rate was 7.8% in the placebo group and 3.2% in the carvedilol group. The reduction in risk attributable to carvedilol was 65%. This finding led the Data and Safety Monitoring Board to recommend termination of the study before its scheduled end. Compared with placebo, carvedilol therapy was accompanied by 27% reduction in the risk of hospitalization for cardiovascular diseases (19.6% vs. 14%), as well as a 38% reduction in the combined risk of hospitalization or death (Figures 3-10 and 3-11). Worsening heart failure as an adverse reaction during treatment was less frequent in the carvedilol-treated patients. Thus, carvedilol, a nonselective β-blocker that also blocks α-1 adrenergic receptors and exerts antioxidant and vasodilative effects, reduces the risk of death as well as the risk of hospitalization for cardiovascular causes in patients with CHF who are receiving treatment with digoxin, diuretics, and an angiotensin-converting enzyme-inhibitor.

Plasma Endothelin-1 Levels Reflect Clinical Response to β-Blockade

Plasma levels of endothelin-1 are elevated in patients with chronic heart failure; however, it is unknown whether changes in plasma endothelin-1 levels accurately reflect clinical response to therapy in these patients. To determine this, Krum and associates[24] from New York, New York, measured plasma endothelin-1 in addition to functional, hemodynamic, and other neurohormonal parameters as part of a double-blind, placebo-controlled study of the β-blocker vasodilator carvedilol in patients with moderate-to-severe chronic heart failure. Patients were assigned (2 : 1 randomization) to receive carvedilol (25 mg twice daily, n = 10) or placebo (n = 5) for 14 weeks, with evaluations made before and after therapy. Compared with patients receiving placebo, patients receiving carvedilol improved significantly as assessed by the parameters described. These changes were paralleled by significant falls in endothelin-1 with carvedilol in comparison to placebo. Changes in endothelin-1 after treatment in both

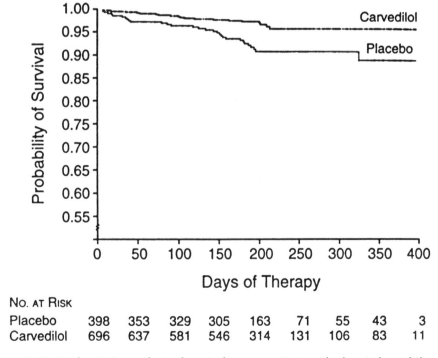

No. at Risk									
Placebo	398	353	329	305	163	71	55	43	3
Carvedilol	696	637	581	546	314	131	106	83	11

FIGURE 3-10. Kaplan-Meier analysis of survival among patients with chronic heart failure in the placebo and carvedilol groups. Patients in the carvedilol group had a 65% lower risk of death than did patients in the placebo group (p <.001). Reproduced with permission from Packer et al.[22]

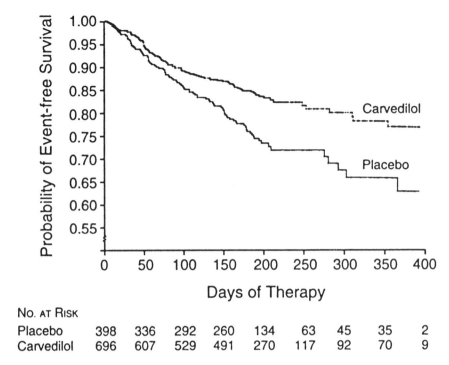

FIGURE 3-11. Kaplan-Meier analysis of survival without hospitalization for cardiovascular reasons (event-free survival) in the placebo and carvedilol groups. Patients in the carvedilol group had a 38% lower risk of death or hospitalization for cardiovascular disease than did patients in the placebo group (p<.001). Reproduced with permission from Packer et al.[22]

groups correlated significantly with changes in symptom severity, New York Heart Association class, 6-minute walk distance, hemodynamic parameters (EF, RA pressure, PA diastolic pressure, PA wedge pressure, and stroke volume index), and neurohormonal parameters (serum aldosterone and plasma norepinephrine). By step-wise regression analysis, change in endothelin-1 was an independent, noninvasive predictor of functional and hemodynamic responses to therapy in these patients. These findings suggest that endothelin-1 accurately reflects functional, hemodynamic, and neurohormonal responses to β-blocker therapy in patients with CHF. Measurement of endothelin-1 may therefore be a useful noninvasive approach to the evaluation of clinical response to drug therapy in these patients.

Metoprolol versus Carvedilol

Gilbert and colleagues[25] compared the effects of carvedilol and metoprolol on adrenergic activity, receptor expression, degree of clinical β-blockade, hemodynamics, and left ventricular function in patients with mild-to-moderate heart failure. The effects of carvedilol versus metoprolol were compared in 2 concurrent, placebo-controlled trials with carvedilol or metoprolol, with common substudies focusing on adrenergic, hemodynamic, and left ventricular functional measurements. All subjects in the substudies had chronic CHF resulting from idiopathic dilated cardiomyopathy. Carvedilol (50 to 100 mg/day) produced reductions in exercise heart rate that were similar to metoprolol (125–150 mg/day) indicating comparable degrees of β-blockade. Compared with metoprolol, carvedilol was associated with greater improvement in New York Heart Association functional class. There were no significant differences in hemodynamic effects between the carvedilol- and metoprolol-active treatment groups, but carvedilol selectively lowered coronary sinus norepinephrine levels, an index of cardiac adrenergic activity, whereas metoprolol did not. Metoprolol was associated with an increase in cardiac β-receptor density, whereas carvedilol did not change this variable. Thus, the third-generation β-blocking agent carvedilol has different effects on adrenergic activity and β-receptor expression and on New York Heart Association functional class than does the second-generation β-blocker metoprolol.

Propranolol versus Metoprolol

Newton and Parker[26] in Toronto, Ontario, Canada, measured cardiac norepinephrine spillover responses in patients with CHF after the acute administration of either propranolol, a nonselected β-blocker, or metoprolol, a $β_1$-selective agent. Eighteen patients were evaluated. Repeated intravenous doses of propranolol (0.5 mg in 9 patients with LVEF of 14%) or metoprolol (1.0 mg in 9 patients with LVEF of 18%) were given until 1 of the following end points was reached: a 15% decrease in heart rate, LV + dP/dt, or mean arterial pressure, or a 5 mm Hg increase in left ventricular end-diastolic pressure. Propranolol (mean dose, 2.0 mg) and metoprolol (mean dose, 3.6 mg) caused similar reductions in heart rate, + dP/dt, and coronary sinus plasma flow. Cardiac norepinephrine spillover was reduced after propranolol, but was increased after metoprolol (Figure 3-12). In comparison of the 2 groups, the decrease in norepinephrine spillover after propranolol was significantly different from the increase seen after metoprolol. Thus, the administration of a $β_1$-selective antagonist was associated with increased cardiac norepinephrine spillover, but the administration of a nonselective β-blocker to similar hemodynamic endpoints caused a reduction in norepinephrine spillover. These data suggest that in patients with CHF, nonselective β-blockade may have favorable inhibitory effects on cardiac sympathetic activity.

Amiodarone

Massie and colleagues[27] in San Francisco, California, determined whether the increase in LVEF after amiodarone administration is associated with an improvement in symptoms and/or physical findings of CHF or a reduction in the number of hospitalizations for CHF. In the Department of Veterans Affairs Cooperative Study of Amiodarone in Congestive Heart Failure, 674 patients with New York Heart Association class II through IV symptoms and LVEF of

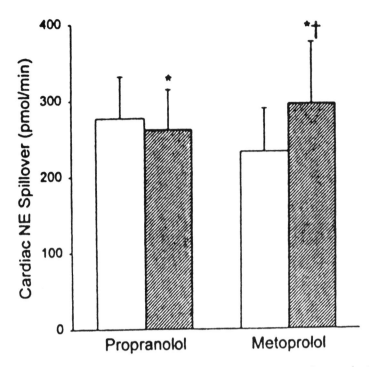

FIGURE 3-12. Bar graph of cardiac norepinephrine spillover at control (open bar) and after administration of either propranolol or metoprolol (hatched bar). *p<.05 vs. control. †p<.01 for between-group comparison of the change in spillover. Reproduced with permission from Newton et al.[26]

40% or less were treated with amiodarone or placebo for a median of 45 months in a randomized, double-blind, placebo-controlled study. Clinical assessments and radionuclide LVEF were performed at baseline and after 6, 12, and 24 months. Compared with the placebo group, LVEF increased more in the amiodarone group at each time point: 8% versus 3% at 6 months, 8% versus 3% at 12 months, and 9% versus 2% at 24 months (Figure 3-13). However, this difference was not associated with greater clinical improvement, fewer diuretic requirements, or fewer hospitalizations for CHF. There was a trend toward a reduction in the combined end point of hospitalizations and cardiac deaths, which was significant in patients with nonischemic etiologies for their CHF but not apparent in the patients with CAD. Thus, although amiodarone therapy results in a substantial increase in LVEF in patients with CHF, this was not associated with clinical benefits in the patients as a whole. Substantial reduction in the combined end points of cardiac death plus hospitalizations for CHF in the nonischemic group suggests possible benefit in these patients.

d-Sotalol

In contrast to Vaughan Williams class I drugs, class III drugs, such as d-sotalol, may not be negative inotropic. These drugs block potassium ion channels and prolong repolarization, theoretically leading to improved contractility. Gottlieb and colleagues[28] from several United States medical centers investigated the hemodynamic action of acute intravenous administration of 1.5 mg/kg of d-sotalol in 28 patients with CHF randomly assigned to receive placebo or active drug in a double-blind study. A Swan-Ganz catheter was placed in all patients at least 16 hours before drug administration. All hemodynamic variables were assessed at baseline at 30 minutes and 1, 2, 4, 8, and 12 hours after administration of the drug. Electrocardiograms were obtained before and 1, 2, 4, and 12 hours after drug administration. The QT interval increased from 370 ± 9 to 426 ± 14 msec at 1 hour, whereas the QTc increased from 433 ± 5 to 470 ± 12 msec. The increase was still statistically significant at 12 hours. There was no change in the placebo group. Although heart rate decreased in the d-sotalol group (84 ± 2 to 76 ± 2 at 1 hour), there were no changes in blood pressure or RA pressure. Cardiac index decreased slightly (2.0 ± 0.2 to 1.9 ± 0.1 mm Hg), consistent with the lower heart rate. Pulmonary artery wedge pressure decreased from 18.9 ± 2.4 to 17.9 ± 1.9 mm Hg at 1 hour despite reduced cardiac index. The authors conclude that in contrast to class I, II, and IV antiarrhythmic drugs, d-sotalol exerts no clinically important acute hemodynamic actions at doses that produce electrophysiologic effects.

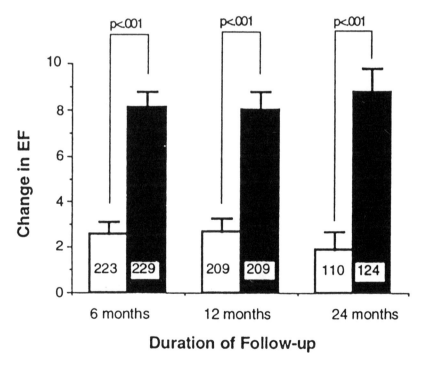

FIGURE 3-13. Change in LVEF. The mean change (± 1 SEM) in EF from baseline to 6, 12, and 24 months is shown for the patients treated with amiodarone (solid bars) and placebo (open bars). The rise in the amiodarone group was significantly greater at each interval, representing an approximate 33% increase over the baseline of 26%. The numbers below each column indicate the number of patients with repeat measurements in whom the change was evaluated. Reproduced with permission from Massie et al.[27]

L-Arginine

Rector and colleagues[29] in Minneapolis, Minnesota, conducted a randomized, double-blind crossover study design to determine whether supplemental oral L-arginine augments peripheral blood flow and improves functional status in patients with moderate-to-severe CHF. Fifteen subjects were given 6 weeks of L-arginine hydrochloride and 6 weeks of matched placebo capsules in random sequence. Compared with placebo, supplemental oral L-arginine significantly increased forearm blood flow during forearm exercise on average from 5 to 7 mL · min^{-1} · dL^{-1}. Functional status was better on L-arginine compared with placebo as indicated by increased distances achieved during a 6-minute walk and lower scores on the Living With Heart Failure questionnaire (Figures 3-14 and 3-15). Oral L-arginine also improved arterial compliance and reduced circulating levels of endothelin. Thus, supplemental oral L-arginine had beneficial effects in patients with CHF in this study. No important adverse effects were identified as a consequence of L-arginine therapy in these patients.

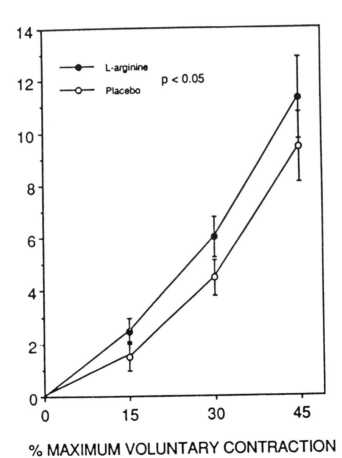

% MAXIMUM VOLUNTARY CONTRACTION

FIGURE 3-14. Effect of oral L-arginine on forearm blood flow during exercise with a hand dynamometer. Increases in forearm blood flow were significantly greater (p<.05) after 6 weeks of L-arginine compared with the placebo. Reproduced with permission from Rector et al.[29]

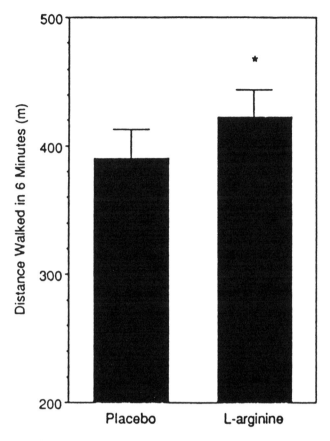

FIGURE 3-15. Mean changes in the 6-minute walk test. Patients walked significantly (*p<.05) greater distances after 6 weeks of oral L-arginine. Reproduced with permission from Rector et al.[29]

Endothelin-Converting Enzyme Inhibitor and Endothelin DT$_A$ Receptor Blockade

Love and colleagues[30] in Glasgow, Scotland, investigated the effects of endothelin-converting enzyme inhibition and endothelin ET$_A$ receptor blockade in patients with CHF treated with ACE inhibitors. The authors compared the function of ET$_A$ and ET$_B$ receptors in healthy subjects and patients with CHF. Locally active doses of study drugs were infused into the nondominant brachial artery while forearm blood flow was measured by venous occlusion plethysmography. In CHF patients (n = 10), phosphoramidon (a combined endothelin-converting enzyme and neutral endopeptidase inhibitor), and BQ-123 (an ET$_A$ receptor antagonist) increased forearm blood flow by 52% ± 10% and 31% ± 6%, respectively, and thiorphan (a selective neutral endopeptidase inhibitor) reduced forearm blood flow by 15% ± 5%. Forearm vasoconstriction to endothelin-1 was significantly blunted in CHF patients compared with control subjects, whereas vasoconstriction to sarafotoxin S6c (an ET$_B$ receptor agonist) was significantly enhanced in CHF patients compared with controls. These data suggest that endothelin-converting enzyme inhibitors and ET_A receptor antagonists may be useful as vasodilator agents in CHF patients already receiving treatment with an ACE inhibitor. Both ET_A and ET_B receptors may mediate agonist-induced vasoconstriction in healthy subjects and patients with CHF, but further studies are required to clarify the contribution of each receptor subtype in mediating the effects of endothelin-1.

Zofenopril

Limited data are available on the effects of ACE inhibitors on the onset and progression of CHF in patients with AMI. Borghi and associates[31] on behalf of the Survival of Myocardial Infarction Long-term Evaluation (SMILE) study investigators performed a substudy of the SMILE trial involving 1/146 patients with anterior wall AMI not undergoing thrombolysis. Patients with prior history or clinical signs of CHF on admission were excluded. Patients were randomly allocated to treatment with zofenopril (7.5 to 30 mg twice daily) or placebo for a cumulative period of 6 weeks. The prevalence of CHF, either mild-to-moderate or severe, has been the main objective and has been evaluated 6 weeks and 1 year after AMI. The overall prevalence of CHF was not reduced by zofenopril after both 6 weeks and 12 months. Conversely the prevalence of severe CHF (1.6% vs. 2.6%: risk reduction 55.5%) and the combined occurrence of death or severe CHF (4.8% vs. 8.2%: risk reduction 59%) were reduced after 6 weeks of treatment with zofenopril. Moreover, the percentage of patients experiencing a deterioration to severe CHF after 1 year was significantly reduced with zofenopril (11.0% vs. 24.3%). In conclusion, the early administration of zofenopril to patients with AMI attenuates the progression of the clinical symptoms of CHF and its clinical consequences, suggesting that ACE inhibitors should be regarded as a suitable strategy for the prevention and treatment of CHF in patients with AMI.

Furosemide

Diuretic therapy is a mainstay for controlling fluid overload in patients with CHF. Dormans and colleagues[32] from Nijmegen, Amsterdam, and Veldhoven, The Netherlands, compared the efficacy of high-dose bolus injection versus continuous infusion of furosemide. In a randomized, crossover trial, they studied the efficacy of a continuous infusion of high-dose furosemide (mean daily dose, 690 mg) versus a single bolus injection of an equal dose in 20 patients with severe CHF. Daily urinary volume and sodium excretion were significantly higher after treatment with continuous infusion than with bolus injection (infusion 2860 mL vs. bolus 2260 mL). Short-term, completely reversible hearing loss was reported after bolus injection in 5 patients. These authors concluded that in patients with severe CHF, high-dose furosemide administered as a continuous infusion is more efficacious than bolus injection and causes fewer ototoxic side effects.

Digitalis

In a double-blind, placebo-controlled, crossover study designed to determine the influence of digitalis on left ventricular response to physical exercise in patients with CHF, Morisco and associates[33] from Naples, Italy, and Pozzilli, Italy, assessed left ventricular function in 10 patients with CHF (EF, 29% ± 2%). The study utilized upright bicycle exercise with an ambulatory radionuclide detector for continuous noninvasive monitoring of cardiac function. Exercise was performed during control conditions and after a 3-week treatment with digoxin (0.25 mg/day orally) or placebo. Ten normal volunteers matched for sex and age constituted the control group. In normal volunteers, exercise ejection fraction and end-diastolic volume increased, while end-systolic volume decreased progressively. In control conditions, patients with CHF had a sharp increase in heart rate during exercise, while EF did not change; both end-diastolic and end-systolic volumes increased significantly during exercise. During digoxin treatment, heart rate response to exercise recorded in patients with CHF was comparable to that recorded in normal subjects. In addition, a significant increase in ejection fraction during exercise was detected, and the increase in end-systolic volume was significantly smaller than that observed in control conditions. When patients received placebo, the responses of left ventricular function to exercise were comparable to those observed in control conditions. These findings demonstrate that digitalis has a favorable influence on left ventricular functional adaptation to exercise in CHF.

Cardiomyoplasty

Dynamic cardiomyoplasty was first performed in 1985 for patients with CHF. Since heart transplantation is appropriate or available for only a small proportion of patients with severe CHF, dynamic cardiomyoplasty is a reasonable alternative for therapy. Furnary and colleagues[34] from Portland, Oregon; Philadelphia, Pennsylvania; and Sao Paulo, Brazil for the American Cardiomyoplasty Group prospectively assessed the effect of dynamic cardiomyoplasty in patients with symptomatic chronic heart failure. Eight centers in North and South America performed 68 cardiomyoplasty procedures between May 1991 and September 1993. Data were prospectively collected every 6 months. The mean age of patients was 57 years, and 78% were male. Sixty-nine percent had idiopathic cardiomyoplasty, and 31% had ischemic heart disease. The in-hospital mortality rate was 12%, and the survival rate at 6 and 12 months was 75% and 68%. Objective improvements were seen at 6 months in left ventricular ejection fraction (23% vs. 25%) and stroke volume (50% vs. 56%). Improvements in mean New York Heart Association functional class (3% vs. 1.8%) and activity of daily living score (59% vs. 80%) were also observed. There were no significant changes at 6 months in peak oxygen consumption, cardiac index, pulmonary capillary wedge pressure, or heart rate. These authors concluded that dynamic cardiomyoplasty has the potential for improving systolic function and reducing the symptoms of heart failure. This improvement occurred without changes in peak exercise capacity, ventricular filling pressure or actuarial survival. Although these results have some promise, it is clear that the ultimate role of this procedure remains uncertain until one can assess the long-term results of this and other trials.

Long-Term Left Ventricular Assist Device

James and colleagues[35] in Cleveland, Ohio, hypothesized that improvement of cardiac function by a left ventricular assist device is associated with the normalization of volume load secondary to normalization of its regulatory substances. They studied 15 patients, including 13 men and 2 women (mean age, 51 years), with end-stage CHF who were cardiac transplant candidates and eligible for HeartMate (Thermo Cardiosystems, Inc, Woburn, MA) left ventricular assist devices. They measured plasma volume and plasma levels of atrial natriuretic peptide, aldosterone, renin, and arginine vasopressin sequentially before HeartMate implantation at baseline, after HeartMate implantation (weeks 4 and 8), and after transplantation. Baseline plasma volume was 123% of normal, but it was 122% at week 4 and decreased to 115% at week 8. Atrial natriuretic peptide (ANP) was 359 pg/mL at baseline, 245 pg/mL at week 4, and 151 pg/mL at week 8. Plasma aldosterone fell from 68 ng/dL at baseline to 17 ng/dL at week 4 and was 32 ng/dL at week 8. Plasma renin activity decreased from 80 ng/dL at baseline to 11 ng/dL at week 4 and 16 ng/dL at week 8. Arginine vasopressin fell from 5 fmol/mL at baseline to 1 fmol/mL at weeks 4 and 8. Thus, the reduction of plasma renin activity, aldosterone, and arginine vasopressin occurs earlier than the reduction of plasma volume and ANP after HeartMate left ventricular assist device implantation, possibly because of decreased pulmonary congestion and improved renal perfusion. The reduction of ANP does not appear to be responsible for the lack of adequate decrease of plasma volume, but its reduction may be a marker of improved congestive symptoms and cardiac pump function.

Hypertrophic Cardiomyopathy

Echocardiographic Features of Left Ventricular Outflow Obstruction

Nakatani and associates[36] from Cleveland, Ohio, examined resting echocardiographic features predictive of latent left ventricular obstruction in 50 consecutive patients with nonobstructive hypertrophic cardiomyopathy (26 provocable, 24 nonprovocable with amyl nitrite inhalation). These findings contributed to better understanding of the pathophysiology of the hypertrophic cardiomyopathy and helped to identify latent left ventricular obstruction without pharmacological provocation. Measurements included wall thickness, type of hypertrophy, left ventricular outflow tract diameter, degree of mitral systolic anterior motion, outflow pressure gradient, and ventricular volume. The direction of the ejection streamline was measured to assess the magnitude of the drag acting on the mitral valve. Thirteen of 16 patients (81%) with proximal septal bulge were provocable, whereas only 3 of 8 patients (38%) with asymmetric septal hypertrophy and 10 of 26 (38%) with concentric hypertrophy were provocable. Left ventricular outflow tract was significantly narrower and the angle between the ejection flow and the mitral valve was larger in provocable patients. The sensitivity for predicting provocable patients by a combination of a narrow outflow tract (≥35°) was 65%, with a specificity of 80% and a positive predictive value of 79%. When these criteria were combined with the presence of septal bulge, the sensitivity was 35%, but the specificity and the positive predictive value were both 100%. Patients with nonobstructive hypertrophic cardiomyopathy with proximal septal bulge, a narrow left ventricular outflow tract, and an oblique angle between the ejection flow and the mitral valve appeared to be predisposed for latent outflow obstruction. These features are consistent with the presence of the large Venturi and drag forces. Thus, the left ventricle, which is capable of increasing both the Venturi and the drag forces on the basis of the morphologic change, contributes to the development of outflow obstruction with amyl nitrite inhalation.

Dual-Chamber Pacing

Dual-chamber pacing has been proposed as an alternative in the symptomatic treatment of patients with hypertrophic obstructive cardiomyopathy. Nishimura and colleagues[37] from Rochester, Minnesota, evaluated the acute hemodynamic effects of dual-chamber pacing. Twenty-nine patients underwent a combined cardiac catheterization and Doppler echocardiographic study during normal sinus rhythm and P-synchronous pacing at various AV intervals. During AV pacing at the shortest delay of 60 msec, there was a significant decrease in cardiac output and peak positive dP/dt and an increase in mean LA pressure and prolongation of relaxation time. During pacing at the optimal AV delay, which was the longest AV interval without pre-excitation, there was a similar trend with deterioration in both systolic and diastolic function, but of lesser magnitude. The deterioration in both systolic and diastolic function was present in 21 patients with and 8 without left ventricular outflow obstruction. There was a modest decrease in left ventricular outflow tract gradient from 73 to 61 mm Hg during dual-chamber pacing at the optimal AV delay, compared with normal sinus rhythm. These authors concluded that further studies of the long-term effects of dual-chamber pacing in carefully performed randomized trials are needed.

Hypertrophic cardiomyopathy is characterized by impaired ventricular diastolic function and, in about 25% of patients, left ventricular outflow tract obstruction. Atrioventricular (AV) pacing diminishes left ventricular outflow tract gradient in hypertrophic cardiomyopathy, but impairs diastolic function in experimental animals and in different categories of patients. To investigate the effects of AV pacing on hemodynamics and left ventricular function in obstructive hypertrophic cardiomyopathy, Betocchi and associates[38] from Naples, Italy, studied 16 patients with hypertrophic cardiomyopathy by cardiac catheterization and simultaneous radionuclide angiography during atrial and

AV pacing. The resting LV outflow tract gradient decreased with AV pacing from 60 ± 34 to 38 ± 37 mm Hg (mean = SD). Regional EF decreased significantly at the septal level, from $0.81\% \pm 0.21\%$ to $0.69\% \pm 0.27\%$. PA wedge pressure increased from 10 ± 5 to 15 ± 6 mm Hg. AV pacing-induced asynchrony (ie, the coefficient of variation of the time to end-systole) increased from $7\% \pm 4\%$ to $14\% \pm 10\%$. The time constant of isovolumetric relaxation (T) increased from 58 ± 24 to 74 ± 33 msec, and peak filling rate decreased from 491 ± 221 to 416 ± 184 mL/s. Thus, AV pacing greatly diminishes resting obstruction through a reduction in septal ejection fraction (ie, an increase in left ventricular outflow tract width in systole), but impairs active diastolic function and increases filling pressures. These latter effects are potentially detrimental in patients with hypertrophic cardiomyopathy in whom diastolic dysfunction is present.

Diltiazem

Hypertrophic cardiomyopathy is characterized by impaired diastolic function and left ventricular outflow tract obstruction in about one fourth of patients. Verapamil improves diastolic properties, but may have dangerous adverse effects. Betocchi and associates[39] from Naples, Italy, investigated the effects of diltiazem on hemodynamics and left ventricular function in 16 patients with hypertrophic cardiomyopathy who were studied with cardiac catheterization and simultaneous radionuclide angiography. Studies were performed during atrial pacing (15 beats above spontaneous rhythm) at baseline and during intravenous diltiazem administration (0.25 mg·kg^{-1} over 2 minutes, and 0.014 mg·kg^{-1} min^{-1}). Diltiazem induced a systemic vasodilation (cardiac index: 3.4 ± 1.0 to 4.0 ± 1.0 L·min^{-1} min^{-2}; aortic systolic pressure: 116 ± 16 to 107 ± 19 mm Hg; systemic resistance index: 676 ± 235 to 532 ± 193 dynes·s·cm^{-5}·m^{-2}), not associated with changes in the left ventricular outflow tract gradient. The end-systolic pressure/volume ratio decreased (30 ± 42 to 21 ± 29 mm Hg·ml^{-1}·m^{-2}). PA wedge pressure (11 ± 5 to 15 ± 6 mm Hg), and peak filling rate increased (4.1 ± 1.3 to 6.0 ± 2.4 stroke counts ·s^{-1}). The time constant of isovolumetric relaxation decreased (74 ± 40 to 59 ± 38 msec). The constant of left ventricular chamber stiffness did not change. Thus, active diastolic function is improved by the acute administration of diltiazem by both direct action and changes in hemodynamics and loading conditions. Left ventricular outflow tract gradient does not increase despite systemic vasodilation. In some patients, however, a marked increase in obstruction and a potentially harmful elevation in pulmonary artery wedge pressure do occur. Passive diastolic function is not affected.

Surgical Treatment

McCully and colleagues[41] in Rochester, Minnesota, obtained clinical, electrocardiographic, echocardiographic, cardiac catheterization, and surgical data in 65 patients 20 to 70 years old with hypertrophic obstructive cardiomyopathy who had surgical intervention between 1986 and 1992. Specific symptoms and overall functional status were evaluated before surgery and at the end of the first postoperative year. Subsequent long-term clinical postoperative follow-up was also obtained. The extent of postoperative improvement was measured by the presence and severity of persistent symptoms, overall New York Heart Association functional class, and patients' self-perception of overall improvement. Among the patients, 95% were in New York Heart Association functional class III or IV before surgery, 95% had dyspnea, 62% had angina, 63% had near-syncope, and 23% had syncope. The overall early mortality rate was 4.6%. There was no mortality among the 45 patients who underwent isolated septal myectomy. At the 1-year postoperative evaluation, 89% of survivors were in New York Heart Association functional class I or II, and 47% believed they had 100% improvement. Significant improvement was seen in 67% of patients with dyspnea, 90% with angina, 86% with near-syncope, and 100% with syncope. The 5-year survival rate was 92%. Thus, the results of the present study reaffirm the efficacy of surgical treatment of hypertrophic obstructive cardiomyopathy in patients who are severely symptomatic despite optimal medical therapy (Figure 3-16).

Dilated Cardiomyopathy

Tumor Necrosis Factor-α and Tumor Necrosis Receptors

Torre-Amione[42] and colleagues in Houston, Texas, examined messenger RNA (mRNA) and protein levels for tumor necrosis factor receptors 1 and 2 and tumor necrosis factor-α in explanted hearts from organ donors, as well as in patients with end-stage dilated cardiomyopathy and CAD. Northern blot analysis revealed that the mRNA for tumor necrosis factor 1 and 2 was present in nonfailing, dilated cardiomyopathic, and coronary heart disease-affected hearts. Tumor necrosis factor 1 and 2 receptor protein levels were decreased 60% in patients with dilated cardiomyopathy and those with coronary heart disease compared with those who had nonfailing hearts. To evaluate a mechanism for the decrease in tumor necrosis factor receptor expression, the authors measured circulating levels of soluble tumor necrosis factor receptors in patients with dilated cardiomyopathy and coronary heart disease. There was a significant 1- to 3-fold increase in soluble tumor necrosis factor receptors in patients with dilated cardiomyopathies and coronary heart disease with heart failure. Thus, the results of this study suggest that tumor necrosis factor receptor proteins may be dynamically regulated in patients with advanced CHF. Tumor necrosis factor-α messenger RNA and tumor necrosis factor-α protein were present in the explanted hearts from patients with dilated cardiomyopathy and coronary heart disease, but not in nonfailing hearts (Figures 3-17 and 3-18). The observation that failing hearts express elevated levels of tumor necrosis factor-α suggests that overexpression of this cytokine may be one of the several different maladaptive mechanisms responsible for progressive cardiac decompensation occurring in advanced heart failure.

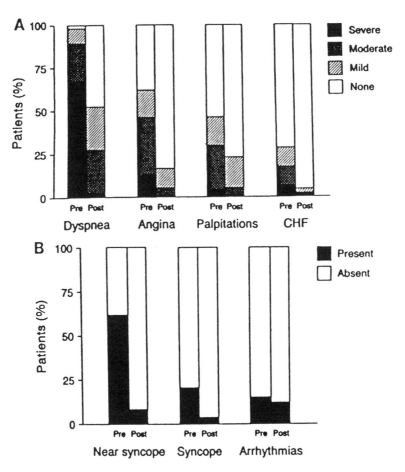

FIGURE 3-16. Symptoms before (Pre) (n = 65) and 1 year after (Post) (n = 61) surgical treatment of adult patients with hypertrophic obstructive cardiomyopathy. **A,** Severity of specific symptoms. **B,** Presence or absence of specific symptoms. The 2 patients with syncope after surgery were free of syncope before surgery. CHF indicates congestive heart failure. Reproduced with permission from McCully et al.[41]

Effects of Long-Term Metoprolol Therapy

Andersson and colleagues[43] in Göteborg, Sweden, conducted a substudy of the international Metoprolol in Dilated Cardiomyopathy Trial to evaluate diastolic function in 77 patients randomly assigned to placebo or metoprolol. The patients were treated for 12 months. Changes in Doppler flow variables in the metoprolol group indicated a less restrictive filling pattern, expressed as an increase in E-wave deceleration time (Figure 3-19). Maximal increase in deceleration time had occurred by 3 months, whereas systolic recovery was achieved gradually and maximal effect was seen by 12 months of treatment (Figure 3-20). Although deceleration time was correlated to heart rate at baseline, changes in deceleration time were not significantly correlated to changes in heart rate during treatment. During the first 3 months of treatment, maximal effects on diastolic variables were reached, whereas the most prominent effect on systolic function was seen late in the study. These data suggest that effects on diastolic left ventricular filling account for subsequent later myocardial systolic recovery. The E-wave deceleration time, which in recent studies has been shown to be a predictor of survival, was improved in the metoprolol-treated patients.

Carvedilol

Recent evidence has shown that β-adrenergic blocking agents improve left ventricular systolic function in patients with New York Heart Association class II to III CHF. The specific effects on left ventricular diastolic function have been subjected to only limited examination. Quaife and associates[44] from Denver, Colorado, and Salt Lake City, Utah, investigated the effects of the combined β blocker/vasodilator carvedilol on systolic and diastolic left ventricular performance in dilated cardiomyopathy. Thirty-six patients with New York Heart Association functional class II to III heart failure and LVEF of 35% or less were entered into either arm of this placebo-controlled, double-blind 4-month trial. Twenty-one subjects were entered into the carvedilol treatment arm, and

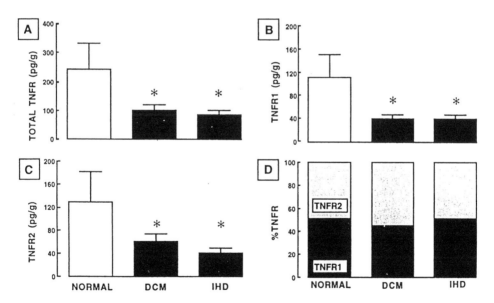

FIGURE 3-17. TNF receptor proteins (picograms of receptor protein per gram of membrane protein) in nonfailing and failing myocardium. **A,** The level of total TNF receptor proteins (TNFR1 + TNFR2) was significantly less (p<.03) in DCM and IHD patients compared with control subjects. **B and C,** The level of TNFR1 and TNFR2 receptor proteins were significantly less (p≤.03) in IHD (B) and DCM (C) hearts compared with nonfailing hearts. **D,** The relative percentages of TNFR1 and TNFR2 proteins were similar (P=.33 by ANOVA) in nonfailing, IHD, and DCM hearts. *p<.05 compared with nonfailing control hearts. Reproduced with permission from Torre-Amione et al.[42]

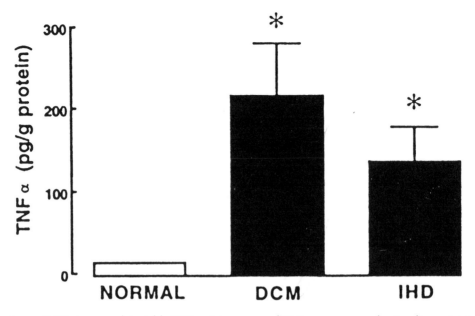

FIGURE 3-18. Immunodetectable TNF-α (picograms of TNF-α per gram of cytosolic protein) in nonfailing and failing myocardium. As shown by the open bar, immunodetectable TNF-α (ie, <5 ng/dL) was not present in nonfailing hearts (n=7), whereas immunodetectable levels of TNF-α were present in both DCM hearts (n=14) and IHD (n=16) hearts. The proportion of patients with elevated TNF-α levels was significantly greater in the DCM and IHD groups compared with nonfailing subjects (*p<.05 compared with control). Levels of intracardiac TNF-α were not significantly different in IHD and DCM hearts. Reproduced with permission from Torre-Amione et al.[42]

15 patients were entered into the placebo arm in a 3:2 ratio. Carvedilol therapy resulted in a significant improvement in LVEF (from 22% ± 2% to 30% ± 2%) when compared with the placebo group (19% ± 2% to 21% ± 2%) at baseline and after 4 months of therapy. However, no significant change in radionuclide parameters of left ventricular diastolic function, including peak filling rate or time to peak filling rate, was observed. Left ventricular end-diastolic volume index did not change with carvedilol therapy, whereas end-diastolic volume index increased in the placebo group, although the difference between groups at 4 months was significant. In conjunction with these changes, end-systolic volume index was smaller at 4 months after carvedilol treatment compared with that of the placebo group. Thus, these results demonstrate that in moderate chronic heart failure, systolic left ventricular performance improves but diastolic left ventricular function does not improve when compared with placebo after treatment with carvedilol.

Growth Hormone in the Treatment of Idiopathic Cardiomyopathy

Fazio and colleagues[45] in Naples, Italy, hypothesized that inducing cardiac hypertrophy with recombinant human growth hormone might be an effective approach to the treatment of idiopathic dilated cardiomyopathy. Seven patients with idiopathic dilated cardiomyopathy and moderate-to-severe CHF were studied at control, after 3 months of therapy with human growth hormone, and 3 months after the discontinuation of growth hormone. Standard therapy for CHF was continued in a constant manner throughout the study. Cardiac function was evaluated with Doppler echocardiography, right heart cardiac catheterization, and exercise testing. When given at a dose of 14 IU per week, growth hormone doubled the serum concentrations of insulin-like growth factor I. Growth hormone increased left ventricular wall thickness and reduced chamber size significantly. Consequently, end-systolic wall stress, a function of both wall thickness and chamber size, fell markedly from a mean of 144 ± 11 to 85 ± 8 dyne per square cm (p<.001). Growth hormone improved cardiac output, especially during exercise from 7.4 to 9.7 L/min (p = .003), and enhanced ventricular work while reducing myocardial oxygen consumption and energy production. Ventricular mechanical efficiency rose from $9\% \pm 2\%$ to $21\% \pm 5\%$ with growth hormone therapy. Growth hormone therapy also improved clinical symptoms, exercise capacity, and the patients' quality of life. The improvements in cardiac size and shape, systolic function and exercise tolerance were partially reversed 3 months after growth hormone was discontinued. These data suggest that recombinant human growth hormone administered for 3 months to patients with idiopathic dilated cardiomyopathy increases myocardial mass and reduces the size of the left ventricular chamber, resulting in improvement in hemodynamics, myocardial energy metabolism, and clinical status.

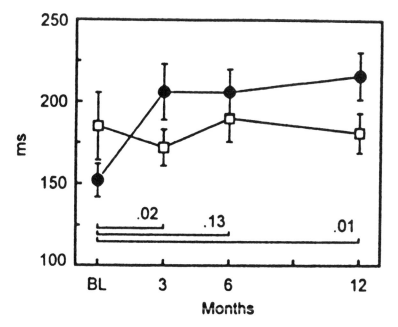

FIGURE 3-19. Effects on transmitral Doppler E-wave deceleration time. Probability values denote intergroup comparison by ANOVA from baseline (BL) to 6 and 12 months of follow-up. Data are mean ± SEM values. Filled circles represent metoprolol; unfilled squares, placebo. Reproduced with permission from Andersson et al.[43]

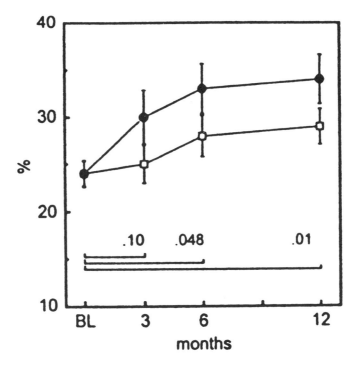

FIGURE 3-20. Effects on radionuclide ejection fraction. Probability values denote intergroup comparison by ANOVA from baseline (BL) to 6 and 12 months of follow-up. Data are mean ± SEM values. Filled circles represent metoprolol; unfilled squares, placebo. Reproduced with permission from Andersson et al.[43]

Diltiazem

Figulla and colleagues[46] in Germany evaluated the effects of adjunct diltiazem (60 to 90 mg, 3 times a day) on standard therapy in patients with idiopathic dilated cardiomyopathy. The Diltiazem in Dilated Cardiomyopathy Trial (DiDi) was a randomized, double-blind, placebo-controlled, multicenter trial of 186 patients with 92 receiving diltiazem and 94 receiving placebo. The patients had idiopathic dilated cardiomyopathy diagnosed by coronary angiography, catheterization of the left side of the heart, and a LVEF of less than 50%. The effect of adjunct diltiazem treatment on transplant listing-free survival, hemodynamics, exercise capacity, and subjective status was investigated. During the 24-month study period, 33 patients dropped out of the study; 153 patients finished the study protocol. Twenty-seven patients died or were placed on the waiting list for heart transplantation: 16 from the placebo group and 11 from the diltiazem group. Transplant listing-free survival rate was 85% for diltiazem and 80% for placebo recipients. After 24 months, only diltiazem significantly increased cardiac index at rest and under workload, systolic and diastolic pressures, stroke volume index, and stroke work index, and decreased pulmonary artery pressure under workload and heart rate. Diltiazem also increased exercise capacity and subjective sense of well being. Adverse reactions were few and distributed evenly in both groups. Thus, in patients with idiopathic dilated cardiomyopathy, adjunctive therapy of diltiazem improves cardiac function, exercise capacity, and subjective status without deleterious effects on transplant listing-free survival (Figure 3-21).

Exercise Training

The aim of this study by Belardinelli and associates[47] from Ancona, Italy, and Gilroy, California, was to determine whether exercise training can augment left ventricular diastolic filling at rest and during exercise in patients with ischemic cardiomyopathy and whether any correlation exists between changes in diastolic filling and changes in exercise tolerance. Forty-three consecutive patients (mean age, 54 ± 8 years) with ischemic cardiomyopathy and severe left ventricular systolic dysfunction (EF <30%) were studied. Group T (29 patients) was exercised on a cycle ergometer 3 times a week for 8 weeks at 60% of peak oxygen uptake. Group C (14 patients) was not exercised. All patients underwent an exercise test and radionuclide ventriculography at baseline and after 8 weeks. At the end, no changes were found in group C. In group T, exercise training increased peak oxygen uptake (15%), work rate (15%), peak early filling rate (10%), and peak filling rate (11%). At submaximal exercise, peak filling rate increased at all matched heart rates. The increase in peak filling rate was correlated with the increase in cardiac index at peak exercise. The independent predictors of the increase in peak oxygen uptake were changes in work capacity and peak early filling rate. These data demonstrate that exercise training can improve the exercise capacity of patients with ischemic cardi-

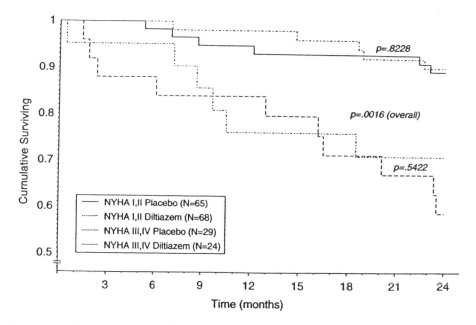

FIGURE 3-21. Heart transplant indication-free survival as classified in terms of study medication and NYHA functional class. Reproduced with permission from Figulla et al.[46]

omyopathy and severe systolic dysfunction. The increase in early diastolic filling at rest and during exercise may contribute to the improvement in peak
oxygen uptake.

Coronary Calcium to Differentiate Ischemic from Nonischemic Cardiomyopathy

Several noninvasive approaches have been investigated for differentiating
dilated cardiomyopathy due to CAD (ischemic cardiomyopathy) from nonischemic cardiomyopathy. There are few data regarding the application of cardiac fluoroscopy for distinguishing between the 2 different types of dilated
cardiomyopathy. The new computed tomographic (CT) methods based on fast
scanning techniques have clearly been superior to fluoroscopy and conventional computerized tomography in detecting calcium in epicardial coronary
arteries. Shemesh and associates[48] from Tel Aviv, Israel, examined the hypothesis that the presence or absence of coronary calcium on double-helix CT represents a useful sign in the differentiation between ischemic and nonischemic
dilated cardiomyopathy. The authors examined 32 patients aged 43 to 71 years
with dilated cardiomyopathy and LVEFs of less than 30%. Of the 19 patients
with ischemic cardiomyopathy, 6 had 2-vessel CAD, and 13 had 3-vessel CAD.
All 19 patients with ischemic cardiomyopathy had coronary calcium on double-
helix CT scanning. Only 1 patient with nonischemic dilated cardiomyopathy
and normal coronary arteries on coronary angiography had calcium, and that
deposit was small. Thus, the detection of coronary calcium on double-helix CT
yielded a sensitivity of 100%, a specificity of 92%, and a total accuracy of 97%
in diagnosis of the ischemic type of dilated cardiomyopathy.

Idiopathic Myocarditis

Left Ventricular Endocardial Surface and Relation to Histological Changes

To examine the feasibility of percutaneous cardioscopy for diagnosis of
idiopathic myocarditis, cardioscopic appearance of the left ventricle and biopsy
findings were compared in 21 such patients in this study by Uchida and associates[49] from Tokyo, Japan. The endocardial surface was milky white, red, pink,
or reddish-brown and edematous at the segments that exhibited histological
changes of acute myocarditis; purplish-red in those that exhibited chronic active myocarditis; and yellow in those that exhibited chronic inactive or healed
myocarditis. Follow-up study by repeated cardioscopy and biopsy in 6 patients
revealed that the milky white surface disappeared and that the red, pink, and
reddish-brown surfaces changed to purplish-red and then to yellow or white.
The results indicate that the endocardial coloration of the left ventricle represents histological changes and that cardioscopy is feasible for macroscopic
pathological diagnosis and for follow-up of idiopathic myocarditis.

TABLE 3-1
Hemodynamics: Group A Versus Group B

	Group A—Increase in PA			Group B—Decrease in PA		
	Initial	Final	p Value (initial vs final)	Initial	Final	p Value (initial vs final)
Right atrial pressure (mm Hg)	7±4	8±5	0.9	11±7	5±4	<0.0001
PA (mm Hg)	39±13	49±15	0.6	57±11	37±11	<0.0001
PA wedge pressure (mm Hg)	17±7	21±9	0.9	25±9	14±7	<0.0001
Pulmonary vascular resistance (Wu)	2.3±1.3	2.5±1.3	0.2	3.5±2.0	2.1±0.8	<0.001
Cardiac output (L/min)	4.5±1.2	4.6±1.2	0.7	3.8±0.9	4.7±1.1	<0.001
Ejection fraction (%)	18±7	24±8	<0.01	18±6	27±11	<0.005
Norepinephrine level (pg/ml)	738±265	661±345	0.2	842±503	710±377	0.1

Values are expressed as mean ± SD.
PA = pulmonary artery.
Reproduced with permission from Levine et al.[23]

Medical Therapy for Pulmonary Hypertension in Patients Awaiting Transplantation

Pulmonary artery hypertension in transplant recipients increases mortality from right-sided heart failure following heart transplantation. Levine and associates[23] from Detroit, Michigan, examined the impact of long-term medical therapy on the severity of PA hypertension in patients with end-stage CHF on a transplant waiting list. The initial and final quarterly right heart catheterization data on 60 patients (50 men, aged 50 ± 9 years, New York Heart Association class III to IV) awaiting heart transplantation were analyzed and the patients divided into 2 groups: group A, those with persistent elevated systolic PA pressures throughout the 10-month follow-up (n=31 of 60), and group B, those who had any decrease in systolic PA pressure during that period (n=29 of 60). Group A had no change in hemodynamics. Group B had a significant decrease (±SD) in right atrial (11 ± 7 to 5 ± 4 mm Hg), PA (57 ± 11 to 37 ± 11 mm Hg), and PA wedge (25 ± 9 to 14 ± 7 mm Hg) pressures, with increases in cardiac output (3.8 ± 0.9 to 4.7 ± 1.1 L/min) and EF (18 ± 6% to 27 ± 11%). The combined endpoint of transplant or death occurred in 28 of 31 patients (90%) in group A versus 14 of 29 (50%) in group B. Ischemic etiology was present in 71% of patients in group A versus 68% with idiopathic dilated cardiomyopathy in group B. The reversibility of PA hypertension, rather than its initial severity, is predictive of patient clinical outcome. Idiopathic, as opposed to ischemic, cardiomyopathy responds better to medical therapy (Table 3-1).

1. Konstam V, Salem D, Pouleur H, Kostis J, Gorkin L, Shumaker S, Mottard I, Woods P, Konstam MA, Yusuf S, for the SOLVD Investigators: Baseline quality of life as a predictor of mortality and hospitalization in 5,025 patients with congestive heart failure. Am J Cardiol 1996 (October 15);78:890–895.
2. Torre-Amione G, Kapadia S, Benedict C, Oral H, Young JB, Mann DL: Proinflammatory cytokine levels in patients with depressed left ventricular ejection fraction: A

report from the Studies of Left Ventricular Dysfunction (SOLVD). J Am Coll Cardiol 1996 (April);27:1201–1206.

3. Haywood GA, Tsao PS, von der Leyen HE, Mann MJ, Keeling PJ, Trindade PT, Lewis NP, Byrne CD, Rickenbacher PR, Bishopric NH, Cooke JP, McKenna WJ, Fowler MB. Expression of inducible nitric oxide synthase in human heart failure. Circulation 1996 (March 15);93:1087–1094.

4. Marmor A, Raphael T, Marmor M, Blondheim D. Evaluation of contractile reserve by dobutamine echocardiography: Noninvasive estimation of the severity of heart failure. Am Heart J 1996 (December);132:1195–1201.

5. Andreas S, Hagenah G, Möller C, Werner GS, Kreuzer H, Cheyne-Stokes respiration and prognosis in congestive heart failure. Am J Cardiol 1996 (December 1);78:1260–1264.

6. Yu CM, Sanderson JE, Chan S, Yeung L, Hung YT, Woo KS. Right ventricular diastolic dysfunction in heart failure. Circulation 1996 (April 15);93:1509–1514.

7. Koilpillai C, Quiñones MA, Greenberg B, Limacher MC, Shindler D, Pratt CM, Benedict CR, Kopelen H, Shelton B, for the SOLVD Investigators: Relation of ventricular size and function to heart failure status and ventricular dysrhythmia in patients with severe left ventricular dysfunction. Am J Cardiol 1996 (March 15);77:606–611.

8. Køber L, Torp-Pedersen C, Pedersen OD, Høiberg S, Camm AJ on behalf of the TRACE Study Group. Importance of congestive heart failure and interaction of congestive heart failure and left ventricular systolic function on prognosis in patients with acute myocardial infarction. Am J Cardiol 1996 (November 15);78:1124–1128.

9. Wilson JR, Groves J, Rayos G. Circulatory status and response to cardiac rehabilitation in patients with heart failure. Circulation 1996 (October 1);94:1567–1572.

10. Meyer K, Schwaibold M, Westbrook S, Beneke R, Hajric R, Gornandt L, Lehmann M, Roskamm H: Effects of short-term exercise training and activity restriction on functional capacity in patients with severe chronic congestive heart failure. Am J Cardiol 1996 (November 1);78:1017–1022.

11. Massie BM, Simonini A, Sahgal P, Wells L, Dudley GA: Relation of systemic and local muscle exercise capacity to skeletal muscle characteristics in men with congestive heart failure. J Am Coll Cardiol 1996 (January);27:140–145.

12. Chati Z, Zannad F, Jeandel C, Lherbier B, Escanye J-M, Robert J, Aliot E. Physical deconditioning may be a mechanism for the skeletal muscle energy phosphate metabolism abnormalities in chronic heart failure. Am Heart J 1996 (March);131:560–566.

13. Eisenhofer G, Friberg P, Rundqvist B, Quyyumi AA, Lambert G, Kaye DM, Kopin IJ, Goldstein DS, Esler MD. Cardiac sympathetic nerve function in congestive heart failure. Circulation 1996 (May 1);93:1667–1676.

14. Adams KF Jr, Dunlap SH, Sueta CA, Clarke SW, Patterson JH, Blauwet MB, Jensen LR, Tomasko L, Koch G: Relation between gender etiology and survival in patients with symptomatic heart failure. J Am Coll Cardiol 1996 (December);28:1781–1788.

15. Andersson B, Sylvén C: The DD genotype of the angiotensin-converting enzyme gene is associated with increased mortality in idiopathic heart failure. J Am Coll Cardiol 1996 (July);28:162–167.

16. Stevenson WG, Stevenson LW, Middlekauff HR, Fonarow GC, Hamilton MA, Woo MA, Saxon LA, Natterson PD, Steimle A, Walden JA, Tillisch JH: Improving survival for patients with atrial fibrillation and advanced heart failure. J Am Coll Cardiol 1996 (November 15);28:1458–1463.

17. Díaz-Velez CR, Garcia-Castineiras S, Mendoza-Ramos E, Hernandez-Lopez E. Increased malondialdehyde in peripheral blood of patients with congestive heart failure. Am Heart J 1996 (January);131:146–152.

18. Carson P, Johnson G, Fletcher R, Cohn J: Mild systolic dysfunction in heart failure (left ventricular ejection fraction >35%): Baseline characteristics, prognosis and response to therapy in the Vasodilator in Heart Failure Trials (V-HeFT). J Am Coll Cardiol 1996 (March 1);27:642–649.

19. Packer M, Colucci WS, Sackner-Bernstein JD, Liang C, Goldscher DA, Freeman I,

Kukin ML, Kinhal V, Udelson JE, Klapholz M, Gottlieb SS, Pearle D, Cody RJ, Gregory JJ, Kantrowitz NE, LeJemtel TH, Young ST, Lukas MA, Shusterman NH, for the PRECISE Study Group. Double-blind, placebo-controlled study of the effects of carvedilol in patients with moderate to severe heart failure. The PRECISE trial. Circulation 1996 (December 1);94:2793–2799.

20. Colucci WS, Packer M, Bristow MR, Gilbert EM, Cohn JN, Fowler MB, Krueger SK, Hershberger R, Uretsky BF, Bowers JA, Sackner-Bernstein JD, Young ST, Holcslaw TL, Lukas MA, for the United States Carvedilol Heart Failure Study Group. Carvedilol inhibits clinical progression in patients with mild symptoms of heart failure. Circulation 1996 (December 1);94:2800–2806.

21. Bristow MR, Gilbert EM, Abraham WT, Adams KF, Fowler MB, Hershberger RE, Kubo SH, Narahara KA, Ingersoll H, Krueger S, Young S, Shusterman N, for the MOCHA Investigators. Carvedilol produces dose-related improvements in left ventricular function and survival in subjects with chronic heart failure. Circulation 1996 (December 1);94:2807–2816.

22. Packer M, Bristow MR, Cohn JN, Colucci WS, Fowler MB, Gilbert EM, Shusterman NH, for the U.S. Carvedilol Heart Failure Study Group. The effect of carvedilol on morbidity and mortality in patients with chronic heart failure. N Engl J Med 1996 (May 23);334:1349–1355.

23. Levine TB, Levine AB, Goldberg AD, Narins B, Goldstein S, Lesch M: Impact of medical therapy on pulmonary hypertension in patients with congestive heart failure awaiting cardiac transplantation. Am J Cardiol 1996 (August 15);78:440–443.

24. Krum H, Gu A, Wilshire-Clement M, Sackner-Bernstein J, Goldsmith R, Medina N, Yushak M, Miller M, Packer M. Changes in plasma endothelin-1 levels reflect clinical response to β-blockade in chronic heart failure. Am Heart J 1996 (February); 131:337–341.

25. Gilbert EM, Abraham WT, Olsen S, Hattler B, White M, Mealy P, Larrabee P, Bristow MR. Comparative hemodynamic, left ventricular functional, and antiadrenergic effects of chronic treatment with metoprolol versus carvedilol in the failing heart. Circulation 1996 (December 1);94:2817–2825.

26. Newton GE, Parker JD. Acute effects of β_1-selective and nonselective β-adrenergic receptor blockade on cardiac sympathetic activity in congestive heart failure. Circulation 1996 (August 1);94:353–358.

27. Massie BM, Fisher SG, Deedwania PC, Singh BN, Fletcher RD, Singh SN, for the CHF-STAT Investigators. Effect of amiodarone on clinical status and left ventricular function in patients with congestive heart failure. Circulation 1996 (June 15);93: 2128–2134.

28. Gottlieb SS, Singh S, Munger M, Eichhorn EJ, Ilgenfritz J, Hanyok J: Hemodynamic effects of the class III antiarrhythmic drug, d-Sotalol, in patients with congestive heart failure. Am J Cardiol 1996 (December 15);78:1411–1415.

29. Rector TS, Bank AJ, Mullen KA, Tschumperlin LK, Sih R, Pillai K, Kubo SH. Randomized, double-blind, placebo-controlled study of supplemental oral L-arginine in patients with heart failure. Circulation 1996 (June 15);93:2135–2141.

30. Love MP, Haynes WG, Gray GA, Webb DJ, McMurray JJV. Vasodilator effects of endothelin-converting enzyme inhibitor and endothelin ET_A receptor blockade in chronic heart failure patients treated with ACE inhibitors. Circulation 1996 (November 1);94:2131–2137.

31. Borghi C, Ambrosioni E, Magnani B, on behalf of the SMILE Study Investigators: Effects of the early administration of zofenopril on onset and progression of congestive heart failure in patients with anterior wall acute myocardial infarction. Am J Cardiol 1996 (August 1);78:317–322.

32. Dormans TPJ, van Meyel JJM, Gerlag PGG, Tan Y, Russel FGM, Smits P: Diuretic efficacy of high dose furosemide in severe heart failure: Bolus injection versus continuous infusion. J Am Coll Cardiol 1996 (August);28:376–382.

33. Morisco C, Cuocolo A, Romano M, Nappi A, Iaccarino G, Volpe M, Salvatore M, Trimarco B: Influence of digitalis on left ventricular functional response to exercise in congestive heart failure. Am J Cardiol 1996 (March 1);77:480–485.

34. Furnary AP, Jessup M, Moreira LP: Multicenter Trial of Dynamic Cardiomyoplasty for Chronic Heart Failure. J Am Coll Cardiol 1996 (November 1);28:1175–1180.

35. James KB, McCarthy PM, Jaalouk S, Bravo EL, Betkowski A, Thomas JD, Nakatani S, Fouad-Tarazi FM. Plasma volume and its regulatory factors in congestive heart failure after implantation of long-term left ventricular assist devices. Circulation 1996 (April 15);93:1515–1519.

36. Nakatani S, Marwick TH, Lever HM, Thomas JD: Resting echocardiographic features of latent left ventricular outflow obstruction in hypertrophic cardiomyopathy. Am J Cardiol 1996 (September 15) 78:662–667.

37. Nishimura RA, Hayes DL, Ilstrup DM, Holmes DR, Tajik AJ: Effects of dual-chamber pacing on systolic and diastolic function in patients with hypertrophic cardiomyopathy: Acute Doppler echocardiographic and catheterization hemodynamic study. J Am Coll Cardiol 1996 (February);27:421–430.

38. Betocchi S, Losi MA, Piscione F, Boccalatte M, Pace L, Golino P, Perrone-Filardi P, Briguori C, Franculli F, Pappone C, Salvatore M, Chiariello M: Effects of dual-chamber pacing in hypertrophic cardiomyopathy on left ventricular outflow tract obstruction and on diastolic function. Am J Cardiol 1996 (March 1);77:498–502.

39. Betocchi S, Piscione F, Losi M-A, Pace L, Boccalatte M, Perrone-Filardi P, Cappelli-Bigazzi M, Briguori C, Manganelli F, Ciampi Q, Salvatore M, Chiariello M: Effects of diltiazem on left ventricular systolic and diastolic function in hypertrophic cardiomyopathy. Am J Cardiol 1996 (August 15);78:451–457.

40. Paz R, Jortner R, Tunick PA, Sclarovsky S, Eilat B, Perez JL, Kronzon I. The effect of the ingestion of ethanol on obstruction of the left ventricular outflow tract in hypertrophic cardiomyopathy. N Engl J Med 1996 (September 26);335:938–941.

41. McCully RB, Nishimura RA, Tajik AJ, Schaff HV, Danielson GK. Extent of clinical improvement after surgical treatment of hypertrophic obstructive cardiomyopathy. Circulation 1996 (August 1);94:467–471.

42. Torre-Amione G, Kapadia S, Lee J, Durand J-B, Bies RD, Young JB, Mann DL. Tumor necrosis factor-α and tumor necrosis factor receptors in the failing human heart. Circulation 1996 (February);93:704–711.

43. Andersson B, Caidahl K, di Lenarda A, Warren SE, Goss F, Waldenström A, Persson S, Wallentin I, Hjalmarson Å, Waagstein F. Changes in early and late diastolic filling patterns induced by long-term adrenergic β-blockade in patients with idiopathic dilated cardiomyopathy. Circulation 1996 (August 15);94:673–682.

44. Quaife RA, Gilbert EM, Christian PE, Datz FL, Mealey PC, Volkman K, Olsen SL, Bristow MR: Effects of carvedilol on systolic and diastolic left ventricular performance in idiopathic dilated cardiomyopathy or ischemic cardiomyopathy. Am J Cardiol 1996 (October 1);78:779–784.

45. Fazio S, Sabatini D, Capaldo B, Vigorito C, Giordano A, Guida R, Pardo F, Biondi B, Saccà L. A preliminary study of growth hormone in the treatment of dilated cardiomyopathy. N Engl J Med 1996 (March 28);334:809–814.

46. Figulla HR, Gietzen F, Zeymer U, Raiber M, Hegselmann J, Soballa R, Hilgers R, for the DiDi Study Group. Diltiazem improves cardiac function and exercise capacity in patients with idiopathic dilated cardiomyopathy. Results of the Diltiazem in Dilated Cardiomyopathy Trial. Circulation 1996 (August 1);94:346–352.

47. Belardinelli R, Georgiou D, Cianci G, Purcaro A. Effects of exercise training on left ventricular filling at rest and during exercise in patients with ischemic cardiomyopathy and severe left ventricular systolic dysfunction. Am Heart J 1996 (July);132:61–70.

48. Shemesh J, Tenenbaum A, Fisman EZ, Har-Zahav Y, Rath S, Apter S, Itzchak Y, Motro M: Coronary calcium as a reliable tool for differentiating ischemic from nonischemic cardiomyopathy. Am J Cardiol 1996 (January 15);77:191–193.

49. Uchida Y, Nakamura F, Hirose J, Oshima T, Morita T, Morizuki S, Sasaki T, Tsubouchi N. Cardioscopic spectrum of the left ventricular endocardial surface and its relation to histologic changes in idiopathic myocarditis. Am Heart J 1996 (January);131:107–114.

4

Hypertension

Hypertension (General Topics)

Influence of Angiotensin-Converting Enzyme and Angiotensin II Type 1 Receptor Gene Polymorphisms on Aortic Stiffness

Benetos and colleagues[1] developed a study to evaluate the contribution of polymorphisms of the angiotensin-converting enzyme (ACE) insertion/deletion (I/D) and angiotensin II type 1 receptor genes on aortic stiffness regulation. The study included 311 untreated hypertensive patients and 128 normotensive subjects. Aortic stiffness was evaluated by measurement of the carotid-femoral pulse-wave velocity. In normotensive subjects, the 2 polymorphisms did not influence the evaluated parameters. In hypertensive subjects, there was a decreasing trend of mean carotid-femoral pulse-wave velocity with the number of ACE D alleles, but this association became significant only after adjustment for blood pressure (Table 4-1). Conversely, the $AGTR_1A$ ^{1166}C polymorphism was independently associated with aortic stiffness. These results suggest that in hypertensive, but not normotensive, subjects the $ABTR_1$ and ACE genotypes are involved in the regulation of aortic stiffness. The presence of the $AGTR_1$ C allele is a strong independent determinant of aortic stiffness.

Factor VII Hyperactivity and Endothelial Cell Damage in Elderly Hypertensives

Kario and co-workers[2] in Hyogo, Japan, studied the relations among albuminuria, factor VII hyperactivity, and endothelial cell damage in 61 elderly hypertensive subjects. The plasma levels of activated factor VII, factor VII coagulant activity, factor VII antigen, von Willebrand factor, and thrombomodulin were measured to assess factor VII hyperactivity and endothelial cell damage; and urinary albumin excretion rate was calculated using 12-hour nighttime urine collection. The investigators performed 24-hour ambulatory blood pressure monitoring in all 61 hypertensive patients and classified them into a white-coat hypertension group and a sustained hypertension group. For the levels of factor VII, von Willebrand factor, and thrombomodulin, there were no differences between the white-coat hypertensive group and normotensive control subjects. In the sustained hypertension group, only the microalbuminuric subgroup showed significant elevation compared with the normotensive group for the level of factor VII(a). In contrast, none of the levels in the normoalbumi-

403

TABLE 4-1
Multiple Regression Analysis of PWV* on the $AGTR_1$ $A^{1166}C$
and ACE I/D Genotypes and Covariables

Independent Variable	Normotensive Subjects		Hypertensive Patients	
	Partial R^2	p	Partial R^2	p
Sex	.021	.07	...	NS
Age	.160	<.0001	.061	<.0001
BMI (kg/m²)	...	NS	.014	<.01
SBP (mm Hg)	.042	<.02	.141	<.0001
DBP (mm Hg)	...	NS	.019	<.004
ACE I/D		NS	.017	<.006
$AGTR_1$ A/C†	...	NS	.116	<.0001
Model R^2†	.222	<.0001	.368	<.0001

* Log-transformed PWV was used as a dependent variable.

† Both polymorphisms were tested as codominant 0, 1, or 2 ordinal variables (presence of 0, 1, or 2 C or D alleles). The interaction term involving both polymorphisms was not statistically significant.

Reproduced with permission from Benetos et al.[1]

nuric hypertensive group differed from those in the normotensive control group. The results suggested that among elderly hypertensives, only those with microalbuminuria show enhancement of factor VII activation and endothelial cell damage, whereas patients with white-coat hypertension and normoalbuminuric hypertensives do not show these accompanying abnormalities. Thus, increased levels of factor VII activity and markers of endothelial cell damage might account for the higher risk of cardiovascular events in essential hypertension with microalbuminuria.

Pathogenesis of Essential Hypertension

Noll and colleagues[3] in Bern, Switzerland, evaluated the pathogenesis of essential hypertension in 10 normotensive offspring of parents with essential hypertension and 8 offspring of normotensive parents by using muscle sympathetic nerve activity recording measured from the peroneal nerve. Measurements were performed under resting conditions, during a 10-minute period of hypoxia, and during a 3-minute mental stress period. The tests were separated by a 30-minute resting period. Plasma samples for determination of norepinephrine and endothelin were collected before and after the tests. Baseline values of muscle sympathetic nerve activity were comparable in offspring of hypertensive and normotensive parents. During hypoxia, muscle sympathetic activity, heart rate, and norepinephrine and endothelin plasma levels increased in offspring of hypertensive and normotensive parents to a comparable degree, but no significant changes in blood pressure and plasma epinephrine levels were observed. However, during mental stress, muscle sympathetic activity and plasma norepinephrine and endothelin increased only in offspring of hypertensive parents. Blood pressure increased in parallel and only in offspring

TABLE 4-2
**Blood Pressure, Heart Rate, Plasma Norepinephrine, and Endothelin-1 During MS
in Offspring of Hypertensive and Normotensive Parents**

	Offspring of Normotensives (n = 8)		Offspring of Hypertensives (n = 10)	
	Before MS	During MS	Before MS	During MS
Systolic blood pressure, mm Hg	115 ± 4	124 ± 5	127 ± 4	139 ± 4‡
Diastolic blood pressure, mm Hg	75 ± 3	82 ± 3	77 ± 5	83 ± 6*
Heart rate, beats per minute	61 ± 4	69 ± 4*	64 ± 4	74 ± 4§
Plasma norepinephrine, pg/mL	200 ± 33	223 ± 31	130 ± 9†	186 ± 17§
Plasma endothelin-1, pg/mL	1.47 ± 0.17	1.52 ± 0.10	1.44 ± 0.12	1.87 ± 0.15‡

MS indicates mental stress.
* p <.05, ‡ p <.001; § p <.001 vs. resting.
† p <.05 vs. offspring of normotensives.
Reprinted with permission from Noll et al.[3]

of hypertensive parents, but heart rate increased in both groups. Thus, sympathetic nervous system activity and plasma norepinephrine and endothelin levels are increased during mental stress in the offspring of hypertensive parents, but the response to hypoxia is similar in offspring in hypertensive and normotensive parents. This suggests genetically determined abnormal regulation of the sympathetic nervous system to selected stressful stimuli in the offspring of hypertensive parents (Figure 4-1 and Table 4-2).

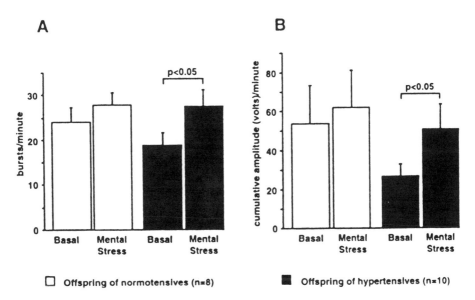

FIGURE 4-1. Muscle sympathetic activity in the peroneal nerve at rest and during mental stress expressed as bursts per minute (A) and cumulative amplitude of bursts (volts per minute) (B) in offspring of normotensive (□) and hypertensive (■) parents. Data are mean ± SEM. Reproduced with permission from Noll et al.[3]

Factors Affecting Blood Pressure

Caffeine

Whether the vasoconstrictive actions of caffeine are enhanced in hypertensive persons has not been demonstrated. Thus, caffeine (3.3 mg/kg) versus placebo was tested by Pincomb and associates[4] from Oklahoma City, Oklahoma, in 48 healthy men (aged 20 to 35 years) selected after screening on 2 separate occasions. Borderline hypertensive men (n = 24) were selected with screening systolic blood pressure of 140 to 160 mm Hg and/or diastolic blood pressure 90 to 99 mm Hg. Low-risk controls (n = 24) reported no parental history of hypertension and had screening less than 130/85 mm Hg. Participants were then tested on 2 occasions after 12-hour abstinence from caffeine in each of 2 protocols; this required a total of 4 laboratory visits. Caffeine-induced changes in diastolic blood pressure were 2 to 3 times larger in borderline subjects than in controls (+ 8.4 vs. + 3.8 mm Hg), and were attributable to larger changes in impedance-derived measures of systemic vascular resistance (+ 135 vs. + 45 dynes·s·cm^{-5}). These findings were consistent and reached significance in both protocols. The percentage of borderline subjects in whom diastolic blood pressure changes exceeded the median control response was 96%. Consequently, whereas all participants exhibited normotensive levels during the resting predrug baseline, 33% of borderline subjects achieved hypertensive blood pressure levels after caffeine ingestion. Thus, in borderline hypertensive men, exaggerated responses to caffeine were as follows: selective for diastolic blood pressure, consistent with greater vasoconstriction, replicated in 2 protocols, and representative of nearly all borderline hypertensives. We suspect that the potential for caffeine to stabilize high-resistance states in susceptible persons may facilitate their disease progression, as well as hinder accurate diagnosis and treatment (Figure 4-2).

Obesity and Lifestyle Factors

Liu and colleagues[5] in the Coronary Artery Risk Development in Young Adults (CARDIA) study evaluated lifestyle and the evolution of cardiovascular disease risk factors in a random sample of young adults ages 18 to 30 years at baseline (1985 to 1986). Data from 4 examinations over 7 years were analyzed by using a method that simultaneously examined cross-sectional and longitudinal relationships of lifestyle factors and blood pressure. This study included 1154 black women, 853 black men, 1126 white women, and 1013 white men. Blacks had higher systolic and diastolic blood pressures than did whites at every examination. Racial differences were greater in women than in men and increased over time. Within each sex-race group, average diastolic blood pressure over 4 examinations was positively associated with baseline age, body mass index, and alcohol intake and negatively associated with physical activity, cigarette use, and intake of potassium and protein. Longitudinal change in diastolic blood pressure was positively associated with changes in body mass index and alcohol intake. After adjustment for obesity and other lifestyle factors, black-white diastolic

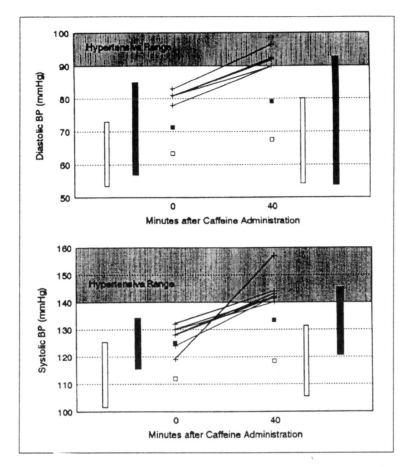

FIGURE 4-2. Occurrences among borderline hypertensive men of a shift from a predrug normotensive level to a hypertensive state after caffeine ingestion. The 3 blood pressure (BP) measurements obtained at the end of the predrug baseline (0 minutes) and again at 40 minutes after the drug were averaged for each subject. The group means for controls (*open squares*) and borderline subjects (*closed squares*) and 90% confidence intervals (*open and closed bars*, respectively) are shown for comparison. All subjects were normotensive during the predrug baseline and 40 minutes after placebo. After caffeine, no controls became hypertensive, but 8 of 24 borderline hypertensive men had hypertensive systolic and/or diastolic blood pressure (*solid lines*). Reproduced with permission from Pincomb et al.[4]

blood pressure was reduced substantially, 21% to 75% in men and 49% to 129% for women. Results for systolic blood pressure were similar. Thus, these data demonstrate differences in obesity and other lifestyle factors in young adults that largely explain the higher baseline blood pressure and greater increase over time in blacks relative to whites.

Appetite Suppressants and the Risk of Primary Pulmonary Hypertension

Abenhaim and colleagues[6] for the International Primary Pulmonary Hypertension Study Group investigated the potential role of anorexic agents and other suspected risk factors for primary pulmonary hypertension. They used a case-control study assessing 95 patients with primary pulmonary hypertension from 35 centers in France, Belgium, the United Kingdom, and The Netherlands and 355 controls recruited from general practice and matched to the patients' sex and age. The use of anorexic drugs, primarily derivatives of fenfluramine, was associated with an increased risk of primary pulmonary hypertension with an odds ratio of any anorexic drug use, 6.3. For the use of anorexic agents in the preceding year, the odds ratio for developing primary pulmonary hypertension was 10.1. When anorexic drugs were used for a total of more than 3 months, the odds ratio was 23. The authors also confirmed an association with several previously identified risk factors, including a family history of pulmonary hypertension, infection with the human immunodeficiency virus, cirrhosis, and the use of cocaine or intravenous drugs. Thus, the use of anorexic drugs was associated with the development of primary pulmonary hypertension. Active surveillance for this disease should be considered, especially since the use of anorexic drugs may increase in the future.

Prevalence and Circadian Variations in ST-Segment Depression and Concomitant Blood Pressure Changes

Myocardial ischemia occurs in many patients with systemic hypertension. Asmar and associates[7] from Paris, France, assessed the prevalence and circadian distribution of ST-segment depression together with concomitant blood pressure and heart rate variations in 100 patients (mean age, 51 ± 8 years). They all underwent ambulatory monitoring with use of the combined AMP 5600 monitor, which simultaneously records a continuous Holter electrocardiogram and intermittent noninvasive blood pressure measurements at 15-minute intervals. Extra measurements are triggered by detection of a horizontal or downsloping ST depression (>1 mm and >60 seconds). Cardiovascular risk factors were fully evaluated in all patients; accurate and reliable echocardiogram enabled left ventricular mass index to be calculated in 52 patients. Twenty-three patients (15 men and 8 women) experienced a total of 72 episodes of ST depression. Duration of such episodes (mean ± SD) was 132 ± 65 seconds, and amplitude was 1.51 ± 0.55 mm. Circadian distribution showed 2 peaks: on awakening and in the late afternoon periods. The mean ambulatory blood pressure load was greater in the patients with ST segment depression for both systolic and diastolic blood pressure than those without (135 ± 14 vs. 129 ± 15 mm Hg and 84 ± 8 vs. 79 ± 10 mm Hg, respectively). Plasma glucose (5.83 ± 0.70 mmol/L vs. 5.46 ± 0.71 mmol/L) and self-rated work-related stress levels (22% vs. 13%) were also higher in patients with ST-segment depression. There were no significant differences between groups for clinical parameters, left ventricular mass index, and other cardiovascular risk factors. During ST depression episodes, systolic BP increased by 9 ± 15 mm Hg, diastolic blood pressure by 7 ± 11 mm Hg, and heart rate by 5 ± 17 beats per minute. Thus, 24-hour Holter electrocardiographic monitoring showed ST depression episodes in 23 of 100 hypertensive patients (23%); ambulatory blood pressure load was greater in these patients. Blood pressure variations, especially elevation, may trigger such episodes of ST-segment depression.

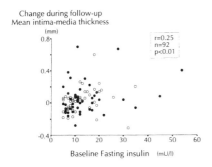

Change during follow-up
Mean intima-media thickness
(mm)

r=0.25
n=92
p<0.01

Baseline Fasting insulin (mU/l)

FIGURE 4-3. Illustration of the relation between fasting insulin at the baseline investigation and the change in mean intima-media thickness recorded during follow-up (r=.25, n=92, p<.01, nondiabetic patients only). In this analysis, all patients have been handled as 1 group, but for illustrative purposes, solid circles refer to patients randomized to the intervention group (n=46) and open circles to the control group (n=46). Fasting insulin was missing in 2 nondiabetic patients at the baseline investigation. Reproduced with permission from Suurkula et al.[8]

Risk Factor Modification

In spite of optimal blood pressure control, available data indicate that the risk of CAD remains high in many patients with hypertension. Multifactorial risk intervention programs have therefore been advocated. The aim of a study by Suurküla and coworkers[8] in Gothenburg, Sweden, was to analyze whether a favorable change in risk factors caused by a comprehensive risk factor modification program (focused mainly on nonpharmacological intervention) might beneficially affect ultrasound-assessed far-wall common carotid intima-media thickness or plaques in the carotid artery in high-risk hypertensive patients in comparison with those undergoing usual care. A further aim was to analyze whether risk factors measured at baseline or follow-up were related to the change recorded in intima-media thickness during follow-up. The results showed a favorable change in the intervention group in LDL cholesterol, in smoking habits (32% of smokers quit smoking) and in HbA$_{1c}$ over the 3.5-year observation period. However, no difference between the 2 randomized groups could be observed for far-wall common carotid intima-media thickness or plaque status during follow-up. Of all tested potential risk factors, only fasting insulin at baseline was significantly related to the change in mean intima-media thickness during follow-up (Figure 4-3). The relation (negative) between follow-up serum HDL and change in mean intima-media thickness during the preceding follow-up was of borderline significance. Patients with moderate-to-large plaques in the carotid artery region at baseline had a significantly larger increase in common carotid artery intima-media thickness during follow-up than did patients with no or only small plaques. The results were disappointing and may have indicated that either the change in risk factors occurred too late in life or that a considerably larger change in concomitant risk factors than the investigators observed is needed to favorably affect intima-media thickness during an observation period of around 3 years in high-risk hypertensive patients.

Influence of Risk Modification on Lipid Profiles in Hypertensive Patients

An abnormal plasma lipid and lipoprotein profile is an independent and strong predictor of mortality and morbidity from CAD. Lakshman and associates[9] for the Department of Veterans Affairs Cooperative Study Group on Antihypertensive Agents reported on plasma lipid and lipoprotein profiles with respect to race, age, obesity, blood pressure, smoking, and alcohol consumption in 1292 male veterans with a diastolic blood pressure of 95 to 109 mm Hg while off antihypertensive medications. Blacks had 24% lower triglycerides than whites. In contrast, the following parameters were higher in blacks than in whites by the indicated percentages: HDL cholesterol, 16%; HDL_2 cholesterol, 36%; apolipoprotein (Apo) A_1, 8%; HDL/LDL, 18%; HDL_2/LDL_3, 21%; and Apo A_1/Apo B, 15%. Triglycerides were unchanged up to age 60, but were lower by 24% in those aged 70 or older. Apo A_1 levels were higher, whereas LDL cholesterol was lower in moderate alcohol consumers versus abstainers. Triglycerides were higher, whereas HDL, HDL_2 cholesterol, and Apo A_1 were lower with increasing obesity. Moderate alcohol consumption had a strong favorable effect on HDL, HDL_2, and HDL_3 cholesterol among subjects of normal weight, but this effect was diminished in obese subjects. Total and LDL cholesterol were higher by 6.4% and 9.4%, respectively, whereas HDL cholesterol remained unchanged in those with diastolic blood pressure of 105 to 109 mm Hg versus those with diastolic blood pressure of 95 to 99 mm Hg. The authors concluded that hypertensive black men have lipid and lipoprotein profiles indicative of less CAD risk than white men. Chronic moderate alcohol consumption correlates with a favorable plasma lipid and lipoprotein profile in normal, but not obese, men. Obesity is associated with an adverse plasma lipid and lipoprotein profile. Thus, race, alcohol intake, and obesity may be important modifiers of CAD in untreated hypertensive men (Table 4-3).

TABLE 4-3
Racial Differences in Plasma Lipid and Lipoprotein Profiles*

Plasma Component	Whites (n = 622)	Blacks (n = 594)	Racial Difference (p Value)
Triglycerides	153 ± 103	116 ± 100	<0.001
Total cholesterol	205 ± 37	204 ± 37	<0.547
LDL cholesterol	130 ± 36	130 ± 38	<0.788
HDL cholesterol	45 ± 11	52 ± 14	<0.001
HDL_2 cholesterol	11 ± 8	15 ± 11	<0.001
Apo A_1	112 ± 23	121 ± 29	<0.001
Apo B	77 ± 19	75 ± 21	<0.069
HDL/LDL	0.4 ± 0.38	0.47 ± 0.61	<0.018
HDL_2/LDL	0.11 ± 0.24	0.15 ± 0.37	<0.031
HDL_2/HDL_3	0.34 ± 0.35	0.41 ± 0.32	<0.001
HDL/TC	0.23 ± 0.07	0.26 ± 0.09	<0.001
Apo A_1/Apo B	1.55 ± 0.52	1.79 ± 1.97	<0.001

* Concentration (mg/100 mL).

After an initial washout period of 4 weeks, plasma lipids and lipoproteins were determined in the plasma samples of the indicated number of veterans, as described in the Methods section. Values are expressed as mean $\pm$ SD.

Apo = apolipoprotein; HDL = high-density lipoprotein; LDL = low-density lipoprotein; TC = total cholesterol.

Reprinted with permission from Lakshman et al.[9]

Coronary Artery Disease in Hypertension

Serum Lipids and Incidence of Coronary Heart Disease (Systolic Hypertension in the Elderly Study)

Frost and colleagues[10] studied the association between serum lipids and CAD in individuals 60 years of age or older in an attempt to identify whether the previously defined association between serum lipids and CAD progression in middle-aged men also is true in older individuals. The Systolic Hypertension in the Elderly Program (SHEP) recruited 4736 persons (mean age, 72 years) of whom 14% were African American and 43% were men. Mean systolic and diastolic blood pressures were 170 and 77 mm Hg, respectively. Baseline mean total serum cholesterol was 6 mmol/L (236 mg/dL); HDL cholesterol, 1.4 mmol/L (54 mg/dL); and non-HDL cholesterol, 4.7 mmol/L (182 mg/dL). Triglyceride levels were 1.6 mmol/L (144 mg/dL) for the fasting participants and 1.8 mmol/L for the total group. LDL cholesterol, estimated in fasting samples with triglycerides of 4.5 mmol/L or less averaged 4 mmol/L (154 mg/dL). Mean follow-up was 4.5 years. By multivariate Cox regression analysis, baseline total, non-HDL and HDL cholesterol levels, and the ratios of total, non-HDL, and LDL to HDL cholesterol were significantly related to CAD presence. HDL cholesterol and triglycerides were not significantly related to CAD presence. In fasting participants with triglyceride levels of less than 4.5 mmol/L, a 1 mmol/L (40 mg/dL) higher baseline total, non-HDL, or LDL cholesterol was associated with a 30% to 35% higher CAD event rate. Thus, the results of this study support the concept that serum lipids are CAD risk factors in older Americans just as they are in younger ones.

Coronary Heart Disease Risk Factors in Men and Women Older than 60 Years of Age (Systolic Hypertension in the Elderly Study)

Frost and colleagues[11] in SHEP recruited 4736 patients with a mean age of 72 years to evaluate coronary heart disease risk factors in older men and women with isolated systolic hypertension. Fourteen percent of these patients were African Americans, and 43% were men. Mean systolic and diastolic blood pressures were 170 and 77 mm Hg, respectively. Approximately 13% of participants were current smokers, 10% had a history of diabetes, 5% had a history of prior myocardial infarction (MI), 5% had angina, 2% had intermittent claudication, and 7% had a carotid bruit. Mean total cholesterol value was 6 mmol/L. Mean follow-up was 4.5 years. In a multivariate Cox regression analysis for coronary heart disease, variables that were significant were the baseline total cholesterol value, smoking, history of diabetes, presence of carotid bruit, and treatment group in the trial. Active treatment yielded a 27% reduction in the coronary heart disease risk. The drug used in treatment was chlorthalidone, and the goals of the study were to reduce systolic blood pressure to less than 160 mm Hg for patients with initial systolic blood pressures of 180 mm Hg or greater and to reduce systolic blood pressure by at least 20 mm Hg in those patients whose initial systolic blood pressures were 160 to 179 mm Hg. For each 1 mmol/L increase in total cholesterol value, there was an increase in risk of approximately 20%. Current smokers had a 73% increase, diabetics a 121% increase, and those with carotid bruit had a 113% increase in coronary heart disease risk. These data support the concept that coronary heart disease risk factors are important in older men and women with isolated systolic hypertension.

Endothelial Dysfunction with Abnormal Coronary Vasodilation in Response to Acetylcholine in Patients with Arterial Hypertension

Endothelial dysfunction with abnormal coronary vasodilation in response to acetylcholine has been reported in patients with arterial hypertension. Frielingsdorf and colleagues[12] from Zurich, Switzerland, evaluated the effects of dynamic exercise on coronary vasomotion in hypertensive patients in the presence and absence of CAD. Coronary artery dimensions of normal and stenotic vessel segments were determined in 64 patients by biplane quantitative coronary arteriography. Patients were classified into 2 groups: 20 patients without evidence of CAD (group 1) and 44 patients with CAD (group 2). Both groups were comparable with regard to clinical characteristics, serum cholesterol levels, body mass index, exercise capacity, and hemodynamic data. Mean aortic pressure was significantly higher in the hypertensive than in the normotensive patients. Exercise-induced vasodilation of the normal vessel segment was similar in normotensive and hypertensive patients without CAD (+19% vs. +20%). However, in hypertensive patients with CAD, exercise-induced vasodilation was significantly less in both normal and stenotic vessel segments than in normotensive subjects (+1% vs. +20% for normal, −20% vs. −5% for stenotic vessels). Administration of sublingual nitroglycerin at the end of exercise led to a normalization of the vasodilator response in normotensive as well as hypertensive patients. However, this response became progressively abnormal in group 2 when CAD was present. These authors concluded that in the absence of CAD, the vasomotor response to exercise is normal in both normotensive and hypertensive patients. However, in hypertensive patients with CAD, an abnormal response of the coronary vessels can be observed with a reduced vasodilator response to exercise in normal arteries but an enhanced vasoconstrictor response in stenotic arteries. This data confirm the fact that all risk factors for CAD appear to have an adverse effect on endothelial function, which may be one of the common pathways for the development of atherosclerosis.

Left Ventricular Mass

Weight Reduction Regresses Left Ventricular Mass

The effects of weight reduction on left ventricular mass in obese normotensive and hypertensive individuals were investigated in this study by Himeno and associates[13] from Kitakyushu, Japan, and Fukuoka, Japan. Previous studies have shown that weight reduction in hypertensive obese patients is associated with decreased left ventricular mass and decreased blood pressure. This study was performed (1) to examine whether weight reduction would also regress left ventricular mass in normotensive obese individuals, and (2) to clarify the mechanisms of these effects if they occurred. A weight-reduction program consisted of mild exercise and mild hypocaloric intake. M-mode echocardiography was performed to estimate the left ventricular mass. After the 12-week intervention, the mean reductions in body weight in the normotensive (n = 11) and hypertensive (n = 11) groups were 4.9 kg and 4.6 kg, respectively. Systolic, diastolic, and mean blood pressures were significantly reduced by 13, 9, and 11 mm Hg, respectively, in the hypertensive group. By contrast, no significant changes in systolic, diastolic, or mean BP were observed in the normotensive group. Left ventricular mass was significantly reduced from 176 ± 26 gm to 159 ± 26 gm in the hypertensive group and from 167 ± 33 gm to 145 ± 34 gm in the normotensive group. These results suggest that weight reduction in obese individuals by mild exercise and mild hypocaloric intake can lead to a reduction in left ventricular mass, regardless of whether the individuals have normal or high blood pressure.

Antihypertensive Treatment in Hypertensive Patients with Normal Left Ventricular Mass

Antihypertensive therapy in hypertensive patients with left ventricular hypertrophy causes hypertrophy regression and improved diastolic filling. Whether similar changes occur in hypertensive patients with left ventricular diastolic dysfunction and no hypertrophy is unknown. Schulman and associates[14] from Pittsburgh, Pennsylvania, determined the effect of antihypertensive therapy on left ventricular geometry and function in hypertensive patients without left ventricular hypertrophy. In 18 mild-to-moderate hypertensive patients without significant hypertrophy, baseline echocardiograms and rest and exercise radionuclide angiograms were performed. Subjects were treated for 8 to 12 months with the calcium channel-blocker felodipine and then restudied 2 weeks after treatment withdrawal. Blood pressure normalized with treatment (165 ± 22/98 ± 9 to 128 ± 12/80 ± 5 mm Hg) and returned to pretreatment levels after therapy withdrawal. Rest ejection fraction and peak oxygen consumption and cardiac outputs were unchanged after treatment, but rest peak filling rate increased (2.63 ± 0.57 to 3.11 ± 0.95 end-diastolic volume/second). Ejection fraction increased with exercise only after treatment (64 ± 5% at rest to 71 ± 8% at peak exercise). Left ventricular mass index was unchanged (97 ± 18 to 101 ± 23 g/m^2), but relative wall thickness declined (0.41 ± 0.05 to 0.37 ± 0.05) and left ventricular end-diastolic dimension increased (4.9 ± 0.4 to 5.2 ± 0.4). Blood pressure control in hypertensive patients without hypertrophy leads to improved peak filling rates and remodeling with decreased relative wall thickness. Improved diastolic function can occur without alterations in left ventricular mass.

Prognostic Value of Left Ventricular Mass and Geometry

To determine the independent prognostic significance of left ventricular mass and geometry (concentric vs. eccentric pattern) in hypertensive subjects with left ventricular hypertrophy at echocardiography, Verdecchia and associates[15] from Perugia, Italy, followed 274 subjects for up to 8.7 years (mean 3.2). All patients had systemic hypertension and left ventricular mass greater than or equal to 125 g/body surface area (BSA) and underwent ambulatory blood pressure monitoring and echocardiography before treatment. Eccentric and concentric hypertrophy were defined by the ratio between left ventricular posterior wall thickness and left ventricular radius at telediastole of less than 0.45 and greater than or equal to 0.45, respectively. Age, sex ratio, body mass index, office blood pressure and serum glucose, cholesterol, and triglycerides did not differ between the groups with eccentric (n = 145) and concentric (n = 129) hypertrophy. Average 24-hour, daytime, and nighttime systolic ambulatory blood pressures were higher in concentric than in eccentric hypertrophy. Left ventricular mass was slightly greater in concentric than in eccentric hypertrophy (157 vs. 149 g/BSA). Endocardial and midwall shortening fraction were lower in concentric than in eccentric hypertrophy (96.5% vs. 106.0% of predicted and 71.4% vs. 89.7% of predicted, respectively). The rate of major cardiovascular morbid events was 2.20 and 3.34 per 100 patient-years in eccentric and concentric hypertrophy, respectively (log rank test). Age greater than 60 years and left ventricular mass above median (145 g/BSA) were significant adverse prognostic predictors, whereas left ventricular geometry (eccentric vs. concentric hypertrophy) and ambulatory blood pressure were not. The event rates per 100 patient-years were 1.38 and 3.98, respectively, in the patients with left ventricular mass below and above median (age-adjusted relative risk 2.70). In hypertensive subjects with established left ventricular hypertrophy, left ventricular mass, but not its geometric pattern, provides important prognostic information independent of conventional risk markers including office and ambulatory blood pressure.

Prediction of Left Ventricular Mass from the Electrocardiogram

Although echocardiography provides a reliable method to determine left ventricular mass, it may not be available in all settings. Numerous electrocardiography criteria for the detection of left ventricular hypertrophy have been developed, but few attempts have been made to predict the left ventricular mass itself from the electrocardiogram. In a community-based survey program in the general population, de Vries and associates[16] from Groningen, The Netherlands, identified 277 subjects with untreated diastolic systemic hypertension (blood pressure 95–115 mm Hg, 3 occasions) or isolated systolic hypertension (diastolic blood pressure <95 mm Hg and systolic blood pressure 160–220 mm Hg, 3 occasions). All subjects underwent electrocardiography and echocardiography on the same date. A multiple linear regression analysis was performed by using a random training sample of the data set (n = 185). The independent

TABLE 4-4

Correlation Between the Echocardiographically Determined Left Ventricular Mass and the Value Predicted by the Regression Model Developed in this Study, Compared With Other Combinations of Electrocardiographic Variables*

	Definition	r	p Value
Present model	See appendix	0.65	0.000
Linear regression model II by Wolf et al[8]	See appendix	0.41	0.000
Linear regression model I by Wolf et al[8]	See appendix	0.40	0.000
Logistic regression model for LV hypertrophy[15]	See Casale et al[15]	0.36	0.001
Cornell voltage[14,15]	RaVL + SV3	0.31	0.004
12-lead QRS voltage-duration product[18,19]	12-lead QRS sum × QRS duration	0.27	0.014
12-lead QRS voltage[17]	12-lead QRS sum	0.16	0.136
RV6/RV5[16]	RV6/RV5	0.15	0.161
Cornell voltage-duration product[18,19]	Cornell voltage × QRS duration†	0.14	0.219
Sokolow-Lyon voltage[1]	SV1 + RV5 or RV6	0.03	0.804
Gubner and Ungerleider[13]	RI + SIII	−0.01	0.921

* Analysis is based on the validation sample data (n = 92; see text).

† Sex-specific Cornell voltage adjusted by increasing 0.8 mV for women.

LV = left ventricular.

Reprinted with permission from de Vries et al.[16]

variables included both electrocardiographic and nonelectrocardiographic. The resulting model was used to predict the left ventricular mass in the remainder of the data set, the validation sample (n = 92). Using sex, age, BSA, the S-voltage in V_1 and V_4, and the duration of the terminal P in V_1 as independent variables, the model explained 45% of the variance in the training sample and 42% in the validation sample. This result exceeded that of 2 existing electrocardiography models for left ventricular mass. The correlations between left ventricular mass and combinations of electrocardiography variables used for the detection of left ventricular hypertrophy, such as the Sokolow-Lyon Voltage and the Cornell Voltage, were comparatively low. In settings where echocardiography is not available or is too expensive and time-consuming, prediction of the left ventricular mass from the electrocardiography may offer a valuable alternative (Table 4-4).

Plasma Angiotensin II, Predisposition to Hypertension, and Left Ventricular Size in Healthy Patients

Harrap and colleagues[17] in Glasgow, United Kingdom, and Newcastle, United Kingdom measured left ventricular mass by echocardiography and blood pressure, heart rate, body dimensions, and plasma concentrations of components of the renin-angiotensin system under resting conditions in 1473 pairs of husbands and wives taken from 2 general group practices in the west of Edinburgh, Scotland. Ventricular mass was similar in individuals predisposed to hypertension on the basis of high personal and parental blood pres-

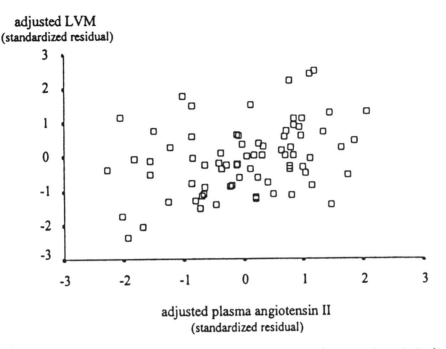

adjusted LVM
(standardized residual)

adjusted plasma angiotensin II
(standardized residual)

Figure 4-4. Partial regression plot of left ventricular mass against plasma angiotensin II after both were adjusted for the linear effects of lean body mass and systolic blood pressure. Adjustments are expressed as standardized residual values for both LV mass and plasma angiotensin II. Positive correlation (r = .35, p < .002) indicates a statistically independent association of plasma angiotensin II and LV mass. Reproduced with permission from Harrap et al.[17]

sures and those with contrasting predisposition, ie, those with personal and parental blood pressures. Regression analysis of the combined groups showed that left ventricular mass correlated with body size, especially lean body mass, and systolic, but not diastolic, blood pressure. Plasma angiotensin II, renin, and ACE showed significant correlations with left ventricular mass. Multiple regression analysis revealed that plasma angiotensin II was the most important component of the renin-angiotensin system and that its effect was independent of systolic blood pressure and body size. These findings provide evidence in humans that angiotensin II exerts a direct effect on myocardial size (Figure 4-4); this association may have important implications for the complications and treatment of left ventricular hypertrophy.

Treatment

Verapamil

Because the risk of cardiovascular events appears to be greatest in the early morning, this period is a time during which adequate blood pressure control appears to be most desirable. In this study by Neutel and associates[18] from Orange, California, and Irvine, California, a controlled-onset extended-release system that delivers verapamil in a manner designed to achieve maximal levels of drug during the early morning surge in blood pressure was compared with placebo. Ninety-five patients with mild-to-moderate hypertension were studied. Of this group, 49 patients (mean age, 58 ± 1.4 years; 35 men and 14 women) were randomly assigned to take verapamil by the controlled-onset extended-release system (240 mg at 10 PM) and 46 individuals (mean age 56 ± 1.5 years; 29 men and 17 women) were randomly assigned to take placebo. Ambulatory blood pressure monitoring was performed after a 4-week initial placebo period and was repeated after 4 weeks of treatment with verapamil or placebo. Verapamil by the controlled-onset extended-release system resulted in significant decreases in mean whole-day systolic and diastolic blood pressure (−8.2/−6.3 mm Hg; baseline 152/93 mm Hg) when compared with placebo (+0.3/−0.9 mm Hg; baseline 150/93 mm Hg). From 6 AM to 12 PM, verapamil by the controlled-onset extended-release system resulted in a change in systolic and diastolic blood pressure of −11.6/−9.0 mm Hg, which was significantly greater than the change that occurred with placebo (−0.5/−1.0 mm Hg) during the same period. In the last 4 hours of the dosing interval (6 PM to 10 PM, verapamil by the controlled-onset extended release system caused significantly greater decreases in blood pressure (−7.4/−4.8 mm Hg) than did placebo (+2.7/+1.0 mm Hg). These data demonstrate that the controlled-onset extended release system, when administered in the late evening, achieves maximal blood pressure reduction during the early morning hours. Moreover, blood pressure reductions were sustained throughout the 24-hour period.

Milrinone

Fixed pulmonary hypertension is a risk factor for right heart failure and death after heart transplantation. Sodium nitroprusside, the agent used most commonly to test for reversibility of pulmonary hypertension before transplantation, requires dose titration and is frequently limited by hypotension. Milrinone is an intravenous phosphodiesterase inhibitor that acts rapidly and exerts both positive inotropic and direct vasodilator effects in patients with heart failure. Givertz and colleagues[19] from Boston, Massachusetts, examined the feasibility of using milrinone to test pulmonary vascular reactivity in patients before heart transplantation. In 27 patients with NYHA function class III or IV heart failure referred for heart transplantation with a pulmonary vascular resistance of greater than 200 dynes-s-cm^{-5}, they measured the hemodynamic response to a single intravenous bolus of milrinone (50 μg/kg body weight) infused over 1 minute. Milrinone decreased pulmonary vascular resistance in all patients. The effect was maximal 5 to 10 minutes after the bolus and persisted for at least 20 minutes. The reduction in pulmonary vascular resistance (PVR) at 5 minutes was associated with a 42% increase in cardiac output and a decrease of 12% and 16% in mean pulmonary artery (PA) and PA wedge pressures, respectively. There was no effect on heart rate or systemic blood pressure. The magnitude of the decrease in PVR correlated inversely with the milrinone-induced increase in cardiac output. These authors concluded that bolus milrinone consistently decreases PVR in patients with pulmonary hypertension secondary to severe congestive heart failure (CHF). This effect is rapid in onset and well tolerated, even by patients with low systemic blood pressure. They believe that an intravenous bolus of milrinone can be used to test for the reversibility of pulmonary hypertension in patients with CHF undergoing evaluation for heart transplantation.

Prostacylin

Raffy and colleagues[20] in Clamart, France, attempted to evaluate in a nonselected population of patients with primary pulmonary hypertension the degree of vasodilatation achieved during short-term infusion of prostacyclin. They also examined whether these patients might differ with regard to baseline characteristics and prognoses, depending on the level of vasodilatation achieved with the prostacyclin. Between 1984 and 1992, 91 consecutive patients with primary pulmonary hypertension underwent catheterization of the right side of the heart with a short-term vasodilator trial with prostacyclin. Patients were divided into 3 groups: 1) nonresponding (n = 40); 2) moderately responding (n = 42); and 3) highly responding (n = 9) patients. The 3 groups were defined by a decrease in total pulmonary vascular resistance of less than 20%, between 20% and 50%, and greater than 50%, respectively, related to the control values. Prolonged oral vasodilator therapy was started only in moderately and highly responsive patients. All patients had long-term oral anticoagulant therapy. The survival rate at 2 years was significantly higher in highly responsive patients, compared with nonresponsive and moderately responsive ones (62% vs. 38% and 47% survivors) (Figure 4-5). Comparisons between groups showed no significant differences in baseline hemodynamics or clinical characteristics except for a longer time between onset of symptoms and diagno-

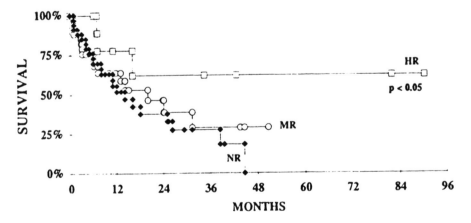

FIGURE 4-5. Plot showing survival curves of the 3 groups of patients (transplant recipients excluded; Kaplan-Meier life table analysis). Survival rates between groups were compared with the log-rank test. No MR patient was followed for longer than 50 months at the time of the study. NR, nonresponding; MR, moderately responding; HR, highly responding. Reproduced with permission from Raffy et al.[20]

sis of primary pulmonary hypertension in highly responsive patients. Thus, these data indicate that patients with primary pulmonary hypertension exhibiting a decrease in total pulmonary vascular resistance of greater than 50% during short-term prostacyclin administration had longer disease evolutions and better prognoses than did patients with a lower vasodilator response.

Barst and colleagues[21] conducted a 12-week prospective, randomized, multicenter open trial comparing the effects of the continuous intravenous infusion of epoprostenol (prostacyclin) and conventional therapy with those of conventional therapy alone in 81 patients with severe primary pulmonary hypertension who were in New York Association functional class III or IV. In this study, exercise capacity was improved in the 41 patients treated with epoprostenol, with a median distance walked in 6 minutes of 362 meters at 12 weeks versus 315 meters at control, but it decreased in the 40 patients treated with conventional therapy alone, being 204 meters at 12 weeks versus 270 meters at baseline (p<.002 for the comparison of the treatment groups). Indexes of the quality of life were improved only in the epoprostenol-treated group. Hemodynamics improved at 12 weeks in the epoprostenol-treated patients. The changes in mean pulmonary artery pressure for the epoprostenol and control groups were −8% and +3%, respectively, and the mean changes in pulmonary vascular resistance for the epoprostenol and control groups were −21% and +9%, respectively. Eight patients died during the study, all of whom had been randomly assigned to conventional therapy (p=.003). Serious complications included 4 episodes of catheter-related sepsis and 1 thrombotic event. These data suggest that, as compared with conventional therapy, the continuous intravenous infusion of epoprostenol produces symptomatic and hemodynamic improvement, as well as improved survival in patients with severe pulmonary hypertension.

Calcium Antagonists

Frielingsdorf and colleagues[22] in Zürich, Switzerland, evaluated coronary vasomotor responses to dynamic exercise in patients with coronary artery disease (CAD), with and without arterial hypertension, and determined the effect of calcium antagonists on that vasomotion. Cross-sectional areas of a normal and a stenotic coronary artery segment were examined in 79 patients with CAD at rest and during supine bicycle exercise. Changes in luminal area after acute administration of a calcium antagonist (diltiazem or nicardipine) during exercise and after sublingual nitroglycerin were assessed by biplane quantitative coronary arteriography. Patients were divided into 2 groups: group 1 (control) consisted of 48 patients without pretreatment with a calcium antagonist and group 2 of 31 patients with (normotensive subjects, n=15; hypertensive subjects, n=16) pretreatment with a calcium antagonist immediately before exercise. The groups did not differ with regard to clinical characteristics or hemodynamic data measured during exercise. Mean aortic pressure at rest, however, was increased in hypertensive patients compared with normotensive subjects in groups 1 and 2. In group 1, exercise-induced vasomotor responses were different between normotensive and hypertensive subjects in both normal and

Coronary Vasomotor Response: Normotensive Patients

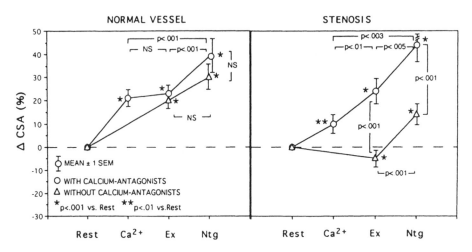

FIGURE 4-6. Luminal area change in percent of resting cross-sectional area (ΔCSA) after treatment with calcium antagonists (Ca^{2+}) and during exercise (Ex), as well as after 1.6 mg sublingual nitroglycerin (Ntg) in normotensive patients. The normal vessel shows normal behavior during exercise with or without Ca^{2+} treatment. However, the stenotic vessel shows an abnormal response (vasoconstriction) to exercise that is reversed after pretreatment with calcium channel blockers. There is an additive effect of Ca^{2+} and nitroglycerin on maximal vasodilation of the stenotic, but not the normal, vessel. Values are mean ± SEM. Reproduced with permission from Frielingsdorf et al.[20]

stenotic vessels. However, in group 2, there was a coronary vasodilatation in normotensive and hypertensive patients for both normal and stenotic segments. Thus, abnormal coronary vasomotion during exercise may be observed in hypertensive patients with reduced vasodilator responses in normal arteries and enhanced vasoconstriction in stenotic arteries. Calcium antagonists prevent the abnormal response of normal and stenotic coronary arteries to exercise in hypertensive patients and may compensate for endothelial dysfunction with reduced vasodilator response to exercise (Figure 4-6 and 4-7).

Amlodipine

Kloner and associates[23] for the Amlodipine Cardiovascular Community Trial Study Group assessed whether there were age, sex, or racial differences in response to amlodipine (5–10 mg once daily) in patients with mild-to-moderate essential hypertension. This prospective, open-label trial had a 2-week placebo period, a 4-week upward drug titration/efficacy period, and a 12-week drug maintenance period. There were 1084 evaluable patients (mean age 55.5 years; 65% men and 35% women; 79% white and 21% black; 75% <65 and 25% ≥65 years old). At the end of the titration/efficacy phase, the mean ± SD blood pressure decreased by −16.3 ± 12.3/−12.5 ± 5.9 mm Hg. Amlodipine produced a goal blood pressure response (sitting diastolic blood pressure ≤ 90 mm Hg, or a 10 mm Hg decrease) in 86.0% of patients overall. The blood pressure response was greater in women (91.4%) than in men (83.0%), and greater in those older than 65 years old (91.5%) than in those younger than 65 years old (84.1%); however, it was similar between whites and blacks (86.0% vs. 85.9%), respectively). The sex difference in blood pressure response could not be fully explained by differences in age, weight, dose (mg/kg), race, baseline blood pressure, or compliance, and there were no differences among women based on use of hormone replacement therapy. Amlodipine was well tolerated; mild-to-moderate edema was the most common adverse effect. Thus, amlodipine was effective and safe as once-a-day monotherapy in the treatment of mild to moderate hypertension in a community-based population. Women had a greater blood pressure response to amlodipine.

Doxazosin

The Hypertension and Lipid Trial (HALT) was undertaken by Levy and associates[24] from Boston, Massachusetts, and New York, New York, to assess the efficacy and safety of doxazosin, a selective α_1-adrenergic blocker, in patients with hypertension in a clinical practice setting. The effects of doxazosin on office blood pressure, changes in lipid profiles, and theoretical coronary disease risk were studied. In an open, noncomparative, multicenter trial, 851

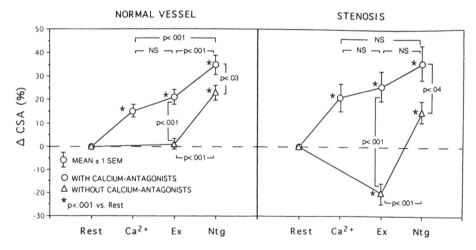

Coronary Vasomotor Response: Hypertensive Patients

FIGURE 4-7. Luminal area change in percent of resting cross-sectional area (ΔCSA) after treatment with calcium antagonists (Ca^{2+}) and during exercise (Ex), as well as after 1.6 mg sublingual nitroglycerin (Ntg) in hypertensive patients. The reaction of the normal vessel to exercise is abnormal in hypertensive patients but is normalized after administration of Ca^{2+}. The same response can be observed in the stenotic vessel, although the abnormal response to exercise is even more pronounced than in the normal vessel. Again, the vasoconstrictive response is eliminated by calcium channel blockers, and there is an additive effect between Ca^{2+} and nitroglycerin, not only in the stenotic but also in the normal vessel. Values are mean ± SEM. Reproduced with permission from Frielingsdorf et al.[20]

patients were studied for a maximum of 16 weeks. Doxazosin significantly reduced mean sitting systolic blood pressure and diastolic blood pressure by 15/13 mm Hg and standing systolic blood pressure and diastolic blood pressure by 16/13 mm Hg in the total study population (n = 807) with no significant effect on heart rate. Mean total cholesterol levels were significantly reduced by 2.7% LDL cholesterol levels by 2.4%, and mean triglyceride levels by 3.4%. HDL cholesterol levels were essentially unchanged. The mean ratio of total to HDL cholesterol was significantly reduced. Mean predicted 5-year coronary disease risk was significantly reduced with doxazosin therapy by 15% in previously untreated patients and by 1.7% in patients who were previously receiving antihypertensive therapy. The drug was well tolerated. This study demonstrates that antihypertensive therapy with doxazosin can favorably affect coronary disease risk factors and reduce predicted coronary disease risk.

1. Benetos A, Gautier S, Ricard S, Topouchian J, Asmar R, Poirier O, Larosa E, Guize L, Safar M, Soubrier F, Cambien F. Influence of angiotensin-converting enzyme and angiotensin II type 1 receptor gene polymorphisms on aortic stiffness in normotensive and hypertensive patients. Circulation 1996 (August 15);94:698–703.
2. Kario K, Matsuo T, Kobayashi H, Matsuo M, Sakata T, Miyata T, Shimada K: Factor VII hyperactivity and endothelial cell damage are found in elderly hypertensives only when concomitant with microalbuminuria. Arterioscler Thromb Vasc Biol 1996 (March);16:455–461.
3. Noll G, Wenzel RR, Schneider M, Oesch V, Binggeli C, Shaw S, Weidmann P, Lüscher TF. Increased activation of sympathetic nervous system and endothelin by mental stress in normotensive offspring of hypertensive patients. Circulation 1996 (March 1);93:866–869.
4. Pincomb GA, Lovallo WR, McKey BS, Sung BH, Passey RB, Everson SA, Wilson MF: Acute blood pressure elevations with caffeine in men with borderline systemic hypertension. Am J Cardiol 1996 (February 1);77:270–274.
5. Liu K, Ruth KJ, Flack JM, Jones-Webb R, Burke G, Savage PJ, Hulley SB. Blood pressure in young blacks and whites: Relevance of obesity and lifestyle factors in determining differences. The CARDIA study. Circulation 1996 (January);93:60–66.
6. Abenhaim L, Moride Y, Brenot F, Rich S, Benichou J, Kurz X, Higenbottam T, Oakley C, Wouters E, Aubier M, Simonneau G, Bégaud B, for the International Primary Pulmonary Hypertension Study Group. Appetite-suppressant drugs and the risk of primary pulmonary hypertension. N Engl J Med 1996 (August 29);335: 609–616.
7. Asmar R, Benetos A, Pannier B, Agnes E, Topouchian J, Laloux B, Safar M: Prevalence and circadian variations of ST-segment depression and its concomitant blood pressure changes in asymptomatic systemic hypertension. Am J Cardiol 1996 (February 15);77:384–390.
8. Suurküla M, Agewall S, Fagerberg B, Wendelhag I, Wikstrand J, on behalf of the Risk Intervention Study Group: Multiple risk intervention in high-risk hypertensive patients: A 3-year ultrasound study of intima-media thickness and plaques in the carotid artery. Arterioscler Thromb Vasc Biol 1996 (March);16:462–470.
9. Lakshman MR, Reda D, Materson BJ, Cushman WC, Kochar MS, Nunn S, Hamburger RJ, Freis ED, for the Department of Veterans Affairs Cooperative Study Group on Antihypertensive Agents. Comparison of plasma lipid and lipoprotein profiles in hypertensive black versus white men. Am J Cardiol 1996 (December 1); 78:1236–1241.
10. Frost PH, Davis BR, Burlando AJ, Curb JD, Guthrie GP Jr, Isaacsohn JL, Wasser-theil-Smoller S, Wilson AC, Stamler J, for the Systolic Hypertension in the Elderly Research Group. Serum lipids and incidence of coronary heart disease. Findings from the Systolic Hypertension in the Elderly Program (SHEP). Circulation 1996 (November 15);94:2381–2388.

11. Frost PH, Davis BR, Burlando AJ, Curb JD, Guthrie GP Jr, Isaacsohn JL, Wasser-theil-Smoller S, Wilson AC, Stamler J, for the Systolic Hypertension in the Elderly Research Group. Coronary heart disease risk factors in men and women aged 60 years and older. Findings from the Systolic Hypertension in the Elderly Program. Circulation 1996 (July 1);94:26–34.

12. Frielingsdorf J, Kaufmann P, Seiler C, Vassalli G, Suter T, Hess OM: Abnormal coronary vasomotion in hypertension: Role of coronary artery disease. J Am Coll Cardiol 1996 (October);28:935–941.

13. Himeno E, Nishino K, Nakashima Y, Kuroiwa A, Ikeda M. Weight reduction regresses left ventricular mass regardless of blood pressure level in obese subjects. Am Heart J 1996 (February);131:313–319.

14. Schulman DS, Flores AR, Tugoen J, Dianzumba S, Reichek N: Antihypertensive treatment in hypertensive patients with normal left ventricular mass is associated with left ventricular remodeling and improved diastolic function. Am J Cardiol 1996 (July 1);78:56–60.

15. Verdecchia P, Schillaci G, Borgioni C, Ciucci A, Gattobigio R, Zampi I, Santucci A, Santucci C, Reboldi G, Porcellati C: Prognostic value of left ventricular mass and geometry in systemic hypertension with left ventricular hypertrophy. Am J Cardiol 1996 (July 15);78:197–202.

16. de Vries SO, Heesen WF, Beltman FW, Kroese AH, May JF, Smit AJ, Lie KI: Prediction of the left ventricular mass from the electrocardiogram in systemic hypertension. Am J Cardiol 1996 (May 1);77:974–978.

17. Harrap SB, Dominiczak AF, Fraser R, Lever AF, Morton JJ, Foy CJ, Watt GCM. Plasma angiotensin II, predisposition to hypertension, and left ventricular size in healthy young adults. Circulation 1996 (March 15);93:1148–1154.

18. Neutel JM, Alderman M, Anders RJ, Weber MA. Novel delivery system for verapamil designed to achieve maximal blood pressure control during the early morning. Am Heart J 1996 (December);132:1202–1206.

19. Givertz MM, Hare JM, Loh E, Gauthier DF, Colucci WS: Effect of bolus milrinone on hemodynamic variables and pulmonary vascular resistance in patients with severe left ventricular dysfunction: A rapid test for reversibility of pulmonary hypertension. J Am Coll Cardiol 1996 (December);28:1775–1780.

20. Raffy O, Azarian R, Brenot F, Parent F, Sithon O, Petitpretz P, Hervé P, Duroux P, Dinh-Xuan AT, Simonneau G. Clinical significance of the pulmonary vasodilator response during short-term infusion of prostacyclin in primary pulmonary hypertension. Circulation 1996 (February);93:484–488.

21. Barst RJ, Rubin LJ, Long WA, McGoon MD, Rich S, Badesch DB, Groves BM, Tapson VF, Bourge RC, Brundage BH, Koerner SK, Langleben D, Keller CA, Murali S, Uretsky BF, Clayton LM, Jöbsis MM, Blackburn SD, Shortino D, Crow JW, for the Primary Pulmonary Hypertension Study Group. A comparison of continuous intravenous epoprostenol (prostacyclin) with conventional therapy for primary pulmonary hypertension. N Engl J Med 1996 (February 1);334:296–301.

22. Frielingsdorf J, Seiler C, Kaufmann P, Vassalli G, Suter T, Hess OM. Normalization of abnormal coronary vasomotion by calcium antagonists in patients with hypertension. Circulation 1996 (April 1);93:1380–1387.

23. Kloner RA, Sowers JR, DiBona GF, Gaffney M, Wein M, for the Amlodipine Cardiovascular Community Trial Study Group: Sex- and age-related antihypertensive effects of amlodipine. Am J Cardiol 1996 (April 1);77:713–722.

24. Levy D, Walmsley P, Levenstein M. Principal results of the Hypertension and Lipid Trial (HALT): A multicenter study of doxazosin in patients with hypertension. Am Heart J 1996 (May);131:966–973.

5

Valvular Heart Disease

Valvular Heart Disease (General Topics)

Aspirin and Oral Anticoagulants in Mechanical Heart Valve Replacement

Altman and colleagues[1] in Buenos Aires, Argentina, compared the use of aspirin (100 mg/day vs 650 mg/day) in the prevention of systemic embolism and vascular death in patients with heart valve replacement who were being treated with oral anticoagulants, with a target international normalized ratio (INR) of 2.0 to 3.0. Four hundred and nine of 416 consecutive patients who had cardiac valve replacement were randomized in open allocation into 1 of 2 groups: both groups were treated with oral anticoagulant therapy with a target INR of 2.0 to 3.0. Two hundred and seven patients who received 100 mg/day of aspirin for an average of 24 months were compared with 202 patients who received 650 mg/day of aspirin for an average of 22 months in a randomized-treatment, open-allocation study. There were no significant differences in systemic embolism, vascular death, or total death rates between the low- and high-dose aspirin treatment groups. The total number of hemorrhagic events was 13 per 100 patients in the high-dose aspirin group and 8 per 100 patients in the low-dose aspirin group, but the rate of bleeding was influenced by dipyridamole in the 650 mg aspirin group. Thus, in patients with mechanical heart valve replacement, low-dose aspirin (100 mg per day) in conjunction with oral anticoagulants at an INR of 2.0 to 3.0 is as effective as the use of high-dose aspirin (650 mg/day) in the prevention of systemic embolism.

Multicenter Comparison of Low-Dose versus Standard-Dose Anticoagulation for Mechanical Heart Valves

Acar and colleagues[2] from Paris, France, compared moderate oral anticoagulation (INR of 2.0 to 3.0) with the usual regimen (INR of 3.0 to 4.5) after a single-valve replacement with a mechanical prosthesis, either Omnicarbon or St. Jude. Patients included were between 18 and 75 years of age, they were in sinus rhythm, and they had a left atrial diameter of 50 mm or less by echocardiography. Patients were randomized for INR after surgery. From 1991 to 1994, 433 patients had valve replacement (aortic, 414; mitral, 19) with 353 St. Jude and 80 Omnicarbon prostheses. Three hundred and eighty patients were randomized for INR: 188 for INR 2.0 to 3.0, and 192 for INR 3.0 to 4.5. The mean follow-up was 2 years, with a range of 1 to 4 years. Analysis of 18,001 INR samples showed that the mean of the median of INR was 2.74 ± 0.35 in the

2.0 to 3.0 group and 3.2 ± 0.33 in the 3.0 to 4.5 group. Thromboembolic events as assessed from clinical data and CT brain scans occurred in 10 patients in the 2.0 to 3.0 INR group and 9 patients in the 3.0 to 4.5 INR group. Hemorrhagic events occurred in 34 patients in the 2.0 to 3.0 INR group and 56 patients in the 3.0 to 4.5 INR group (p<.01), with 13 and 19 major hemorrhagic events, respectively. Thus, in selected patients with mechanical prostheses, moderate anticoagulation prevents thromboembolic events as effectively as conventional anticoagulation and reduces the incidence of hemorrhagic events.

Transthoracic and Transesophageal Echocardiography in Suspected Endocarditis

Lindner and colleagues[3] in Charlottesville, Virginia, evaluated transthoracic echocardiography (TTE) in the diagnosis of endocarditis by using TTE and TEE (TEE) in 105 consecutive patients with suspected endocarditis. Patients were classified as having either low, intermediate, or high probability of endocarditis on the basis of clinical criteria and separately on the basis of both TTE and TEE findings. TTE and TEE classified the majority of the 67 patients with a low clinical probability of endocarditis as having a low likelihood of the disease (82% and 85%, respectively). Among the 14 patients with intermediate clinical probability, 12 had technically adequate TTE studies, and 10 of these (83%) were classified as either high or low probability. All patients with intermediate clinical probability were classified as high or low probability by TEE. The majority of the 24 patients with high clinical probability were placed in the low-likelihood category by echocardiography. There was concordance between TTE and TEE in 83% of the cases. TEE was useful for the diagnosis of endocarditis in patients with prosthetic valves and in those in whom TTE indicated an intermediate probability. The course of antibiotic therapy was influenced only by the clinical profile and not by the echocardiographic results. Thus, echocardiography should not be used to make a diagnosis of endocarditis in those with a low clinical probability of the disease. In those with an intermediate or high probability, TTE should be the diagnostic procedure of choice, and TEE should be reserved for patients who have prosthetic valves or in whom TTE is either technically inadequate or indicates an intermediate probability of endocarditis (Figures 5-1–5-3).

Valvular Heart Disease in Pregnancy

Pregnant patients with prosthetic heart valves require long-term anticoagulant therapy. To avoid increased incidence of fetal morbidity and mortality with the use of coumarin agents in such patients, anticoagulation with subcutaneous heparin has been suggested. Salazar and colleagues[4] from Mexico City, Mexico, evaluated the use of an anticoagulant regimen of adjusted doses of subcutaneous heparin during pregnancy in women with cardiac valve

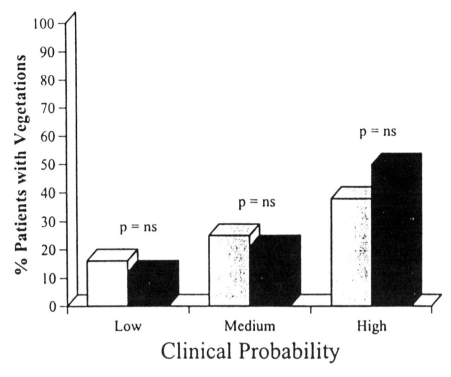

FIGURE 5-1. Bar graph showing detection of vegetations by transthoracic echocardiography (TTE) and TEE (TEE) according to the clinical likelihood of endocarditis. Vegetations include those classified as definite, probable, and possible. Probability values are for the comparison between the 2 echocardiographic techniques. There is a significant increase in the presence of vegetations for low versus high clinical probability by TTE (p<.05) and TTE (p<.001). Reproduced with permission from Lindner et al.[3]

prostheses. Forty pregnancies in 37 women with prosthetic heart valves were prospectively followed up. Subcutaneous heparin was administered from the 6th until the end of the 12th week and then the last 2 weeks of gestation. Heparin was given every 8 hours in the first 36 cases and every 6 hours in the last 4 cases, and the dose was adjusted to maintain the activated partial thromboplastin time (aPTT) at 1.5 to 2.5 times the control level. A coumarol derivative was used at the other times. The incidence rate of spontaneous abortions was 37.5%, with 1 neonatal death due to cerebral hemorrhage. No signs of coumarin-induced embryopathy were found in any of the 16 live-born infants. One mother died of gastrointestinal bleeding while receiving oral anticoagulant agents. There were 2 cases of fatal massive thrombosis of a mitral tilting-disk prostheses during heparin therapy. This study was interrupted after the last of these 2 cases. These authors concluded that the regimen of adjusted doses of subcutaneous heparin was not effective in preventing thrombosis of mechanical valve prostheses during pregnancy. The use of heparin from the 6th to the 12th week of gestation does not decrease the high incidence of fetal wastage associated with anticoagulant therapy.

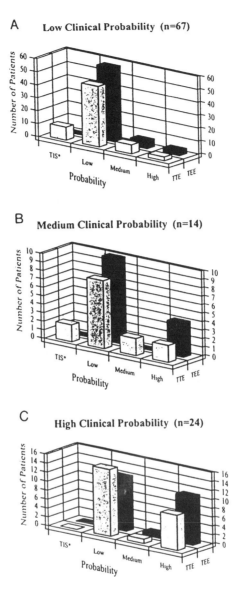

Figure 5-2. Bar graph showing likelihood of endocarditis by transthoracic echocardiography (TTE) and TEE (TEE) in patients with low, intermediate, and high clinical probability of the disease. TIS* indicates technically inadequate study. Reproduced with permission from Lindner et al.[3]

Mitral Valvular Disease

Mitral Regurgitation and Prognosis of Mitral Valve Prolapse

Kim and associates[5] from Tochigi, Japan, investigated the relationship between the severity of mitral regurgitation (MR) and the development of complications and cardiac events by using 2-dimensional and color Doppler echocardiography in 229 consecutive patients with mitral valve prolapse (MVP). The frequency of moderate and severe MR was significantly higher in patients with a prolapsed posterior leaflet (61%) than in patients with a prolapsed anterior leaflet (25%), and the older the patient, the greater the severity of MR. The occurrence of complications, such as atrial fibrillation (AF), congestive heart failure (CHF), and chordal rupture, was significantly greater in prolapsed posterior leaflet cases than in prolapsed anterior leaflet cases, and the occurrence was closely associated with the degree of severity of MR. Multiple logistic regression showed that the severity of MR is a strong prognostic indicator for developing complications. Furthermore, in a subgroup of 49 patients tracked for a mean of 4.8 years, the new development of complications was significantly higher in those who showed a progression in the severity of MR (52%) than in those without progression in severity (8%). The initial severity of MR was related to the occurrence of cardiac events (MVR, infective endocarditis, cerebral embolism, and death). These data indicate that the progression of MR is closely associated with the development of complications and cardiac events and suggest that the severity of MR is an important prognostic indicator for the development of complications and cardiac events in patients with MVP.

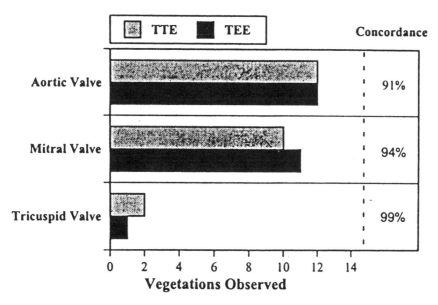

FIGURE 5-3. Bar graphs showing detection of possible, probable, or definite vegetations by transthoracic echocardiography (TTE) and transesophageal echocardiography (TEE) according to valve location. Neither technique identified a vegetation of the pulmonary valve. The bars depict the number of valves with vegetations by TTE and TEE, and the concordance numbers reflect agreement for both presence and absence of vegetations. Reproduced with permission from Lindner et al.[3]

Balloon Mitral Commissurotomy: Long-Term Results

Treviño and associates[6] from Monterrey, Mexico, and Chicago, Illinois, examined the immediate results and 2-year follow-up of percutaneous transvenous mitral commissurotomy using the Inoue balloon and double-balloon techniques. Short-term comparisons have been described, but long-term comparisons have not been available. Percutaneous transvenous mitral commissurotomy was performed in 208 adult patients with symptomatic mitral stenosis and a mitral valve area of 0.94 ± 0.2 cm^2, by use of the Inoue balloon in 157 (73%) and the double balloon technique in 56 (26%). Procedures were performed successfully and without complications in 198 (93%) cases. Adequate mitral dilatation (mitral valve area ≥ 1.6 cm^2) without significant regurgitation was obtained in 179 (86%) of 192 patients. The final mitral valve area was 2.0 ± 0.43 cm^2 after Inoue balloon and 2.06 ± 0.51 cm^2 after double-balloon. Technical difficulties and complications were more frequent with double-balloon (16% vs. 3.8%). Severe MR (grade III-IV) occurred in 4.6% of the Inoue balloon procedures and 4.1% of the double-balloon procedures, whereas grade I MR was greater with the Inoue balloon (21% vs. 10%). A total of 172 patients were monitored for an average of 24 ± 11 months, with 83% in New York Heart Association functional class I, with an echocardiographic mitral valve area of 1.84 ± 44 cm^2, and a restenosis rate of 22% at 36 months. Percutaneous transvenous mitral commissurotomy was a safe, effective treatment for symptomatic mitral stenosis. Results of both Inoue balloon and double-balloon techniques were similar, but the Inoue balloon was simpler and safer. Long-term clinical improvement was maintained, although the restenosis rate seems to be progressive and related to inadequate immediate results.

In 1987, the NHLBI established the multicenter balloon valvuloplasty registry to assess both short- and long-term safety and efficacy of percutaneous balloon mitral commissurotomy. Dean and colleagues[7] for this multicenter registry reported the long-term outcome of patients undergoing percutaneous balloon mitral commissurotomy in the registry. Between November 1987 and October 1989, 736 patients older than 18 years of age underwent percutaneous balloon mitral commissurotomy at 23 registry sites in North America. The maximal follow-up period was a little more than 5 years. The actuarial survival rate was 93%, 90%, 87%, and 84% at 1, 2, 3 and 4 years, respectively. Eighty percent of the patients were alive and free of mitral surgery or repeat balloon mitral commissurotomy at 1 year. The event-free survival rate was 80% at 1 year, 71% at 2 years, 66% at 3 years, and 60% at 4 years. Important univariable predictors of actuarial mortality at 4 years included age greater than 70 years, New York Heart Association functional class IV, and baseline echocardiographic score greater than 12. These authors concluded from analysis of this registry data that percutaneous balloon mitral commissurotomy has a favorable effect on the hemodynamic variables of MS, and long-term follow-up data suggest that it is a viable alternative with respect to surgical commissurotomy in selected patients.

Iung and colleagues[8] from Paris, France, evaluated the late functional results after successful percutaneous mitral commissurotomy. Between 1986 and 1992, 528 patients underwent successful commissurotomy. The survival rate for patients in NYHA functional class I or II with no cardiac-related deaths or need for mitral surgery or repeat dilation was 76% at 5 years. Independent predictors of a good functional result included echocardiographic data, functional class, cardiothoracic index before the procedure, and valve area after the procedure. Good functional results were observed 5 years after successful percutaneous mitral commissurotomy.

Multiplane Transesophageal Echocardiography to Assess Mitral Regurgitation

Pieper and associates[9] from Amsterdam in Utrecht, The Netherlands, designed a study to examine the accuracy of multiplane transesophageal echocardiography (TEE) color Doppler measurements in comparison with monoplane or biplane measurements in estimating the severity of MR. Multiplane TEE potentially increases diagnostic accuracy of transesophageal examinations; it is unknown whether multiplane is more accurate in assessing the severity of MR than monoplane or biplane TEE. Left ventricular cineangiograms of 91 patients with MR (40 no or mild, 30 moderate, and 21 severe) were compared with systolic pulmonary venous flow reversal and transesophageal color Doppler measurements, jet area and length in the transverse and longitudinal plane, maximal and average of those 2 planes (biplane), and maximal and average of 11 different planes (multiplane). Flow reversal (16 patients) identified severe MR, with a specificity of 96% and a sensitivity of 62%; these were 96% and only 10% to 43%, respectively, for color Doppler measurements. In the absence of flow reversal, multiplane maximal jet area predicted severe MR with a sensitivity of 88% and a specificity of 75%, which were 85% and 76%, respectively, for no or mild MR; this did not differ significantly from results obtained by monoplane or biplane measurements. Color Doppler measurements of eccentric jets were not reliable for identification of severe MR. Systolic pulmonary venous flow reversal identifies 2 of 3 patients with severe MR with high accuracy. In patients without flow reversal, multiplane color Doppler TEE is very capable of assessing MR severity, but biplane and monoplane TEE are equally accurate.

Mitral Valve Annulus Displacement to Assess Septal Contractility

To determine whether mitral valve annulus displacement can be used to assess septal contractility in patients with paradoxical septal motion, Silva and associates[10] from New Orleans, Louisiana, assessed 4 atrioventricular (AV) regions (septum, lateral wall, anterior wall, and inferior wall) by mitral valve annulus displacement in 80 consecutive patients. The patients were divided into 5 groups: group 1 (control) (n = 20), normal left ventricular systolic function group; group 2 (n = 15), paradoxical septal motion resulting from left BBB and normal segmental and global LV systolic function; group 3 (n = 19), paradoxical septal motion as a result of cardiac surgery, and normal segmental and global LV systolic function; group 4 (n = 11), paradoxical septal motion resulting from left BBB, dilated cardiomyopathy, and severely depressed left ventricular systolic function; group 5 (n = 15), septal hypokinesis with either normal or mildly depressed global left ventricular systolic function. In groups 1, 2, and 3, 80% to 100% of patients had septal and other regional mitral valve annulus displacement of 1.0 cm or greater. The average mitral valve annulus displacement in group 4 (dilated cardiomyopathy), was significantly decreased (≤0.8 cm) in all 4 regions. In group 5 (septal hypokinesis), the septal mitral valve annulus displacement was 1.0 cm or greater in only 13% of the patients. In conclusion, patients with paradoxical septal motion caused by left BBB or cardiac surgery have preserved septal contractility when evaluated by mitral valve annulus displacement.

Echocardiographic Predictors of Survival after Mitral Valve Surgery

The objective of this study by Fleischmann and associates[11] from Boston, Massachusetts, was to identify echocardiographic and clinical predictors of survival after mitral valve surgery when mitral repair is an option. In 132 patients undergoing mitral valve repair or replacement for the diagnosis of MR, preoperative echocardiograms were analyzed quantitatively and reviewed by 2 independent observers for structural abnormalities of the mitral valve. In Cox regression analysis, clinical factors such as age and New York Heart Association class IV, and echocardiographic factors including morphologic evidence of endocarditis or myxomatous disease were significant predictors of overall survival, although valve repair itself was not. End-systolic dimensions and volumes were not significant predictors, likely related to the small number of patients with markedly increased end-systolic dimensions or volumes (5 patients [4%] with end-systolic dimension >5.5 cm, 12 patients [9%] with end-systolic volume index >60 mL/m^2). New York Heart Association class IV, age, and the presence of calcification were independent predictors of survival in multivariate analysis. In this contemporary cohort of patients undergoing repair or replacement for MR, factors such as echocardiographically determined cause of disease and presence of calcification predicted survival; traditional measurements such as end-systolic dimensions and volumes were less predictive, most likely because patients underwent surgery before their ventricles became markedly enlarged. Clinical factors such as age and functional status remained the most potent predictors of survival after surgery for MR.

Reduction of Mitral Valve Systolic Anterior Motion after Ventricular Septal Myomectomy

To determine the mechanism of reduction of mitral valve systolic anterior motion by myectomy, Nakatani and associates[12] from Boston, Massachusetts, and Cleveland, Ohio, examined 33 patients with obstructive HC echocardio-graphically before and after myectomy. Measurements included outflow tract diameter, the direction of ejection streamline (the angle between the ejection flow and the mitral valve), midventricular fractional area change, and papillary muscle inward excursion in the short-axis image. After myectomy, the outflow tract was enlarged (from 1.2 ± 0.3 cm to 2.1 ± 0.4 cm), and the ejection flow became more parallel to the mitral leaflets (from 51° ± 10° to 28° ± 8°), whereas hyperdynamic midventricular fractional area change was reduced (81% ± 14% to 62% ± 14%), and papillary muscle excursion decreased (1.3 ± 0.3 cm to 0.8 ± 0.3 cm). Outflow enlargement and reduced ventricular contraction would decrease the Venturi force. Change of ejection streamline and reduced contraction would decrease the drag force onto the mitral leaflets. Blunted papillary motion would increase the mitral leaflet tension and decrease the effect of drag force on both leaflets. Thus, myectomy decreases Venturi and drag forces and appears to reduce systolic anterior motion of the mitral valve.

Aortic Valvular Disease

Determination of Aortic Valve Area

Quantitative assessment of aortic stenosis (AS) is subject to the limitations of all current noninvasive and invasive methods. The ability to obtain a direct measurement of aortic valve area with high resolution by intracardiac echocardiography could be of great benefit to catheterized patients. To provide a fixed AS area as an ideal standard for comparison, Jiang and associates[13] from Boston, Massachusetts, performed intracardiac echocardiography in 12 sheep hearts with experimentally created AS and 5 human AS hearts from autopsies. Intracardiac echocardiography catheters were passed retrograde across the aortic valve, and the minimal orifice area on pullback was planimetered and compared with calibrated video imaging. The entire orifice circumference could be successfully recorded in 16 (94%) hearts. Orifice area from intracardiac echocardiography correlated well with actual values. To illustrate the applicability *in vivo*, 2 canine models and 10 patients with AS were studied. The limiting orifice could be imaged in both animals and in 8 of 10 patients, in whom values agreed well with invasive data. Intracardiac echocardiography can therefore accurately measure AS orifice area *in vitro;* it can be applied *in vivo* as well. These validation studies provide the foundation for subsequent clinical studies and applications.

Measurements of valve orifice area in AS are based on the assumption that orifice area remains constant throughout ejection and is independent of transvalvular gradients and flow. Recent studies, however, have suggested that the calculated valve area in AS may change in different flow conditions. Badano and associates[14] from Genoa and La Spezia, Italy, tested the hypothesis that *in vivo* effective orifice area of a stenotic aortic valve changes continuously during ejection, which would make a single area measurement a potentially inadequate indicator of the severity of the stenosis. Doppler measurements of flow velocity in the ascending aorta and in the left ventricular outflow tract at peak velocity, at half-peak velocity during acceleration (midacceleration), and at half-peak velocity during deceleration (middeceleration) were obtained in 26 patients with AS (mean gradient, 50 ± 19 mm Hg; effective aortic orifice, $0.7 ± 0.3$ cm^2) and in 14 normal subjects of similar age and gender, to calculate instantaneous effective aortic orifice area at midacceleration, at peak velocity, and at middeceleration. In the 26 patients with AS, aortic valve area at midacceleration was 84% ± 15% of valve area at peak velocity, and valve area at middeceleration was 113% ± 17% of that measured at peak velocity. Conversely, in normal subjects, aortic valve area remained constant during ejection and was 97% ± 5% and 99% ± 6% of valve area at peak velocity at midacceleration and middeceleration. In addition, in patients with AS, the percentage of change in effective aortic valve area from midacceleration to middeceleration varied widely, from −17% to +49% (mean change, +26 ± 14%). There was no relationship between the percentage of change in effective valve area and mean transaortic gradient or effective valve area at peak velocity. Our results indicate that effective aortic valve continues to change during ejection in patients with AS, and that the magnitude of this change is independent of the usual indexes of severity of the stenosis. Conversely, effective aortic valve area remains constant during ejection in normal subjects (Figures 5-4 and 5-5).

Two-dimensional TEE has been shown to be an accurate method of measuring aortic valve area in patients with AS. The accuracy of Doppler TEE for this purpose is unknown. Thus, in this study by Stoddard and associates[15] from Louisville, Kentucky, 86 consecutive adult patients (mean age, 68 ± 11 years) with calcific (n = 79) or congenital bicuspid (n = 7) AS were studied by biplane

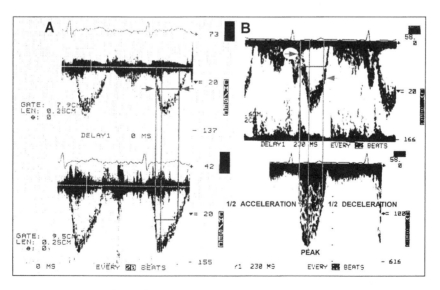

FIGURE 5-4. Left ventricular outflow tract flow velocity (*top*) and aortic flow velocity (*bottom*) in a normal control subject (**A**), and in a patient with aortic stenosis (**B**). The 3 *vertical lines* indicate the 3 points at which Doppler-derived aortic valve area was measured. The horizontal lines show the half-peak velocity. Reproduced with permission from Badano et al.[14]

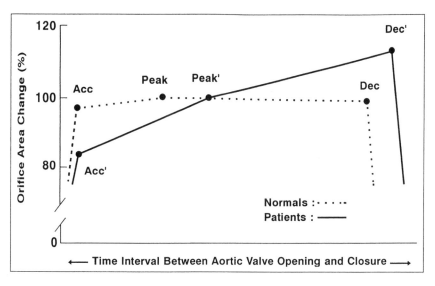

FIGURE 5-5. Valve area at midacceleration and mid-deceleration in normal control subjects (Acc and Dec, on the *dotted line*) and in patients with aortic stenosis (Acc' and Dec', on the *continuous line*), expressed as a percentage of their respective valve area at peak flow velocity in normals (Peak), and in patients (Peak'). Reproduced with permission from Badano et al.[14]

or multiplane TEE. From the transgastric long-axis view, continuous wave Doppler of peak aortic valve velocity and pulsed Doppler of left ventricular outflow tract velocity were determined. Left ventricular outflow tract diameter was measured from a TEE long-axis view, and cross-sectional area was calculated. Aortic valve area was calculated by the continuity equation. Two-dimensional TEE was used to measure directly aortic valve area by planimetry of the minimal orifice from a short-axis view. Aortic valve area determination was less feasible by Doppler (62 of 86 patients, or 72%) versus 2-dimensional TEE (81 of 86 patients, or 94%) because of the inability to align the continuous wave Doppler beam with the aorta in 24 patients. The feasibility of obtaining aortic valve area by Doppler TEE improved from the first 43 patients (24 of 43 patients, or 56%) to the latter 43 patients (38 of 43 patients, or 88%) and suggests a significant learning curve. In 62 patients, aortic valve area by Doppler and 2-dimensional TEE did not differ (1.30 ± 0.54 cm^2 vs. 1.23 ± 0.46 cm^2) and correlated well. Absolute and percentage differences between aortic valve area measured by Doppler and 2-dimensional TEE were small (0.18 ± 0.20 cm^2 and $15\% \pm 15\%$, respectively). Mild, moderate, and severe AS by 2-dimensional TEE was correctly identified in 93% (28 of 30), 79% (15 of 19), and 77% (10 of 13) of patients by Doppler TEE, respectively. Doppler TEE is an accurate method to measure aortic valve area in patients with AS and should complement 2-dimensional TEE. The feasibility of Doppler TEE for aortic valve area determination has a significant learning curve.

In this study by Kim and associates[16] from Los Angeles, California, the correspondence of aortic valve area measurements from TEE, transthoracic echocardiography (TTE), and cardiac catheterization was determined in 100 patients with severe AS (aortic valve area ≤0.75 cm^2), moderate AS (aortic valve area >0.75 to 1.2 cm^2), mild AS (aortic valve area >1.2 to ≤2.0 cm^2), and nonstenotic aortic valves (aortic valve area >2.0 cm^2). Because high correlation does not require high agreement, data were assessed by analysis of agreement. Aortic valve areas determined by TTE (1.43 ± 0.76 cm^2), TEE (1.40 ± 0.79 cm^2), and cardiac catheterization (1.47 ± 0.82 cm^2) were similar. Correlations between methods were excellent. Limits of agreement between the 3 comparisons did not differ significantly. Similar levels of agreement when comparing these independent methods for determining the aortic valve area indicate that direct planimetry by TEE, the continuity equation with TTE, the continuity equation with TTE, and the Gorlin formula are equally accurate and may be used interchangeably. Clinical important discrepancies between methods are uncommon and are readily settled by adding a third method.

Hemodynamic Assessment of Aortic Stenosis

In AS, conventional indexes of severity vary with changes in transvalvular flow. It is important to determine the true severity of obstruction because AS in the presence of low cardiac output and low valvular gradient is associated with high mortality during AVR. Blitz and Herrmann[17] from Philadelphia, Pennsylvania, compared 3 indexes of AS severity at different transvalvular flow rates in patients with low-flow, low-gradient, critical AS. Eight patients with critical AS (valve area ≤0.7 cm^2), low cardiac output (<4.0 L/min), and low mean transvalvular gradient (≤40 mm Hg) underwent hemodynamic assessment at baseline, after transvalvular flow was augmented with dobutamine, and after the valve opening was increased with percutaneous balloon aortic valvuloplasty. Severity of obstruction was assessed by using 3 different measures: Gorlin formula-calculated valve area, valvular resistance, and percentage left ventricular stroke work loss. Dobutamine infusion increased cardiac output by 35% and mean transvalvular gradient by 27%. The mean Gorlin formula-calculated aortic valve area increased from 0.5 to 0.6 cm^2. Percentage LV stroke work loss increased from 23% to 28%. Valve resistance was unchanged by dobutamine (350 to 310 dynes · sec · cm^{-5}). Balloon valvuloplasty increased cardiac output 13% and decreased the gradient 31%; this resulted in an increase in the calculated valve area from 0.6 to 0.9 cm^2. Percentage LV stroke work loss decreased from 310 to 181 dynes · sec · cm^{-5} after valvuloplasty. We conclude that in patients with low-flow, low-gradient critical AS, valve resistance is the most flow-independent measures of severity of stenosis. All measures improve with percutaneous balloon aortic valvuloplasty.

Apoproteins B, (a), and E in Degenerative Valvular AS

Nonrheumatic AS of trileaflet aortic valves has been considered to be a "degenerative" process, but the early lesion of AS contains the chronic inflammatory cells, macrophages, and T lymphocytes. Because lipoprotein deposition is prominent in atherosclerosis, another chronic inflammatory process, a study by O'Brien and coinvestigators[18] in Seattle, Washington, examined whether lipoproteins accumulate in aortic valve lesions. Immunohistochemical studies were performed to detect apolipoprotein B, apolipoprotein (a), apolipoprotein E, macrophages and α-actin-expressing cells on 18 trileaflet aortic valves that ranged from normal to stenotic. All 3 apolipoproteins were detected in early through end-stage lesions of AS, but not in histologically normal regions. Comparison with oil red O staining suggested that most of the extracellular neutral lipid in these valves was associated with either plasma-derived or locally produced apolipoproteins. Thus, in early through end-stage aortic valve lesions, apolipoproteins accumulate and are associated with the majority of extracellular valve lipid. These results are consistent with the hypothesis that lipoprotein accumulation in the aortic valve contributes to pathogenesis of AS.

Surgery for Aortic Regurgitation

Klodas and colleagues[19] in Rochester, Minnesota, evaluated indications and results for surgical correction of aortic regurgitation (AR) in women. Baseline characteristics and postoperative outcomes were compared in 51 women and 198 men who underwent surgery for isolated AR between 1980 and 1989 at the Mayo Clinic. Compared with men, women rarely had surgery for severe left ventricular enlargement (systolic diameter ≥55 mm in 11% versus 27% in men, and diastolic diameter ≥80 mm in 0% versus 16% in men) and more often with class III to IV symptoms (59% versus 32% in men). Operative mortalities were similar in men and women (4% and 5%, respectively). Among operative survivors, 10-year survival was poorer for women than for men (39 ± 9% vs 72 ± 4%, respectively), and was worse than expected for women (Figure 5-6). Independent predictors of late survival were different for men (age and LVEF) and women (age and concomitant CABG). Multivariate analysis indicated that the female sex was an independent predictor of worse late survival (Figure 5-7 and 5-8). Thus, after surgery for AVR, women exhibit an excess late mortality, suggesting that surgical correlation of AR should be considered at an earlier stage in women.

Echocardiographic Follow-Up after Aortic Valve Reconstruction

Eighty-six patients (mean age, 29 ± 15 years), underwent aortic valve reconstruction with bovine or autologous pericardial tissue in this study by Bjørnstad and colleagues[20] from Riyadh, Saudi Arabia. Mean clinical follow-up was 35 months. Echocardiographic data were assessed in 65 patients with a follow-up of 6 months or more. There were 2 in-hospital deaths and 3 late deaths. Warfarin was not given, and no thromboembolic events occurred. Five

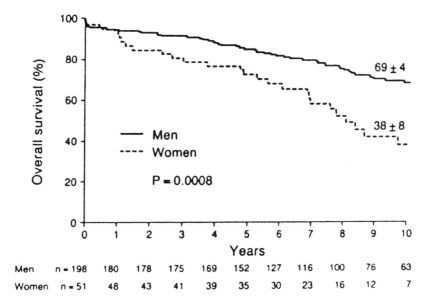

FIGURE 5-6. Overall survival (including operative mortality) in men and women after AVR for AR. Reproduced with permission from Klodas et al.[19]

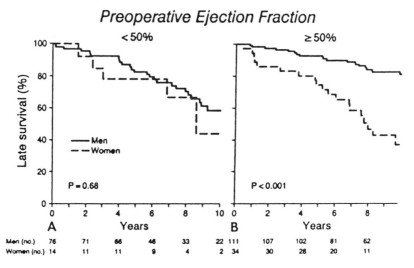

FIGURE 5-7. Late survival comparison in men and women stratified according to preoperative ejection fraction: **A,** <50% and **B,** ≥50%. Women with ejection fractions ≥50% had a significantly worse survivial rate than did men with ejection fractions ≥50%. No significant difference was noted in survival rates between women with ejection fractions <50% and men with ejection fractions <50%. Reproduced with permission from Klodas et al.[19]

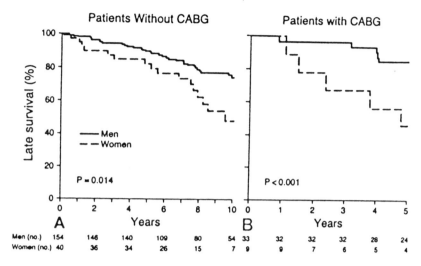

FIGURE 5-8. Late survival comparison in men and women stratified according to concomitant CABG: **A,** without CABG, and **B,** with CABG. Men requiring concomitant CABG at the time of AVR had superior survival rates compared with women requiring concomitant CABG at the time of AVR. Even in patients not undergoing CABG, women displayed significantly worse survival rates than did men. Reproduced with permission from Klodas et al.[19]

(6%) patients needed reoperation because of severe AR. Peak aortic valve gradients remained low (26 ± 14 mm Hg for the bovine group, and 16 ± 16 mm Hg for the autologous group). One patient is awaiting surgery for AS after 76 months. Leaflet thickening at latest follow-up was marked in 6 (9%) patients. Left ventricular dimensions normalized postoperatively and showed only an insignificant increase during follow-up. This technique is a promising alternative to valve prostheses in selected patients; however, longer follow-up is necessary to assess long-term results.

Pulmonary Valvular Disease

Pulmonic Valvuloplasty

Chen and colleagues[21] in Washington, D.C., performed percutaneous pulmonic valvuloplasty with a single Inoue balloon catheter in 53 adolescent or adult patients (age 13 to 55 years; mean, 26 years). Follow-up studies were performed 0.2 to 9.8 years after the procedure by Doppler echocardiography in all the patients and by cardiac catheterization and angiography in 9 of the patients. Pulmonary balloon valvuloplasty is the accepted first-line treatment for congenital pulmonic stenosis in children, but its efficacy in adolescents and adults is not well established. After balloon valvuloplasty in this study, the systolic pressure gradient across the pulmonic valve decreased from 91 ± 46 mm Hg to 38 ± 32 mm Hg (p<.001), and the diameter of the pulmonic valve orifice increased 8.9 ± 3.6 mm to 17.4 ± 4.6 mm (p<.001). In the 9 patients catheterized at follow-up, the systolic gradient decreased from 107 ± 48 mm Hg before valvuloplasty to 50 ± 29 mm Hg after valvuloplasty, and to 30 ± 16 mm Hg at follow-up (p<.001). In the same 9 patients, the diameter of the pulmonic valve as measured by right ventricular angiography increased from 8.3 ± 1.4 mm before valvuloplasty to 17 ± 2 mm after valvuloplasty (p<.001), and to 18 ± 1.4 mm at follow-up (p=.08). Regurgitation across the pulmonic valve was found in 7 of the 53 patients (13%) after balloon valvuloplasty, but it had disappeared at follow-up in all of them. These data indicate that patients with congenital pulmonic stenosis who present in late adolescence or adult life may be treated with percutaneous balloon valvuloplasty with excellent short-term and long-term results similar to those obtained in young children.

1. Altman R, Rouvier J, Gurfinkel E, Scazziota A, Turpie AGG. Comparison of high-dose with low-dose aspirin in patients with mechanical heart valve replacement treated with oral anticoagulant. Circulation 1996 (November 1);94:2113–2116.
2. Acar J, Iung B, Boissel JP, Samama MM, Michel PL, Teppe JP, Pony JC, Le Breton H, Thomas D, Isnard R, de Gevigney G, Viguier E, Sfihi A, Hanania G, Ghannem M, Mirode A, Nemoz C, and the AREVA Group. AREVA: Multicenter randomized comparison of low-dose versus standard-dose anticoagulation in patients with mechanical prosthetic heart valves. Circulation (November 1);94:2107–2112.
3. Lindner JR, Case RA, Dent JM, Abbott RD, Scheld WM, Kaul S. Diagnostic value of echocardiography in suspected endocarditis. An evaluation based on the pretest probability of disease. Circulation 1996 (February);93:730–736.
4. Salazar E, Izaguirre R, Verdejo J, Mutchinick O: Failure of adjusted doses of subcutaneous heparin to prevent thromboembolic phenomena in pregnant patients with mechanical cardiac valve prostheses. J Am Coll Cardiol 1996(June);27:1698–1703.
5. Kim S, Kuroda T, Nishinaga M, Yamasawa M, Watanabe S, Mitsuhashi T, Ueda S, Shimada K. Relation between severity of MR and prognosis of mitral valve prolapse: Echocardiographic follow-up study. Am Heart J 1996 (August);132:348–355.
6. Trevino AJ, Ibarra M, Garcia A, Uribe A, de la Fuente F, Bonfil MA, Feldman T. Immediate and long-term results of balloon mitral commissurotomy for rheumatic mitral stenosis: Comparison between Inoue and double-balloon techniques. Am Heart J 1996 (March);131:530–536.
7. Dean LS, Mickel M, Bonan R, Holmes DR, O'Neill WW, Palacios IF, Rahimtoola S, Slater JN, Davis K, Kennedy JW: Four-year follow-up of patients undergoing percutaneous balloon mitral commissurotomy: A report from the National Heart, Lung, and Blood Institute Balloon Valvuloplasty Registry. J Am Coll Cardiol 1996 (November 15);28:1452–1457.
8. Iung B, Cormier B, Ducimetiere P, Porte JM, Nallet O, Michel PL, Acar J, Vahanian A: Functional results 5 years after successful percutaneous mitral commissurotomy in a series of 528 patients and analysis of predictive factors. J Am Coll Cardiol 1996 (February);27:407–414.
9. Pieper EPG, Hamer HPM, Sluijs RAP, Ravelli ACJ, Tijssen JGP, Crijns HJGM, Lie KI, Visser CA: Usefulness of multiplane TEE to improve the assessment of severity of MR. Am J Cardiol 1996 (November .15);78:1132–1139.
10. Silva JA, Khuri B, Barbee W, Fontenot D, Cheirif J. Systolic excursion of the mitral annulus to assess septal function in paradoxic septal motion. Am Heart J 1996 (January);131:138–145.
11. Fleischmann KE, Wolff S, Lin C-M, Reimold SC, Lee TH, Lee RT. Echocardiographic predictors of survival after surgery for MR in the age of valve repair. Am Heart J 1996 (February);131:282–288.
12. Nakatani S, Schwammenthal E, Lever HM, Levine RA, Lytle BW, Thomas JD. New insights into the reduction of mitral valve systolic anterior motion after ventricular

septal myectomy in hypertrophic obstructive cardiomyopathy. Am Heart J 1996 (February);131:294–300.

13. Jiang L, Vazquez de Prada JA, Lee M-Y, He J, Padial LR, Fallon JT, King ME, Palacios IF, Weyman AE, Levine RA. Quantitative assessment of stenotic aortic valve area by using intracardiac echocardiography: In vitro validation and initial in vivo illustration. Am Heart J 1996 (July);132:137–144.

14. Badano L, Cassottana P, Bertoli D, Carratino L, Lucatti A, Spirito P: Changes in effective aortic valve area during ejection in adults with aortic stenosis. Am J Cardiol 1996;(November)8:1023–1028.

15. Stoddard MF, Hammons RT, Longaker RA. Doppler transesophageal echocardiographic determination of aortic valve area in adults with aortic stenosis. Am Heart J 1996 (August);132:337–342.

16. Kim C-J, Berglund H, Nishioka T, Luo H, Siegel RJ. Correspondence of aortic valve area determination from TEE, transthoracic echocardiography, and cardiac catheterization. Am Heart J 1996 (December);132:1163–1172.

17. Blitz LR, Herrmann HC: Hemodynamic assessment of patients with low-flow, low-gradient valvular aortic stenosis. Am J Cardiol 1996 (September 15);78:657–661.

18. O'Brien KD, Reichenbach DD, Marcovina SM, Kuusisto J, Alpers CE, Otto CM: Apolipoproteins B, (a), and E accumulate in the morphologically early lesion of 'degenerative' valvular aortic stenosis. Arterioscler Thromb Vasc Biol 1996 (April); 16:523–532.

19. Klodas E, Enriquez-Sarano M, Tajik AJ, Mullany CJ, Bailey KR, Seward JB. Surgery for aortic regurgitation in women. Contrasting indications and outcomes compared with men. Circulation 1996 (November 15);94:2472–2478.

20. Bjornstad K, Duran RM, Nassau KG, Gometza B, Hatle LK, Duran CMG. Clinical and echocardiographic follow-up after aortic valve reconstruction with bovine or autologous pericardium. Am Heart J 1996 (December);132:1173–1178.

21. Chen C-R, Cheng TO, Huang T, Zhou Y-L, Chen J-Y, Huang Y-G, Li H-J. Percutaneous balloon valvuloplasty for pulmonic stenosis in adolescents and adults. N Engl J Med 1996 (July 4);335:21–25.

6

Arrhythmias

Premature Ventricular Contractions

To evaluate whether the identification of the different relations between premature ventricular contractions (PVCs) and the preceding sinus cycle length will help to predict the effect of β-blockers on the PVCs themselves, 55 patients (43 men, 12 women, mean age 53 ± 16 years) with different cardiac diseases, and greater than 30 PVCs/hr characterized by stability and the same relation at 2 Holter monitoring periods were studied by Pitzalis and associates[1] from Bari, Italy. The relation was tachycardia-enhanced (the shorter the preceding cycle length, the higher the incidence of PVCs) in 23 patients (group 1); indifferent (no correlation between the preceding cycle length and PVCs incidence) in 21 (group 2); and bradycardia-enhanced (the longer the preceding cycle length, the higher the incidence of PVCs) in 11 (group 3). A third Holter monitoring was performed 6 days after nadolol administration (80 mg/day) to evaluate its effect on the 3 types of PVCs. In group 1, nadolol caused a reduction in the PVC incidence in all patients (− 88%). In group 2, it caused a reduction in the majority of patients (− 60%) but an increase in 5. In group 3, it caused a reduction in only half of the patients (45%) and a 91% increase in the remainder. The difference in the effect of nadolol in the 3 groups was highly significant. The relation between the incidence of PVCs and the preceding cycle length was a useful means of identifying subsets of patients with PVCs who will benefit from β-blockers.

Ventricular Arrhythmias

Pattern of Occurrence

Peters and colleagues[2] in Baltimore, Maryland, examined the septadian distribution of life-threatening ventricular arrhythmias in 683 consecutive patients receiving a third-generation implantable defibrillator with an event recorder. There was a prominent Monday peak, with a midweek decline and a secondary peak later in the week (Figure 6-1). A marked trough was apparent on both weekend days. The observed pattern was independent of age, sex, left ventricular ejection fraction (LVEF), New York Heart Association functional class, type of heart disease, and the use of antiarrhythmic drugs, but was not observed in patients receiving β-blockers. Thus, these data suggest that potentially lethal arrhythmias are not random events, but occur in a daily pattern, suggesting a relationship to the beginning and end of the work week. The ab-

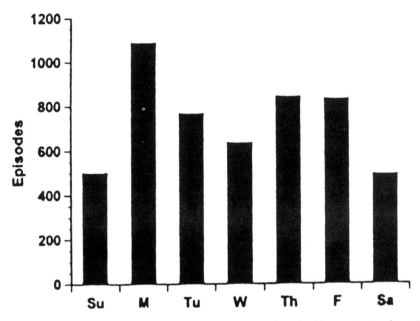

FIGURE 6-1. Daily distribution of device activations. Reproduced with permission from Peters et al.[2]

sence of a Monday peak in patients receiving β-blockers suggests that the pattern may be influenced by β-blockers.

Recurrent Arrhythmias Detected by Defibrillators in Sudden Death Survivors

This retrospective study by Zaim[3] and associates from Philadelphia, Pennsylvania; St. Louis, Missouri; Sunnyvale, California; and Houston, Texas, characterized the recurring ventricular arrhythmias with an electrogram-storing defibrillator in survivors of sudden cardiac death who had no inducible sustained ventricular arrhythmias at baseline electrophysiological testing. The study group comprised 24 selected patients with documented ventricular fibrillation (VF) without need of revascularization or chronic antiarrhythmic therapy. The electrophysiological testing protocol usually consisted of 3 extrastimuli at 2 drive cycles at 2 right ventricular sites. Nonischemic cardiomyopathy was the most frequent structural abnormality (n = 11) followed by CAD (n = 7). The mean ejection fraction (EF) was 0.37 ± 0.13. Cardiac status did not appear to change during a mean follow-up period of 16 ± 13 months, and 8 (33%) patients received appropriate shocks in that time period. On the basis of intracardiac electrograms, 7 (88%) patients experienced VF and 1 (12%) patient had ventricular tachycardia (VT) as the first recurring arrhythmia. Four patients had additional recurrences and all were VF episodes. VF was usually present from the onset of the arrhythmia. In addition, 9 (38%) patients had nonsustained ventricular arrhythmias that were solely VF in 6 (67%). In conclusion, VF of sudden onset was the most frequent recurring sustained ventricular arrhythmia in this group.

Transthoracic Defibrillation

Kerber and associates[4] from 3 United States medical centers examined in a prospective, multicenter trial the feasibility and advantage of current-based, transthoracic defibrillation. Current-based, damped, sinusoidal waveform shocks of 18, 25, 30, 35, or 40 amperes (A) were administered beginning with 25 A for polymorphic VT and VF, or 18 A for monomorphic VT; success rates were compared with those of energy-based shocks beginning at 200 J for VF/polymorphic VT and 100 J for VT. The current-based shocks were delivered from custom-modified defibrillators that determined impedance in advance of any shock using a "test-pulse" technique; the capacitor then charged to the exact energy necessary to deliver the operator-selected current against the impedance determined by the defibrillator. Three hundred sixty-two patients received more than 1 shock for VF; polymorphic VT, or monomorphic VT: 569 current-based shocks and 420 energy-based shocks. Current-based shocks of 35/40 A achieved success rates of up to 74% for VT/polymorphic VT; 30 A shocks terminated 88% of monomorphic VT episodes. Energy-based shocks of 300 J terminated 72% of VT/polymorphic VT; 200-J shocks terminated 89% of monomorphic VT. The authors could not demonstrate a significant increase in the success rate of current-based shocks over energy-based shocks for patients with high transthoracic impedance; this may be due to inadequate sample size. Thus, current-based defibrillation is clinically feasible and effective. A larger study will be needed to test whether current-based defibrillation is superior to energy-based defibrillation.

Nonsustained VT in Sudden Death

Doval and colleagues[5] in Capital Federal, Argentina, studied 516 patients from the GESICA trial in an attempt to determine the prognostic value of nonsustained VT in total mortality in patients with severe CHF. Patients were initially studied with a 24-hour Holter and 2 years of follow-up. Within 2 years, there were 87 deaths among 173 patients with nonsustained VT, and 106 deaths among 343 patients without nonsustained VT. Relative risk was 1.69, and Cox proportional hazard analysis was 1.62. Sudden death increased from 8.7% to 23.7% in patients with nonsustained VT. Progressive CHF death was also increased from 17.5% to 20.8%. Quantitative analysis of 24-hour Holter demonstrated that couplets had a similar RR to that of nonsustained VT for both total mortality and sudden death. Couplets and/or nonsustained VT were even more predictive for sudden death. Thus, in patients with CHF, nonsustained VT is an independent marker for increased overall mortality rate and sudden death.

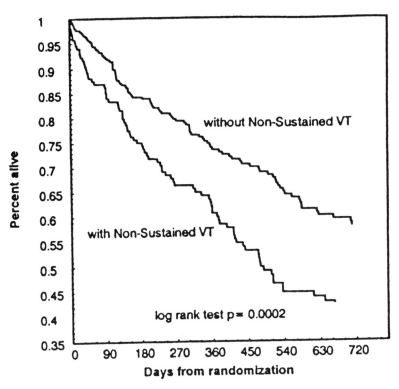

FIGURE 6-2. Nonsustained VT and total mortality. Reproduced with permission from Doval et al.[5]

The absence of nonsustained VT and ventricular repetitive beats in a 24-hour Holter indicates a low probability of sudden death (Figure 6-2).

Procainamide versus Lidocaine

Efficacy of procainamide and lidocaine in terminating spontaneous mono-morphic VT was assessed by Gorgels and associates[6] from Maastricht, The Netherlands, in a randomized parallel study. Patients with acute myocardial infarction (AMI) and those with poor hemodynamic tolerance of VT were excluded. Procainamide (10 mg/kg) was given intravenously with an injection speed of 100 mg/min, and lidocaine was administered at an intravenous dose of 1.5 mg/kg in 2 minutes. Fourteen patients were randomized to lidocaine, and 15 were randomized to procainamide. Termination occurred in 3 of 14 patients after lidocaine and in 12 of 15 patients after procainamide. Procainamide stopped 8 of 11 VTs not responding to lidocaine, and lidocaine stopped 1 of 1 not responding to procainamide. Of a total of 41 VT episodes, 4 of 15 responded to lidocaine and 20 of 26, to procainamide. Because of VT recurrences, 16 patients could be studied repeatedly with drugs given in the reverse order. This resulted in a total of 55 trials of 79 drug injections. Lidocaine terminated 6 of 31 VTs and procainamide, 38 of 48. The protocol was stopped in 4 cases because of adverse effects. A comparison of the QRS width and QT interval before and at the end of the injection revealed significant lengthening of these values after procainamide, but no change after lidocaine. In conclusion, procainamide is superior to lidocaine in terminating spontaneously occurring monomorphic VT.

Treatment of Idiopathic Right Ventricular Outflow Tract Tachycardia

Pace mapping used to locate the site for ablation of idiopathic right ventricular outflow tract VT remains difficult and time consuming. A method to facilitate pace mapping and the most common site of ablation of this tachycardia is reported in this study carried out by Movsowitz and associates[7] from Philadelphia, Pennsylvania. In 18 consecutive patients with right ventricular outflow tract VT, electrocardiographic criteria based on the QRS orientation in lead 1 and the R wave progression in the precordial leads were used to find pace maps matching the arrhythmia. Identical pace maps were obtained on the septum of the right ventricular outflow tract in 16 patients and resulted in successful ablations. These sites were concentrated in the anterior-superior aspect of the right ventricular outflow tract as determined by fluoroscopic imaging. In the remaining 2 cases, identical pace maps could not be found in this area. The results of this study narrow the anatomic location for radiofrequency ablation of idiopathic right ventricular outflow tract VT. This is the first description of an electrocardiographic approach to finding an identical pace map in the right ventricular outflow tract.

Sotalol

The efficacy and safety of sotalol therapy for ventricular arrhythmias was evaluated by Lee and associates[8] from San Francisco, California, in 133 patients with drug-refractory ventricular arrhythmias. All patients had baseline electrophysiologic studies before and after oral sotalol therapy. Sixty-six patients were discharged home, treated with sotalol (52 patients without inducible VT or VF, and 14 patients with hemodynamically stable inducible VT). The mean follow-up period was 41 ± 27 months for the 14 patients with hemodynamically stable VT. Sotalol was effective in 8 of these 14 patients. Recurrent nonlethal VT occurred in 3 patients: 2 patients had sudden death; and 1 patient had adverse side effects. The 52 patients without inducible VT were followed for a mean period of 36 ± 30 months. Thirty-five of 52 patients were successfully treated. Two patients had recurrent VT; both of these episodes of VT occurred within the 1st year. Four patients had sudden cardiac death; 3 of these deaths occurred within the first month, and the last episode of sudden death occurred after 8 years of sotalol therapy. The actuarial incidence of sotalol efficacy was 76% at 1 year, 72% at 2 years, 64% at 4 years, and 52% at 5 years. Approximately 46% of patients receiving long-term sotalol treatment reported side effects. Side effects severe enough to warrant withdrawal of sotalol occurred in 7 (11%) patients. The results of this study suggest that sotalol is effective for selected patients with drug-refractory ventricular arrhythmias. Although the incidence of side effects was high, patients appeared to tolerate long-term sotalol therapy well.

d,l-*Sotalol and Implantable Defibrillators*

Böcker and colleagues[9] from Münster, Germany, compared the long-term efficacy of *d,l*-sotalol and implantable cardioverter defibrillators (ICD) in patients with coronary artery disease (CAD) in a case-control study of 50 individuals treated with oral *d,l*-sotalol matched with 50 patients treated with ICDs. Both groups were matched for sex, age, LVEF (40 ± 12%), extent of CAD, presenting arrhythmia, and year that treatment began. In all patients in the sotalol group, VT/VF was inducible in the drug-free electrophysiological study. Induction of sustained VT/VF was suppressed by *d,l*-sotalol. In the ICD group, either VT/VF was not inducible (n = 5) or inducible sustained VT/VF was refractory to antiarrhythmic drug treatment (n = 5). Sotalol led to a marked reduction in arrhythmic events. Whereas 83% of the patients in the sotalol group were free of sudden death and nonfatal VT at 3 years, only 33% of the ICD patients did not receive appropriate ICD therapies. Actuarial rates for absence of sudden death at 3 years were 85% in the sotalol group and 100% in the ICD group. Actuarial rates for overall survival at 3 years were 75% in the sotalol group and 85% in the ICD group (Figure 6-3). Thus, these data demonstrate that in this case-control study, ICD therapy was more effective than electrophysiologi-

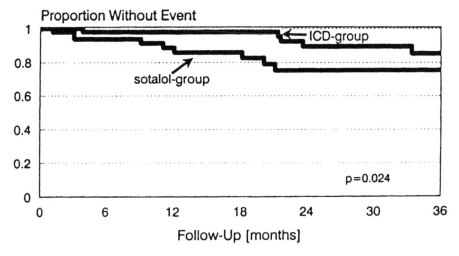

FIGURE 6-3. Actuarial curves for the total mortality in patients treated with oral *d,l*-sotalol (88%, 74%, and 74% at 1, 2, and 3 years, respectively) vs. ICDs (98%, 89%, and 84%, respectively). Reproduced with permission from Böcker et al.[9]

cally guided antiarrhythmic therapy with *d,l*-sotalol in prevention of sudden death and reduction of total mortality in patients with CAD.

Propafenone

An important issue regarding the long-term use of antiarrhythmic drugs concerns the safety of these agents, particularly with regard to cardiac toxicity. Propafenone is an effective drug for preventing supraventricular tachyarrhythmia, but the incidence of side effects during long-term therapy in patients with such arrhythmias has not been adequately reported. Podrid and Anderson for the Propafenone Multicenter Study Group[10] reported results in 480 patients who received oral propafenone as therapy for symptomatic atrial fibrillation (AF), atrial flutter, or supraventricular tachycardia (SVT). During the follow-up (mean 14.4 months), 290 patients (60%) discontinued propafenone therapy, but in only 70 patients (15%) was the reason for discontinuation an adverse drug reaction. Overall, 284 patients (59%) experienced at least 1 adverse reaction, and the incidence was related to dose and age greater than 65 years. The overall incidence of side effects was not related to structural heart disease; however, cardiovascular toxicity, including arrhythmia aggravation, congestive heart failure, and serious conduction disturbances occurred more often in those with heart disease (20% vs. 13%). Sixteen patients died during drug therapy, but in only 1 case was the drug considered contributory. For patients with a supraventricular arrhythmia, propafenone was well tolerated and was infrequently discontinued because of side effects. The incidence of serious cardiac toxicity when propafenone was used to treat supraventricular arrhythmia was low, and these side effects were more frequent in patients with structural heart disease.

Amiodarone

Several small retrospective reports have suggested that intravenous amiodarone is useful in refractory ventricular tachyarrhythmias. Levine and colleagues[11] organized a multicenter trial that enrolled 273 patients with recurrent hypotensive ventricular tachyarrhythmias refractory to lidocaine, procainamide, and bretylium. They were randomly assigned to receive 1 of 3 doses of intravenous amiodarone: 524, 1050, or 2100 mg per 24 hours. Forty percent of the patients survived 24 hours without another hypotensive ventricular tachyarrhythmic event while being treated with intravenous amiodarone as a single agent. Although there was no clear dose-response relation observed in this trial, the number of supplemental infusions of intravenous amiodarone given during hours 0 to 6 was greater in the low-dose group than in the high-dose group. Thus, intravenous amiodarone appears to be a relatively safe therapy for ventricular arrhythmias refractory to other medications.

Comorbidity and Outcome

Hallstrom and colleagues[12] in Seattle, Washington, determined the influence of comorbidity on the outcome of patients treated with out-of-hospital VF. They defined a comorbidity index, constructed from histories of chronic conditions as well as a number of recent symptoms in 282 victims of out-of-hospital VF Table 6-1. The presence of comorbidity was strongly associated with ultimate outcome. When analyzing a comprehensive set of predictors of survival after out-of-hospital VF, including the index of co-morbidity, the authors could identify only about one-fourth of the variation that one might hope to account for by this type of analysis. Thus, co-morbidity appears to be an important predictor of survival from out-of-hospital VF. However, most of the statistical variability in predicting survival remains unexplained, even when co-morbidity is considered.

Torsades de Pointes

Lehmann and colleagues[13] in Detroit, Michigan, tested the hypothesis that women are more prone than men to develop torsades de pointes in a defined cohort of patients exposed to the QT-prolonging antiarrhythmic drug, *d,l*-sota-

TABLE 6-1
Histories and Recent Symptoms in 282 Patients Treated for Out-of-Hospital Cardiac Arrest With Ventricular Fibrillation the First Recorded Rhythm

Variable*	Yes, %	No, %	Unknown, %
History of			
Use of heart medications	69.1	24.1	6.7
Congestive heart failure	26.2	59.6	14.2
Heart attack	50.0	44.3	5.7
Diabetes	20.6	75.5	3.9
Hypertension	49.3	38.7	12.1
Chest pain/angina	50.0	44.3	5.7
Lung disease	8.5	84.4	7.1
Gastrointestinal disorders	24.5	63.5	3.9
Cancer	7.1	86.9	6.0
Other chronic conditions	54.3	17.7	28.0
Heart surgery	16.3	81.9	1.8
Symptoms			
Chest pain	21.3	72.0	6.7
Dizziness	19.1	74.5	6.4
Indigestion	24.8	67.0	8.2
Dyspnea	39.7	55.0	5.3
Nausea	16.0	78.7	5.3
Tiredness	58.2	39.4	2.5
Recent physician visit	14.5	81.6	3.9

* Variables: Lung disease indicates history consistent with emphysema, chronic pulmonary disease, or chronic bronchitis; Symptoms, symptoms reported to have occurred within 2 days of the arrest; and Recent physician visit, visit to physician or medical facility within 2 days before arrest.
Reproduced with permission from Hallstrom et al.[12]

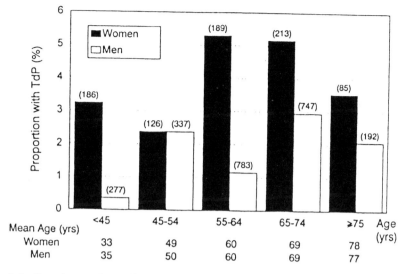

FIGURE 6-4. Prevalence of torsades de pointes (TdP) by sex in each of 5 age groups. Numbers of women and men in each age group are shown in parentheses above bars. Reproduced with permission from Lehmann et al.[13]

lol. In a database derived from 22 clinical trials involving 3135 adult patients receiving oral *d,l*-sotalol with a median follow-up of 164 days, torsades de pointes developed in 44 (2%) of 2336 men and in 33 (4%) of 799 women. Logistic regression analysis identified female sex, presenting arrhythmia of sustained VT or VF, history of CHF, and *d,l*-sotalol dose greater than 320 mg/day as factors most predictive of the development of torsades de pointes (Figure 6-4). A serum creatinine greater than 1.4 mg/dL in women and greater than 1.6 mg/dL in men was also predictive of the development of torsades de pointes. After adjustment for risk factors, women had a 3-fold greater risk of developing torsades de pointes than did men. The sex differences in torsades de pointes risk were age-independent and could not be explained by differential dose-related bradycardic responses in women as compared with men. Thus, women are at increased risk of developing torsades de pointes during administration of *d,l*-sotalol, and greater caution should be used in giving this antiarrhythmic agent to women.

Syncope

Sheldon and colleagues[14] in Alberta, Canada, identified patients at high risk for recurrence of syncope mediated by neural mechanisms after a positive isoproterenol/tilt-table test. A cohort of 101 drug-free patients at a university hospital outpatient clinic with syncope and a positive isoproterenol/tilt-table test underwent baseline assessment of demographic variables, symptoms, and hemodynamic and clinical responses to tilt testing. The primary outcome measure was the time to the first recurrent syncopal spell. The probabilities of remaining syncope-free after 1 and 2 years were 72% and 60%. Multivariate

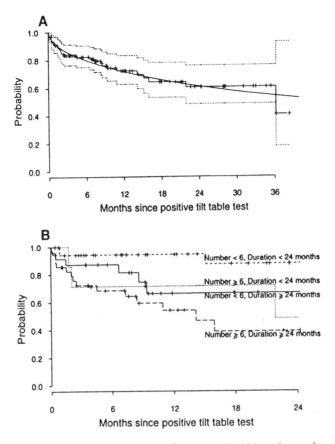

FIGURE 6-5. A, Probability of remaining free of syncope in 101 patients after a positive tilt-table test. The step functions indicate the Kaplan-Meier estimate of the survival function with 95% confidence intervals. The smooth curve indicates the survival function for the Weibull function. **B,** Kaplan-Meier estimate of the probability of remaining free of syncope after a tilt-table test in patients who have fewer than 6 and 6 or more spells and had symptoms for <24 or ≥24 months. Reproduced with permission from Sheldon et al.[14]

proportional hazards analysis demonstrated that the most powerful predictor of recurrence of syncope was a logarithm of the number of preceding syncopal spells (Figure 6-5). Other predictive variables included the duration of syncope, tilt-test symptomatic outcome, and trough heart rate. The probability of recurrence of syncope also varied with the logarithm of the frequency of the preceding spells. The median frequency of pretest spells was 0.3 per month. After the tilt test, the median frequency dropped approximately 90% to 0.03 per month. Thus, the risk of a recurrence of syncope after a positive tilt-table test can be predicted with simple pretest and intratest variables.

Long QT Syndrome

Compton and colleagues[15] in Salt Lake City, Utah, studied 7 patients with chromosome 7-linked long QT syndrome and 5 normal control subjects to determine whether an increase in serum potassium normalizes repolarization in these patients. Repolarization was measured by electrocardiography and body surface potential mapping during sinus rhythm, exercise, and atrial pacing, before and after serum potassium was increased. Potassium administration improved repolarization of the long QT syndrome. At baseline, long QT subjects differed from control subjects: resting corrected QT interval (QT_c, 627 ± 90 vs. 425 ± 25 msec, p=.0007), QT_c dispersion (133 ± 62 vs. 36 ± 9 msec, p=.009), QT/RR slope (0.35 ± 0.08 vs. 0.24 ± 0.07, p=.04), and global root-mean-square QT interval (RMS-QT_c; 525 ± 68 vs. 393 ± 22, p=.002). All long QT subjects had biphasic or notched T waves. After administration of potassium, the long QT group had a 24% reduction in the resting QT_c interval. The reduction was significantly greater in patients with a long QT than among control subjects. QT dispersion became normal in long QT subjects and did not change in control subjects. Thus, an increase in serum potassium corrects abnormalities and repolarization duration, T-wave morphology, and QT dispersion in patients with chromosome 7-linked long QT.

The primary goal of the investigation by Pratt and associates[16] from Houston, Texas; Kansas City, Missouri; Miami Florida; Philadelphia Pennsylvania; and Boston, Massachusetts, was to describe the effect of terfenadine on the QT interval corrected for heart rate (QT_c) of the scalar electrocardiogram. The design was double-blind, 4-period crossover, dose escalation, which involved 28 normal healthy volunteers and 28 patients with stable cardiovascular disease. At baseline, the normal individuals had a mean QT_c interval of 407 msec, whereas the patients with cardiovascular disease had a mean QT_c interval of 417 msec. The largest increase in mean QT_c on terfenadine was 24 msec in a normal individual and 28 msec in a patient with cardiovascular disease. The longest average QT_c observed was 449 msec and 501 msec in any normal individual and patients with cardiovascular disease, respectively. Compared with baseline, terfenadine (60 mg twice daily) was associated with a QT_c increase of 6 msec in normal individuals and a 12-msec increase in patients with cardiovascular disease. Although the QT_c increases from baseline were statistically significant, the magnitude of the spontaneous variability in QT_c in the same patients was much greater. Because 40 electrocardiograms were obtained while taking placebo in each participant, the spontaneous variability in QT_c interval with placebo was also described. Only 1 of the 28 normal individuals had a mean baseline QT_c of 440 msec or greater, yet 14 of the 28 normal individuals had a least 1 of the 40 placebo electrocardiograms with a QT_c of 440 msec or greater. The 28 patients with cardiovascular disease had a mean QT_c at baseline of 417 msec; yet 20 of 28 had at least 1 electrocardiogram on placebo with a QT_c interval of 440 msec or greater. On the average, the QT_c fluctuated 56 msec in each patient during placebo administration. From the observed placebo variability, the authors calculated that an increase in QT_c of 35 msec or greater while receiving drug therapy is likely to represent a drug effect at the 95% confidence interval.

Implantable Cardioverter-Defibrillators

Survey in the United States (Pacemakers and ICDs)

Bernstein and Parsonnet[17] from Newark, New Jersey, conducted a survey of implanters of permanent cardiac pacemakers and ICDs in the United States

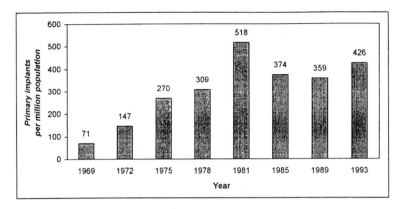

FIGURE 6-6. Trend in primary pacemaker implantation over a 24-year period. The decrease between 1981 and 1985 is attributed in part to effects of concerns expressed by the federal government regarding fraud and abuse in the pacemaker industry and the development by the American College of Cardiology, the American Heart Association, and the North American Society of Pacing and Electrophysiology of guidelines for identifying valid indications for antibradycardia pacing. Reproduced with permission from Bernstein and Parsonnet.[17]

during 1993 to identify present and changing patterns in indications for pacing, implantation techniques, pacing-mode selection, follow-up, and opinions regarding pacing- and ICD-related issues. Five major pacemaker manufacturers also provided estimates of the numbers of pacemakers and ICDs implanted in the United States from 1990 through 1993. In 1993, approximately 133,000 new rhythm-management devices, including 112,000 primary pacing systems and 16,000 ICDs, were implanted, an increase of 18% for pacemakers and 113% for ICDs since 1990. In 1993, pacemaker implantations were performed by about 8700 physicians working in 3300 hospitals and 1000 independent "surgicenters." Since the last survey, which addressed pacing practices in 1989, respondents' use of dual-chamber pacemakers increased from 32% to 68% of the total, and adaptive-rate systems from 29% to 48%. Significant differences were found among subcategories of implanters and among complications encountered in different circumstances. Surgeons tended be the older and more experienced implanters, but used a smaller proportion of active-fixation leads, dual-chamber systems, and adaptive-rate pulse generators, and tended to rely more heavily on a pacemaker manufacturer's representative in operative and follow-up procedures. Complications were more common with bipolar leads, with leads implanted by means of an introducer, and with passive-fixation ventricular leads. The survey provided useful insights into trends and differences in pacemaker and defibrillator practice. Future surveys would be facilitated if a standardized implant registry such as that used in Europe were established in the United States. (Figures 6-6, 6-7, 6-8).

Clinical Significance of High-Energy Discharge

Villacastín and colleagues[18] in Madrid, Spain, evaluated 80 consecutive patients with an automatic ICD who were followed for up to 82 months. Thirty-

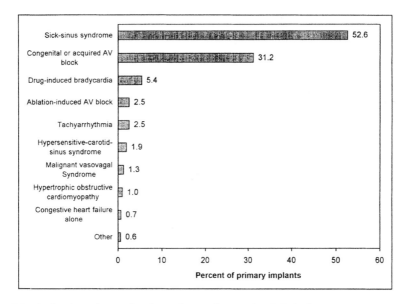

FIGURE 6-7. Indications for pacing in patients who received their first permanent pacemaker in 1993. "Other" indications included ablation-induced atrioventricular block, malignant vasovagal syndrome, and hypertrophic obstructive cardiomyopathy. Reproduced with permission from Bernstein and Parsonnet.[17]

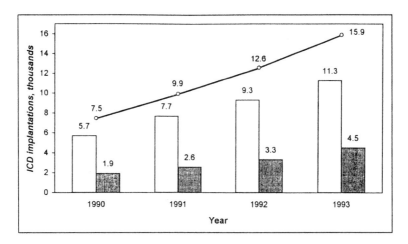

FIGURE 6-8. Volume of primary (unshaded bars), replacement (shaded bars), and total (line) implantable cardioverter/defibrillator (ICD) implantations in the United States over a 3-year period, as estimated by the pacemaker manufacturers. Reproduced with permission from Bernstein and Parsonnet.[17]

eight patients had survived an out-of-hospital cardiac arrest, and 42 had recurrent VT. During follow-up, 16 patients had appropriate, consecutive, high-energy discharges (group A), 26 patients had episodes of single appropriate discharges (group B), and 38 patients had no appropriate discharges (group C). Patients in group A had a poorer left ventricular functional status, lower LVEF, and shorter survival rates than the remaining 2 groups of patients. Cox analysis showed LVEF to be an independent predictor of the presence of multiple, appropriate, consecutive, high-energy discharges. Independent predictors of death or heart transplantation were the presence and frequency of these discharges, female sex, age, history of cardiac arrest, and functional status. The only independent predictor of total mortality was female sex. Independent predictors of cardiac death were the presence of multiple, appropriate, consecutive, high-energy discharges, and female sex. Independent predictors of arrhythmic death were age, female sex, and multiple, appropriate, consecutive, high-energy discharges (Figures 6-9 and 6-10). Thus, in patients with an ICD, development of multiple, appropriate, consecutive, high-energy discharges during follow-up is an independent predictor of cardiac and arrhythmic mortality.

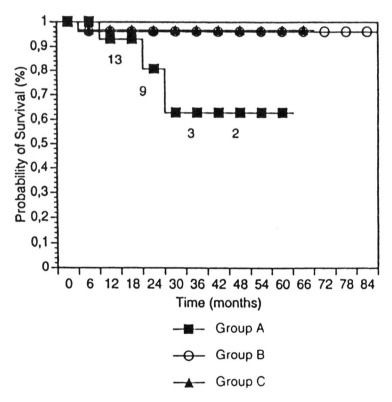

FIGURE 6-9. Actuarial analysis depicting survival free of death or heart transplant among the 3 groups: patients who experienced MCDs (group A), those who experienced single ICD discharges (group B), and those who did not have appropriate ICD discharges (group C). Note that during follow-up, group B and C patients have similarly better survival than group A patients. There were statistically significant differences among the actuarial curves of the 3 groups of patients (p = .0001). Reproduced with permission from Villacastin et al.[18]

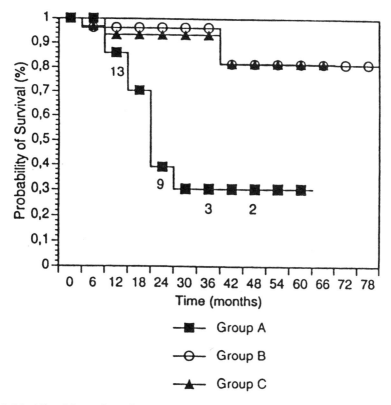

FIGURE 6-10. Life-table analysis depicting survival from arrhythmic mortality in the 3 groups of patients. Note that during follow-up, group B and group C patients have similarly better survival than group A patients. This difference did not reach statistical significance (p = .09). Reproduced with permission from Villacastin et al.[18]

Undetected VF

Natale and colleagues[19] in Durham, North Carolina, prospectively analyzed redetection problems after unsuccessful shock with different lead systems and devices in transvenous ICDs. Monophasic and biphasic transvenous ICDs were included. Subthreshold shocks were intentionally delivered, and redetection of VF was assessed before discharge and at 1, 3, 6, and 12 months after patient hospitalization. Sensing of VF resulted from antitachycardia pacing and low-energy cardioversion of 2 J or less was also analyzed. Each patient underwent subthreshold shock testing at 3 different time intervals for inclusion in this study. Among the 160 ICDs with standard bipolar sensing, 530 VF inductions were analyzed. After the failed shocks, undersensing was more frequent (3% vs. 20%), but did not remarkably prolong redetection. Among the 201 ICDs with integrated bipolar sensing, 80 were connected to a CPI device and 121 to the Ventritex defibrillator. After 252 failed shocks, redetection was prolonged with the CPI system (3 vs. 5 seconds) but did not change after 396 failed shocks with the Ventritex system. These differences may reflect different nominal settings for detection and redetection. In 9 of 121 patients with the Ventritex and 1 of 80 with the CPI ICDs, the devices failed to redetect VF. However, redetection malfunction was never observed in patients with integrated bipolar systems with more than 6-mm electrode separation. After antitachycardia pacing in 1 patient and a 2-J shock in 1 patient, VT turned into VF, which was undetected. Both patients used the Endotak 60 series-Cadence combination. None of the patients showing VF undersensing had sudden death at follow-up. Only 3 of the 12 patients with sensing malfunction were on antiarrhythmic drugs at the time of testing. Analysis of endocardial electrograms showed that failure to redetect VF is not associated with a uniform reduction, but with a rapid and repetitive change of electrogram amplitude. These data suggest that standard bipolar sensing redetects VF more effectively than does integrated bipolar sensing. Endocardial electrogram analysis provides insights into the understanding of the mechanism of undersensing and certain lead-device combinations, resulting in a higher occurrence of VF undersensing.

Sudden Death

Of the 733 patients with ICDs from 1982 to 1995 in the study center of Li and associates[20] from Milwaukee, Wisconsin, 20 died suddenly while the ICD was activated. This number included 16 men and 4 women (mean age, 60 ± 8 years) with EFs of 24% ± 8.6%. ICDs were implanted for drug-refractory VT in 13 patients and for resuscitated cardiac arrest in 7 patients. The clinical VT was associated with syncope in 7 of 13 patients. VT was induced in 18 patients and was hemodynamically unstable in 12 patients. Shock therapies associated with syncope were delivered in 7 of 15 patients during the follow-up. This subgroup of patients survived a median of only 18 months after ICD implant. VF-defibrillation was found to surround death in 9 patients. It was concluded that 1) sudden death victims of the ICD population are characterized by poor left ventricular function and hemodynamically unstable ventricular tachyarrhythmias; and 2) ventricular tachyarrhythmias are the major cause of sudden death in ICD patients.

Use in High-Risk Asymptomatic Patients

In this study by Levine and associates[21] from Roslyn, New York; Cincinnati, Ohio; and Chicago, Illinois, 27 patients with asymptomatic, nonsustained VT whose evaluation suggested they were at high risk for sustained ventricular arrhythmias were treated with ICDs. The option of conventional therapy (including the option of no therapy) was presented to each patient and rejected in favor of defibrillator implantation on an experimental basis. Eighteen patients had CAD and inducible sustained VT, 8 had idiopathic dilated cardiomyopathy, and 1 had hypertrophic cardiomyopathy (HC) and a family history of sudden cardiac death. The mean ejection fraction was 27% ± 10%. Operative morbidity (3%) and mortality (3%) were low. Mean overall survival was 92% and 88% at 1 and 2 years, respectively. Sixteen (59%) of the 27 patients had appropriate defibrillator discharges during a mean follow-up of 35 ± 15 months. The mean time to first appropriate discharge was 18 ± 17 months, and mean follow-up after first discharge was 17 ± 20 months. In conclusion, ICD placement in high-risk patients without symptoms is a feasible approach that may have resulted in benefit in selected patients. Large-scale randomized trials currently underway will determine the risk/benefit ratio of this management approach.

Cost Effectiveness

Wever and colleagues[22] in Utrecht, The Netherlands, evaluated the cost effectiveness of early implantation of the ICD in postinfarct sudden death survivors. Sixty consecutive postinfarct survivors of cardiac arrest caused by VT or VF were randomly assigned either ICD as first choice (n = 29) or a tiered therapy starting with antiarrhythmic drugs and guided by electrophysiological pacing (n = 31). Median follow-up was 729 days. Fifteen patients died, 4 in the early ICD group and 11 in the electrophysiology-guided strategy group (Figure 6-11). For quantitative assessment, the cost-effectiveness ratio was calculated for both groups and expressed as median total costs per patient per day alive. Cost-effectiveness aspects other than mortality were not incorporated in this ratio, but other factors related to quality of life were used as qualitative measures of cost-effectiveness. Cost-effectiveness ratios were $63 and $94 for the early ICD and electrophysiology-guided strategy groups, respectively, per patient per day alive. This amounts to a net cost-effectiveness of $11,315 per patient per year alive saved by early ICD implantations. Costs in the early ICD group were

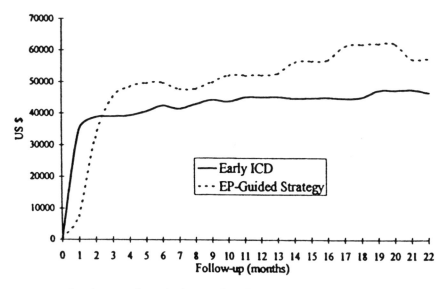

Figure 6-11. Plot showing the calculation of medians of total costs per patient at monthly intervals for survivors in each strategy arm to correct for the difference in follow-up duration between the early ICD group and the EP-guided strategy (median duration, 871 vs. 676 days) and the higher mortality in the EP-guided group. Dips in the curves are due to deaths of patients with high costs. Reproduced with permission from Wever et al.[22]

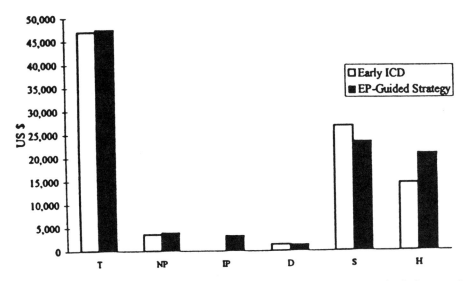

FIGURE 6-12. Bar graph showing total costs (1992 cost scenario) per patient in both therapeutic strategies (T) and costs for noninvasive procedures (NP); invasive procedures (IP, eg, catheterizations, EP studies); drugs including antiarrhythmic drugs (D); surgical procedures, including map-guided surgery and ICD implantation and costs of the ICD device (S); and hospitalization (H). All values are medians. Reproduced with permission from Wever et al.[22]

higher only during the first 3 months of follow-up. Costs in the electrophysiology-guided strategy became higher later. Patients discharged with antiarrhythmic drugs as the sole therapy had the lowest costs. However, this subset also showed the highest mortality, resulting in a poor cost-effectiveness ratio. Invasive therapies and hospitalizations were the major contributors to costs (Figure 6-12). Recurrent cardiac arrest and cardiac transplantation occurred in the electrophysiology-guided strategy group only, whereas exercise tolerance, total hospitalization duration, number of invasive procedures, and antiarrhythmic therapy changes were significantly in favor of early ICD implantation. Thus, early ICD implantation is superior to the electrophysiology-guided therapeutic strategy in postinfarct sudden death survivors.

Outcomes in Thoracotomy Versus Nonthoracotomy Treatment

Kim and associates[23] from the Bronx, New York, compared thoracotomy approaches in 87 patients to nonthoracotomy approaches in 106 patients treated with implantable defibrillators. Long-term outcomes of the 2 groups were compared by the intention-to-treat analysis. Surgical mortality (30-day mortality) rates were 5.7% in the thoracotomy group and 0% in the nonthoracotomy group. Six of 106 patients who underwent nonthoracotomy implantation had a high defibrillation threshold and did not receive nonthoracotomy defibrillators. The duration of follow-up was 52 ± 31 months in the thoracotomy group. Actuarial survival rates of 6 and 24 months were, respectively, 90% and 81% in nonthoracotomy patients and 89% and 80% in the thoracotomy patients. In patients with LVEF less than 30%, surgical mortality was 0% by the nonthoracotomy approach and 10% by the thoracotomy approach. Despite the 10% difference in 30-day mortality, survival rates at 6 months were 85% in nonthoracotomy patients and 81% in thoracotomy patients. At 24 months, they were 73% in nonthoracotomy patients and 74% in thoracotomy patients. Thus, this nonrandomized study suggests that while short-term survival is better in nonthoracotomy patients, the difference in survival diminishes quickly during the first few months and disappears by 6 months. The results were similar in patients with severe left ventricular dysfunction. Several important ICD trials initially utilized thoracotomy ICDs. Although questions may be raised with regard to applicability of such a trial in the era of nonthoracotomy ICDs, this study suggests that the results of such ICD trials will be largely applicable to patients treated with nonthoracotomy ICDs.

Improved Survival

Moss and colleagues[24] for the Multicenter Automatic Defibrillator Implantation Trial Investigators (MADIT Trial) evaluated 196 patients in New York Heart Association functional class I, II, or III with prior myocardial infarction (MI) and LVEFs of 35% or less, a documented episode of asymptomatic sustained VT, and inducible, nonsuppressible ventricular arrhythmia on an electrophysiological study to determine whether an implanted defibrillator reduces mortality in these patients. Unsustained VT in patients with prior MI and left ventricular dysfunction is known to be associated with a 2-year mortality rate of approximately 30%. The authors used a 2-sided sequential design with death from any cause as the primary end point. The baseline characteristics of the 2 treatment groups were similar. During an average follow-up of 27 months, there were 15 deaths in the defibrillator group (11 from cardiac causes) and 39 deaths in the conventional therapy group (27 from cardiac causes) (hazard ratio for overall mortality, 0.46; 95% confidence interval, 0.26 to 0.82; p = 0.009) (Figure 6-13). In this study, even though the numbers of patients treated were relatively small, there was no clear evidence that amiodarone, β-blockers, or other antiarrhythmic therapy had a significant influence in prolonging survival. Thus, the data obtained from the MADIT study in patients with prior MI, left ventricular dysfunction, and at high risk for ventricular arrhythmia, suggest that prophylactic therapy with an implanted defibrillator leads to improved survival as compared with conventional medical therapy.

Radiofrequency Catheter Ablation

Recurrent Arrhythmias

Bubien and colleagues[25] in Birmingham, Alabama, used a measure of general health status and an Activities of Daily Living questionnaire to assess quality of life in 161 patients before radiofrequency catheter ablation for arrhyth-

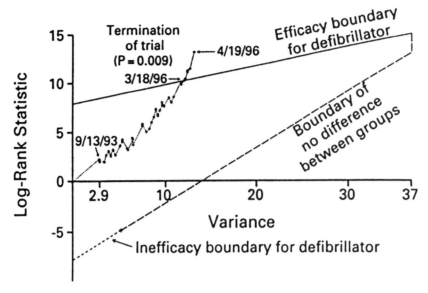

FIGURE 6-13. Sequential monitoring in the triangular design. The vertical axis is a measure of the accumulated differences in survival between the 2 treatments (log-rank statistic). The horizontal axis is the variance of the log-rank statistic and is closely related to the number of deaths. A positive value of the log-rank statistic indicates superiority of the defibrillator relative to conventional medical treatment, and negative values indicate inferiority of the defibrillator. The upper stopping boundary indicates defibrillator efficacy, whereas the lower boundary indicates defibrillator inefficacy or no difference between treatments. The solid circles reflect weekly analyses, which were initiated after 10 deaths had been recorded (September 13, 1993). The trial was stopped shortly after the path crossed the upper boundary (March 18, 1996), indicating the superiority of the defibrillator over conventional medical therapy in reducing mortality. The trajectory of the path provides evidence of the rejection of the null hypothesis at p = .009 (two-sided), with a hazard ratio of 0.46 (95% confidence interval, 0.26 to 0.82) in favor of the defibrillator. The path continues upward after the termination of the trial as a result of a lag in reporting three additional deaths that occurred before the stopping date but were uncovered during the close-out procedure (April 19, 1996). Reproduced with permission from Moss et al.[24]

mias. These same instruments were used to measure quality of life 1 and 6 months after ablation with complete data in 159 of the original 161 patients. Prior to ablation, the questionnaires evaluating general health status and quality of life were low compared with the United States normative database reflecting significant impairment in physical functioning and well being. The lowest scores were reported by patients with AF and atrial flutter. Catheter ablation was associated with significant improvement in quality of life that was sustained more than 6 months after ablation. Improvements were measured in both the general health questionnaire and the disease-specific Symptom Checklist. Catheter ablation was followed by improved performance of activities of daily living and a marked decrease in the number of visits to physicians and emergency rooms in the 6 months after ablation compared with the 6 months before. Thus, this study suggests that radiofrequency catheter ablation improves the health-related quality of life for patients with a variety of different cardiac arrhythmias.

Atrial Tachycardia

Atrial tachycardias are frequently unresponsive to medical therapy. His bundle ablation has been proposed as a palliative treatment for symptoms and as preventive treatment for development of tachycardia-mediated cardiomyopathy. Experience with catheter ablation directed at the atrial origin of the tachycardia remains limited. Poty and associates[26] from Rouen, France, and Bordeaux, France, reviewed the initial success rate and long-term follow-up of radiofrequency ablation of atrial tachycardias. Thirty-six patients underwent electrophysiological study and radiofrequency ablation of atrial tachycardias, excluding atrial flutter. The suspected mechanism of the clinical arrhythmias was automatic in 16 patients, intraatrial reentrant in 15, sinoatrial reentrant in 3, and unknown in 2. One or 2 ablation catheters with a 4-mm distal electrode were used to find: 1) the earliest local atrial activation time compared to P wave onset in the bipolar recording mode, and 2) a QS pattern in the unipolar mode. When 2 ablation catheters were used, an encircling approach was taken. Pace-mapping during sinus rhythm and entrainment techniques were occasionally used for mapping. Tachycardia rose from the right atrium in 33 of 36 patients and from the left atrium in the remaining 3. Three patients showed multiple foci during the procedure. Successful ablation was obtained in 31 (86%) of 36 patients, with a median of 2 radiofrequency applications (range 1 to 32) at 10 to 50 W for 10 to 60 seconds. Failure occurred in 5 patients (including the 3 patients with multiple atrial foci). Late follow-up (18 ± 15 months) showed recurrence of atrial tachycardia in 2 patients, each of whom underwent a successful second ablation. Emergence of another atrial tachycardia was noted in 2 other patients, and an uncommon atrial flutter was noted in 1 patient with repaired atrial septal defect (ASD). No late sinus or atrioventricular (AV) nodal dysfunction was observed. In conclusion, radiofrequency catheter ablation is a safe and reasonable alternative for atrial tachycardias that do not respond to drugs. However, as previously suggested by surgical experience, the success rate of ablation appears less satisfactory in patients with multiple sites of origin of ectopic atrial tachycardia.

Complications

Predictors and comparisons of complications in patients with electrophysiological study or radiofrequency ablation have been assessed in a number of published reports. A report by Chen and associates[27] from Taiwan, Republic of China, prospectively evaluated the procedure-specific complications and investigated the possible causes and predictors of complications in electrophysiologic study and radiofrequency ablation. Data of diagnostic electrophysiologic studies and radiofrequency ablation were prospective and included 3966 procedures. The present study showed that a significantly higher complication rate occurred in radiofrequency ablation than in electrophysiologic study (3.1% vs. 1.1%, respectively) and a significantly higher complication rate occurred in elderly than in young patients with electrophysiologic study (2.2% vs. 0.5%) or radiofrequency ablation (6.1% vs. 2.0%). Multiple logistic analysis found that older age and systemic disease in elderly patients were the independent predictors of complications in both procedures. Furthermore, there was no

TABLE 6-2
Indications for Clinical Electrophysiological Studies in 1643 Patients
Undergoing 2524 Procedures

	Number of Patients/Number of Proc.
Diagnostic study	
Sinus node dysfunction	206/206
AV conduction dysfunction	155/155
Preexcitation syndrome with tachyarrhythmias	80/80
Paroxysmal supraventricular tachycardia	322/322
Ventricular tachycardia	151/151
Tachycardia or palpitation of uncertain types	254/254
Syncope of unknown cause	20/20
Survivors of cardiac arrest	5/5
Evaluation of drug effects:	
Immediately after diagnostic study	746/*
In days after diagnostic study	310/386
Follow-up after radiofrequency ablation	450/945
Total	1,643/2,524

* These procedures belonged to the same session of diagnostic procedures.
AV = atrioventricular; Proc. = procedures.
Reproduced with permission from Chen et al.[27]

temporal trend in the incidence of complication. We conclude that the incidence of complication was higher in radiofrequency ablation, and elderly patients had a higher incidence of complications in both electrophysiological study and radiofrequency ablation. These procedures, when performed by experienced personnel in an appropriately staffed and equipped laboratory, can be undertaken with an acceptable risk (Tables 6-2–6-4).

AV Accessory Pathways/Ebstein's Anomaly

Cappato and colleagues[28] in Hamburg, Germany, studied 21 patients with Ebstein's anomaly and reentrant atrioventricular tachycardias who underwent

TABLE 6-3
Tachyarrhythmias Induced During Diagnostic Electrophysiologic Study

Tachyarrhythmia	Number of Patients
Sinus node reentrant tachycardia	6
Atrial tachycardia	67
Atrial flutter	50
Atrial fibrillation	133
Accessory pathway-mediated tachyarrhythmias	191
AV node reentrant tachycardia	142
Sustained ventricular tachycardia	131
Nonsustained ventricular tachycardia	24
Ventricular fibrillation	12
Negative finding	86

AV = atrioventricular.
Reproduced with permission from Chen et al.[27]

TABLE 6-4
Analysis of Factors Related to Complications in Radiofrequency Ablation

Related Factors	Complications		p Values
	Present	Absent	
Types of arrhythmias			0.1759
WPW	28	672	
AVNRT	16	509	
IST	0	4	
AT	0	60	
AF	0	39	
A. fib.	0	90	
VT	0	24	
Ablation sites in WPW syndrome			0.7704
Lt H	16	426	
Rt H	11	220	
Lt + Rt H	1	26	
Ablation sites of all arrhythmias			0.5020
Lt H	17	429	
Rt H	26	944	
Lt + Rt H	1	25	
Associated systemic diseases			
Young patients (<65 yr)			0.2159
Present	2	41	
Absent	20	1,021	
Elderly patients (≥65 yr)			0.0022
Present	9	45	
Absent	13	291	

AF = atrial flutter; A. fib. = atrial fibrillation; AT = atrial tachycardia; AVNRT = atrioventricular node reentrant tachycardia; IST = inappropriate sinus tachycardia; Lt H = left-sided heart; Rt H = right-sided heart; VT = ventricular tachycardia; WPW = Wolff-Parkinson-White syndrome.
Reproduced with permission from Chen et al.[27]

electrophysiological evaluation and subsequent attempts at radiofrequency catheter ablation. Thirty-four right-sided accessory pathways were found, with 30 located along the atrialized ventricle. Local electrograms in this region were normal in 10 patients, but fragmented in 11. Fragmented electrograms prevented the clear distinction between atrial and ventricular activation potentials, as well as the identification of accessory pathway potentials. Right coronary artery mapping was performed in 7 patients. Abolition of all 26 accessory pathways was achieved in the 10 patients with normal local electrogram and in 6 of 11 patients with abnormal electrograms. Right coronary artery mapping allowed accessory pathway localization and ablation in 5 patients. In the 5 patients with abnormal electrograms and a total of 8 accessory pathways, 6 accessory pathways could not be ablated. Unsuccessfully treated patients received antiarrhythmic drugs. During 22 months of follow-up, 5 patients had clinical recurrences, including 4 who had undergone a successful radiofrequency procedure. Thus, in patients with Ebstein's anomaly and reentrant atrioventricular tachycardias, factors likely to account for failure of radiofrequency catheter ablation include an accessory pathway located along the atrialized right ventricle and the abnormal morphology of endocardial activation potentials generated in this region.

AV Nodal Reentrant Tachycardia

Age of Onset Comparison

AV nodal reentrant tachycardia and accessory pathway-mediated tachycardia may be associated with different ages of tachycardia onset. In this study by Goyal and associates[29] from Ann Arbor, Michigan, symptom onset data were obtained in 519 patients (AV nodal reentrant tachycardia, 231; accessory pathway-mediated tachycardia, 288). The mean age of the patients at the time of evaluation was 47 ± 17 years (AV nodal reentrant tachycardia) and 37 ± 15 years (accessory pathway-mediated tachycardia). The mean age of symptom onset was 32 ± 18 years for AV nodal reentrant tachycardia and 23 ± 14 years for accessory pathway-mediated tachycardia. A significantly greater proportion of patients with A-V nodal reentrant tachycardia had the initial onset of symptoms after the age of 20 years (AV nodal reentrant tachycardia, 67%; accessory pathway-mediated tachycardia, 41%). In summary, there is a different mean age of symptom onset for patients with AV nodal reentrant tachycardia and accessory pathway-mediated tachycardia.

Significance of Slow Potentials in Dual AV Node Physiology

AV nodal reentrant tachycardia is now routinely cured by selective radiofrequency ablation of slow AV node pathway conduction. However, debate remains concerning the optimum method for localizing the site at which radiofrequency energy should be delivered to eliminate slow-pathway conduction. Some investigators have proposed simple anatomy-guided ablations posteriorly near the ostium of the coronary sinus, whereas others suggest an electrophysiology-guided ablation using either recorded slow potentials or mapping of the retrograde atrial exit site of slow AV node pathway conduction when possible. To examine these issues, Kuo and associates[30] from Stanford, California, systematically studied slow potentials recorded in the AV junction of patients undergoing radiofrequency catheter ablation for medically refractory AV nodal reentrant tachycardia. In 67 patients with the slow-fast form of AV nodal reentrant tachycardia, the investigators performed detailed atrial mapping along the tricuspid annulus within the triangle of Koch. Two types of slow potentials were identified. Low-amplitude, low-frequency potentials, found in 48% of patients, were localized to the mid to posterior portions of the triangle of Koch, whereas high-amplitude, high-frequency potentials, observed in 22% of patients, were located only posteriorly near the ostium of the coronary sinus. In response to a bolus infusion of adenosine or incremental atrial pacing-induced AV nodal Wenckebach periodicity, the low-amplitude, low-frequency potentials showed an increased duration and further reduction in amplitude and frequency, which often totally disappeared. In contrast, in spite of these maneuvers, the high-amplitude and high-frequency potentials remained unchanged. Of the 25 (37%) of 67 patients in whom the earliest retrograde atrial activation during ventriculoatrial slow AV nodal pathway conduction could be recorded, no patient exhibited low-amplitude, low-frequency potentials; and only 7 (28%) of 25 of these patients showed high-amplitude, high-frequency potentials. High-amplitude, high-frequency potentials persisted after successful radiofrequency ablation of slow pathway conduction. Fewer applications of radiofrequency energy were required for successful elimination of slow-pathway conduction in patients in whom the retrograde atrial exit site of slow-pathway conduction could be localized, compared with those patients who only exhibited retrograde fast AV nodal pathway conduction. The investigators concluded that high-amplitude, high-frequency potentials are part of atrial activity, whereas the origin of low-amplitude, low-frequency potentials is unclear and may represent either true intranodal biophysical electrical activity or merely artifact or far-field potentials. Regardless, the recording of high-amplitude or low-amplitude potentials is not required for successful ablation of slow-pathway conduction, although the ability to localize the retrograde atrial exit of slow-pathway conduction may assist in the ablation procedure.

Comparison of Atrial-His Intervals: Dual AV Node Physiology and AV Node Reentrant Tachycardia

The purpose of this study by Bogun and associates[31] from Ann Arbor, Michigan, was to compare the atrial-His intervals generated during programmed stimulation in patients with and without inducible AV nodal reentrant tachycardia. Programmed atrial stimulation at a basic- drive cycle length of 500 to 600 msec was performed in 180 patients. The minimum atrial-His interval was defined as the atrial-His interval of the basic-drive beats. The maximum atrial-His interval was defined as the longest A_2H_2 interval. The criterion for dual AV nodal physiology was an increment of 50 msec in the A_2H_2 interval in association with a 10-msec decrement in the A_1A_2 interval. The minimum atrial-His interval was significantly shorter (106 ± 34 msec vs. 116 ± 29 msec), and the maximum atrial-His interval was significantly longer (304 ± 101 msec vs. 222 ± 56 msec) in the 87 patients who had AV nodal reentry than in the 93 patients who did not. Among the 87 patients who had AV nodal reentry, the maximum atrial-His interval was significantly longer in 53 patients who had dual AV nodal physiology than in 34 patients who did not (340 ± 105 msec vs. 249 ± 62 msec). Among the 66 patients who had dual AV nodal physiology, the maximum atrial-His interval was significantly longer in 53 patients who had AV nodal reentry than in 13 patients who did not (340 ± 105 msec vs. 268 ± 61 msec). The insensitivity of the conventional dual AV nodal physiology criterion for the detection of dual AV nodal pathways is in part attributable to a lesser degree of slowing of conduction in the slow pathway relative to the fast pathway in some patients who have AV nodal reentry. The inability to demonstrate AV nodal reentry despite the presence of dual AV nodal physiology in some persons may be attributable in part to an inadequate degree of conduction delay in the slow pathway.

The study by King and associates[32] from Taiwan, Republic of China, examined the incidence and significance of catheter-induced AV nodal block during a radiofrequency ablation procedure that uses stiff large-tip steerable ablation catheters. AV nodal block was noted in 10 (1.6%) of 613 consecutive patients undergoing radiofrequency ablation therapy for AV nodal reentrant tachycardia (592 patients) or AV reentry tachycardia incorporating a midseptal accessory pathway (21 patients). Of these 10 patients, 9 underwent AV nodal modification for AV nodal reentrant tachycardia and 1 for ablation of a midseptal accessory pathway. One patient had 2 episodes of AV nodal block during 2 sessions undertaken because of recurrence of tachycardia. No patient had a preexisting conduction defect before the study. In all 10 patients, AV nodal block was transient, and it lasted for a mean of 9.1 ± 19 minutes. It occurred during positioning of the ablation catheter in the junctional area before (8 patients) or after (2 patients) the start of radiofrequency current applications. Complete AV nodal block was noted on 6 occasions, second-degree AV nodal block on 4 occasions, and first-degree AV nodal block on 1 occasion. All blocks were associated with narrow QRS ventricular beats and with a site of block proximal to the His bundle. The mean ventricular heart rate during AV nodal block was 60 ± 23 beats/min. Two patients had transient asystole, with 1 having loss of consciousness. No patient required special treatment for heart block. One-to-one conduction resumed after repositioning of the catheters, and the subsequent ablation procedure was successfully completed in 8 of the 10 patients. During a follow-up of 20 ± 12 months, none of the patients had severe dizziness or syncope, and none required implantation of a permanent pacemaker. In conclusion, transient AV nodal block due to mechanical injury occurs during positioning of a stiff large-tip steerable ablation catheter in the junctional area. Delivery of radiofrequency current to the site that provokes catheter-induced AV nodal block should be avoided.

Left Bundle Branch Block

Natural History

Fahy and associates[33] from Cleveland, Ohio, and Dublin, Ireland, determined a long-term outcome of patients with BBB who have no clinical evidence of cardiovascular disease. Among 110,000 participants in a screening program, 310 subjects with BBB without apparent or suspected heart disease were identified. Their outcome after a mean follow-up of 9.5 years was compared with that of 310 similarly screened age- and sex-matched controls. Among the screened population, isolated right BBB was more prevalent than isolated left BBB (0.18% vs 0.1%, respectively), and the prevalence of each abnormality increased with age. Total actuarial survival was no different for those with left BBB or right BBB and their respective controls. Cardiac mortality, however, was increased in the left BBB group when compared with their controls (log rank test). Left BBB, but not right BBB, was associated with an increased prevalence of cardiovascular disease at follow-up (21% vs. 11%). In the absence of clinically overt cardiac disease, the presence of left BBB or right BBB is not associ-

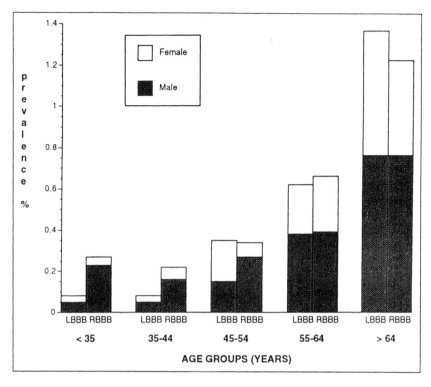

Figure 6-14. Prevalence of left BBB (LBBB) and right BBB (RBBB) according to age. The prevalence of each abnormality increased with age (p<.001). Reproduced with permission from Fahy et al.[33]

ated with increased overall mortality. Isolated left BBB is associated with an increased risk of developing overt cardiovascular disease and increased cardiac mortality (Figure 6-14, Table 6-5).

Pharmacological Stress Testing

Patients with left BBB often have septal perfusion defects during exercise perfusion tomography that mimic defects caused by CAD. These defects may be less frequent during pharmacological stress using adenosine or dipyridamole. Vaduganathan and colleagues[34] from Houston, Texas, evaluated the role of dobutamine tomography in these patients as a diagnostic test. They studied 383 consecutive patients with left BBB who were referred for perfusion scintigraphy. Perfusion tomography was performed in conjunction with exercise in 206 patients, adenosine in 127, and dobutamine in 50. Coronary angiography was performed within 1 month of the stress test in 77, 50, and 27 patients, respectively. Results showed that exercise, adenosine and dobutamine tomography had similar sensitivity and specificity for the detection of stenosis greater than 50% in the LC (74% and 96%; 50% and 100%; 63% and 91%, respectively)

TABLE 6-5
Causes of Death

	Left BBB Cases (n=112)	Left BBB Controls (n=112)	Right BBB Cases (n=198)	Right BBB Controls (n=198)	Total
Myocardial infarction	5	2	1	5	13
Heart failure	1	0	1	1	3
Sudden death	2	0	0	0	2
Stroke	0	0	1	4	5
Nonvascular	3	6	7	4	20
Unknown	1	0	0	5	6
Total	12	8	10	19	49

Reproduced with permission from Fahy et al.[33]

and right coronary artery (96% and 86%; 82% and 91%; 79% and 100%, respectively) and similar sensitivity for LAD coronary artery stenosis (88%, 79%, and 100%, respectively). However, the false-positive rate for septal defects was higher by exercise tomography (46%) than by pharmacologic methods (10%), and there was no significant difference between adenosine and dobutamine. The specificity and predictive value of a positive test response for LAD coronary artery stenosis were 36% and 51% for exercise, compared with 81% and 85% for adenosine and 80% and 90% for dobutamine, respectively. These authors concluded that in patients with left BBB, pharmacologic stress is more specific than exercise tomography in the diagnosis of LAD coronary artery stenosis. Dobutamine and adenosine tomography were equally specific in these patients. These data help to define a specific circumstance where one type of imaging may be preferable to others.

Diagnosis of AMI by Electrocardiography in Patients with Left Bundle-Branch Block

Sgarbossa and colleagues[35] from the Cleveland Clinic, Cleveland, Ohio, and for the Global Utilization of Streptokinase and Tissue Plasminogen Activator for Occluded Coronary Arteries (GUSTO-1) investigators tested electrocardiographic criteria for the diagnosis of AMI in the presence of left BBB. Baseline electrocardiograms of patients enrolled in the GUSTO-1 trial who had left BBB and AMI confirmed by enzyme studies were blindly compared with the electrocardiograms of control patients who had chronic CAD and left BBB. The electrocardiographic criteria for the diagnosis of AMI were tested in an independent sample of patients presenting with chest pain and left BBB. Among 26,003 North American patients, 131 (0.5%) with AMI had left BBB. The 3 electrocardiographic criteria with independent value in the diagnosis of AMI in these patients were ST-segment elevation of 1 mm or more that was concordant with (in the same direction as) the QRS complex; ST-segment depression of 1 mm or more in leads V_1, V_2, or V_3, and ST-segment elevation of 5 mm or more that was discordant with (in the opposite direction from) the

QRS complex. These 3 criteria were used to develop a scoring system of 0 to 5, which allowed a highly specific diagnosis of AMI to be made. This study suggests that a clinical prediction rule based on a set of electrocardiographic criteria for the diagnosis of AMI may be used in patients with chest pain and left BBB.

Miscellaneous

Pacemaker Dysfunction Caused by Digital Mobile Phones

Electromagnetic fields may interfere with normal pacemaker function. Naegeli and colleagues[36] from Basel, Switzerland, evaluated possible interactions between digital mobile telephones and implanted pacemakers. In 39 patients with an implanted pacemaker, 4 mobile telephones with different levels of power output (2 and 8 W) were tested in the standby, dialing, and operating modes. During continuous electrocardiographic monitoring, 672 tests were performed in each mode, with the telephones positioned over the pulse generator. In 18%, a reproducible interference was induced during 26 of 672 tests with the operating telephones in close proximity to the pacemaker. When the bipolar and unipolar pacing modes were compared in the same patients, ventricular inhibition was induced only in the unipolar mode. Interference was more likely to occur at high power output of the telephone at a maximal sensitivity of the pacemakers. These authors concluded that digital mobile telephones in close proximity to implanted pacemakers may cause intermittent pacemaker dysfunction with inappropriate ventricular tracking and potentially dangerous pacemaker inhibition.

Sex Differences in Cardiac Arrest Survivors

Albert and colleagues[37] in Boston, Massachusetts, evaluated 355 consecutive survivors of out-of-hospital cardiac arrest, including 84 women and 271 men referred for electrophysiologically guided therapy. These individuals were analyzed retrospectively for sex differences, underlying pathology, and predictors of outcome. Women were significantly less likely to have underlying CAD than men and were more likely to have other forms of heart disease or structurally normal hearts (Figures 6-15, 6-16). The mean LVEF was higher in women (46% vs. 41%), and women were more likely to have no inducible arrhythmia at baseline electrophysiological testing (46% vs. 27%), although when the patients were stratified by CAD status, these sex differences were no longer present. The independent predictors of outcome differed between men and women. In men, an LVEF of less than 40% was the most powerful independent predictor of total and cardiac mortality, but in women, the presence of CAD was the only independent predictor of total and cardiac mortality (Figure 6-17). Thus, female survivors of cardiac arrest are less likely to have underlying CAD. The

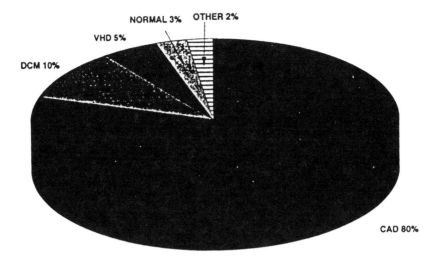

FIGURE 6-15. Pie chart illustrating the proportions of various types of underlying structural heart disease in the male survivors of cardiac arrest. CAD, coronary artery disease; DCM, dilated cardiomyopathy; VHD, valvular heart disease. Reproduced with permission from Albert et al.[37]

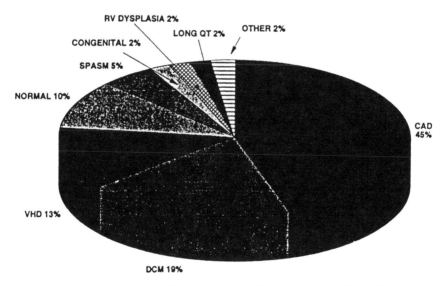

FIGURE 6-16. Pie chart illustrating the proportions of various types of underlying structural heart disease in the female survivors of cardiac arrest. CAD, coronary artery disease; DCM, dilated cardiomyopathy; VHD, valvular heart disease; SPASM, coronary vasospasm; RV, right ventricular. Reproduced with permission from Albert et al.[37]

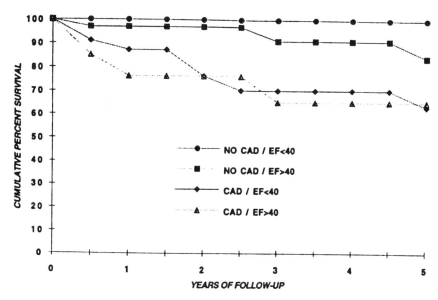

FIGURE 6-17. Plot of total mortality in women with and without coronary artery disease (CAD) stratified by left ventricular ejection fraction (EF). Reproduced with permission from Albert et al.[37]

predictors of total and cardiac mortality differ between male and female survivors. CAD status is the most important predictor in women, and impaired LVEF is the most important predictor in men.

Sudden Death in Athletes

Sudden cardiac death during athletic activities is a highly visible event. Maron and colleagues[38] from Minneapolis, Minnesota, attempted to assess the relative risks associated with marathon running. The prevalence of sudden death was assessed in 2 groups of endurance runners competing in the annual Marine Corps (1976 to 1994) and Twin Cities (1982 to 1994) marathons, held over a cumulative 30-year period. A total of 215,413 runners completed the races, and 4 exercise-related sudden deaths occurred, each due to unsuspected structural cardiac disease. Three deaths occurred during the race and the other immediately after its completion. Three were due to atherosclerotic coronary disease and 1 to anomalous origin of the left main coronary artery from the right sinus of Valsalva. None of the 4 runners had prior documentation of heart disease or apparent prodromal symptoms. These authors concluded that although highly trained athletes such as marathon runners may harbor underlying and potentially lethal cardiovascular disease, the risk for sudden cardiac death associated with such intense physical effort is exceedingly small (1 in 50,000). They further concluded that the low risk for sudden death identified in long distance runners suggests that routine screening for cardiovascular disease in such athletic populations may not be justifiable.

Ambulatory Electrocardiography in the Elderly

Functional, ambulatory, community-dwelling subjects (n = 423, aged 75 to 85 years) underwent baseline 24-hour ambulatory electrocardiography examinations as part of the Bronx Aging Study, a 10-year prospective cohort study carried out by Frishman and associates[39] from the Bronx, New York. It is designed to identify risk factors and disease markers for cardiovascular, cerebrovascular, and dementia illnesses in older people. VPCs were the most commonly observed arrhythmias (93% of individuals), with a low prevalence of nonsustained VT (5%), paroxysmal atrial tachycardia (13%), AF (4%), and A-V nodal block (4%). A 24-hour sinus rate of less than 60 beats/min was noted in 13% of individuals, and 11% of individuals were noted to have transient episodes of severe bradycardia (<40 beats per minute). In a multivariate analysis, nonsustained VT was an independent predictor of death. Transient AV block was an independent predictor of stroke, as was sinus bradycardia over a 24-hour period. Ventricular tachycardia approached significance as an independent predictor of multiinfarct dementia. Episodes of paroxysmal AF, atrial tachycardia, and severe bradycardia were not associated with adverse outcomes. Some arrhythmias found on the ambulatory electrocardiogram in very old individuals can predict an increased risk for subsequent death, myocardial infarction, stroke, and multiinfarct dementia.

Gender Differences in Autonomic Modulation of Heart Rate

Huikuri and colleagues[40] in Oulu, Finland, studied sex-related differences in the autonomic modulation of heart rate in middle-aged subjects without known heart disease. Baroreflex sensitivity and heart rate variability were studied in randomly selected, age-matched populations of middle-aged women (n = 186; mean age, 50 years) and men (n = 188; mean age, 50 years) without hypertension, diabetes, or clinical or echocardiographic evidence of heart disease. Baroreflex sensitivity measured from the overshoot phase of the Valsalva maneuver was significantly lower in women than in men, and the low frequency component of heart rate variability measured from electrocardiographic recordings was also lower in women, whereas the high frequency component was higher in women than in men. The ratio between low- and high-frequency oscillations was lower in women. The increase in heart rate and decrease in high-frequency component of heart rate variability in response to upright posture were smaller in magnitude in women than in men. After adjustment for differences in the baseline variables, such as blood pressure, heart rate, smoking, alcohol consumption, and psychosocial score, the sex-related differences in baroreflex sensitivity and heart rate variability remained significant. Women with estrogen replacement (n = 46) had significantly higher baroreflex sensitivity and total heart rate variance than did age-matched women without hormone therapy. The baroreflex sensitivity and heart rate variability of women with estrogen therapy did not differ from those of the age-matched men. Thus, baroreflex responsiveness is attenuated in middle-aged women compared with men, but the tonic vagal modulation of heart rate is augmented. Hormone replacement therapy appears to have favorable effects on the cardiovascular autonomic regulation in postmenopausal women.

Atrial Fibrillation/Flutter

Prevalence

An increasing prevalence of AF recently noted in hospital discharge data has not been verified in a population-based sample. Wolf and associates[41] from Boston, Massachusetts, determined the prevalence of AF from 1968 to 1989 in the Framingham Study cohort aged 65 to 84 years. AF prevalence was evaluated by sex and in the presence of valvular disease, prior AMI, and CHF. AF prevalence increased significantly in men overall, but not in women, and in men with and without valvular disease and AMI, but not CHF. In men with prior AMI, age-adjusted prevalence rose from 4.9% to 17.4%. Multivariate analysis confirmed the increase in AF prevalence in men, when age, valvular disease, and prior AMI were taken into account. The basis for the increased AF prevalence in men is unexplained but may relate to recent improved AMI survival. In an aging U.S. population, this trend raises the concern of future increases in stroke incidence.

Fourier Analysis of Mechanical Function

The aim of this study by Grimm and associates[42] from Cleveland, Ohio, was to characterize left atrial (LA) appendage mechanical function in AF and atrial flutter by Fourier analysis to analyze frequency and regularity of flow. LA appendage function is central to a patient's risk for thromboembolism. Although the function of the appendage can be analyzed by Doppler echocardiography in sinus rhythm, its mechanical function in AF and atrial flutter has not been well characterized. This lack of adequate definition is caused by the complexity and temporal variability of the Doppler flow profiles. These investigators assessed LA appendage function in 21 cases of AF (n = 11) and atrial flutter (n = 10) and 5 in sinus rhythm with transesophageal Doppler echocardiography. Doppler profiles were examined by Fourier analysis, and the power spectra compared and analyzed between patients with AF and atrial flutter. LA appendage Doppler flow in AF produced Fourier spectra over a narrow band of frequencies with a peak frequency of 6.2 ± 1.0 Hz, significantly higher than in atrial flutter (3.9 ± 0.6 Hz). Additionally, a significant difference in subharmonic modulation (spectral power below the peak frequency) was observed between atrial appendage flow in AF and atrial flutter, because 37% ± 16% of the total spectral power was achieved before the dominant frequency in AF compared with 20% ± 14% in atrial flutter. Conversely, patients in sinus rhythm exhibited broad-banded Fourier spectra with most of the power in discrete frequency spikes at harmonics above the fundamental frequency with very little subharmonic modulation. LA appendage function in AF and atrial flutter can be well characterized by Fourier analysis of Doppler flow. AF has higher dominant frequencies and greater subharmonic modulation compared with atrial flutter. Moreover, AF demonstrated quasiperiodic contraction patterns typically found in chaotic systems. Fourier analysis of LA appendage contraction patterns may therefore have significant promise in providing insights into mechanisms of AF and thromboembolism.

Hemodynamic Assessment: MRI versus Invasive Measurements

Currently available invasive and noninvasive techniques for the determination of left ventricular end-diastolic and end-systolic volumes, EF, and cardiac output are more time consuming and potentially less accurate in patients with AF than in those with sinus rhythm. Although MRI (MRI) can rapidly and accurately measure these variables in patients with sinus rhythm, its ability to do so in subjects with AF is not known. To determine whether LV volumes, EF, and cardiac output can be accurately measured in patients with AF by use of MRI, Hundley and associates[43] from Dallas, Texas, performed MRI followed immediately thereafter by invasive measurements of these indexes in 26 subjects (13 women and 13 men: age, 15–76 years) in sinus rhythm (n = 13) or AF (n = 13). For those in AF, MRI measurements of left ventricular end-diastolic volume, end-systolic volume, stroke volume, EF, and cardiac output correlated well with catheterization measurements. In addition, the mean difference between MRI and catheterization measurements was similar in subjects with AF and in those with sinus rhythm. Compared with standard invasive measurements, MRI provides an accurate noninvasive determination of left ventricular volumes, EF, and cardiac output in patients with AF.

Doppler-Measured Blood Flow Velocity

Doppler measurement of LA appendage blood velocity during TEE has been proposed as a method of assessing LA appendage contractile function and thromboembolic risk. Clinical and echocardiographic determinants of 5 LA appendage Doppler blood velocity patterns were examined by Fatkin and Feneley[44] from Sydney, Australia, in 40 patients with a history of AF, in 10 control, and in 5 patients aged 60 years or younger having sinus rhythm and LV hypertrophy. In sinus rhythm, 2 blood-velocity patterns were differentiated by the extent of passive emptying of the LA appendage, which was related to age and left ventricular early diastolic filling properties. In AF, 3 blood-velocity patterns were differentiated by the relative preservation of LA appendage mechanical function during fibrillatory activity. LA appendage contractile function is an important, but not the sole, determinant of blood flow in the normal and fibrillating human LA appendage.

Predictors of AF after Coronary Artery Surgery

Aranki and colleagues[45] in Boston, Massachusetts, determined the current incidence of atrial fibrillation after CABG surgery and attempted to identify its clinical predictors and examine its impact on resource utilization. During a 12-month period ending July 31, 1994, a CABG procedure was performed on 570 consecutive patients (mean age, 67 years): 175 were women, 173 were diabetics, 364 required nonelective surgery, and 86 had a prior CABG. AF occurred in 189 patients (33%). The median age for patients with AF was 71 years; for patients with AF, it was 66 years. Multivariate without logistic regression analysis was used to identify the following independent predictors of postoperative AF: increasing age (age 70 to 80 years), age greater than 80 years, male gender, hypertension, need for intraoperative intraaortic balloon pump, postoperative pneumonia, ventilation for more than 24 hours, and need to return to the intensive care unit (Table 6-6). The mean length of hospital stay after surgery was 15 days for patients with AF, compared with 9 days for patients without AF. The adjusted length of hospital stay attributable to AF was 5 days corresponding to $10,055 or more in hospital charges. Thus, atrial fibrillation remains the most common complication after CABG and consequently is a relative drain on hospital resources.

AF After Valve Replacement

Chronic AF occurs often in the setting of mitral and aortic valve disease. Eventually, patients with chronic AF require valve replacement, which improves cardiac function but does not prevent AF. Crijns and associates[46] from Groningen, The Netherlands, investigated which patients may benefit from additional surgery performed in combination with valve surgery for the cure of AF. Seventy-four patients were retrospectively included from our prospective database of patients referred for serial cardioversion therapy between 1986 and 1993. All these patients had chronic AF after valve replacement. After the first electrical cardioversion, patients did not receive antiarrhythmic drugs. Relapses were managed by repeated cardioversions, and then antiarrhythmic drugs were instituted. After a median follow-up of 7 years (range, 1.3 to 23),

TABLE 6-6
Multivariate Predictors of AF

Predictor	OR	p	95% CI
Age 70 to 80 y	2.0	.002	1.3–3.0
Age >80 y	3.0	.0007	1.6–5.8
Male gender	1.7	.01	1.1–2.7
Hypertension	1.6	.03	1.0–2.3
Intraoperative IABP	3.5	.03	1.2–10.9
Pneumonia	3.9	.01	1.3–11.5
Ventilation >24 h	2.0	.003	1.3–3.2
Return to intensive care unit	3.2	.03	1.1–8.8

Reproduced with permission from Aranki et al.[45]

TABLE 6-7
**Comparison of Baseline Characteristics Known at Surgery in Patients with Successful
Versus Unsuccessful Serial Cardioversion (SR)**

	AF (n = 39)	SR (n = 35)	p Value
Age at surgery*	53 ± 15	57 ± 11	NS
Men/women	12/27	18/17	0.10
History of chronic atrial fibrillation before surgery	26 (67%)	12 (34%)	0.01
Duration of last episode of AF (mos)†	6	2	0.03
Rheumatic heart disease	26 (67%)	15 (43%)	0.02
Coronary artery disease	6 (15%)	9 (26%)	NS
Systemic hypertension	2 (5%)	2 (6%)	NS
NYHA Class at surgery			
I	2 (5%)	3 (14%)	NS
II	9 (23%)	7 (17%)	
III	20 (51%)	20 (55%)	
IV	8 (21)	5 (14%)	
Mitral valve replacement/aortic valve replacement	29/10	16/19	0.02
Left atrial size (mm)	51 ± 9	53 ± 8	NS
Left ventricular end-diastolic diameter (mm)	51 ± 10	54 ± 11	NS
Left ventricular end-systolic diameter (mm)	37 ± 11	35 ± 15	NS
Fractional shortening (%)	32 ± 11	38 ± 17	0.14

* Mean ± SD; † median value.
AF = atrial fibrillation; NYHA = New York Heart Association.

39 patients had intractable AF. Multivariate analysis revealed that patients with a history of chronic AF before surgery had a poor arrhythmia outcome. In addition, Kaplan-Meier survival analysis demonstrated a lower success rate in patients with mitral valve disease than in those with aortic valve disease. CHF (41% vs. 6%) and cardiovascular mortality (23% vs. 9%) were seen most often in patients with an unsuccessful cardioversion strategy. Thus, patients scheduled for mitral valve surgery with a history of chronic AF should be considered candidates for concomitant surgery for AF. (Table 6-7, Figure 6-18).

Tricuspid Annulus as Anterior Barrier in AF

Kalman and colleagues[47] in Melbourne, Australia, have evaluated the hypothesis that the tricuspid annulus forms a continuous anterior barrier to the atrial flutter circuit. Thirteen patients with typical atrial flutter were studied. A 20-pole halo catheter was situated around the tricuspid annulus. A mapping catheter was used for activation, and entrainment mapping was studied from 7 sequential sites around the tricuspid annulus and from 3 additional sites, including the tip of the right atrial appendage, at the fossa ovalis, and in the distal coronary sinus. Sites were considered to be within the circuit when the postpacing interval minus the flutter cycle length and the stimulus time minus the activation time were 10 msec or less. Sites were considered to be outside the circuit when these intervals were greater than 10 msec. All 7 annular sites

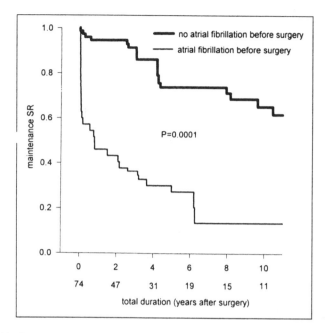

Figure 6-18. Kaplan-Meier curves depicting the probability of maintenance of sinus rhythm (SR) after serial electrical cardioversion therapy. Patients with and without a history of chronic atrial fibrillation before surgery are compared. The numbers below the figure indicate numbers of patients at risk. Reproduced with permission from Crijns et al.[46]

were within the circuit. Activation occurred sequentially around the annulus and accounted for 100% of the flutter cycle length. The fossa ovalis, distal coronary sinus, and the right atrial appendage were outside the circuit. Thus, these data indicate that closely spaced sites around the tricuspid annulus are activated sequentially, and all are within the flutter circuit according the entrainment criteria. This demonstrates that the tricuspid annulus constitutes a continuous anterior barrier constraining the reentrant wave front of human counterclockwise atrial flutter (Figure 6-19).

Radiofrequency Catheter Ablation

Catheter ablation of atrial flutter can be performed with different techniques. Chen and colleagues[48] from Tapei, Taiwan, and Kaoshiung, Taiwan, compared the electrophysiologically guided focal ablation technique and linear ablation technique in patients with atrial flutter in a prospective randomized trial. Sixty patients with drug-refractory common atrial flutter were randomly assigned to undergo radiofrequency catheter ablation with 1 of the 2 techniques. Successful elimination of the flutter was achieved in 28 of 30 patients with the focal ablation technique and in 29 of 30 patients with the linear ablation technique. More atrial premature beats and episodes of short run atrial tachyarrhythmias in the early period were seen with the linear ablation tech-

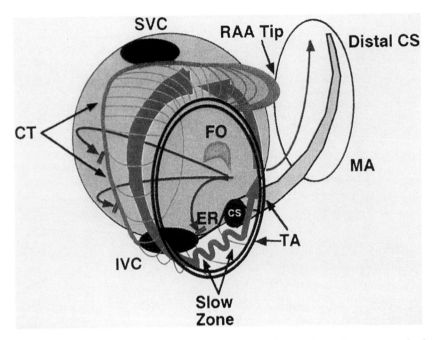

FIGURE 6-19. Schematic depicting the entire flutter circuit in red rotating counterclockwise around the TA. Blue arrows represent passive activation outside the circuit. Note that the crista terminalis and the ER act as lines of block preventing activation from "short circuiting" the annulus. Reproduced with permission from Kalman et al.[47]

nique. Recurrence rate (2 of 28 in focal ablation vs. 3 of 21 in the linear ablation technique) and incidence of new, sustained atrial tachyarrhythmias were similar in the 2 groups. These authors concluded that both techniques were safe and effective in ablating the atrial flutter circuit. However, the linear ablation technique was time-saving.

Electrophysiological Effects of Catheter Ablation

The study by Cauchemez and colleagues[49] from Bordeaux-Pessac, France, studied 20 patients with common atrial flutter. All had inducible atrial flutter, and 8 had both common and reverse atrial flutter (Figure 6-20). Right atrial activation sequences were investigated during pacing from sites proximal (low lateral right atrium) and distal (proximal coronary sinus) to the inferior vena cava-tricuspid annulus isthmus during both entrainment of common or reverse atrial flutter and during pacing in sinus rhythm. This was repeated after ablation. During pacing in sinus rhythm from the low lateral right atrium, the septum was activated by caudocranial and craniocaudal wave fronts. During pacing from the proximal coronary sinus, the lateral right atrium was activated by 2 wave fronts. Catheter ablation of the inferior vena cava-tricuspid annulus isthmus induced marked changes in mapping due to the loss of cranialcaudo wave front in all but 1 patient. The septum and the lateral right atrium were

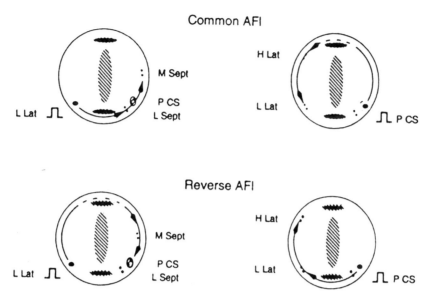

FIGURE 6-20. Diagrammatic illustration of right atrial activation during atrial flutter (AFl) entrainment. Openings of the superior and inferior venae cavae and coronary sinus are shown for reference. Shaded area in posterior (intercaval) right atrial represents a zone of block. Last paced beat that is entrained but not fused is represented. Thus, the orthodromic wave front is the only 1 schematized. **Top,** Entrainment of common AFl is a model of unidirectional counterclockwise RA activation. During pacing from the low lateral RA, conduction times to the lower septum (L Sept), proximal coronary sinus (PCS), and His bundle region (M Sept) are representative of activation by a single "anterograde" caudal input. During pacing from the PCS, conduction times to the high- and low-lateral RA (H, L Lat) are a model of activation via a single "retrograde" cranial input. **Bottom,** Entrainment of reverse AFl is a model of unidirectional clockwise RA activation. In this circumstance, conduction times are a reference for activation by a single "anterograde" cranial input when pacing the low lateral RA and a single "retrograde" caudal input when pacing the PCS. Dotted lines express uncertainty concerning upper part of circuit that was not studied. Reproduced with permission from Cauchemez et al.[49]

activated by a single craniocaudal front during entrainment of reverse or common atrial flutter, respectively. During a follow-up period of 8 months, common or reverse atrial flutter occurred in 4 patients. Two had no or only unidirectional change in the isthmus conduction induced by ablation. The other 2 had a late recovery of conduction. Thus, the data obtained in this study provide evidence that the mechanism of successful atrial flutter ablation targeting the inferior vena cava-tricuspid annulus isthmus is local, bidirectional conduction block. This change can be used as an electrophysiological end point for the procedure. Atrial flutter recurrences appear to be associated with failure to achieve a permanent block.

Atrial Pacing

Daoud and colleagues[51] assessed the local and left atrial response to pacing at the high right atrium during type I AF in humans. Pacing was performed at the high right atrium during type I AF in 24 patients in the electrophysiology laboratory. The response to pacing was assessed at cycle lengths 10, 20, 30, 40, and 50 msec less than the mean baseline atrial cycle length. Digitized tracings of the baseline tachycardia and the response to pacing were recorded from the high right atrium and from the distal coronary sinus. Computer analysis of these signals was used to calculate a left atrial electrogram density before, during, and after pacing. Two hundred eighty-eight segments of AF with a duration of 3.9 seconds were analyzed. Local capture of the right atrium during AF was demonstrated for at least 1 pacing cycle length in each patient. The left atrial electrogram density was significantly greater than baseline at each pacing cycle length that resulted in local capture, except when pacing at 50 msec less than the mean AF cycle length. There was no significant change in baseline left atrial electrogram density compared with baseline when pacing did not result in capture of AF. Thus, local right atrial capture is often possible by pacing during type I AF and consistently influences the left atrial electrograms recorded in the coronary sinus.

AF and its recurrence after cardioversion is an increasingly common arrhythmia treated by practicing physicians. Saksena and colleagues[51] from Passaic, New Jersey, and Minneapolis, Minnesota, developed and applied a novel technique of dual-site right atrial pacing in an unselected group of consecutive patients with AF requiring demand pacing. A prospective crossover study design was used to evaluate single- and dual-site right atrial pacing modes. The frequency of AF during 3 months after pacemaker implantation was analyzed. Consecutive consenting patients underwent insertion of 2 atrial leads and 1 ventricular lead with a DDDR pulse generator. Patients were placed in a dual-site pacing mode for the first 3 minutes and subsequently, mode-switched to single-site pacing for 3 minutes. Mode switching was repeated at 6-month intervals thereafter. They showed that atrial pacing resulted in a marked decline in recurrences of atrial fibrillation. During dual-site pacing with an optimal drug regimen, there was no AF recurrence in any patient, compared with 5 recurrences in 12 patients during single-site pacing. The mean arrhythmia-free interval before pacing (14 days) was prolonged with dual- (89 days) and single-site pacing (76 days). Symptomatic episodes of AF showed a declining trend during dual- and single-site pacing compared with those during the pre-implantation period. Mean anti-arrhythmic drug use for all classes declined from an average of 4 drugs before implantation to 1.5 drugs after implantation. Twelve (80%) of 15 patients remained in an atrial-paced rhythm for an average of 13 months. These authors concluded that multi-site right atrial pacing is feasible, effective, and safe for long-term application. Atrial pacing significantly prolonged arrhythmia-free intervals in patients with drug-refractory paroxysmal AF. Dual-site right atrial pacing may offer additional benefits and should be considered either as the primary mode or in patients unresponsive to single-site pacing.

Cardioversion in the Elderly

Carlsson and associates[52] for the ALKK-Study Group investigated cardioversion success rate, frequency of complications of cardioversion, and current treatment practices in patients aged 65 years or older with AF, and compared these results with those in patients younger than 65 years. The investigation was a prospective multicenter observational study with 61 participating cardiology clinics. Consecutive patients in whom cardioversion of AF was planned had to be prospectively registered. Of 1,152 patients registered, 570 (49.5%) were younger than 65 years (group 1), and 582 (50.5%) were aged 65 years or older. (group 2). The overall success rate of cardioversion on an intention-to-treat basis was 76.1% in group 1 and 72.7% in group 2. In multivariate analysis, left atrial size and New York Heart Association functional class before cardioversion were identified as predictors of success, respectively. These clinical factors were not equally distributed between the age groups: LA size was larger in the elderly than in younger patients (44.0 ± 6.4 mm vs. 42.8 ± 6.4 mm); and a New York Heart Association functional class of II or higher was more prevalent in group 2 than in group 1 (48.6% vs. 29.6%). The overall complication rates were not significantly different between the 2 groups (4.2% in group 1 vs. 5.3% in group 2). The frequency of patients who were adequately anticoagulated for cardioversion was 56.9% in age group 1 and 39.6% in age group 2. In chronic AF, the same trend for age-dependent underuse of anticoagulation was observed. Age itself was not a predictor of cardioversion success and did not predispose to higher complication rates. Therefore, cardioversion should be considered in older patients with the same criteria and emphasis as in younger patients. Anticoagulation and antithrombotic medication is underused for cardioversion and in treating chronic AF, especially in elderly patients.

Autonomic Blockade and β-Adrenergic Stimulation Effects of Ventricular Rate

Strickberger and colleagues[53] determined the effects of slow-pathway ablation on ventricular rate in AF during autonomic blockade and sympathetic stimulation in patients with AV nodal reentrant tachycardia. Thirty-five patients underwent slow-pathway radiofrequency ablation for AV nodal reentrant tachycardia and were assigned to autonomic blockade with propranolol and atropine or isoproterenol. AF was induced before and after slow-pathway radiofrequency ablation. During autonomic blockade, the mean ventricular cycle length and maximum ventricular cycle length were prolonged after ablation, whereas the minimum ventricular cycle length did not change significantly. During isoproterenol infusion, the mean ventricular cycle length, maximal ventricular cycle length, and minimum ventricular cycle length did not change significantly after slow-pathway ablation. Thus, slow-pathway ablations slow the ventricular rate during AF under conditions of autonomic blockade, but not during sympathetic stimulation. Therefore, slow-pathway ablation alone cannot account for the clinical results obtained with radiofrequency modification of AV conduction in patients with AF (Figures 6-21, 6-22).

Slow Pathway Ablation

Kreiner and colleagues[54] investigated whether selective ablation of the posterior AV nodal input can provide a sufficient reduction in heart rate during

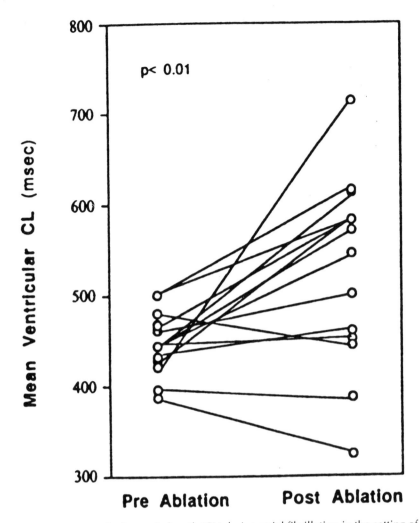

FIGURE 6-21. Mean ventricular cycle length (CL) during atrial fibrillation in the setting of autonomic blockade before and after slow-pathway ablation. Reproduced with permission from Strickberger et al.[53]

atrial fibrillation in 30 patients with AV nodal reentrant tachycardia. Conduction properties of AV nodal pathway were determined before and after slow pathway ablation. AF was induced by burst pacing at baseline and after ablation, and the mean ventricular cycle length was determined. After slow pathway ablation, the mean ventricular cycle length during atrial fibrillation increased from 449 to 515 msec, a highly significant change. At baseline, the mean ventricular cycle length correlated with the Wenckebach cycle length of both the slow and fast pathways. After ablation, the mean ventricular cycle length was determined by the Wenckebach cycle length of the fast pathway. The slope of the regression line was significantly steeper compared with baseline, thereby illustrating that the reduction in ventricular rate was not as evident if the fast pathway had a short Wenckebach cycle length. These data indicate that selec-

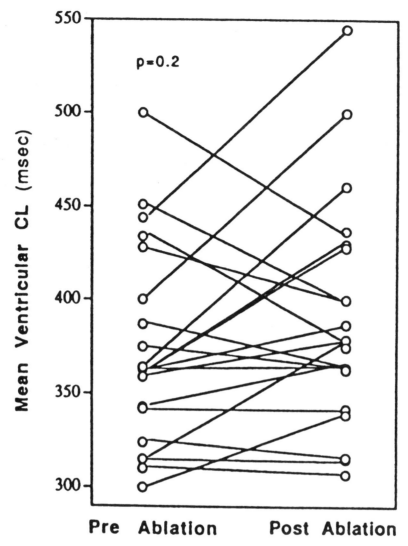

FIGURE 6-22. Mean ventricular cycle length (CL) during atrial fibrillation in the setting of sympathetic stimulation before and after slow-pathway ablation. Reproduced with permission from Strickberger et al.[53]

tive elimination of the slow pathway reduces ventricular rate in patients with atrial fibrillation. However, in patients with a short Wenckebach cycle length of anterior AV nodal input that causes a more rapid atrial fibrillation, this effect may be insufficient to provide adequate control of heart rate.

Diltiazem

Blackshear and associates[55] from several United States and Canadian medical centers tested whether patients presenting with AF or atrial flutter with a rapid ventricular response could maintain control of heart rate while transferring from a bolus and continuous infusion of intravenous diltiazem to oral diltiazem. Forty patients with AF or atrial flutter and a sustained ventricular rate of 120 beats per minute or greater received intravenous diltiazem "bolus" (20 to 25 mg for 2 minutes) and "infusion" (5 to 15 mg/h for 6 to 20 hours). Oral long-acting diltiazem (diltiazem CD 180, 300, or 360 mg/24 hours) was administered in patients in whom stable heart rate control was attained during constant infusion. Intravenous diltiazem infusion was discontinued 4 hours after the first oral dose, and patients were monitored during 48 subsequent hours of "transition" to oral therapy. Response to diltiazem was defined as heart rate of less than 100 beats per minute, a 20% or greater decrease in heart rate from baseline, or conversion to sinus rhythm. Other rate control or antiarrhythmic medications were not allowed during the study period. Thirty-seven of 40 patients maintained heart rate control during the bolus, and 35 of the remaining 37 maintained control during the infusion of intravenous diltiazem. Of the 35 patients achieving heart rate control with intravenous diltiazem who entered the transition to oral therapy, 27 maintained heart rate control (response rate of 77%, 95% confidence interval, 63% to 91%). The median infusion rate of intravenous diltiazem was 10 mg/hour, and the median dose of oral diltiazem CD was 300 mg/day. Oral, long-acting diltiazem was 77% effective in controlling ventricular response over 48 hours in patients with AF or atrial flutter in whom ventricular response was initially controlled with intravenous diltiazem.

Ibutilide

Stambler and colleagues[56] in West Roxbury, Massachusetts, determined the efficacy and safety of repeated doses of intravenous ibutilide, a class III antiarrhythmic drug, in terminating atrial fibrillation or flutter in 266 patients with sustained AF (n = 133) or flutter (n = 133) with an arrhythmia duration of 3 hours to 45 days. They were randomized to receive up to 2 10-minute infusions, separated by 10 minutes of ibutilide (1.0 and 0.5 mg or 1.0 and 1.0 mg) or placebo. The conversion rate was 47% after ibutilide and 2% after placebo (Figure 6-23). The 2 ibutilide dosing regimens did not differ in conversion efficacy (44% and 49%, respectively). Efficacy was higher in atrial flutter than in fibrillation (63% vs. 31%). In patients with atrial fibrillation but not flutter, conversion rates were higher with a shorter arrhythmia duration or a normal LA size. Arrhythmia termination occurred a mean of 27 minutes after the start of the infusion. Among 180 ibutilide-treated patients, 15 (8%) developed polymorphic VT during or soon after the infusion. The arrhythmia required cardioversion in 3 patients and was nonsustained in 12. Thus, intravenous ibutilide given in repeated doses is effective in terminating atrial fibrillation and flutter and is an alternative to cardioversion options in some patients.

Amiodarone

Amiodarone is an effective antiarrhythmic agent with activity in both supraventricular and ventricular tachyarrhythmias. Galve and colleagues[57] from

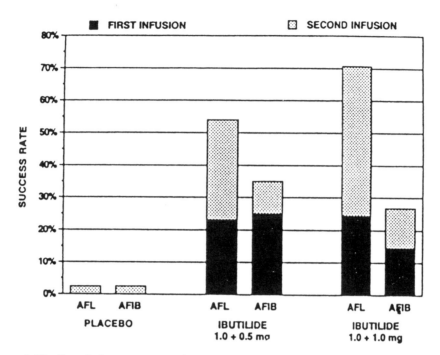

FIGURE 6-23. Cumulative percentage of patients converting after two infusions of placebo, 1.0 mg/0.5 mg ibutilide or 1.0 mg/1.0 mg ibutilide, in patients with atrial flutter (AFL) or atrial fibrillation (AFIB). Conversion efficacy was significantly higher after ibutilide than after placebo (p<.0001) and was higher in AFL than in AFIB (p<.0001) but did not differ significantly between the 2 ibutilide dosing regimens. Reproduced with permission from Stambler et al.[56]

Barcelona, Spain, evaluated the efficacy of intravenous amiodarone in the management of recent onset AF. One hundred consecutive patients with recent onset (<1 week) AF who were not taking antiarrhythmic agents were randomized to receive either intravenous amiodarone (5 mg/kg in 30 minutes followed by 1200 mg over 24 hours) or an identical amount of saline. Both groups received intravenous digoxin (0.5 mg initially, followed by .25 mg at 2 hours and .25 mg every 6 hours to complete 24 hours while the ventricular rate was >100 beats per minute). At the end of 24 hours, 68% in the amiodarone group and 60% in the control group had returned to sinus rhythm. Amiodarone was associated with a slower ventricular rate (82 beats per minute) than the rate in the control group (91 beats per minute). After restoration of sinus rhythm, AF recurred during the 15-day follow-up period in 12% of the amiodarone group versus 10% of the control group. These authors concluded that, at the doses used in this study, there was not a significant benefit of intravenous amiodarone in converting acute AF to sinus rhythm.

1. Pitzalis MV, Mastropasqua F, Massari F, Totaro P, Di Maggio M, Rizzon P. Holter-guided identification of premature ventricular contractions susceptible to suppression by β-blockers. Am Heart J 1996 (March);131:508–515.
2. Peters RW, McQuillan S, Resnick SK, Gold MR. Increased Monday incidence of

life-threatening ventricular arrhythmias. Experience with a third-generation implantable defibrillator. Circulation 1996 (September 15);1346–1349.

3. Zaim S, Zaim B, Rottman J, Mendoza I, Nasir N Jr, Pacifico A. Characterization of spontaneous recurrent ventricular arrhythmias detected by electrogram-storing defibrillators in sudden cardiac death survivors with no inducible ventricular arrhythmias at baseline electrophysiologic testing. Am Heart J 1996 (August);132: 274–279.

4. Kerber RE, Kieso RA, Kienzle MG, Olshansky B, Waldo AL, Carlson MD, Wilber DJ, Aschoff AM, Birger S, Charbonnier F: Current-based transthoracic defibrillation. Am J Cardiol (November 15) 1996;78:1113–1118.

5. Doval HC, Nul DR, Grancelli HO, Varini SD, Soifer S, Corrado G, Dubner S, Scapin O, Perrone SV, for the GESICA-GEMA Investigators. Nonsustained ventricular tachycardia in severe heart failure. Independent marker of increased mortality due to sudden death. Circulation 1996 (December 15);94:3198–3203.

6. Gorgels APM, van den Dool A, Hofs A, Mulleneers R, Smeets JLRM, Vos MA, Wellens HJJ: Comparison of procainamide and lidocaine in terminating sustained monomorphic ventricular tachycardia. Am J Cardiol 1996 (July 1);78:43–46.

7. Movsowitz C, Schwartzman D, Callans DJ, Preminger M, Zado E, Gottlieb CD, Marchlinski FE. Idiopathic right ventricular outflow tract tachycardia: Narrowing the anatomic location for successful ablation. Am Heart J 1996 (May);131:930–936.

8. Lee RJ, Wong M, Sisu A, Namekawa-Wong M, Epstein LM, Fitzpatrick AP, Grogi HR, Scheinman MM, Lesh MD. Long-term results of electrophysiologically guided sotalol therapy for life-threatening ventricular arrhythmias. Am Heart J 1996 (November);132:973–978.

9. Böcker D, Haverkamp W, Block M, Borggrefe M, Hammel D, Breithardt G. Comparison of d,l-sotalol and implantable defibrillators for treatment of sustained ventricular tachycardia or fibrillation in patients with coronary artery disease. Circulation 1996 (July 15);94:151–157.

10. Podrid PJ, Anderson JL, for the Propafenone Multicenter Study Group: Safety and tolerability of long-term propafenone therapy for supraventricular tachyarrhythmias. Am J Cardiol 1996 (August 15);78:430–434.

11. Levine JH, Massumi A, Scheinman MM, Winkle RA, Platia EV, Chilson DA, Gomes JA, Woosley RL: Intravenous amiodarone for recurrent sustained hypotensive ventricular tachyarrhythmias. J Am Coll Cardiol 1996 (January);27:67–75.

12. Hallstrom AP, Cobb LA, Yu BH. Influence of comorbidity on the outcome of patients treated for out-of-hospital ventricular fibrillation. Circulation 1996 (June 1);93: 2019–2022.

13. Lehmann MH, Hardy S, Archibald D, Quart B, MacNeil DJ. Sex difference in risk of torsades de pointes with d,l-sotalol. Circulation 1996 (November 15);94:2535–2541.

14. Sheldon R, Rose S, Flanagan P, Koshman ML, Killam S. Risk factors for syncope recurrence after a positive tilt-table test in patients with syncope. Circulation 1996 (March 1);93:973–981.

15. Compton SJ, Lux RL, Ramsey MR, Strelich KR, Sanguinetti MC, Green LS, Keating MT, Mason JW. Genetically defined therapy of inherited long-QT syndrome. Correction of abnormal repolarization by potassium. Circulation 1996 (September 1);94: 1018–1022.

16. Pratt CM, Ruberg S, Morganroth J, McNutt B, Woodward J, Harris S, Ruskin J, Moye L. Dose-response relation between terfenadine (Seldane) and the QTc interval on the scalar electrocardiogram: Distinguishing a drug effect from spontaneous variability. Am Heart J 1996 (March);131:472–480.

17. Bernstein AD, Parsonnet V: Survey of cardiac pacing and defibrillation in the United States in 1993. Am J Cardiol 1996 (July 15);78:187–196.

18. Villacastín J, Almendral J, Arenal A, Albertos J, Ormaetxe J, Peinado R, Bueno H, Merino JL, Pastor A, Medina O, Tercedor L, Jiménez F, Delcán JL: Incidence and clinical significance of multiple consecutive, appropriate, high-energy discharges in patients with implanted cardioverter-defibrillators. Circulation 1996 (February); 93:753–762.

19. Natale A, Sra J, Axtell K, Akhtar M, Newby K, Kent V, Geiger MJ, Brandon MJ,

Kearney MM, Pacifico A: Undetected ventricular fibrillation in transvenous implantable cardioverter-defibrillators. Prospective comparison of different lead system-device combinations. Circulation 1996 (January);93:91–98.

20. Li H, Axtell K, Biehl M, Deshpande S, Dhala A, Blanck Z, Sra J, Jazayeri M, Akhtar M: Sudden death in patients with implantable cardioverter-defibrillators. Am Heart J 1996 (November);132:986–988.

21. Levine JH, Waller T, Hoch D, Greenberg S, Goldberger J, Kadish A: Implantable cardioverter defibrillator: Use in patients with no symptoms and at high risk. Am Heart J 1996 (January);131:59–65.

22. Wever EFD, Hauer RNW, Schrijvers G, van Capelle FJL, Tijssen JGP, Crijns HJGM, Algra A, Ramanna H, Bakker PFA, Robles de Medina EO: Cost-effectiveness of implantable defibrillator as first-choice therapy versus electrophysiologically guided, tiered strategy in postinfarct sudden death survivors. A randomized study. Circulation 1996 (February);93:489–496.

23. Kim SG, Pathapati R, Fisher JD, Rameneni A, Nagabhairu R, Ferrick KJ, Roth JA, Ben-Zur U, Gross J, Brodman R, Furman S: Comparison of long-term outcomes of patients treated with nonthoracotomy and thoracotomy implantable defibrillators. Am J Cardiol 1996 (November 15);78:1109–1112.

24. Moss AJ, Hall WJ, Cannom DS, Daubert JP, Higgins SL, Klein H, Levine JH, Saksena S, Waldo AL, Wilber D, Brown MW, Heo M, for the Multicenter Automatic Defibrillator Implantation Trial Investigators. Improved survival with an implanted defibrillator in patients with coronary disease at high risk for ventricular arrhythmia. N Engl J Med 1996 (December 26);335:1933–40.

25. Bubien RS, Knotts-Dolson SM, Plumb VJ, Kay GN: Effect of radiofrequency catheter ablation on health-related quality of life and activities of daily living in patients with recurrent arrhythmias. Circulation 1996 (October 1);94:1585–1591.

26. Poty H, Saoudi N, Haissaguerre M, Daou A, Clementy J, Letac B: Radiofrequency catheter ablation of atrial tachycardias. Am Heart J 1996 (March);131:481–489.

27. Chen SA, Chiang CE, Tai CT, Cheng CC, Chiou CW, Lee SH, Ueng KC, Wen ZC, Chang MS: Complications of diagnostic electrophysiologic studies and radiofrequency catheter ablation in patients with tachyarrhythmias: An eight-year survey of 3,966 consecutive procedures in a tertiary referral center. Am J Cardiol 1996 (January 1);77:41–1946.

28. Cappato R, Schlüter M, Weiß C, Antz M, Koschyk DH, Hofmann T, Kuck K-H: Radiofrequency current catheter ablation of accessory atrioventricular pathways in Ebstein's anomaly. Circulation 1996 (August 1);94:376–383.

29. Goyal R, Zivin A, Souza J, Shaikh SA, Harvey M, Bogun F, Daoud E, Man KC, Strickberger SA, Morady F: Comparison of the ages of tachycardia onset in patients with atrioventricular nodal reentrant tachycardia and accessory pathway-mediated tachycardia. Am Heart J 1996 (October);132:765–767.

30. Kuo C-T, Lauer MR, Young C, Hou CJ, Liem LB, Yu J, Sung RJ: Electrophysiologic significance of discrete slow potentials in dual atrioventricular node physiology: Implications for selective radiofrequency ablation of slow pathway conduction. Am Heart J 1996 (March);131:490–498.

31. Bogun F, Daoud E, Goyal R, Harvey M, Knight B, Weiss R, Bahu M, Man KC, Strickberger SA, Morady F: Comparison of atrial-His intervals in patients with and without dual atrioventricular nodal physiology and atrioventricular nodal reentrant tachycardia. Am Heart J 1996 (October);132:758–764.

32. King A, Wen M-S, Yeh S-J. Wang C-C, Lin F-C, Wu D: Catheter-induced atrioventricular nodal block during radiofrequency ablation. Am Heart J 1996 (November); 132:979–985.

33. Fahy GJ, Pinski SL, Miller DP, McCabe N, Pye C, Walsh MJ, Robinson K: Natural history of isolated BBB. Am J Cardiol 1996 (June 1);77:1185–1190.

34. Vaduganathan P, He ZX, Raghavan C, Marmarian JJ, Verani MS: Detection of left anterior descending coronary artery stenosis in patients with left BBB: Exercise, adenosine or dobutamine imaging? J Am Coll Cardiol 1996 (September);28: 543–550.

35. Sgarbossa EB, Pinski SL, Barbagelata A, Underwood DA, Gates KB, Topol EJ, Califf

RM, Wagner GS, for the GUSTO-1 (Global Utilization of Streptokinase and Tissue Plasminogen Activator for Occluded Coronary Arteries) Investigators. Electrocardiographic diagnosis of evolving acute myocardial infarction in the presence of left bundle-branch block. N Engl J Med 1996 (February 22);334:481–487.

36. Naegeli B, Osswald S, Deola M, Burkart F: Intermittent pacemaker dysfunction caused by digital mobile telephones. J Am Coll Cardiol 1996 (May);27:1471–1477.

37. Albert CM, McGovern BA, Newell JB, Ruskin JN: Sex differences in cardiac arrest survivors. Circulation 1996 (March 15);93:1170–1176.

38. Maron BJ, Poliac LC, Roberts WO: Risk for sudden cardiac death associated with marathon running. J Am Coll Cardiol 1996 (August);28:428–431.

39. Frishman WH, Heiman M, Karpenos A, Ooi WL, Mitzner A, Goldkorn R, Greenberg S: Twenty-four-hour ambulatory electrocardiography in elderly subjects: Prevalence of various arrhythmias and prognostic implications (report from the Bronx Longitudinal Aging Study). Am Heart J 1996 (August);132:297–302.

40. Huikuri HV, Pikkujämsä SM, Airaksinen KEJ, Ikäheimo MJ, Rantala AO, Kauma H, Lilja M, Kesäniemi YA: Sex-related differences in autonomic modulation of heart rate in middle-aged subjects. Circulation 1996 (July 15);94:122–125.

41. Wolf PA, Benjamin EJ, Belanger AJ, Kannel WB, Levy D, D'Agostino RB: Secular trends in the prevalence of atrial fibrillation: The Framingham study. Am Heart J 1996 (April);131:790–795.

42. Grimm RA, Chandra S, Klein AL, Stewart WJ, Black IW, Kidwell GA, Thomas JD: Characterization of left atrial appendage Doppler flow in atrial fibrillation and flutter by Fourier analysis. Am Heart J 1996 (August);132:286–296.

43. Hundley WG, Meshack BM, Willett DL, Sayad DE, Lange RA, Willard JE, Landau C, Hillis LD, Peshock RM: Comparison of quantitation of left ventricular volume, ejection fraction, and cardiac output in patients with atrial fibrillation by cine MRI versus invasive measurements. Am J Cardiol 1996 (November 15);78:1119–1123.

44. Fatkin D, Feneley MP: Patterns of Doppler-measured blood flow velocity in the normal and fibrillating human left atrial appendage. Am Heart J 1996 (November);132:995–1003.

45. Aranki SF, Shaw DP, Adams DH, Rizzo RJ, Couper GS, VanderVliet M, Collins JJ Jr., Cohn LH, Burstin HR: Predictors of atrial fibrillation after coronary artery surgery: Current trends and impact on hospital resources. Circulation 1996 (August 1);94:390–397.

46. Crijns HJGM, Van Gelder IC, Van der Woude HJ, Grandjean JG, Tieleman RG, Brügemann J, De Kam PJ, Ebels T: Efficacy of serial electrical cardioversion therapy in patients with chronic atrial fibrillation after valve replacement and implications for surgery to cure atrial fibrillation. Am J Cardiol 1996 (November 15);78:1140–1144.

47. Kalman JM, Olgin JE, Saxon LA, Fisher WG, Lee RJ, Lesh MD: Activation and entrainment mapping defines the tricuspid annulus as the anterior barrier in typical atrial flutter. Circulation 1996 (August 1);94:398–406.

48. Chen SA, Chiang CE, Wu TJ, Tai CT, Lee SH, Cheng CC, Chiou CW, Ueng KC, Wen ZC, Chang MS: Radiofrequency catheter ablation of common atrial flutter: Comparison of electrophysiologically guided focal ablation technique and linear ablation technique. J Am Coll Cardiol 1996 (March 15);27:860–868.

49. Cauchemez B, Haissaguerre M, Fischer B, Thomas O, Clementy J, Coumel P: Electrophysiological effects of catheter ablation of inferior vena cava-tricuspid annulus isthmus in common atrial flutter. Circulation 1996 (January);93:284–294.

50. Daoud EG, Pariseau B, Niebauer M, Bogun F, Goyal R, Harvey M, Man KC, Strickberger SA, Morady F: Response of type I atrial fibrillation to atrial pacing in humans. Circulation 1996 (September 1);94:1036–1040.

51. Saksena S, Prakash A, Hill M, Krol RB, Munsif AN, Mathew PP, Mehra R: Prevention of recurrent atrial fibrillation with chronic dual-site atrial pacing. J Am Col Cardiol 1996 (September);28:687–694.

52. Carlsson J, Tebbe U, Rox J, Harmjanz D, Haeten K, Neuhaus K-L, Seidel F, Niederer W, Miketić S, for the ALKK-Study Group: Cardioversion of atrial fibrillation in the elderly. Am J Cardiol 1996 (December 15);78:1380–1384.

53. Strickberger SA, Weiss R, Daoud EG, Goyal R, Bogun F, Man KC, Morady F: Ventricular rate during atrial fibrillation before and after slow-pathway ablation. Effects of autonomic blockade and β-adrenergic stimulation. Circulation 1996 (September 1);94:1023–1026.

54. Kreiner G, Heinz G, Siostrzonek P, Gössinger HD: Effect of slow pathway ablation on ventricular rate during atrial fibrillation. Dependence on electrophysiological properties of the fast pathway. Circulation 1996 (January);93:277–283.

55. Blackshear JL, Stambler BS, Strauss WE, Roy D, Dias VC, Beach CL, Ebener MK: Control of heart rate during transition from intravenous to oral *diltiazem* in atrial fibrillation or flutter. Am J Cardiol 1996 (December 1);78:1246–1250.

56. Stambler BS, Wood MA, Ellenbogen KA, Perry KT, Wakefield LK, VanderLugt JT, and the Ibutilide Repeat Dose Study Investigators: Efficacy and safety of repeated intravenous doses of ibutilide for rapid conversion of atrial flutter or fibrillation. Circulation 1996 (October 1);94:1613–1621.

57. Galve E, Ruis T, Ballester R, Artaza MA, Arnau JM, Garcia-Dorado D, Soler-Soler J: Intravenous amiodarone in treatment of recent-onset atrial fibrillation: Results of a randomized, controlled study. J Am Coll Cardiol 1996 (April);27:1079–1082.

7

Peripheral Vascular Disease

Deep Venous Thrombosis

Risk Factors in the Elderly

Peripheral vascular disease as measured by the ankle-brachial blood pressure index is associated with increased risk of mortality and morbidity. Few sources of data on the relation of risk factors to ankle-brachial blood pressure are available for the elderly, especially those older than 80 years of age and those in minority populations. Curb and coworkers[1] in Honolulu, Hawaii, examined the ankle-brachial blood pressure measurements from the Honolulu Heart Program for reexamination of 3450 ambulatory, elderly Japanese-American men. The study indicated the prevalence of an abnormal ankle-brachial index (defined as a ratio less than 0.9) was 14%, increasing from 8% in those 71 to 74 years of age to 27% in those 85 to 93 years of age. Associations that were U- or J-shaped were present for a number of risk factors in those in the lowest and highest risk factors in a cross-sectional analysis. Risk factors measured at baseline were also predictive of an abnormal ankle-brachial blood pressure index 25 years later, even after adjustment for multiple risk factors. The odds ratio for an ankle-brachial blood pressure index less than 0.9 at the 80th percentile of cholesterol compared with that at the 20th percentile was 1.4; the odds ratio for a 1-hour post-load glucose was 1.3 and for alcohol intake, 1.2. The odds ratio associated with hypertension was 1.8 and that for smoking, 2.9. These findings are consistent with ankle-brachial blood pressure index being a marker for generalized atherosclerotic disease in old and very old Japanese-American men.

Hyperhomocysteinemia as a Risk Factor

den Heijer and colleagues[2] in The Hague, The Netherlands, assessed the risk of venous thrombosis associated with hyperhomocysteinemia by studying homocysteine levels in patients with a first episode of deep-vein thrombosis and in normal control subjects. They measured plasma homocysteine levels in 269 patients with a first, diagnosed episode of deep-vein thrombosis and in 269 healthy controls matched to the patients according to age and sex. Hyperhomocysteinemia was defined as a plasma homocysteine level above the 95th percentile in the control group, i.e., 18.5 μmol/L. Among the 269 patients, 28 (10%) had plasma homocysteine levels above the 95th percentile as compared with 13% (5%) in the control group. The association between elevated plasma homocysteine levels and venous thrombosis was stronger among women than among men and increased with age. The exclusion of subjects with other established risk factors for thrombosis, including deficiencies of protein C, protein S, or antithrombin, resistance to activated protein C, pregnancy or recent childbirth, or oral-contraceptive use did not substantially affect the risk estimates described above. Thus, high plasma homocysteine levels are a risk factor for deep-vein thrombosis.

Epidemiological Characteristics, Management, and Outcome in a Tertiary-Care Hospital

Entry into clinical trials of treatment for deep venous thrombosis involves a screening process that excludes many patients with this condition. Therefore, to obtain a profile of patients with deep venous thrombosis that reflects actual day-to-day clinical practice, Piccioli and associates[3] from Padua, Italy, and Boston, Massachusetts, initiated a prospective registry of 150 consecutive patients with deep venous thrombosis at Brigham and Women's Hospital, Boston. They reviewed the medical records of all patients who received a diagnosis of deep venous thrombosis from November 1, 1994, through March 31, 1995, and did not exclude any patients. Of the 150 patients, 120 (80%) were symptomatic and 30 (20%) were asymptomatic. Frequent baseline characteristics included surgery within the preceding 6 months (47%), cancer (26%), and previous venous thromboembolism (23%). Deep venous thrombosis was diagnosed by ultrasonography (n=145), contrast venography (n=3), or clinical evaluation (in 2 patients who had technically unsatisfactory ultrasound results). Overall, 133 (89%) patients received anticoagulation; 5 (3%) received thrombolysis; and 27 (18%) underwent placement of an inferior vena caval filter. In 3 patients, major hemorrhage developed from anticoagulation or thrombolysis. The 3-month mortality rate was 19%, including 10 patients who died during the index hospitalization. In no case was pulmonary embolism thought to be the cause of death. Ten patients had recurrent venous thrombosis during the initial 3 months after diagnosis. The most surprising findings in the deep venous thrombosis registry were the high rates of cancer and surgery, the high rate of filter placement, and the high mortality rate. These registry results differ substantially from findings in randomized controlled trials of deep venous thrombosis treatment.

Intravenous Heparin versus Low-Molecular-Weight Heparin

Koopman and colleagues[4] in Amsterdam, The Netherlands, randomly assigned patients to adjusted-dose intravenous standard heparin in the hospital (n = 198 patients) or fixed-dose subcutaneous low molecular weight heparin administered at home when feasible (n = 202 patients) in the treatment of patients with deep-vein thrombosis. They compared the treatments with respect to recurrent venous thromboembolism, major bleeding, quality of life, and costs. Seventeen of the 198 patients who received standard heparin (8.6%) and 14 of the 202 patients who received low molecular weight heparin (6.9%) had recurrent thromboembolism. Major bleeding occurred in 4 patients assigned to standard heparin (2%) and 1 patient assigned to low molecular weight heparin (0.5%). Quality of life improved in both groups. Physical activity and social functioning were better in the patients assigned to low molecular weight heparin. Among the patients in that group, 36% were not admitted to the hospital and 40% were discharged early. The subcutaneous administration of low molecular weight heparin was associated with a mean reduction in hospital days of 67%, ranging from 29% to 86% in the various study centers. Thus, in patients with proximal vein thrombosis, treatment with low-molecular-weight heparin at home is feasible, effective, and safe.

Low-Molecular-Weight Heparin at Home versus Unfractionated Heparin in the Hospital

Levine and colleagues[5] in Canada compared hospital-administered intravenous standard (unfractionated) heparin with the low molecular weight heparin given subcutaneously and usually at home in the treatment of patients with acute proximal deep-vein thrombosis. These patients were randomly assigned to receive either intravenous standard heparin in the hospital (n = 253) or low molecular weight heparin (enoxaparin, 1 mg/kg/body weight subcutaneously, twice daily) administered primarily at home (n = 247 patients). The study design allowed outpatients taking low molecular weight heparin to go home immediately and hospitalized patients taking low molecular weight heparin to be discharged early. All the patients received warfarin starting on the second day. Thirteen of the 247 patients receiving low molecular weight heparin (5%) had recurrent thromboembolism, as compared with 17 of the 253 patients receiving standard heparin (6.7%). Five patients receiving low molecular weight heparin had major bleeding, as compared with 3 patients receiving standard heparin. After randomization, the patients who received low molecular weight heparin spent a mean of 1.1 days in the hospital as compared with 6.5 days for the standard heparin group. One hundred and twenty patients in the low molecular weight heparin group did not need to be hospitalized. Thus, low molecular weight heparin can be used safely and effectively to treat patients with proximal deep-vein thrombosis at home.

Bolus Recombinant Urokinase versus Heparin

Bolus urokinase is effective for initial treatment of deep venous thrombosis but is associated with a high rate of rigors. This randomized controlled trial by Goldhaber and associates[6] from Boston, Massachusetts, was undertaken among patients with deep venous thrombosis to evaluate the efficacy and safety of a novel thrombolytic agent, recombinant urokinase, administered as 3 bolus infusions of 1 million U over a 24-hour period versus heparin alone. Of 361 patients with deep venous thrombosis screened, 17 (5%) were enrolled. Recent surgery was the most common reason for exclusion (n=113, 31%). Images of the patients were obtained at baseline, 24 to 48 hours after randomization, and before hospital discharge. Two patients in each treatment group had minor clot progression. One patient in the heparin group had no change; all other patients showed mild (<50%; n=5 in each group) or moderate (>50%; n=1 in each group) improvement. No bleeding complications or rigors developed in patients randomly assigned to recombinant urokinase. Mean bleeding times among patients given recombinant urokinase were not significantly different from mean values of patients given heparin at any of the measured time points available for comparison (331 vs. 387 seconds at baseline and 381 vs. 416 seconds at 24 hours). However, mean fibrinogen levels declined with successive urokinase boluses and were significantly lower than levels in patients treated with heparin at 24 (233 mg/dL vs. 466 mg/dL) and 48 hours (270 mg/dL vs. 474 mg/dL). Although bolus recombinant urokinase had a favorable safety profile, recombinant urokinase was no more effective than heparin in achieving clot lysis at the doses used in this trial.

Low Molecular Weight Heparin after Hip Replacement

Prevention of Thromboembolism after Hip Replacement

Bergqvist and colleagues[7] determined whether 1 month of anticoagulant therapy with the low molecular weight heparin enoxaparin is more effective than enoxaparin therapy given only during the hospitalization for surgery. Two hundred and sixty-two patients undergoing total hip replacement received enoxaparin during their hospitalizations during an average stay of 10 to 11 days. They were randomly assigned to receive enoxaparin or placebo (131 patients each). Blinded outpatient therapy (or placebo) was continued long enough that the total treatment period, inpatient plus outpatient, was 1 month for each patient. Bilateral ascending phlebography was performed 19 to 23 days after discharge, with deep-vein thrombosis as the primary end point. Distal and proximal thrombosis, pulmonary embolism, and hemorrhage were also recorded, as were deaths. Venography was adequate in 116 patients in the placebo group and 117 in the enoxaparin group. The authors observed 43 episodes of deep-vein thrombosis and 2 episodes of pulmonary embolism in the placebo group, but only 21 episodes of deep-vein thrombosis and no episodes of pulmonary embolism in the enoxaparin group for an incidence of thromboembolism of 39% and 18%, respectively, p<.001. The difference in incidence of proximal deep-vein thrombosis was also significant (24% and 7% in the placebo and enoxaparin groups, respectively, p<.001). Six patients in the enoxaparin group and 1 patient in the placebo group had hematomas at their injection sites. No patients died or had major complications. Thus, there were significantly fewer venous thromboembolic complications in patients undergoing elective hip replacement when prophylaxis with enoxaparin was given for a total of 1 month rather than only during the hospitalization.

Gent and colleagues[8] in Hamilton, Ontario, Canada, determined the relative efficacy and safety of a low molecular weight heparinoid (orgaran) compared with aspirin for the prevention of postoperative venous thromboembolism in patients undergoing surgery for hip fracture. A double-blind randomized, controlled trial was used to study 251 consecutive eligible and consenting patients undergoing surgery for hip fracture in 7 participating hospitals. In this study, patients received either fixed-dose orgaran by subcutaneous injection (every 12 hours) or aspirin (100 mg orally, twice daily). Both regimens were begun 12 to 24 hours after surgery and continued for 14 days or until discharge, if discharge was sooner. All patients had postoperative ^{125}I-fibrinogen leg scanning and impedance plethysmography. If the results of 1 or both tests were positive, then venography was performed. Venography was done at day 14, or sooner, if the patient was ready for discharge. Pulmonary embolism in symptomatic patients was diagnosed on the basis of a high probability perfusion/ventilation lung scan, a positive angiogram, or a clinically significant embolism detected at autopsy. Venograms were obtained in 90 of the 125 patients randomly assigned to receive orgaran and 87 of the 126 patients assigned to receive aspirin. Venous thromboembolism was detected in 25 patients in the orgaran group (28%) and in 39 (44%) of the patients in the aspirin group. This represented a relative risk reduction of 37% with orgaran. Six of 88 patients in the orgaran group and 12 of 84 in the aspirin group developed proximal deep-vein thrombosis or pulmonary embolism; this represented a relative risk reduction of 52% with orgaran. Hemorrhagic complications occurred in 2 patients given orgaran and 8 given aspirin. There was 1 major bleed in the orgaran group compared with 4 in the aspirin group. These data suggest that orgaran is significantly more efficacious than aspirin in treating postoperative venous thromboembolism in patients undergoing surgery for hip fractures.

After Major Trauma

Geerts and colleagues[9] compared low-dose heparin and a low molecular weight heparin with regard to efficacy and safety in a randomized clinical trial in patients with major trauma at a high risk for venous thromboembolism. Consecutive adult patients admitted to a trauma center who had Injury Severity Scores of at least 9 and no intracranial bleeding were randomly assigned to heparin (5000 U) or enoxaparin (30 mg), each given subcutaneously every 12 hours in a double-blind manner, beginning 36 hours after their injury. The primary outcome was deep-vein thrombosis as assessed by contrast venography performed on or before day 14 after randomization. Among 344 randomized patients, 136 who received low-dose heparin and 129 who received enoxaparin had venograms adequate for analysis. Sixty patients given heparin (44%) and 40 patients given enoxaparin (31%) had deep-vein thrombosis (p = .014).

The rates of proximal-vein thrombosis were 15% and 6%, respectively (p = .01). The reductions in risk with enoxaparin as compared with heparin were 30% for all deep-vein thrombosis and 58% for proximal-vein thrombosis. Only six patients had major bleeding, 1 in the heparin group and 5 in the enoxaparin group, p = NS. Thus, low molecular weight heparin was more effective than low-dose heparin in preventing venous thromboembolism after major trauma, and both interventions were safe.

Long-Term Follow-Up of Clinical and Hemodynamic Sequelae

Franzeck and colleagues[10] in Zürich, Switzerland, studied 58 low-risk patients with deep venous thrombosis in a prospective study to evaluate the natural history of the post-thrombotic syndrome. Clinical and hemodynamic examinations were performed at the time of admission, after 3, 6, and 12 months, and after the 2nd, 3rd, 4th, 5th, and 12th years. All patients received heparin initially and oral anticoagulants subsequently. After 12 years, 64% of the patients exhibited normal findings. Mild skin changes were found in 28%, marked trophic changes in 5%, and only 1 venous ulcer occurred. The regular use of compression stockings was reported by 54% of the patients with multilevel thrombosis. Mean maximum venous outflow was significantly reduced from the acute event to 12 years later compared with outflow in the contralateral leg, but significant improvement was observed after 6 months of therapy. Recanalization of calf vein thrombosis was detected by Doppler sonography after 3 months. Sixty-four percent of the multilevel thromboses were recanalized completely or in part after 1 year, but in 69% valvular incompetence was found. Thus, this prospective study for 12 years after deep vein thrombosis demonstrates a low incidence of postthrombotic syndrome associated with administration of heparin initially and oral anticoagulants subsequently with regular compression therapy. However, the adverse clinical event rate, including a mortality of 14% and a recurrence rate of 24%, shows that prognosis after deep vein thrombosis is not favorable even in low-risk patients.

Pulmonary Embolism and Deep Venous Thrombosis During Pregnancy or Oral Contraceptive Use

Activated protein C resistance caused by factor V Leiden mutation is the most common inherited cause of an underlying predisposition to pulmonary embolism and deep venous thrombosis. Hirsch and associates[11] from Boston, Massachusetts, and Lund, Sweden, studied the frequency of the factor V Leiden mutation in 50 women who had pulmonary embolism and/or deep venous thrombosis during or after pregnancy or during oral contraceptive use. Ten of the 50 women were heterozygous for the mutation. First-trimester pulmonary embolism of deep venous thrombosis developed in 6 of the 10 women with the mutation compared with 3 of 40 women without the mutation. These data indicate that the factor V Leiden mutation is an important risk factor for pulmonary embolism or deep venous thrombosis during pregnancy (especially the first trimester), after pregnancy, or during oral contraceptive use.

Shortened Hospitalization after Adjusted-Dose Subcutaneous Heparin

In the study by Hirsch and colleagues[12] from Boston, Massachusetts, adjusted-dose subcutaneous unfractionated heparin was used in the initial management of deep venous thrombosis to allow shortened hospital stay. Of 78 patients screened, 41% were eligible and 18 (23%) were enrolled. Follow-up venous ultrasound examination was performed 6 weeks after discharge. Of enrolled patients, 16 (89%) completed the protocol. Hospital length of stay was 2 days in protocol patients compared with 5 days for patients receiving conventional inpatient heparin with a continuous intravenous infusion. Very high heparin doses (mean 42,000 to 62,000 U daily, given in 3 divided doses every 8 hours) and a median time of 21 hours were required initially to achieve a target aPTT greater than 55 seconds. Subsequently, many patients had supratherapeutic levels, yet there were no bleeding complications. Four patients (25%) did not show improvement at follow-up ultrasound despite aPTT greater than 55 seconds after the second injection. Clot regression was evident in the remaining patients. Hospital cost savings were offset partially by the need for time- and labor-intensive outpatient monitoring after hospital discharge.

Vascular Surgery

Bayesian Model for Perioperative Risk Assessment

Patients who require surgical treatment of peripheral vascular disease are at increased risk of perioperative cardiac morbidity and mortality. L'Italien and colleagues[13] at 5 medical centers sought to develop and validate a Bayesian risk prediction model for vascular surgery candidates. They evaluated 1081 consecutive vascular surgery candidates. Of those, 567 patients from 2 centers were used to develop the model and 514 patients from 3 centers were used to validate it. Risk scores were developed by using logistic regression for clinical variables: advanced age (>70 years); angina; history of acute myocardial infarction AMI, diabetes mellitus; history of CHF; and prior coronary revascularization. A second model was developed from dipyridamole thallium predictors of myocardial infarction (ie, fixed and reversible myocardial defects and ST changes). Model performance was assessed by comparing observed event rates with risk estimates. The postoperative cardiac event rate was 8% for both groups. Prognostic accuracy was 74% for the clinical and 81% for the clinical and dipyridamole thallium models. Observed and estimated rates were comparable for both sets. These authors concluded that simple clinical markers, weighted according to prognostic impact, can reliably stratify risk in vascular surgery candidates referred for dipyridamole thallium testing, thus obviating the need for the more expensive testing. The prediction model retained its prognostic accuracy when applied to the validation sets.

Corcordance of Angiographic Severity of CAD with Preoperative Clinical Risk

Paul and colleagues[14] in Boston, Massachusetts, performed a prospective study of 878 consecutive patients to determine the concordance of clinical risk with severity of coronary artery disease (CAD) and to validate a preoperative clinical index to exclude the presence of significant coronary stenosis in patients undergoing vascular surgery.

"Severe" stenosis was defined as 3-vessel 50% or greater stenosis in each vessel, 2-vessel 50% or greater stenosis in 1 while the other had 70% or greater stenosis of the left anterior descending (LAD), or left main disease 50% or greater. "Critical" stenosis was 3-vessel (more than 70% stenosis in each) and/or left main stenosis more than 70%. A preoperative clinical index, including the presence of diabetes mellitus, prior myocardial infarction (MI) angina, age older than 70 years, and CHF was used to stratify patients. A gradient of risk for severe stenosis was seen with increasing numbers of clinical markers. The following prediction rules were developed from this study: the absence of severe coronary stenoses can be predicted with a positive predictive value of 96% for patients who have no 1) history of diabetes; 2) prior angina; 3) previous MI, or 4) history of CHF. The absence of critical coronary stenoses can be predicted with a positive predictive value of 94% for those who have no 1) prior angina; 2) previous MI; or 3) history of CHF. This study suggests that by identifying a large proportion of patients with a low likelihood of significant stenoses, prediction rules can be developed that help reduce health-care costs associated with preoperative cardiac risk assessment for noncardiac surgery (Figure 7-1).

Risk Stratification by Meta-analysis: Intravenous Dipyridamole-Thallium 201 Imaging and Dobutamine Echocardiography

Numerous studies have demonstrated the prognostic value of dipyridamole-thallium-201 myocardial perfusion and dobutamine echocardiography in vascular surgery candidates. Shaw and colleagues[15] from Durham, North Carolina; Ann Arbor, Michigan; Washington, D.C.; and St. Louis, Missouri, systematically reviewed published reports on preoperative pharmacological stress from the MEDLINE data base (1985 to 1994). They identified 10 reports on dipyridamole-thallium-201 myocardial perfusion (1994 patients) and 5 on dobutamine stress echocardiography (445 patients). Summary odds ratios for death or AMI and secondary cardiac end points were greater for dobutamine echocardiography dyssynergy than for dipyridamole-thallium-201 redistribu-

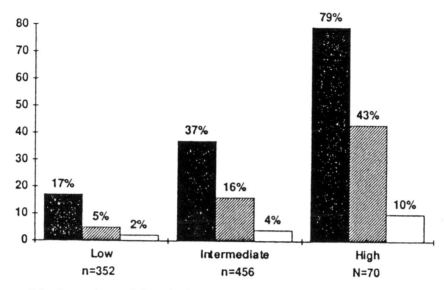

Figure 7-1. Concordance of clinical risk and severity of coronary stenoses on coronary angiography. Bars represent proportions of patients with severe multivessel disease (shaded bars), critical vessel and/or left main disease (hatched bars), and left main stenosis 70% or more (open bars) within each clinical risk group. Reproduced with permission from Paul et al.[14]

tion. Pretest CAD probability was correlated with the positive predictive value of a reversible thallium-201 defect, increasing 6-fold from low-to high-risk patient subsets. Cardiac event rates were low in patients without a history of CAD (1%) compared with patients with CAD and a normal or fixed-defect pattern (4.8%) and 1 or more thallium-201 redistribution abnormalities (18.6%). This meta-analysis of 15 studies demonstrated that the prognostic value of noninvasive stress imaging abnormalities for perioperative ischemic events is comparable among available techniques, but the accuracy varies with CAD prevalence.

Thallium Imaging for Prediction of Late Cardiac Events

Emlein and associates[16] from Worcester, Massachusetts, hypothesized that left ventricular cavity size measured on dipyridamole thallium scintigraphy identifies patients at risk for late nonfatal AMI and cardiovascular death. Accordingly, they retrospectively evaluated the predictive value of clinical and scintigraphic variables, including transendocardial left ventricular cavity measurement performed on formatted images, in 335 vascular surgery patients. A nonhomogeneous perfusion pattern and enlarged left ventricular cavity size were the most significant predictors of late events, and the interaction between these 2 variables was more predictive than was either variable alone. Life-table analysis demonstrated that patients with normal perfusion patterns had the lowest incidence of late events regardless of cavity size. Conversely, patients with a non-homogeneous perfusion pattern and the largest left ventricular cavity measurements were at the highest risk for late cardiac events. Therefore, this study demonstrated that a measurement of left ventricular scintigraphic cavity size can provide important risk stratification for late cardiac events.

Miscellaneous

Concomitant CAD often occurs in patients with peripheral vascular disease, but it may be asymptomatic. Despite being asymptomatic, cardiovascular events are the main source of morbidity and mortality in this group of patients. Dipyridamole thallium scintigraphy has been shown to be of prognostic value in patients with peripheral vascular disease and symptomatic CAD, but its effect on the long-term outcome in the asymptomatic group of patients is less defined. Darbar and associates[17] from Dundee, Scotland, evaluated 84 consecutive patients with peripheral vascular disease and no symptoms of CAD by clinical assessment, dipyridamole thallium imaging, radionuclide ventriculography, and cardiac catheterization and followed them for a mean of 66 months. Abnormal perfusion patterns were found on thallium scintigraphy in 48 patients (57%); fixed, mixed, and reversible defects were present in 14 (17%), 11 (13%), and 23 (27%) patients, respectively. Significant CAD was present in 52 patients (69%), and mean LVEF was 44%. During the follow-up period, 23 patients had a cardiac event (nonfatal AMI or cardiac death). Univariate analysis of 15 clinical, scintigraphic, radionuclide, and angiographic variables revealed that age, angiographic extent of CAD, and an abnormal thallium scan were significant predictors of subsequent cardiac events. Multivariate stepwise logistic regression analyses selected fixed and mixed thallium defects and diffuse CAD as the only significant independent predictors of outcome. Thus, the present study shows the value of dipyridamole thallium scintigraphy as a valuable prognostic indicator for long-term event-free survival in a cohort of patients with peripheral vascular disease and no history or symptoms of CAD (Figures 7-2 and 7-3).

Dipyridamole thallium-201 myocardial imaging can provide information regarding risk of perioperative cardiac events in patients being considered for vascular surgery. The value for this purpose of myocardial imaging with technetium-99m sestamibi, a radiotracer with biokinetic and imaging properties different from thallium-201, has not been established. To this end, the prognostic value of dipyridamole technetium-99m sestamibi tomography for perioperative and late cardiac events was evaluated in 229 consecutive patients being considered for elective vascular surgery in this study performed by Stratmann and associates[18] from St. Louis, Missouri. Vascular surgery was done within 3 months after testing in 197 of these patients. Perioperative cardiac events (cardiac death, nonfatal myocardial infarction, unstable angina, or ischemic pulmonary edema) occurred in 9 (5%) patients. The rate of such events was 3% in patients with normal technetium-99m sestamibi results, 5% in those with abnormal results, and 6% in patients with a reversible technetium-99m sestamibi defect. When patients with abnormal technetium-99m sestamibi results who had preoperative cardiac interventions (coronary revascularization or an increase in antiischemic medical therapy) were compared with those who did not, no significant differences in the occurrence of perioperative car-

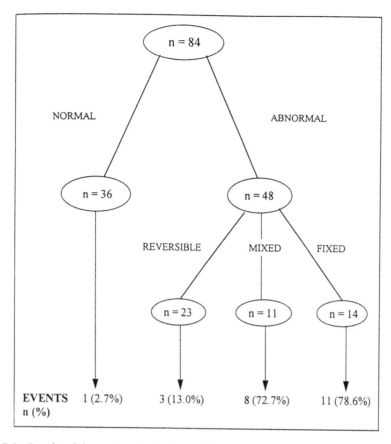

FIGURE 7-2. Results of dipyridamole thallium scintigraphy in patients with peripheral vascular disease and no clinical indications of CAD. The late event rate with regard to scan findings is also displayed. Reproduced with permission from Darbar et al.[17]

diac events were found between these 2 groups. A group of 172 medically treated patients who survived vascular surgery and did not have a nonfatal perioperative cardiac event was then monitored (mean 21 ± 14 months) for the occurrence of a serious late cardiac event (nonfatal myocardial infarction or cardiac death). Event-free survival was significantly less in patients with abnormal studies than in those with normal scan results. Late cardiac events occurred in 26 (15%) patients, with those having an abnormal technetium-99m sestamibi result showing a significantly greater event rate than those with normal results (26% vs. 4%). The rate of late cardiac events was 33% in patients with a reversible technetium-99m sestamibi defect and 23% in those with a fixed defect. Independent Cox multivariable predictors of increased risk of late cardiac events were a history of diabetes mellitus, an abnormal technetium-99m sestamibi study, and a reversible technetium-99m sestamibi defect. It was concluded that, although its ability to assess increased perioperative cardiac risk remains uncertain, dipyridamole technetium-99m sestamibi tomography does provide important prognostic information regarding the risk of serious late cardiac events in patients having vascular surgery. The presence of an

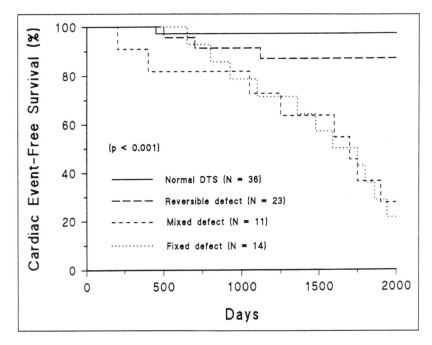

FIGURE 7-3. Incidence of cardiac events (death or nonfatal myocardial infarction) in 84 asymptomatic patients with peripheral vascular disease, stratified by dipyridamole thallium scintigraphy results. A fixed or mixed thallium defect significantly increased the risk of this end point (p<.001); N = number of patients at entry. DTS = dipyridamole thallium scintigraphy. Reproduced with permission from Darbar et al.[17]

abnormal technetium-99m sestamibi result, specifically 1 demonstrating a reversible perfusion defect, is associated with significantly increased risk.

Arterial Gene Transfer for Limb Ischemia

Isner and colleagues[19] in Boston, Massachusetts, treated a 71-year-old woman with an ischemic right leg with 2000 μg human plasmic phVEGF$_{165}$ (vascular endothelial growth factor) that was applied to a hydrogel polymer coating of an angioplasty balloon. By inflating the balloon, plasmid DNA was transferred to the distal popliteal artery. Digital subtraction angiography 4 weeks after gene therapy showed an increase in collateral vessels at the knee, mid-tibial, and ankle levels, which persisted at a 12-week review. Intra-arterial Doppler-flow studies showed increased resting and maximal flow by 82% and 72%, respectively. Three spider angiomas developed on the right foot/ankle about a week after gene transfer. One lesion was excised and revealed proliferative endothelium; the other 2 regressed. The patient developed edema in the right leg that was successfully treated. Thus, in this 1 patient with an ischemic right leg, the administration of endothelial cell mitogens promoted angiogenesis.

Fibroblast Growth Factor in Limb Ischemia

Basic fibroblast growth factor, a prototypic member of a family of heparin-binding growth factors, is angiogenic both *in vitro* and *in vivo*. Increased levels and activity of basic fibroblast growth factor have been documented in a variety of diseases, including tumors. Rohovsky and associates[20] from Boston, Massachusetts, sought to determine whether basic fibroblast growth factor might be similarly elevated in patients with clinical evidence of limb ischemia. Serum was obtained at the time of percutaneous revascularization from patients with symptomatic peripheral vascular disease (46 procedures were performed on 40 patients). An enzyme-linked immunoassay specific for basic fibroblast growth factor was used (limit of detection, 1 pg/mL; range in normal individuals, 0 to 5 pg/mL). Among the 40 patients (28 men, 12 women, mean age 70 years) studied, elevated circulating basic fibroblast growth factor ($\geq$10 pg/mL) was detected in 36 samples (78%); levels ranged from 10 to 310 pg/mL. In 16 (89%) of 18 patients with both rest pain and nonhealing ischemic ulcers, serum basic fibroblast growth factor levels were elevated up to 30 times normal values. In conclusion, circulating levels of basic fibroblast growth factor are elevated in patients with vascular insufficiency and may reflect a physiological response to limb ischemia.

L-*Arginine and Nitric Oxide-Dependent Vasodilation in Limb Ischemia*

Bode-Böger and colleagues[21] in Hannover, Germany, evaluated the effects of 1 intravenous infusion of L-arginine (30 g, over 60 minutes) or PGE_1 (40 μg, over 60 minutes) versus those of placebo on blood pressure, peripheral hemodynamics, and urinary NO_3^- and cGMP excretion rates in patients with critical limb ischemia, including patients with peripheral arterial occlusive disease stages Fontaine III or IV. Blood flow in the femoral artery was significantly increased by L-arginine by 42% and by PGE_1 by 31%, but not by placebo (Figure 7-4). Urinary NO_3^- excretion increased by 132% after L-arginine but by only 32% after PGE_1. Urinary cGMP excretion increased by 199% after L-arginine and by 94% after PGE_1. These data suggest that intravenous L-arginine induces NO-dependent peripheral vasodilation in patients with severe limb ischemia. These improvements in blood flow were paralleled by increased urinary NO_3^- and cGMP excretion, indicating an enhanced systemic NO production.

Endothelin Receptor Blockade Decreases Pulmonary Vascular Resistance and Blood Pressure

Haynes and colleagues[22] in Edinburgh, Scotland, evaluated the cardiovascular effects of a potent peptide endothelin $ET_{A/B}$ receptor antagonist (a combined inhibitor of the endothelin A and B receptors) in healthy men. Two randomized, placebo-controlled, crossover studies were performed. In 9 subjects,

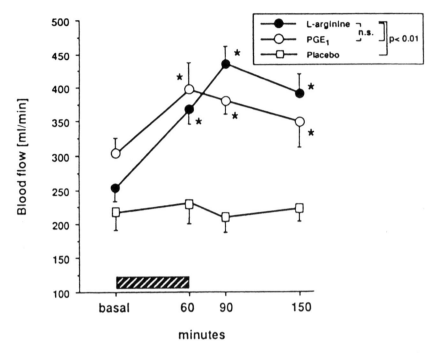

Figure 7-4. Plot of blood flow in the superficial femoral artery determined by image-directed duplex sonography before (basal) and after the infusion of L-arginine (30 g, 60 minutes), PGE$_1$ (40 μg, 60 minutes), or placebo (150 mL 0.9% saline, 60 minutes) in patients with peripheral arterial occlusive disease. Values are mean ± SEM of 10 patients (L-arginine, PGE$_1$) or 6 patients (placebo). *$p<.05$ vs. baseline in multiple ANOVA. Striped bar indicates the duration of the infusions. Reproduced with permission from Bode-Böger et al.[21]

the receptor antagonist (given as 10-1000 mg intravenously during a 15-minute period) caused sustained dose-dependent peripheral vasodilation and hypotension. Four hours after infusion of the highest dose (1000 mg), there were decreases in mean arterial pressure of 18 mm Hg and total peripheral resistance of 665 units and increases in heart rate of 8 beats per minute and cardiac index of 0.9 L/min^{-1}/m^{-2} compared with placebo. The receptor antagonist for ET$_{A/B}$ receptors caused a rapid, dose-dependent increase in the plasma immunoreactive endothelin. In a second study in 8 subjects, intravenous administration of the ET$_{A/B}$ receptor antagonist at doses of 30, 250, and 750 mg caused peripheral vasodilatation, and all 3 doses abolished local forearm vasoconstriction to brachial artery infusion of endothelin-1. Thus, these data suggest that an endothelin ET$_{A/B}$ receptor antagonist decreases peripheral vascular resistance and blood pressure while increasing circulating endothelin concentrations (Figure 7-5). The data also are consistent with the hypothesis that endogenous generation of endothelin-1 plays a physiological role in maintenance of peripheral vascular tone and blood pressure.

Cellular Proliferation in Stenotic Lesions—Arteriovenous Fistulas and Bypass Grafts

Hofstra and colleagues[23] in Maastricht, The Netherlands, studied the proliferation patterns of 35 anatomically intact human stenotic lesions derived

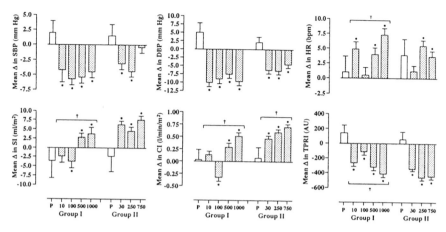

FIGURE 7-5. Mean hemodynamic changes (Δ) over 24 hours after dosing with TAK-044 in study 1. For the placebo columns (open), mean change from predose is shown. For the active treatment columns (stippled), placebo-corrected changes from predose are shown (change from predose [active] minus mean change from predose [placebo]). *$p \leq .05$ for comparison with predose; †$p \leq .05$ for linear contrast test of trend with dose. SBP indicates systolic blood pressure; SI, stroke index; DBP, diastolic blood pressure; CI, cardiac index; HR, heart rate; TPRI, total peripheral resistance index. Reproduced with permission from Haynes et al.[22]

from either peripheral bypasses (normal flow) or hemodialysis atrioventricular (AV) fistulas (high flow) with the use of Ki-67, a cell proliferation marker. Low-flow variables were assessed with ultrasound. Proliferation patterns were similar in the AV fistula and bypass stenoses. In the intima, proliferation was highest in the area just below the endothelium. In adjacent nonstenotic vessel segments that were used as controls, proliferation rate in the intima was 0.3%. Double-labeling studies revealed that subendothelial-intimal proliferation consisted mainly of vascular smooth muscle cells (90%), whereas proliferation in the other layers of the vessel wall also consisted of endothelial cells and macrophages. Blood flow velocity was negatively correlated with subendothelial-intimal proliferation. The endothelial cell coverage of the lumen was positively correlated with proliferation. Thus, these data suggest enhanced cellular proliferation in human stenotic tissue derived from AV fistulas and peripheral bypass grafts. In addition, high proliferation rates appear to be associated with endothelial cell coverage of the lumen and low local flow velocities.

1. Curb JD, Masaka K, Rodriguez BL, Abbott RD, Burchfiel CM, Chen R, Petrovitch H, Sharp D, Yano K: Peripheral artery disease and cardiovascular risk factors in the elderly; The Honolulu Heart Program. Arterioscler Thromb Vasc Biol 1996 (December);16:1495–1500.
2. den Haijer M, Koster T, Blom HJ, Bos GMJ, Briët E, Reitsma PH, Vandenbroucke JP, Rosendaal FR. Hyperhomocysteinemia as a risk factor for deep-vein thrombosis. N Engl J Med 1996 (March 21);334:759–762.
3. Piccioli A, Prandoni P, Goldhaber SZ. Epidemiologic characteristics, management, and outcome of deep venous thrombosis in a tertiary-care hospital: The Brigham and Women's Hospital DVT Registry. Am Heart J 1996 (November);132:1010–1014.
4. Koopman MMW, Prandoni P, Piovella F, Ockelford PA, Brandjes DPM, van der Meer J, Gallus AS, Simonneau G, Chesterman CH, Prins MH, Bossuyt PMM, de Haes H, van den Belt AGM, Sagnard L, d'Azemar P, Büller HR, for the Tasman

Study Group. Treatment of venous thrombosis with intravenous unfractionated heparin administered in the hospital as compared with subcutaneous low-molecular-weight heparin administered at home. N Engl J Med 1996 (March 14);334: 682–687.

5. Levine M, Gent M, Hirsh J, Leclerc J, Anderson D, Weitz J, Ginsberg J, Turpie AG, Demers C, Kovacs M, Geerts W, Kassis J, Desjardins L, Cusson J, Cruickshank M, Powers P, Brien W, Haley S, Willan A. A comparison of low-molecular-weight heparin administered primarily at home with unfractionated heparin administered in the hospital for proximal deep-vein thrombosis. N Engl J Med 1996 (March 14); 334:677–681.

6. Goldhaber SZ, Hirsch DR, MacDougall RC, Polak JF, Creager MA. Bolus recombinant urokinase versus heparin in deep venous thrombosis: A randomized controlled trial. Am Heart J 1996 (August);132:314–318.

7. Bergqvist D, Benoni G, Björgell O, Fredin H, Hedlundh U, Nicolas S, Nilsson P, Nylander G. Low-molecular-weight heparin (enoxaparin) as prophylaxis against venous thromboembolism after total hip replacement. N Engl J Med 1996 (Sept. 5);335:696–700.

8. Gent M, Hirsh J, Ginsberg JS, Powers PJ, Levine MN, Geerts WH, Jay RM, Leclerc J, Neemeh JA, Turpie AGG. Low-molecular-weight heparinoid orgaran is more effective than aspirin in the prevention of venous thromboembolism after surgery for hip fracture. Circulation 1996 (January);93:80–84.

9. Geerts WH, Jay RM, Code KI, Chen E, Szalai JP, Saibil EA, Hamilton PA. A comparison of low-dose heparin with low-molecular-weight heparin as prophylaxis against venous thromboembolism after major trauma. N Engl J Med 1996 (Sept. 5);335: 701–707.

10. Franzeck UK, Schalch I, Jäger KA, Schneider E, Grimm J, Bollinger A. Prospective 12-year follow-up study of clinical and hemodynamic sequelae after deep vein thrombosis in low-risk patients (Zürich Study). Circulation 1996 (January);93: 74–79.

11. Hirsch DR, Mikkola KM, Marks PW, Fox EA, Dorfman DM, Ewenstein BM, Goldhaber SZ. Pulmonary embolism and deep venous thrombosis during pregnancy or oral contraceptive use: Prevalence of factor V Leiden. Am Heart J 1996 (June);131: 1145–1148.

12. Hirsch DR, Lee TH, Morrison HB, Carlson W, Goldhaber SZ. Shortened hospitalization by means of adjusted-dose subcutaneous heparin for deep venous thrombosis. Am Heart J 1996 (February);131:276–280.

13. L'Italien GJ, Paul SD, Hendel RC, Leppo JA, Cohen MC, Fleisher LA, Brown KA, Zarich SW, Cambria RP, Cutler BS, Eagle KA: Development and validation of a Bayesian model for perioperative cardiac risk assessment in a cohort of 1,081 vascular surgical candidates. J Am Coll Cardiol 1996 (March 15);27:779–786.

14. Paul SD, Eagle KA, Kuntz KM, Young JR, Hertzer NR. Concordance of preoperative clinical risk with angiographic severity of coronary artery disease in patients undergoing vascular surgery. Circulation 1996 (October 1);94:1561–1566.

15. Shaw LJ, Eagle KA, Gersh BJ, Miller DD: Meta-analysis of intravenous dipyridamole-thallium-201 imaging (1985 to 1994) and dobutamine echocardiography (1991 to 1994) for risk stratification before vascular surgery. J Am Coll Cardiol 1996 (March 15);27:787–798.

16. Emlein G, Villegas B, Dahlberg S, Leppo J: Left ventricular cavity size determined by preoperative dipyridamole thallium scintigraphy as a predictor of late cardiac events in vascular surgery patients. Am Heart J 1996 (May);131:907–914.

17. Darbar D, Gillespie N, Main G, Bridges AB, Kennedy NSJ, Pringle TH, McNeill GP: Prediction of late cardiac events by dipyridamole thallium scintigraphy in patients with intermittent claudication and occult coronary artery disease. Am J Cardiol 1996 (October 1);78:736–740.

18. Stratmann HG, Younis LT, Wittry MD, Amato M, Miller DD. Dipyridamole technetium-99m sestamibi myocardial tomography in patients evaluated for elective vascular surgery: Prognostic value for perioperative and late cardiac events. Am Heart J 1996 (May);131:923–929.

19. Isner JM, Pieczek A, Schainfeld R, Blair R, Haley L, Asahara T, Rosenfield K, Razvi S, Walsh K, Symes JF. Clinical evidence of angiogenesis after arterial gene transfer of phVEGF$_{165}$ in patient with ischemic limb. Lancet 1996 (August 10);348:370–374.
20. Rohovsky S, Kearney M, Pieczek A, Rosenfield K, Schainfeld R, D'Amore PA, Isner JM. Elevated levels of basic fibroblast growth factor in patients with limb ischemia. Am Heart J 1996 (November);132:1015–1019.
21. Bode-Böger SM, Böger RH, Alfke H, Heinzel D, Tsikas D, Creutzig A, Alexander K, Frölich JC. L-arginine induces nitric oxide-dependent vasodilation in patients with critical limb ischemia. A randomized, controlled study. Circulation 1996 (January); 93:85–90.
22. Haynes WG, Ferro CJ, O'Kane KPJ, Somerville D, Lomax CC, Webb DJ. Systemic endothelin receptor blockade decreases peripheral vascular resistance and blood pressure in humans. Circulation 1996 (May 15);93:1860–1870.
23. Hofstra L, Tordoir JHM, Kitslaar PJEHM, Hoeks APG, Daemen MJAP. Enhanced cellular proliferation in intact stenotic lesions derived from human arteriovenous fistulas and peripheral bypass grafts. Does it correlate with flow parameters? Circulation 1996 (September 15);94:1283–1290.

8

Aortic Inflammation, Atherosclerosis, and Aneurysms

Takayasu's Arteritis

Eichhorn and colleagues[1] examined the sera of 19 patients with Takayasu's arteritis for antineutrophil cytoplasmic antibodies (ANCA), antinuclear antibodies (ANA), anti-DNA antibodies, antibodies to extractable nuclear antigens (ENA), anti-Ro antibodies, anticardiolipin antibodies, circulating immune complexes, and anti-endothelial cell antibodies. They used enzyme-linked immunoassays, immunofluorescence, counterimmunoelectrophoresis, fluorescent-activated cell sorter analysis, and confocal microscopy in these studies. They found that although no patient had positive ANCA, ANA, anti-DNA antibodies, ENA antibodies, anti-Ro antibodies, or anticardiolipin antibodies, 18 of the 19 patients had anti-endothelial cell antibodies. The anti-endothelial cell antibodies titers of the patients were 2561 ± 1458 compared with 126 ± 15 arbitrary units in a normal group of control subjects (Figure 8-1). In order to verify the specificity of anti-endothelial cell antibodies, they performed cytofluorimetry on human endothelial cells with the sera from patients and control subjects. Two entirely separate patterns of fluorescence intensity were identified. They next performed immunocytochemistry and confocal microscopy with human endothelial cells subjected to patients' sera and to sera from normal subjects. The cells subjected to sera from patients with Takayasu's arteritis demonstrate specific immunofluorescent staining of their plasma membrane and cytosol. Thus, anti-endothelial cell antibodies are frequently present in patients with Takayasu's arteritis, and they may play a role in the pathogenesis of this disease.

Atherosclerosis of the Thoracic Aorta

Atherosclerosis of the thoracic aorta has been shown to be associated with a risk for embolic events, but the natural history of the disease has not been investigated. Montgomery and colleagues[2] from Atlanta, Georgia, and Decatur, Georgia, evaluated 191 of 264 patients over a 20-month period who had adequate transesophageal echocardiographic (TEE) visualization of the aorta to

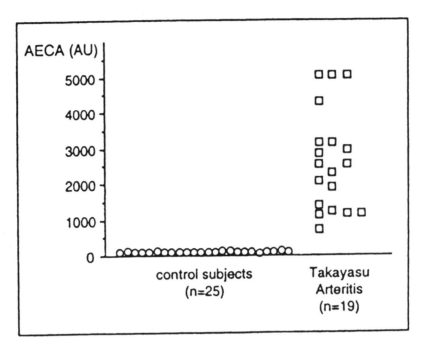

Figure 8-1. Anti-endothelial cell antibodies in 25 control subjects (mean ± SD, 126 ± 15 AU) compared with 19 patients (mean ± SD, 2561 ± 1458) with Takayasu's arteritis. The 20-fold difference was significant (p<.01). Reproduced with permission from Eichhorn et al.[1]

grade the severity of atherosclerosis. Grade I was normal; grade II showed intimal thickening; grade III showed atheroma of less than 5 mm; and grade IV showed atheroma greater than 5 mm. Grade V showed a mobile lesion. Follow-up TEE on 22 patients with grade III, IV, and V was performed about 1 year later. Twenty of the 30 patients had no change in atherosclerotic severity grade. Seven patients showed a severity progression of 1 grade, and 3 showed a decrease with resolved mobile lesions. Eight of 33 patients with grade IV or V disease died during the study period, and 1 had a clinical embolic event. Thus, the presence of severe atherosclerotic disease of the thoracic aorta seen on TEE is associated with a high mortality rate. A dynamic morphology of some lesions during a 1-year period was also noted in this study.

Thoracic Aortic Aneurysms

Milewicz and colleagues[3] in Houston, Texas, tested the hypothesis that mutations in the fibrillin-1 gene cause thoracic aortic aneurysms or dissections in patients who do not have the Marfan syndrome. Previous work done by Milewicz's group has established that mutations in the fibrillin-1 gene are the cause of the Marfan syndrome. The fibrillin-1 gene was screened for mutations by use of genomic DNA from 2 patients with thoracic aortic aneurysms who did not have the Marfan syndrome. Individual fibrillin-1 exons were amplified with intron-based exon-specific primers. The DNA fragments were screened for mutations by using single-stranded conformational polymorphism analysis. Aberrantly migrating bands were sequenced directly. The authors identified a missense mutation in 1 patient. Dermal fibroblasts from the affected individual were used to study the effect of the missense mutation on fibrillin-1 cellular processing. The mutation decreased the amount of fibrillin-1 deposited into the pericellular matrix. A second putative fibrillin-1 mutation was identified in the second patient in exon 44. Although this alteration was not observed in 234 chromosomes from unrelated individuals, the alteration may represent a rare polymorphism. Thus, the results of these studies support the hypothesis that fibrillin-1 mutations may cause thoracic aortic aneurysms in patients who do not have the Marfan syndrome.

Risk Factors for Abdominal Aortic Aneurysms

B-mode ultrasound examinations of the abdominal aorta were performed by Alcorn and colleagues[4] in Pittsburgh, Pennsylvania, from 1990 to 1992, to evaluate the prevalence of abdominal aortic aneurysm in a subgroup of the Pittsburgh Cohort (656 participants, aged 65 to 90 years) of the Cardiovascular Health Study. In this pilot study, the investigators evaluated various definitions of aneurysms and the reproducibility of the measurements. In year 5 (1992-1993), the entire cohort (4,471 participants) was examined. Abdominal aortic aneurysm was defined as an infrarenal aortic diameter of 3.0 cm or greater, or a ratio of infrarenal to suprarenal diameter of 1.2 cm or greater, or a history of abdominal aortic aneurysm repair. For the entire health study cohort, prevalence of aneurysms was 9.5% overall, with a prevalence among men of 14.2% and a prevalence among women of 6.2%. Variables significantly related to abdominal aortic aneurysms were older age; male sex; history of angina, coronary heart disease and myocardial infarction; lower ankle-arm blood pressure ratios; higher maximum carotid stenosis; greater intima-media thickness of the internal carotid arteries; higher creatinine; HDL level and higher LDL level; and cigarette smoking The study has documented the strong association of cardiovascular risk factors in measures of clinical and subclinical atherosclerosis and cardiovascular disease and prevalence of aneurysms. The investigators used a definition that is more sensitive than previously reported (diameter or ratio), which allowed the detection of smaller aneurysms and possibly those at an earlier stage of development. Follow-up of this cohort may lead to new criteria for determining the risk factors for progression of aneurysms.

Aortic Dissection

Because survivors of thoracic aortic dissection require follow-up to detect prognostic factors such as intimal tears, persistent flow in the false lumen, and complications associated with grafts, Masani and colleagues[5] undertook a prospective study to compare transeosophageal echocardiography (TEE) with magnetic resonance imaging (MRI) in 14 patients 1 year after their initial examination. Residual dissection was identified by both techniques in 11 patients. Flow and/or thrombus in the false lumen were detected by TEE in 10 (91%) and 6 (55%) patients, respectively, and by MRI in 9 (82%) and 5 (45%), respectively; more tears were detected by TEE (2.5 ± 1.4 per patient vs. 0.2 ± 0.4). Satisfactory delineation of a graft in the ascending aorta was noted in all 8 (100%) of the surgically treated patients by TEE compared with 4 (50%) by MRI. The upper ascending aorta was clearly visualized in fewer patients by TEE than by MRI (7 [50%] vs. 13 [93%]), as were the origins of the head and neck vessels (10 [71%] vs. 13 [93%]). It was concluded that TEE and MRI are both suitable techniques for the follow-up of patients with aortic dissection. TEE is more sensitive in identifying prognostic factors. MRI has a complementary role, particularly in visualization of the upper ascending aorta and the head and neck vessels.

1. Eichhorn J, Sima D, Thiele B, Lindschau C, Turowski A, Schmidt H, Schneider W, Haller H, Luft FC. Anti-endothelial cell antibodies in Takayasu arteritis. Circulation 1996 (November 15);94:2396–2401.
2. Montgomery DH, Ververis JJ, McGorisk G, Frohwein S, Martin RP, Taylor WR: Natural history of severe atheromatous disease of the thoracic aorta: A transesophageal echocardiographic study. J Am Coll Cardiol 1996 (January);27:95–101.
3. Milewicz DM, Michael K, Fisher N, Coselli JS, Markello T, Biddinger A. Fibrillin-1 (FBN1) mutations in patients with thoracic aortic aneurysms. Circulation 1996 (December 1);94:2708–2711.
4. Alcorn HG, Wolfson SK, Jr., Sutton-Tyrrell K, Kuller LH, O'Leary D: Risk factors for abdominal aortic aneurysms in older adults enrolled in the cardiovascular health study. Arterioscler Thromb Vasc Biol 1996 (August);16:963–970.
5. Masani ND, Banning AP, Jones RA, Ruttley MST, Fraser AG. Follow-up of chronic thoracic aortic dissection: Comparison of TEE and MRI. Am Heart J 1996 (June); 131:1156–1163.

9

Cerebrovascular Disease

Intracranial Bleeding

Shatos and colleagues[1] in Burlington, Vermont, wished to identify potential factors that may contribute to the risk of cerebrovascular bleeding in patients receiving thrombolytic agents. Therefore, they characterized the elaboration of plasminogen activator inhibitor-1 (PAI-1) and measured PAI-1 mRNA levels from human brain endothelial cells. When human cerebral microvascular endothelial cells, pial arterial endothelial cells, and middle meningeal arterial endothelial cells were exposed to 10 to 1000 ng/mL recombinant tissue-type plasminogen activator (rTPA), urokinase-type plasminogen activator (UPA), or streptokinase/plasminogen for 24 hours, they exhibited concentration-dependent decreases in the elaboration of PAI-1 (Figures 9-1 and 9-2). The urokinase and streptokinase/plasminogen elicited decreases of 33% and 35% that were specific. No decrease in PAI-1 elaboration from the cerebral microvascular endothelial cells was induced by coagulation factor Xa. A 2.7-fold increase was induced by α-thrombin. PAI-1 secretion from these cells decreased within 4 hours of exposure to 100 ng/mL of RTPA. In these cells exposed to RTPA for 8 hours, PAI-1 decreased from 176 to 43 pg/μg RNA. These results indicate that brain endothelial cells exposed to RTA exhibit paradoxically diminished elaboration of PAI-1. This property may render brain vasculature vulnerable to attack by serine proteases, thereby predisposing to injury and subsequent intracerebral hemorrhage in patients given plasminogen activators for treatment of coronary thrombosis.

Stroke

Stroke Prevention in Atrial Fibrillation

The Stroke Prevention in Atrial Fibrillation Investigators[2] attempted to identify an alternative that would be safer and easier to administer than adjusted-dose warfarin to patients with atrial fibrillation (AF) who are at high risk for thromboembolism and ischemic stroke. One thousand forty-four patients with AF and at least 1 thromboembolic risk factor, including congestive heart failure or left ventricular fractional shortening of 25% or less, previous

515

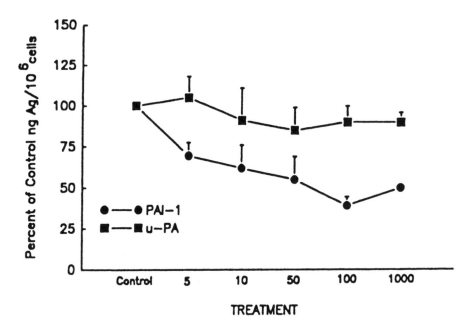

FIGURE 9-1. Secretion of UPA (u-PA in figure) and PAI-1 by HCMEC exposed to RTPA. HCMEC were cultured and grown to confluence in serum-containing medium, rinsed twice with PBS, and fed again for 24 hours with serum-free medium containing concentrations of RTPA ranging from 5 to 1000 ng/mL. The conditioned medium was collected and assayed for UPA and PAI-1 antigen by ELISA. Results are given in nanograms of UPA and PAI-1 antigen per 1×10^6 cells (mean ± SD), percent of control, for n = 9 samples. Reproduced with permission from Shatos et al.[1]

thromboembolism, systolic blood pressure of more than 160 mm Hg at study enrollment, or being a woman 75 years of age or older, were randomly assigned to either a combination of low-intensity, fixed-dose warfarin with an international normalized ratio (INR, 1.2–1.5 for initial dose adjustment and aspirin 325 mg/day) or adjusted-dose warfarin (INR, 2.0–3.0). These drugs were given in an open-labeled form. The mean INR during follow-up of patients taking combination therapy (n = 521) was 1.3, compared with 2.4 for those taking adjusted-dose warfarin (n = 523). During follow-up, 54% of INRs in patients taking combination therapy were 1.2–1.5, and 34% were less than 1.2. The trial was stopped after a mean follow-up of 1.1 years when the rate of ischemic stroke and systemic embolism in patients given combination therapy (7.9% per year) was significantly higher than in those given adjusted-dose warfarin (1.9% per year) at an interim analysis (p = .0001). This represented an absolute reduction of 6% per year by adjusted-dose warfarin. Annual rates of disabling stroke (5.6% vs. 1.7%, p = .0007) and of primary event or vascular death (11.8% vs. 6.4%, p = .002) were also higher with combination therapy. The rates of major bleeding were similar in the 2 treatment groups. Thus, low-intensity, fixed-dose warfarin plus aspirin is insufficient for stroke prevention in patients with nonvalvular AF at high risk for thromboembolism. Adjusted-dose warfarin with the target INR of 2.0 to 3.0 reduces the risk of stroke in high-risk patients.

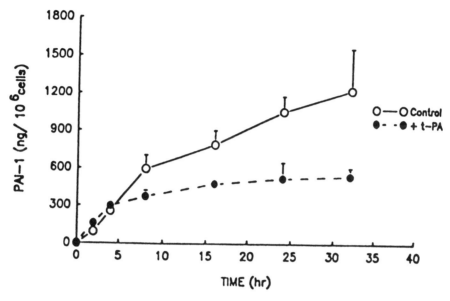

FIGURE 9-2. The time course of PAI-1 elaboration by HCMEC after exposure to RTPA (t-PA in figure). HCMEC were cultured and grown in serum-containing medium, rinsed twice with PBS, and fed again for 0 to 48 hours with serum-free medium containing 100 ng/mL RTPA. The conditioned medium was then collected and assayed for PAI-1 antigen by ELISA. Results are expressed as nanograms of PAI-1 antigen per 1×10^6 cells (mean $\pm$ SD) for n = 9 samples. Reproduced with permission from Shatos et al.[1]

Risk of Stroke with Low-Dose Oral Contraceptives

Petitti and colleagues[3] in Pasadena, California, identified fatal and nonfatal strokes in female members of the California Kaiser Permanente Medical Care Program who were 15 through 44 years of age. Matched controls were randomly selected from female members who had not had strokes. Information about the use of oral contraceptives, which was essentially limited to low-estrogen preparations, was obtained in interviews. A total of 408 confirmed strokes occurred in a total of 1.1 million women during 3.6 million woman-years of observation. The incidence of stroke was 11 per 100,000 woman-years. From data obtained in 295 women with strokes who were interviewed and their controls, the odds ratio for ischemic stroke among current users of oral contraceptives, as compared with former users and women who had never used such drugs, was 1.18 (95% confidence interval, 0.54 to 2.59) after adjustment for other risk factors for stroke. The adjusted odds ratio for hemorrhagic stroke was 1.14 (95% confidence interval, 0.60 to 2.16). With respect to the risk of hemorrhagic stroke, there was a positive interaction between the current use of oral contraceptives and smoking (odds ratio for women with both of these influences, 3.64; 95% confidence interval, 0.95 to 13.87). These data suggest that strokes are rare among women of childbearing age. Low-estrogen oral-contraceptive preparations do not appear to increase the risk of stroke.

Atherosclerosis of the Aortic Arch as a Risk Factor

The French Study of Aortic Plaques in Stroke Group[4] determined whether atherosclerotic plaques in the aortic arch are a risk factor for recurrent brain infarction and for vascular events in general among a cohort of 331 patients 60 years of age or older who were consecutively admitted to the hospital with brain infarction. All patients underwent TEE to determine whether atherosclerotic plaques were present in the aortic arch proximal to the ostium of the left subclavian artery. The patients were divided into 3 groups according to the thickness of the wall of the aortic arch: less than 1 mm, 1 to 3.9 mm, and 4 mm or greater. Recurrent brain infarction occurred in 11.9 per 100 person-years in patients with an aortic-wall thickness of 4 mm or greater, as compared with 3.5 per 100 person-years in patients with a wall thickness of 1 to 3.9 mm and 2.8 per 100 person-years in patients with a wall thickness of less than 1 mm (p<.001). The overall incidence of vascular events was 26, 9, and 5.9 per 100 person-years of follow-up in the respective groups (p<.001). After adjustment for the presence of carotid stenosis, AF, peripheral arterial disease, and other risk factors, aortic plaques 4 mm thick or greater, including the thickness of the aortic wall, were independent predictors of recurrent brain infarction, with a relative risk of 3.8 and a 95% confidence interval of 1.8 to 7.8 (p=.0012), and of all vascular events with a relative risk of 3.5, 95% confidence interval, 2.1 to 5.9 (p<.001). Thus, atherosclerotic plaques 4 mm or greater in the aortic arch are significant predictors of recurrent brain infarction and other vascular events.

Decreased Serum Testerone in Men with Acute Ischemic Stroke

Jeppesen and coworkers[5] in Copenhagen, Denmark, determined serum levels of total and free testosterone and 17 β-estradiol in 144 men with acute ischemic stroke and 47 healthy male control subjects. Blood samples from patients were drawn a mean of 3 days after stroke onset and also 6 months after admission in a subgroup of 45 patients. Initial stroke severity was assessed on the Scandinavian Stroke Scale and infarct size by computed tomographic scan. Mean total serum testosterone was 13.8 nmol/L in stroke patients and 16.5 nmol/L in control subjects; the respective values for free serum testosterone were 41 and 51 pmol/L. Both total and free testosterone were significantly inversely associated with stroke severity and 6-month mortality, and total testosterone was significantly inversely associated with infarct size (Figure 9-3). The differences in total and free testosterone levels between patients and control subjects could not be explained by 10 putative risk factors for stroke, including age, blood pressure, diabetes, ischemic heart disease, smoking, and atrial fibrillation. Total and free testosterone levels tended to normalize 6 months after the stroke. There was no difference between patients and control subjects in serum estradiol-17β levels. These results supported the idea that testosterone affects the pathogenesis of ischemic stroke in men.

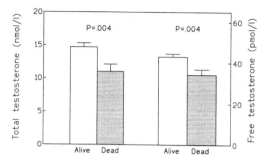

FIGURE 9-3. Bar graph shows total (left) and free (right) testosterone levels in 34 patients who died within 6 months and 110 patients who were alive 6 months after stroke. Values are mean ± SEM. Reproduced with permission from Jeppesen et al.[5]

Deletion Polymorphism in the Angiotensin-Converting Enzyme Gene in Patients with a History of Ischemic Stroke

Margaglione and colleagues[6] in Napoli, Italy, evaluated the genotypes of the angiotensin-converting enzyme gene in 101 subjects with and 109 subjects without a history of ischemia stroke. All were attending a metabolic ward. The 2 groups were compared for major risk factors for ischemic events. The genotypes were determined by polymerase chain reaction, with oligonucleotide primers flanking the polymorphic region in intron 16 of the angiotensin converting enzyme gene. Deletion polymorphism of the angiotensin gene (DD genotype) was shown to be more common in subjects with a history of stroke than in those without. A positive family history of ischemic complications of atherosclerosis was also more common in subjects with documented events. DD genotype and a positive family history were strong independent discriminators of cerebral ischemia. Plasma levels of tissue-type plasminogen activator and plasminogen activator inhibitor-1 helped identify subjects with a history of cerebral ischemic episodes. When such fibrinolytic variables were included in the analysis, the DD genotype still strongly and independently discriminated subjects with a stroke history and significantly interacted with tPA levels greater than 10 ng/mL in such identification. The investigators concluded that in subjects attending a metabolic ward, homozygosity for a deletion polymorphism of the angiotensin-converting enzyme gene consistently discriminated patients with a stroke history. Interaction with tPA improved such identification.

AF with Left Atrial Spontaneous Contrast Detected by Transesophageal Echocardiography as a Risk Factor

Nonrheumatic AF frequently coexists with other risk factors for cerebral ischemia. Jones and associates[7] from Melbourne, Australia, designed a study to determine which combinations of clinical and echocardiographic abnormalities were most closely associated with the risk of cerebral ischemic events.

Patients with cerebral ischemic events. Patients with cerebral ischemic events (n = 214) and community-based control (n = 201) underwent TEE and carotid artery imaging. Adjusted odds ratios were determined by using multiple logistic regression analysis. Independent risk factors for cerebral ischemia included diabetes, carotid stenosis, aortic sclerosis, left ventricular dysfunction, left ventricular hypertrophy, LA spontaneous contrast, and proximal aortic atheroma. Nonrheumatic AF in combination with LA spontaneous contrast and LA enlargement showed a strong association with cerebral ischemic events (adds ratio, 33.7). In subjects with sinus rhythm or nonrheumatic AF, LA enlargement was not associated with an increased risk of cerebral ischemic events in the absence of left atrial spontaneous contrast. However, only 2 patients and 1 control subject had nonrheumatic AF without LA spontaneous contrast or LA enlargement. Therefore, study of a larger number of subjects is required to address the issue of whether nonrheumatic AF itself carries increased risk. The combination of nonrheumatic AF with LA spontaneous contrast is a potent risk factor for cerebral ischemia. Ascertaining the risk factor in nonrheumatic AF requires adequate examination for underlying cardiac, aortic, and carotid vascular disease. Transesophageal echocardiography may contribute to this assessment.

1. Shatos MA, Doherty JM, Penar PL, Sobel BE. Suppression of plasminogen activator inhibitor-1 release from human cerebral endothelium by plasminogen activators. A factor potentially predisposing to intracranial bleeding. Circulation 1996 (August 15);94:636–642.
2. Stroke Prevention in Atrial Fibrillation Investigators. Adjusted-dose warfarin versus low-intensity, fixed-dose warfarin plus aspirin for high-risk patients with atrial fibrillation: Stroke Prevention in Atrial Fibrillation III randomized clinical trial. Lancet 1996 (Sept. 7);348:633–638.
3. Petitti DB, Sidney S, Bernstein A, Wolf S, Quesenberry C, Ziel HK. Stroke in uses of low-dose oral contraceptives. N Engl J Med 1996 (July 4);335:8–15.
4. The French Study of Aortic Plaques in Stroke Group. Atherosclerotic disease of the aortic arch as a risk factor for recurrent ischemic stroke. N Engl J Med 1996 (May 9);334:1216–1221.
5. Jeppesen LL, Jørgensen HS, Nakayama H, Raaschou HO, Olsen TS, Winther K: Decreased serum testosterone in men with acute ischemic stroke. Arterioscler Thromb Vasc Biol 1996 (June);16:749–754.
6. Margaglione M, Celentano E, Grandone E, Vecchione G, Cappucci G, Giuliani N, Colaizzo D, Panico S, Mancini FP, Di Minno G: Deletion polymorphism in the angiotensin-converting enzyme gene in patients with a history of ischemic stroke. Arterioscl Thromb Vasc Biol 1996 (February);16:304–309.
7. Jones EF, Calafiore P, McNeil JJ, Tonkin AM, Donnan GA: Atrial fibrillation with left atrial spontaneous contrast detected by TEE is a potent risk factor for stroke. Am J Cardiol 1996 (August 15);78:425–429.

10

Pericardial Heart Disease

Nugue and colleagues[1] in Lille Cedex, France, assessed the benefits and risks of surgical pericardioscopy in 141 consecutive patients with unexplained pericardial effusion who underwent 142 pericardioscopies with a rigid mediastinoscope. For each patient, the etiologic data obtained by pericardioscopy, which included visualization of the pericardium, guided biopsies, subxiphoid window biopsy, and fluid analysis were compared with the results that would have been obtained with only conventional surgical drainage and biopsy. After complete work-up, a specific cause was found in 69 cases (48.6%); the other 73 were considered idiopathic effusions (51%). Procedural and in-hospital mortality occurred in 8 of 141 patients (5.6%). No death was directly attributable to pericardioscopy. During long-term follow-up, with a median duration of 24 months, a previously unrecognized cause was discovered in 6 patients (4%). By comparing the area under the receiver-operating characteristic curves, the diagnostic advantages of pericardioscopy were significant in the whole series with an increase in sensitivity for diagnosis being most marked in etiologies, including neoplastic (21%), radiation-induced (100%), or purulent (83%) effusions (Table 10-1). Thus, the data obtained in this study demonstrate that pericardioscopy increases the diagnostic sensitivity of surgical pericardial drainage and biopsy without major addition to the risk.

Pericardial Effusion

Pericarditis

Hurrell and colleagues[2] in Rochester, Minnesota, and Scottsdale, Arizona studied the accuracy of dynamic respiratory changes of left ventricular and right ventricular pressures in arriving at a diagnosis of constrictive pericarditis at cardiac catheterization. High-fidelity manometric catheters and respirometry were used to study 36 patients, including 15 patients with surgically proven constrictive pericarditis (group 1) and 21 patients with other causes of heart failure (group 2). Conventional cardiac catheterization variables used to establish the diagnosis of constrictive pericarditis lacked sensitivity and specificity and failed to distinguish between these groups. The finding of discordance between right ventricular and left ventricular pressures during inspiration, a sign of increased ventricular interdependence, accurately distinguished patients in group 1 from those in group 2 in this study (Figure 10-1). Thus, examination of dynamic respiratory changes indicating increased

TABLE 10-1
Comparison of the Diagnostic Categories After Complete Workup With PCS
and at the End of Follow-up

Cause of Pericardial Effusions	After Complete Workup With PCS		After Follow-up	
	n	%	n	%
No specific cause	73	51.4	70	49.3
Idiopathic	56	39.4	51	35.9
Paraneoplastic	16	11.2	19	13.4
Hemopericardium of unknown origin	1	0.7	...	...
Specific causes	69	48.6	72	50.7
Malignant	22	15.5	24	16.9
Radiation-induced*	10	7.0	10	7.0
Viral	8	5.6	8	5.6
Hemopericardium due to coagulation disorders or after chest trauma	6	4.2	6	4.2
Tuberculous	6	4.2	6	4.2
Purulent†	6	4.2	6	4.2
Collagen disease‡	5	3.5	5	3.5
Congestive heart failure	3	2.1	3	2.1
Benign pericardial tumor§	1	0.7	1	0.7
Chronic aortic dissection‖	...	...	1	0.7
Chronic renal failure	1	0.7	1	0.7
Fungal	1	0.7	1	0.7
Total	142		142	

* Including one case previously published.
† Including 1 HIV-positive patient.
‡ Including 1 patient with Still's disease.
§ Cystic lymphangioma.
‖ Including 1 case previously published.
Reproduced with permission from Nugue et al.[1]

ventricular interdependence may be useful in the diagnosis of constrictive pericarditis in the cardiac catheterization laboratory. In this study, increased ventricular interdependence was assessed by comparing left ventricular systolic pressure and right ventricular systolic pressure during respiration. Figure 10-2 displays a representative pressure tracing from a patient in group 1, along with a left ventricular/right ventricular graph demonstrating the 4 beats of the respiratory cycle for this patient. During peak inspiration (beat 2), there was an increase in right ventricular systolic pressure and a decrease in left ventricular systolic pressure. The bottom portion of Figure 10-2 displays a representative pressure tracing and analysis from a patient in group 2. There is a concordant decrease in both right ventricular systolic pressure and left ventricular systolic pressure during peak inspiration. Figure 10-3 demonstrates the raw data for the percentage assigned to the right ventricular systolic pressure at peak inspiration, the right ventricular index. Right ventricular systolic pressure was at its maximum in all patients in group 1, but all but 1 patient in group 2 had right ventricular systolic pressure concordant with left ventricular systolic pressure and did not reach maximum systolic pressure until peak expiration.

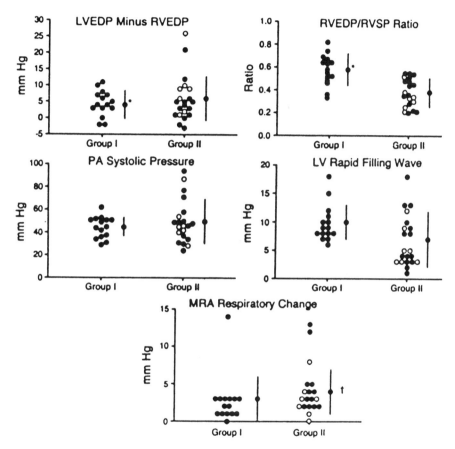

Figure 10-1. Conventional hemodynamic criteria used in an attempt to differentiate constrictive pericarditis from restrictive cardiomyopathy. Individual patient data for group 1, constrictive pericarditis, and group 2, other causes of heart failure. Open circles are from those patients in group 2 identified as having a restrictive cardiomyopathy. The overlap between individuals in each group is apparent. Values are mean ± SD. LV indicates left ventricle; MRA, mean right atrial pressure; and PA, pulmonary artery. *p<.05. †n=19. Reproduced with permission from Hurrell et al.[2]

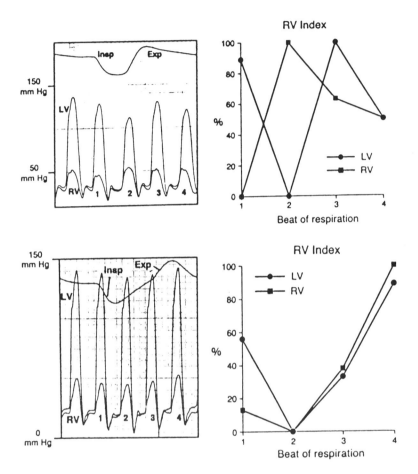

FIGURE 10-2. Respiratory changes in left ventricular (LV) and right ventricular (RV) systolic pressures. **Left,** Sample tracings of LV and RV pressures with respirometry in a patient with constrictive pericarditis (group 1) on the top and in a patient with another form of heart failure (group 2) on the bottom. **Right,** For these specific examples depicted on the left, the percentages of maximal LV and RV systolic pressures recorded are plotted for the 4 beats of the respiratory cycle, as identified in the figure. The RV index is defined as the percentage assigned to the RV pressure for beat number 2. In patients with constrictive pericarditis, LV and RV pressures have a reciprocal relationship throughout the respiratory cycle, whereas patients with heart failure are seen to have concordant changes in their pressures. Insp indicates inspiration; Exp, expiration. Reproduced with permission from Hurrell et al.[2]

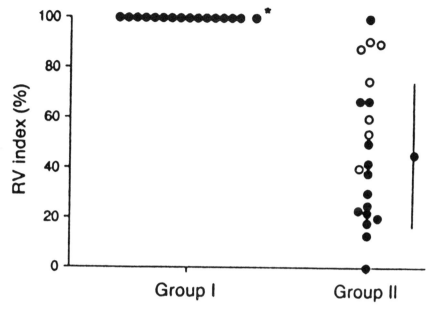

FIGURE 10-3. Right ventricular (RV) index. The individual patient data for the RV index are defined as the percentage assigned to the RVSP of beat number 2. Both group 1, constrictive pericarditis, and group 2, other forms of heart failure, are displayed with mean ± SD. Open circles are for those patients in group 2 identified as having a restrictive cardiomyopathy. Reproduced with permission from Hurrell et al.[2]

1. Nugue O, Millaire A, Porte H, de Groote P, Guimier P, Wurtz A, Ducloux G. Pericardioscopy in the etiologic diagnosis of pericardial effusion in 141 consecutive patients. Circulation 1996 (October 1);94:1635–1641.
2. Hurrell DG, Nishimura RA, Higano ST, Appleton CP, Danielson GK, Holmes DR Jr., Tajik AJ. Value of dynamic respiratory changes in left and right ventricular pressures for the diagnosis of constrictive pericarditis. Circulation 1996 (June 1);93: 2007–2013.

11
Cardiovascular Disease in the Young

Kawasaki Disease

Dobutamine stress echocardiography is a safe and accurate method for detection of coronary artery stenosis in Kawasaki disease. Noto and associates[1] from Tokyo, Japan, examined the effectiveness of dobutamine stress echocardiography in 50 patients in the convalescent stage of Kawasaki disease, including 26 patients with coronary sequelae documented by previous coronary angiography and 24 patients with normal coronary arteries documented by echocardiography, who underwent quantitative angiography on a separate day. Left ventricular regional wall motion, divided into 16 segments, was assessed in relation to the extent of coronary artery disease. A positive response was defined as a new or worsened wall motion abnormality. Significant coronary artery disease was present in 21 patients in the sequelae group. There were self-limiting side effects in 10 patients; however, there were no serious complications from stress-induced ischemia. New wall motion abnormalities, which corresponded to the extent of coronary artery disease, were detected in 19 of 21 patients in the sequelae group, whereas no wall motion abnormalities were detected in the normal group. The usefulness of dobutamine stress echocardiography for detection of coronary artery stenosis in Kawasaki disease deserves further study.

Muzik and associates[2] from Detroit, Michigan, and Ann Arbor, Michigan, assessed myocardial blood flow and flow reserve at rest and during adenosine stress with nitrogen-13 ammonia and position emission tomography in 10 children with a history of Kawasaki disease and in 10 healthy young adult volunteers. All children had acute Kawasaki disease 4 to 15 years before the study, and none had epicardial coronary artery anomalies at the acute stage of disease or during follow-up, as assessed by echocardiography. Rest blood flows were normalized to the rate-pressure product and were similar in both Kawasaki patients and volunteers. Hyperemic blood flows however, were significantly lower in Kawasaki patients than in the controls. As a result, estimates of myocardial flow reserve were lower in patients with Kawasaki disease than in the healthy young adult volunteers (3.2 vs 4.6). In addition, total coronary resistance was higher in the patients with Kawasaki disease than in the adult volunteers (33 ± 11 vs. 24 ± 5). Quantitative analysis of perfusion images demonstrated no regional perfusion abnormalities. These data indicate possible reduced coronary vasodilator reserve in patients with apparently normal coronary arteries by echocardiographic assessment and suggest that all Kawasaki patients deserve long-term follow-up. Whether these findings will prove clinically significant remains unclear.

Ino and colleagues[3] in Tokyo, Japan, retrospectively evaluated the effectiveness of percutaneous transluminal coronary angioplasty (PTCA) in 5 patients with coronary arterial stenosis resulting from Kawasaki disease. The patients ranged in age from 2 to 16 years with a median of 8 years. They underwent conventional PTCA for localized stenosis. The lesion targeted for PTCA was located in the middle right coronary artery of 3 patients and in the left anterior descending (LAD) coronary artery in 2 patients. In 4 of the 5 patients, PTCA was angiographically effective, with stenosis rates improving from 84% to 33%. When the previously reported cases of 6 similar patients were considered, the only predictor of successful PTCA appeared to be the time that elapsed between the onset of Kawasaki disease and the performance of this procedure. Thus, in patients with significant localized stenosis as a result of Kawasaki disease, PTCA should be considered within 6 to 8 years of the onset of the disease. In this study, ultrasound imaging was found to be a useful tool for evaluating internal morphology before and after PTCA (Figures 11-1 and 11-2).

Kato and associates[4] from Kurume, Japan, identified 594 consecutive children with acute Kawasaki disease between 1973 and 1983 and followed these patients for 10 to 21 years, with a mean of 13.6 years. In all patients, coronary lesions were evaluated by coronary angiography just after the acute stage, and coronary aneurysms were diagnosed in 25%. Repeat angiography was performed 1 to 2 years later in all patients who previously had aneurysms, demonstrating that 49% had regression in the aneurysm. Third angiography was performed for 62 patients, fourth for 29, and fifth for 17 patients. By 10 to 21 years after the onset of the illness, stenosis in the coronary aneurysms had developed in 28 patients, myocardial infarction had occurred in 11 patients, and 5 patients had died. In the 26 patients with giant coronary aneurysms, stenotic lesions developed in 12, and no regression occurred. The 448 patients with normal findings at first angiography subsequently never developed any abnormal cardiac findings. Systemic artery aneurysms developed in 2.2%, and valvular heart disease appeared in 1.2%. The incidence of coronary aneurysm in acute Kawasaki was 25%, and 55% of these showed regression. During follow-up, ischemic heart disease developed in 4.7% and myocardial infarction in 1.9%. These data were all obtained from patients seen and managed in the pre-gammaglobulin treatment era. The very low rates of coronary ischemia and myocardial infarction are reassuring, as is the lack of development of coronary or myocardial problems in patients with normal coronary arteries at their initial assessment. Patients with giant aneurysms are another story and need long term follow-up, because their risk of developing ischemia is significant. All patients with coronary involvement at any stage require long-term follow-up.

Coarctation of the Aorta

Quantitative echocardiographic analysis of the aortic arch may be beneficial in predicting outcomes of balloon angioplasty of native coarctation of the aorta. Kaine and associates[5] from Houston, Texas, and Boston, Massachusetts,

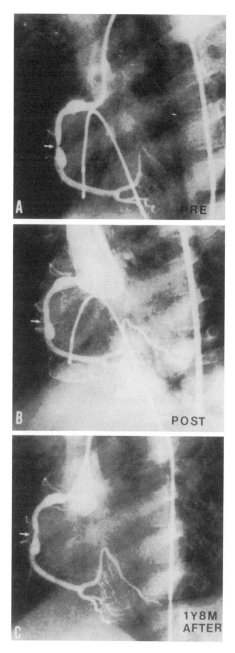

FIGURE 11-1. Right coronary arteriograms in patient 1. **A,** A localized stenosis of the middle right coronary artery was observed at a site just proximal to the aneurysm. **B,** The stenosis was sufficiently dilated by percutaneous transluminal coronary angioplasty (PTCA) with no residual stenosis. **C,** The lesion remained unobstructed 5 months after PTCA. The arrows in A, B, and C indicate the lesion. PRE indicates pre-PTCA; POST, post-PTCA; and 1Y8M AFTER, angiography performed 1 year 8 months after PTCA. Reprinted with permission from Ino et al.[3]

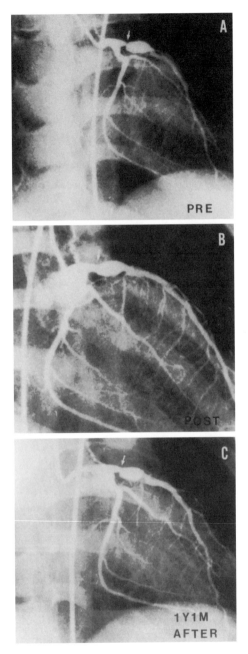

FIGURE 11-2. Left coronary arteriograms in patient 2. **A,** A localized stenosis (arrow) can be seen at a site just proximal to the aneurysm of the left anterior descending artery. **B,** The stenosis was sufficiently dilated by conventional percutaneous transluminal coronary angioplasty (PTCA). **C,** Follow-up angiography performed at 1 year 1 month after (1Y1M AFTER) the initial PTCA revealed no significant restenosis. PRE indicates pre-PTCA; POST, post-PTCA. Reprinted with permission from Ino et al.[3]

studied preangioplasty echocardiograms of 105 patients (aged 3 days to 17 years). Native angioplasty was considered successful if the residual coarctation gradient was less than 20 mm Hg, and no intervention for recoarctation occurred. Univariate analysis identified young age at angioplasty, presence of a patent ductus arteriosus (PDA), and diameters of the aortic isthmus, distal transverse arch, and aortic valve as predictors of early and late outcomes. Multivariate analysis showed that the preangioplasty aortic isthmus z value was the best independent predictor of outcome, eliminating the effect on outcome of age and associated cardiac defects. An isthmus z value of less than or equal to 2.16 predicted early failure with 91% sensitivity and 85% specificity. Kaplan-Meier analysis demonstrated that 90% of patients with an isthmus z value greater than −1.0 remained free of recoarctation at late follow-up, whereas 89% of patients with preangioplasty isthmus z value less than or equal to −2.0 developed recoarctation within 36 months (Figure 11-3). Quantitative echocardiography arch analysis may improve selection of angioplasty candidates who are likely to benefit from the procedure.

Rao and associates[6] from Madison, Wisconsin; Riyadh, Saudi Arabia; and St. Louis, Missouri, report experience with balloon angioplasty for native aortic coarctation in 67 neonates, infants, and children. Angioplasty produced a reduction in peak-to-peak gradient from 46 ± 17 to 11 ± 9 mm Hg. No patient required immediate surgical intervention. At intermediate follow-up at an average of 14 months in 60 patients, a residual gradient of 16 ± 15 mm Hg was found. When individual results were scrutinized, 15 of 60 had recoarctation, defined as peak gradient greater than 20 mm Hg. Recoarctation was higher in neonates (5 of 6, 83%) and infants (7 of 18, 39%) than in children (3 of 36, 8%). Surgical resection of recoarctation was performed with excellent results in 2 infants in the early experience. Three patients with gradients had no discrete narrowing but had normal arm blood pressure and no intervention. The remaining 10 patients had repeat angioplasty with reduction in gradient from 52 ± 13 to 9 ± 8 mm Hg. Re-examination at 31 ± 18 months after repeat angioplasty revealed a residual gradient of 11 ± 6 mm Hg. Aneurysms developed in 3 of 58 patients who underwent follow-up angiography, and detailed

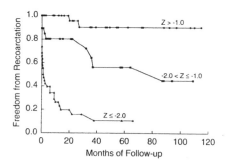

FIGURE 11-3. Kaplan-Meier curves depicting the proportion of patients remaining free of recoarctation over time for three groups stratified by aortic isthmus size: group 1, aortic isthmus z value > −1.0; group 2, −2.0<aortic isthmus z value ≤ −1.0; group 3, aortic isthmus z value ≤ −2.0. p<.01, group 1 vs. group 2; p<.001, group 1 vs. group 3. Reprinted with permission from Kaine et al.[5]

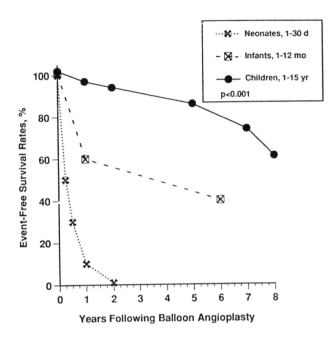

FIGURE 11-4. Actuarial event-free survival curves of neonates (<30 days old), infants (1 to 12 months old) and children (1 to 15 years old) undergoing balloon angioplasty for treatment of aortic coarctation. Note that event-free survival rates are better for children than for the neonatal and infant groups. Reprinted with permission from Rao et al.[6]

evaluation of the femoral artery in 51 of 58 patients at follow-up catheterization revealed patency of the femoral artery in 86%. Femoral artery occlusion was complete in 3 and partial in 4, all with excellent collateral flow. Blood pressure, echocardiography, and repeat angiography or MRI data 5 to 9 years after angioplasty revealed no new aneurysms and minimal late recoarctation (2%). On the basis of these data, it is concluded that balloon angioplasty is safe and effective in the treatment of native aortic coarctation, but prone to early failure in neonates (Figure 11-4). It is not recommended for neonates or young infants unless there are no good alternatives.

Taussig-Bing Anomaly

Mavroudis and associates[7] from Chicago, Illinois, report intracardiac repair of Taussig-Bing anomaly in 20 patients with a mean age of 17 months (range, 1 week to 9 years). Prior palliation included pulmonary artery (PA) band in 15, coarctation repair in 8, and atrial septectomy in 1. Arterial switch with ventricular septal defect (VSD) closure was performed in 16 patients, 10 with anteroposterior great arteries. Kawashima ventricular repair was performed in 4 patients, all with side-by-side great arteries. After arterial switch, there was 1 operative death (6%) due to myocardial ischemia and 3 late deaths (19%) due to pulmonary hypertension, gastrointestinal bleeding, and acute

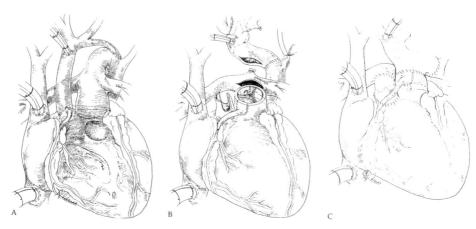

FIGURE 11-5. Arterial switch, ventricular septal defect closure, and aortic relocation: one-stage neonatal repair of **(A)** the Taussig-Bing heart with subaortic obstruction, small ascending aorta, and coarctation of the aorta. **(B)**, After great artery transection and coronary artery transfer are accomplished, the coarctation is repaired under circulatory arrest by coarctectomy with end-to-end anastomosis between the "proximal" ascending and descending aorta. A longitudinal incision is made in the lateral ascending aorta, which is now oriented in a transverse position for anastomosis to the neoaorta. **C**, Completed repair showing the neopulmonary artery reconstruction with a valved homograft after subvalvular resection. Reprinted with permission from Mavroudis et al.[7]

leukemia. There were no deaths in the Kawashima group. After arterial switch, 9 patients underwent 11 operations for residual coarctation in 3, residual PA stenosis in 2, aortic valve replacement, aortic valvuloplasty, unrecognized VSD, mitral valvuloplasty, mediastinitis, and pacemaker insertion. After Kawashima repair, 1 patient underwent reoperation for baffle stenosis and 1 for an unrecognized VSD. The Kawashima repair preserves the native aortic valve and avoids coronary dysfunction. It is particularly useful for patients with side-by-side great arteries. The arterial switch with VSD closure can be applied without ventriculotomy to all great artery relationships and allows neonatal repair with or without concomitant coarctation repair. Both procedures yield excellent early and intermediate results despite high rates of prerepair palliation and postrepair operation for both groups (Figures 11-5 and 11-6).

Transposition of the Great Arteries

van Son and associates[8] from San Francisco, California, report 5 patients with previous Senning or Mustard operations for transposition of the great arteries (TGA) and failing systemic ventricles in whom banding of the PA was performed as an interim step toward an arterial switch. The rise in the ratio of left to right systolic ventricular pressure from 0.35 before operation to 0.9 during operation and 0.8 on the first postoperative day caused a shift of the ventricular septum from a leftward to a midline or nearly midline position. This shift was associated with a reduction of tricuspid regurgitation. At a

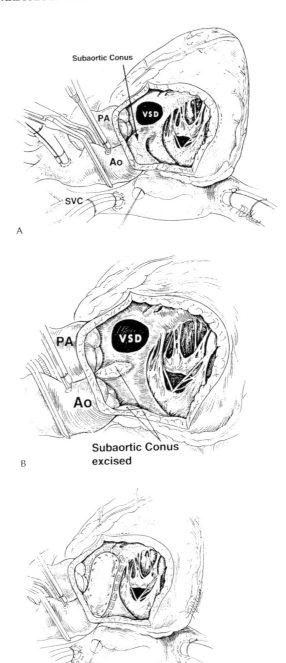

FIGURE 11-6. Kawashima intraventricular repair. Artist's cut-away view of the Taussig-Bing heart with side-by-side great arteries. **A**, The subpulmonic ventricular septal defect (VSD) and subaortic conus are represented in relationship to the great arteries and semilunar valves. **B**, The excised subaortic conus is shown in preparation for (C) the left ventricle-to-aorta intraventricular tunnel, shown here constructed with a Dacron patch and interrupted pledgeted sutures. (Ao = aorta; PA = pulmonary artery; SVC = superior vena cava.) Reprinted with permission from Mavroudis et al.[7]

median interval 5 months after banding, the mean left ventricular posterior wall thickness had increased to 8.2 mm versus 5 mm before operation, and the mean left ventricular myocardial mass index had increased to 90 gm/m^2 versus 56 gm/m^2 before operation. After the arterial switch operation was performed in 4 patients, the tricuspid regurgitation (TR) decreased to a trivial amount or disappeared completely. This report suggests that the TR often associated with systemic right ventricular failure following atrial repair of TGA is primarily related to the afterload which the right ventricle faces. Thus, it appears that even severe TR is not a contraindication to this difficult staged treatment for the failing systemic ventricle following Mustard or Senning operation.

Nakanishi and associates[9] from Tokyo, Japan, measured annular diameters of the old aortic and neopulmonary valves from cineangiograms in patients who underwent cardiac catheterization both before and more than 1 year after the arterial switch operation for TGA. Of 71 patients, 13 (18%) had either a small annulus (<70% of expected normal) or no significant growth of the annulus after the arterial switch operation, and 4 (6%) had a pressure gradient greater than 30 mm Hg. The small annulus, or no growth of the neopulmonary valve, was more frequent in patients with a history of pulmonary artery banding. After the arterial switch operation, the valve diameter in patients with a VSD was 80% ± 15% of normal, and the valve was significantly larger in patients with an intact ventricular septum, 91% ± 11%. In all patients with an intact ventricular septum who underwent a 1-stage arterial switch operation, the valve diameters before and after the operation were within normal limits, and a significant increase in the pulmonary valve annulus was observed. These data indicate that not only supravalvular pulmonary stenosis, but also pulmonary annular stenosis, can occur in TGA, especially in patients with a history of VSD and pulmonary artery banding.

Bonnet and associates[10] from Paris, France, report selective coronary arteriography in 64 children (mean age, 8 years) who had undergone previous arterial switch operation for TGA. Selective coronary angiography was possible in 58 patients, and 5 patients showed occlusion or stenosis of the coronary artery. The prevalence of late coronary artery complications was 8%. The 3 patients with occlusion of 1 coronary artery had perioperative ischemic complications, with associated electrocardiographic evidence of ischemia, left ventricular dysfunction, and mitral regurgitation (MR). Of 2 patients with stenosis of the left main coronary, neither had evidence of an anomaly before catheterization. Although the prevalence of late coronary artery complications after the arterial switch operation was low, these authors suggest screening for late coronary patency because even patients who remain symptom-free may have significant coronary anomalies.

Meijboom and associates[11] from Rotterdam, The Netherlands, conducted a follow-up study on 99 patients who underwent a Mustard repair for TGA between 1973 and 1980. Patients who underwent operations in the first 4 years had a significantly higher mortality rate and higher prevalence of sinus node dysfunction than did patients undergoing procedures in the subsequent years (25% vs. 2% and 41% vs. 3%, respectively). In contrast, the prevalence of baffle obstruction necessitating reoperation was significantly higher in the second group. There were no significant differences in echocardiographic findings and exercise capacity between patients undergoing procedures in the first 4 years and in the subsequent 4 years. None of the patients had right ventricular failure, but a mild degree of baffle leakage or obstruction was seen in 22% of the patients, and the mean exercise capacity was decreased to 84% ± 16% of normal. There was an overall 60% of moderate tricuspid regurgitation (TR) present. The survival curve for the patient group from the earlier time period showed continued decline. These patients not only have rhythm disturbances but also ventricular dysfunction.

Serraf and associates[12] from Le Plessis-Robinson, France, discuss operative management for 34 patients with double outlet right ventricle (n = 15) or TGA (n = 19) with isolated straddling tricuspid valve (n = 17), isolated straddling mitral valve (n = 9), both mitral and tricuspid straddling (n = 2) or abnormal insertion of tricuspid (n = 7) or mitral chordae (n = 2) in the left ventricular outflow precluding an adequate tunnel reconstruction. Straddling was characterized according to the location of the papillary muscle insertion in the opposite ventricular septum: type A, on the edge of the ventricular septal defect (n = 14); type B, on the opposite side of the ventricular septum away from the edge of the defect (n = 8); type C, on the free wall of the opposite ventricular chamber (n = 8). Three types of chordal distribution were identified: on the aortic conus, on the pulmonary conus crossing the VSD, or around the defect closing it like a curtain. All but 3 patients had 2 ventricles of adequate size. Palliative procedures were performed in 16 patients, and median age at definitive operation was 7 months, with a range of 1 to 130 months. Biventricular repair was performed in 30 patients, and univentricular repair was performed in 4. Biventricular repair was achieved by an arterial switch operation in 18 patients and by tunnel construction of the left ventricle to the aorta in 12. In isolated straddling of types A and B, the VSD was closed by adjusting the septal patch on the ventricular side above the straddle papillary muscle. In type C, the patch was sewn over the papillary muscle by applying it on the septum. Curtain-like chordae were a contraindication of biventricular repair in double-outlet right ventricle and not in TGA. Four early deaths and 1 late death all occurred in the group having biventricular repair. Moderate-to-severe postoperative atrioventricular (AV) valve incompetence was present in 2 and was caused by a cleft to the mitral valve in 1. Reoperation for subaortic stenosis in 1, PS in 1, and MR in 1 was required. Mean follow-up was 30 ± 19 months, and all but 1 patient were without symptoms and without AV valve incompetence. Actuarial survival at 4 years was 85% ± 3%. This report details excellent results in some very complex patients. Figures (11-7, 11-8, and 11-9) of this article should be studied by all physicians dealing with complex congenital heart disease in infancy.

Truncus Arteriosus

Lacour-Gayet and associates[13] from Paris, France, report 56 consecutive patients who underwent total repair of truncus arteriosus with median age at repair 41 days (range, 2 days to 8 months). The truncal root was transected, which provided a clear exposure of the coronary ostia. The aorta was recon-

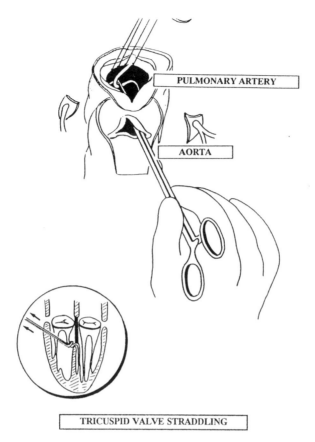

FIGURE 11-7. Surgical technique for intraoperative management of straddling tricuspid valve in TGA. After section of the great arteries, the intracardiac anatomy is explored through the semilunar valves. The chordae or the papillary muscle crossing the VSD into the left ventricular cavity is retracted toward the right ventricle by a hook passed through the native aortic valve. The VSD is then closed through the native pulmonary valve in the usual manner. Sometimes it is necessary to complete this procedure through the right atrium. Reprinted with permission from Serraf et al.[12]

structed with direct end-to-end anastomosis, and the truncal valve was preserved in every case. Several different techniques were used for pulmonary reconstruction, including 3 types of anatomic reconstruction of the pulmonary valve with a tri-sigmoid leaflet system and 2 types of nonanatomic reconstruction. The anatomic techniques included use of 33 Dacron-valved conduits, 8 homograft-valved conduits, and 1 porcine aortic root prosthesis. The nonanatomic reconstructions included direct anastomosis to the right ventricle in 9 patients and insertion of autologous pericardial valve conduits in 5. The hospital mortality was 16% (95% confidence limits: 2% to 30%). Incremental risk factors for hospital death include nonanatomic pulmonary valve reconstruction techniques in infants younger than 1 month of age. The hospital mortality was 6% in those older than 1 month of age versus 30% in those younger than 1 month. There were 2 late deaths; actuarial freedom from reoperation and angioplasty at 7 years was 100% for patients receiving pericardial conduits,

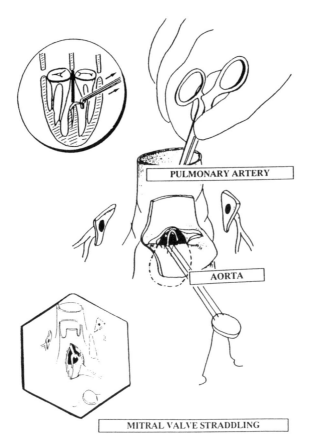

PULMONARY ARTERY

AORTA

MITRAL VALVE STRADDLING

FIGURE 11-8. Surgical technique for intraoperative management of straddling mitral valve in TGA. The chordae or the papillary muscle is retracted into the left ventricle with a hook passed through the native pulmonary artery. The VSD is then closed either through the native aortic valve or through a right ventriculotomy. It is sometimes necessary to complete this procedure through the right atrium. Reprinted with permission from Serraf et al.[12]

80% for those undergoing direct anastomosis, 77% for those receiving Dacron conduits, and only 43% for those receiving homografts. These authors present interesting results with various techniques for truncus repair. These patients remain difficult to treat and, unfortunately, these authors still show a high mortality for the young infant. In the authors' experience, an operation is virtually always needed in early infancy to prevent significant mortality, which occurs all too commonly with prolonged medical management (longer than several days to several weeks).

Single Ventricle

Tweddell and associates[14] from Milwaukee, Wisconsin, report 46 consecutive patients undergoing single ventricle palliation using cardiopulmonary by-

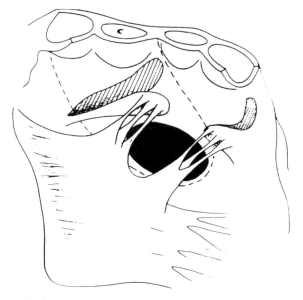

FIGURE 11-9. Surgical technique for tailoring of the myocardial flap in the presence of abnormal attachments of the tricuspid valve on the outlet septum in double-outlet right ventricle. Reprinted with permission from Serraf et al.[12]

pass. Aprotinin, a serine protease inhibitor that inhibits the contact, neutrophil, and platelet activation system during cardiopulmonary bypass, was used in 8 of 30 bidirectional cavopulmonary shunts and in 10 of 16 Fontan procedures. Aprotinin use was associated with a decrease in early postoperative transpulmonary gradient among patients undergoing these procedures. The bidirectional cavopulmonary shunt/aprotinin group had a higher oxygen saturation and a decrease in quantity and duration of thoracic damage. Among patients receiving aprotinin, there were no episodes of mediastinitis, thrombus formation, or renal failure. Aprotinin may have a favorable impact on the early postoperative period of complex patients undergoing cardiopulmonary bypass. This drug deserves further evaluation.

Delius and associates[15] from London, United Kingdom, report 34 patients with AV concordance or discordance, ventriculoarterial discordance, VSD, and PS or atresia who have undergone biventricular repair. Another group of 16 patients with the same diagnoses underwent a single ventricular repair consisting of a total cavopulmonary connection because of either a straddling AV valve or an uncommitted VSD. The mean length of follow-up was 4 years in group 1 and 3 years in group 2. Freedom from reoperation at 7 years was 46% in group 1 and 100% in group 2. The actuarial estimate of survival at 7 years was 68% in group 1 and 94% in group 2. Short and intermediate-term morbidity and mortality was greater in patients undergoing a biventricular repair than in a similar group of patients undergoing total cavopulmonary connection. The question as to when to attempt a complex intraventricular tunnel and/or a valved conduit in patients with abnormal ventricular arterial connection and a large VSD continues to be an important one. The answer to this question varies among institutions. In patients with uncommitted VSD and a partially straddling AV valve, a Fontan type of total cavopulmonary connection appears to be a favored approach and is associated with a better outcome.

In functional single ventricle with pulmonary overcirculation, PA banding is frequently used to alleviate symptoms and to prepare for staged repair. At subsequent cavopulmonary anastomosis or Fontan procedure, the PA may be ligated at the site of the pulmonary band. The article by Oski and associates[16] from Baltimore, Maryland, and St. Louis, Missouri, describes the association of embolic stroke and thrombus in a ligated or divided PA stump in 3 patients with functional single ventricle. These events occurred from 1990 through 1992 among 1700 pediatric cardiology admissions at 2 institutions. The patients, ranging in age from 15 months to 9 years, had cerebral infarctions documented by computed axial tomography or MRI associated with the echocardiographic finding of thrombus in the proximal PA stump after the embolic strokes. The strokes occurred 5 days to 5 years after surgery. Two patients had a second infarction within 2 to 5 weeks of the initial stroke. It is concluded that the presence of the ligated PA stump may place patients at risk for embolic stroke. Surgical approaches to reduce the risk of thrombus formation should be considered prospectively in this patient group.

Double-Outlet Right Ventricle

Belli and associates[17] from Le Plessis-Robinson, France, reviewed 180 patients who underwent biventricular repair of double-outlet right ventricle, with 9 requiring reoperation because of subaortic stenosis. In addition, 2 other patients, who had initial operations at another institution, had reoperation for subaortic stenosis. The median age at biventricular repair was 4 months. Repair consisted of tunnel construction from the left ventricle to the aorta in 9 patients, with arterial switch and VSD closure in 2 patients. Subaortic stenosis developed with time; left ventricle to aorta gradient after repair was 10 ± 20 mm Hg and increased to 84 ± 27 mm Hg during a mean follow-up of 45 ± 66 months. At reoperation, the obstruction was caused by protrusion of the inferior rim of VSD into the left ventricular outflow tract associated with subaortic hypertrophied muscle and membrane. There were 11 patients who underwent 15 reoperations. Surgical technique consisted of an extended septoplasty in 6 reoperations. There were no early or late deaths. At 115 ± 85 months after biventricular repair, all patients were asymptomatic or had mild symptoms, and the mean left ventricular to aortic gradient was 20 ± 24 mm Hg. These authors favor an aggressive approach by an extended septoplasty to avoid multiple reoperations. (See Figure 11-10).

Atrioventricular Canal

Cohen and associates[18] from Philadelphia, Pennsylvania, retrospectively reviewed the echocardiograms of 103 patients with complete AV canal and apportioned left and right components. The ventricular cavity ratio between

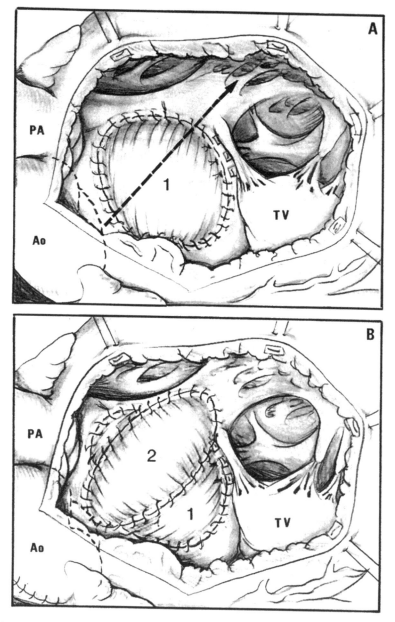

FIGURE 11-10. **A** and **B,** Extended septoplasty viewed through right ventriculotomy. **Arrow** is oriented toward apex of heart. Ao, Aorta; PA, pulmonary artery; TV, tricuspid valve; 1, previous tunnel patch; 2, new patch. Reprinted with permission from Belli et al.[17]

the 2 ventricles was estimated as left ventricular length times width divided by right ventricular length times width. All patients previously categorized as having balanced AV canals had AV valve indices greater than 0.67. Of the 26 patients with unbalanced canal defect, 11 had ductal-dependent circulation and underwent Norwood palliation (AV valve index, 0.21 ± 0.13), and 15 had two-ventricular repair (AV valve index, 0.51 ± 0.12.) Of the latter 15 patients, 9 have survived with no difference in mean AV valve index between survivors and nonsurvivors. For all 103 patients, AV valve index correlated with ventricular cavity ratio. However, of the unbalanced canal group who underwent 2-ventricular repair, 3 nonsurvivors had a discrepancy between AV valve index and ventricular cavity ratio (low AV valve index but normal ventricular size). A large VSD was present in all 6 nonsurvivors and in only 4 of 9 survivors. Echocardiographic morphometry is useful in defining unbalance in complete AV canal defects. If AV valve index is less than 0.67 in the presence of a large VSD, a single-ventricle approach to repair should be considered.

Ventricular Septal Defect

Ueda and associates[19] from Fukuoka, Japan, studied 44 patients requiring surgical repair of VSD during early infancy. Repair was within the first 6 months in 29 patients and during the second 6 months in 15 patients. The left-to-right shunts were significantly greater in the early closure group, whereas the left ventricular end-diastolic volume was significantly greater in the late closure group. The step-up in blood saturation in the lower right atrium was significantly more in the early closure group, suggesting increased shunting across a patent foramen ovale. Right ventricular volume overload caused by left-to-right shunting across the patent foramen ovale, as well as through the VSD during diastole, may be a useful indicator for the likelihood for early repair in infants with large VSD.

Du and associates[20] from Nahariya, Israel, report color Doppler echocardiography performed on (live-birth) preterm neonates from January 1995 to October 1995. The study included 159 infants whose gestational ages ranged from 26 to 36 weeks (mean, 33 weeks) and birth weight from 860 to 2940 g (mean, 2034). At the first examination, the neonates were 12 to 120 hours of age (mean, 46 hours); and in 77 neonates with respiratory diseases or persistent pulmonary hypertension, echocardiography was repeated at an interval of 3 to 5 days until the diagnosis of VSD was confirmed or excluded. Neonates with muscular VSDs were followed at an interval of 2 to 3 months until spontaneous closure was confirmed. Isolated muscular VSD was identified in 9 neonates, a prevalence of 57 per 1000 livebirths. Associated defects were coarctation of the aorta with a perimembranous VSD in 1, pulmonary atresia and large subaortic VSD in 1, and possible ASD in 3. Of 9 neonates with muscular VSDs, 8 had 1 VSD and 1 had multiple defects. Single muscular defects were 1 to 3 mm with a mean of 1.6 mm located at midseptum in 4, apical septum in 3, and posterior trabecular septum in 1. In 7 cases, the defect was detectable only by color Doppler imaging. There were 8 cases followed for 6 to 11 months, or until spontaneous closure occurred. The defect closed in 2 of 6 within 1 to 2 months, 5 of 7 or 71% within 3 to 6 months, and 7 of 8 or 88% within 7 to 11 months. The multiple defects closed at 10 months of age. The reported prevalence of VSD varies from 0.3 to 3.3 per 1000 livebirths, an incidence that is markedly exceeded in this study. Spontaneous closure rates are similar to that of full-term infants.

Pulmonary Atresia

Acherman and associates[21] from Toronto, Ontario, Canada, used 2-dimensional echocardiography and color-flow Doppler to assess pulmonary blood supply in patients with pulmonary atresia and VSD. Studies were performed on 42 patients (aged a few hours to 19 months; mean, 29 days) before any intervention other than intravenous prostaglandins. Angiographic confirmation was available in 29 patients, including 18 of 19 with aortopulmonary collateral channels. A patent arterial duct was correctly identified as the sole source of pulmonary supply in 23 patients, whereas aortopulmonary collateral channels were detected in 19, with 1 of these having a small patent ductus arteriosus and collateral channels. The PDA originated from the undersurface of the aorta in 16 of 24 patients and from the base of the brachiocephalic trunk in 8 of 24. All patients with a PDA as the sole source of blood supply had confluent pulmonary arteries. Nonconfluent PAs were present in 6 patients, with all but 1 having aortopulmonary collateral channels as the sole source of pulmonary flow. These collateral channels were direct in 17 of 19 patients, whereas in 2 of 19, both direct and indirect collateral channels were present. Color-flow Doppler was accurate in determining the presence or absence, the side, and the origin of the collateral channels in all patients, with the correct number being determined in 12 of 18. Failure to identify a tiny central PA occurred in 1 patient. High-resolution imaging and color-Doppler provide good appreciation of the source of pulmonary blood supply in neonates and young infants with pulmonary atresia and VSD, but in most of these patients angiography is needed to plan their operative approach. The echo studies are extremely valuable in planning the most useful angiographic studies.

Moritz and associates[22] from Vienna, Austria, report the use of bilateral transverse thoracosternotomy to provide wide access to the heart, both pleural spaces and hilar structures, for total correction of pulmonary atresia with VSD in 6 patients (ages 1 to 19 years). Blalock-Taussig shunts were previously placed in 3 patients, and intrapericardial PAs were absent in all patients but 1, in whom they were hypoplastic. Central PAs were enlarged with pericardial patches or replaced with tube grafts; the number of unifocalized collateral arteries varied between 2 and 8. There was 1 death caused by respiratory failure and sepsis. Oxygen saturation increased from 75% preoperatively to 96% postoperatively. Mean postoperative PA pressure was 30 mm Hg. One patient had to be reoperated, through the same incision, because of scarring and shrinkage of the peripheral anastomoses. All surviving patients have no symptoms or mild symptoms 6 months after repair. The treatment of pulmonary atresia with VSD and multiple major aortopulmonary collateral arteries remains difficult. This operative technique provides much better access to collateral vessels than a median sternotomy, which gives only a limited exposure to dorsally routed aortico-pulmonary collateral arteries. Although there is a theoretical disadvantage of this clamshell incision with regard to reduced pulmonary function caused by the more painful thoracotomy incision, such was not apparent in this small group of patients.

Partial Atrioventricular Septal Defect

Baufreton and associates[23] from Paris, France, report results in 100 con-secutive patients (aged 2 months to 51 years) who underwent surgical repair of a partial atrioventricular septal defect. Congestive heart failure (CHF) oc-curred in 50% of the cases, and preoperative moderate-to-severe left AV valve incompetence was present in 63% of patients. The cleft of the left valve was closed in 76% of cases. Stepwise logistic regression identified infections and severe abnormalities of the left subvalvular apparatus as predictive factors of early death. Preoperative left valvular incompetence is a predictive factor of residual postoperative valve incompetence. Severe abnormality of the left sub-valvular apparatus is a predictive factor of early reoperation. Abnormalities of the subvalvular apparatus, including malformation or malposition of chordae and/or papillary muscles, are of major importance in postoperative outcome. In addition, a small inferior bridging leaflet can also be an important risk factor. When severe regurgitation is present postoperatively, medical therapy is rarely helpful, and repeat operation usually is required.

Tetralogy of Fallot

Kreutzer and associates[24] from Boston, Massachusetts, and Genolier, Switzerland, report clinical catheterization and surgical data in 10 patients with tetralogy of Fallot with diminutive PAs and severe pulmonary stenosis (PS). Initially, the Nakata index ranged from 20 to 98 mm^2/m^2. The pulmonary valve was first dilated with a balloon (mean balloon/annulus ratio of 1.5), and the mean initial valve annulus score increased from -4 to -3. Other interven-tions included branch PA dilation in 7 patients and coil embolization of aorto-pulmonary channels in 8 patients, with 31 channels embolized. At preoperative follow-up catheterization, the mean pulmonary annulus z score -3 and the Nakata index increased to 143 ± 84 mm^2/m^2. All patients underwent complete surgical repair successfully. At a mean follow-up of 3 years, right ventricular pressure was less than 70% systemic in all patients and less than 50% systemic in 7. In patients with tetralogy of Fallot, severe PS, and diminutive PAs, initial pulmonary valve dilation increases the annulus z score and antegrade pulmo-nary blood flow and facilitates simultaneous coiling of aortopulmonary collat-eral channels and access for PA dilation, all of which results in PA growth and simplification of surgical management.

Norgard and associates[25] from London, United Kingdom, studied 95 pa-tients 4 years after repair of tetralogy of Fallot by echocardiograms, electrocar-diograms and chest radiographs. Restrictive right ventricular physiology de-fined by the presence of antegrade pulmonary flow in late diastole was present in 38% of patients. It was more common in patients with transannular patch repair compared with nontransannular (50% vs. 21%). QRS duration at follow-up was 121 ± 18 and 133 ± 12 msec in restrictive and nonrestrictive patients with transannular patch repair, respectively. Restrictive right ventricular physi-ology has been identified at midterm follow-up in a contemporary surgical series. It is associated with less QRS prolongation, regardless of the technique used for outflow repair, and it may be associated with fewer long-term complications. Nonrestrictive physiology is associated with the most marked QRS prolongation. This subgroup is most at risk from the late deleterious consequences of chronic pulmonary regurgitation.

Bigras and associates[26] from Toronto, Canada, compared the efficacy of 3 procedures for repair of tetralogy of Fallot in 61 patients: 24 patients had undergone transannular patch repair with monocuspid valve, 17 had undergone patch repair without a monocuspid valve, and 20 had undergone repair without a transannular patch. Pulmonary insufficiency was estimated by the width of the pulmonary insufficiency jet to PA diameter by color-flow Doppler. Moderate-to-severe insufficiency was arbitrarily defined as a ratio of at least 0.5. There were no differences in this ratio among the 3 groups. In addition, the percentage of patients with moderate-to-severe pulmonary insufficiency did not differ among the 3 groups. These authors conclude that insertion of a monocuspid valve in repair of tetralogy of Fallot does not prevent short-term postoperative pulmonary insufficiency and does not improve immediate postoperative outcome.

Atallah-Yunes and associates[27] from Syracuse, New York, followed 2 patient groups who had undergone different operations for tetralogy of Fallot: group 1 consisted of 20 patients with repair of tetralogy of Fallot with the use of a modified technique with transatrial VSD closure, a short infundibular incision with avoidance of muscle resection, and patch expansion of the right ventricular outflow tract; group 2 (n = 22) received repair of tetralogy of Fallot by the traditional technique, with VSD closure through ventriculotomy with resection of obstructing muscle. Six patients were excluded from further follow-up: 2 patients, 1 in each group, who required right ventricle pulmonary conduit placement at original repair; 1 patient in group 1 who developed a double-chamber right ventricle; and 3 patients, 2 in group 1 and 1 in group 2, who were lost to follow-up. Postoperative findings more than 10 years after repair showed similar residual or outflow stenosis and obligatory pulmonary insufficiency by examination and Doppler echocardiography; RV size was smaller in the modified group, as reflected by right ventricle/left ventricle ratio on echocardiography, cardiothoracic ratio, and QRS duration. Right ventricular systolic function was more impaired in group 2, as reflected by decreased systolic tricuspid annulus excursion on 2-dimensional echocardiography. Exercise endurance time was significantly higher in group 1 patients, and Lown grade 4 ventricular ectopy was present in 3 patients in group 2 and none in group 1. This modified technique appears to result in better right ventricular function at late follow-up despite apparent similar degrees of pulmonary insufficiency.

Atrial Septal Defect

In this investigation by Sideris and colleagues[28] from Athens, Greece; Hong Kong; Wonju, South Korea; Guandong, China; New Delhi, India; Nancy, France; Lille, France; and Bern, Switzerland, a feasibility clinical study was conducted for the transcatheter occlusion of large ostium secundum atrial septal defects (ASDs) with the centering buttoned device. The centering buttoned device is a modification of the regular buttoned device in which a centering counter occluder is sutured at the central 40% portion of the occluder. During centering, it is stretched, forming a parachute-shaped structure and pulling the occluder over the center of the defect. During buttoning, the counter occluder forms a double figure 8, opposing the right atrial side of the atrial septum. Occlusion was performed in 12 patients aged 6 to 56 years. All had been rejected for transcatheter occlusion by the regular buttoned device, because of either their defect size or the lack of adequate septal rim. The defect size varied between 23 and 31 mm, and the device size varied between 45 and 60 mm. Nine patients had immediately effective occlusions of their defects, and 3 had residual shunts. One patient with unbuttoning had hemolysis at 2 weeks and underwent surgery. Early results of the transcatheter occlusion of large ASDs are promising and larger clinical trials are justified.

Ende and associates[29] from Madison, Wisconsin, and St. Louis, Missouri, attempted transcatheter closure of an atrial defect by using a buttoned occluder system for prevention of recurrence of paradoxic embolism. Nine devices were successfully deployed and 1 was unsuccessful, requiring surgical treatment. There was a residual shunt in 4 patients with 2 of these 4 having resolution of shunting at 6 months and the other 2 at 12 months. One patient had development of a small left atrial thrombus after the procedure without evidence of peripheral embolization and with partial resolution with warfarin sodium treatment. There are now a number of devices that can be used to close atrial defects on an experimental basis. A number will probably be commercially available in the next several years. When to close an atrial defect to prevent paradoxic embolism is an important question that may be answered by large-scale studies.

Heller and associates[30] from Paris, France, sought to determine the clinical significance of a "crochetage" pattern (a notch near the apex of the R wave in the electrocardiogram) on inferior limb leads 2, 3, and AVF in secundum ASD. They searched for this pattern in 1560 older children and adults: 532 with secundum ASD, 266 with VSD, 146 with PS, 110 with MS, 47 with cor pulmonale, and 459 normal subjects. This pattern was observed in 73% of patients with ASD, 36% with VSD, 23% with PS, and only 6% to 11% in other groups. In ASD, the incidence of the "crochetage" pattern increased with larger anatomic defects or greater left-to-right shunt. In all groups, the specificity of the sign for ASD diagnosis was remarkably high when present in all 3 inferior limb leads, even when comparison was limited to patients with an incomplete right BBB pattern. Early disappearance of this pattern was observed in 35% of operated patients. This notch pattern on the R wave of inferior limb leads is common in patients with ASD and may help in terms of the use of electrocardiogram as a screening procedure for patients with subtle ASD findings.

Pascoe and associates[31] from Rochester, Minnesota, performed a retrospective study of 25 patients with sinus venosus ASD who had undergone TEE. The defect was clearly defined by prior transthoracic echocardiography in 3 and was suspected in another 11 on the basis of color-flow imaging. There was unexplained dilatation of the right side of the heart in 10 additional patients, which prompted the transesophageal exam. The defect was visualized with

TEE in all 25 patients and ranged in size from 1 to 3 cm. Right-sided anomalous pulmonary venous connections were identified in 23 patients, and no left-sided anomalous connections were detected. Anatomic confirmation was obtained in all 23 surgical patients, and no patient required preoperative catheterization.

Systemic Arterial Hypertension

Mehta and associates[32] from Cleveland, Ohio, undertook an investigation to examine the relationship of left ventricular mass and function with cardiovascular response to exercise in normotensive adolescents at risk for hypertension. They conducted a prospective, cross-sectional study of 47 individuals (aged 10 to 18 years), who underwent dynamic and isometric exercise, 24-hour Holter monitoring, and echocardiography. Twenty-nine had normotensive parents (group 1, controls), and 18 had hypertensive parents (group 2, "at risk"). Both groups were similar for age, race, sex, body mass index, blood pressures, and resting heart rates. Group 2 had a higher E-A ratio (2.3 ± 0.5 vs. 2.0 ± 0.5) and higher heart rates during stage IV of dynamic exercise (188 ± 20 beats per minute vs. 176 ± 18 beats per minute). The left ventricular mass, 24-hour heart rates, and exercise systolic blood pressures were similar in both groups. In group 2, systolic blood pressures at peak dynamic and isometric exercise correlated best with left ventricular mass. It was concluded that altered hemodynamic regulatory mechanisms may exist before the establishment of hypertension in normotensive subjects with parental hypertension.

Pulmonary Hypertension

Saji and associates[33] from Tokyo, Japan, report preliminary results for oral prostacyclin use in 4 patients with primary pulmonary hypertension and 2 with Eisenmenger syndrome. In primary pulmonary hypertension, there was a 24% fall in pulmonary resistance and a 20% increase in cardiac index. In patients with secondary pulmonary hypertension, there was a 24% fall in pulmonary resistance. This acute demonstration of a favorable effect on pulmonary vascular resistance in this group of patients with rather marked elevation of pulmonary resistance suggests that oral prostacyclin may have a role in treating these life-threatening conditions.

Luciani and associates[34] from Los Angeles, California, report arterial switch for TGA in 2 of 45 infants with profound reversed differential saturation and right-to-left shunting at the ductus after balloon atrial septostomy. A diagnosis of persistent pulmonary hypertension was established and preoperative hemodynamic stabilization was achieved in 1 patient with the use of inhaled nitric oxide, whereas the other required extracorporeal membrane oxygenation for severe biventricular dysfunction. Both underwent successful repair 4 to 5 days after admission but received 1 week of inhaled nitric oxide therapy postoperatively for persistent pulmonary hypertension. Follow-up echocardiography 3 months later showed good biventricular function and normal geometry of the ventricular septum, suggesting a low pulmonary artery pressure in both. Persistent pulmonary hypertension of the newborn can be a devastating disease in infants with normal cardiac anatomy, but results in severe biventricular dysfunction in those infants with TGA who have this added physiological insult. Unless it is recognized early and treated promptly, these infants will not survive. This article, as well as the accompanying commentary by Dr. Wernovsky, should be read by all cardiologists and neonatologists who care for these newborns.

Pulmonary hypertension continues to be a cause of postoperative morbidity and mortality in patients undergoing operations for congenital heart disease. Bando and associates[35] from Indianapolis, Indiana, report 880 high-risk patients with congenital heart disease undergoing cardiopulmonary bypass over a period of 14 years, who were analyzed in terms of risk factors for postoperative pulmonary hypertension. Patients with AV canal (n = 182), truncus arteriosus (n = 47), total anomalous pulmonary venous connection (n = 90), TGA (n = 97), hypoplastic left heart syndrome (n = 50), and VSD (n = 414) demonstrated a higher risk of postoperative pulmonary hypertension. By multivariate logistic regression, preoperative pulmonary hypertension, absence of mixed venous saturation monitoring, and absence of prophylactic α-blockade significantly increased postoperative pulmonary hypertension. Preoperative pulmonary hypertension and absence of prophylactic α-blockers were also significant risk factors for in-hospital death related to pulmonary hypertension. Repair at an older age, except for total anomalous pulmonary venous connection, was also a significant risk for postoperative pulmonary hypertension. These authors conclude that mixed venous saturation monitoring and α-receptor blockade reduced the incidence of pulmonary hypertension after operation for congenital heart disease. Nitric oxide can be a major help in evaluating and treating these patients. Mixed venous saturation monitoring alone obviously will not improve mortality, but the response to the monitoring undoubtedly can improve the outlook in these patients.

Anomalous Pulmonary Venous Drainage

Kubota and associates[36] from Tokyo, Japan, report the use of a rotation-advanced flap method in 11 patients with a partial anomalous venous drainage into the superior vena cava (SVC); of those 5 had sinus venous ASD. Follow-up studies were performed in 7 of 11, and all were alive and well. The surgical technique in Figure 11-11 includes the use of a polytetrafluoroethylene flap to direct the pulmonary venous return to the left atrium. All patient had normal sinus node function, normal hemodynamics, and normal pulmonary angiograms postoperatively. This method appears to be useful in avoiding both pulmonary venous obstruction and sinus node dysfunction for repairing partial anomalous pulmonary venous drainage.

Delius and associates[37] from London, United Kingdom, report 20 of 232 patients with total anomalous pulmonary venous drainage who underwent sur-

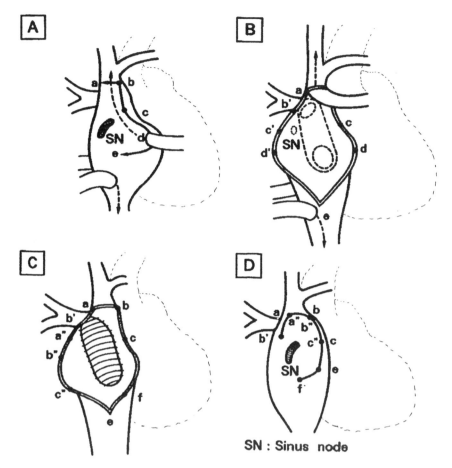

FIGURE 11-11. **A,** Incision is made from a to e. **B,** When original atrial septal defect is small, intraatrial septum in resected to create large atrial septal defect. **C,** Sheet of 0.2 mm polytetrafluoroethylene is sutured so that anomalous pulmonary venous blood is directed into left atrium. **D,** Right atrial wall is used as flap to wider atriocaval channel. Points a-a″, b-b″, and c-c″ are approximated for rotation-advancement of flap. Reprinted with permission from Kubota et al.[36]

gical correction and had a mixed type of drainage. Ages at operation ranged from 1 day to 46 months with a median of 2 months. Both cardiac catheterization and echocardiography were performed before operation in 12 patients, whereas 4 patients underwent only cardiac catheterization, and another 4 underwent only echocardiography. The sensitivity and specificity for diagnosis at catheterization were 94% and 99%; they were 31% and 100%, respectively, for echocardiography. Severe pulmonary venous obstruction was present in 3 patients, all of whom underwent emergency operation. There were 3 deaths (15%), all in patients with preoperative pulmonary venous obstruction who died after operation. There were 2 late deaths: 1 of pulmonary vein stenosis, and the other of probable pulmonary hypertension. The actuarial survival at 10 years was 73% for all patients; patients who survived the initial operation had a 10-year survival of 87%. The diagnosis of mixed total pulmonary venous drainage can be difficult to establish by echocardiography or at the time of operation. For patients in stable condition, cardiac catheterization should be considered if fewer than 3 pulmonary veins are identified by echocardiography. Pulmonary venous obstruction is relatively infrequent in this group but, when present, impacts patient survival significantly.

Total Anomalous Pulmonary Venous Connection

Bando and associates[38] from Indianapolis, Indiana, report risk of early and late mortality and need for reoperation in 105 patients, who underwent surgery for total anomalous pulmonary venous connection between April 1966 and June 1995. Despite increased frequency of neonatal repair in the most recent period, operative mortality declined from 13% in 1966 through 1985 to 0% in 1991 to 1995. The incidence of postoperative pulmonary hypertensive episodes and death related to pulmonary hypertension decreased significantly over the study. By univariate analysis, preoperative pulmonary hypertension and preoperative pulmonary vein obstruction correlated with early mortality, but not in the past 5 years.

Multiple logistic regression analysis showed that only a small pulmonary confluence associated with diffuse pulmonary vein stenosis was an independent risk factor for early or late death, as well as need for reoperation. At a median follow-up of 87 months, late survival was 98% and all were in New York Heart Association class I.

Scimitar Syndrome

Najm and associates[39] from Toronto, Ontario, Canada, report 23 patients with scimitar syndrome, including 11 males and 12 females (median age at diagnosis, 7 months; mean, 8 years; range, 1 day to 70 years). Patients with the diagnosis made during the first year of life (infantile group n = 19) had more severe symptoms, a higher incidence of heart failure (11/19 vs. 0/13) and of pulmonary hypertension (11/19 vs. 1/13) than did the patients in whom the diagnosis was made after age 1 (adult group, n = 13). In 17 patients, the anomalous pulmonary venous drainage was repaired by baffling the vein to the left atrium with median age at this operation of 6 years (mean 15 years, range 6 months to 70%). No deaths occurred in this surgical group during a mean follow-up of 9 years (range 1.6 to 17 years). Pulmonary venous stenosis occurred after repair in 8 patients, or 47%, and 2 required reoperation for this problem. All 6 children in the infantile group had postoperative pulmonary venous stenosis, compared with 2 of 11 older patients. Postoperative quantitative pulmonary perfusion scans performed in 15 patients demonstrated reduced flow to the right lung (mean 24%; range 0% to 59%). The infantile form of this defect is usually associated with hypoplastic right lung, sequestration, and systemic blood supply to the right lung, and pulmonary hypertension with resultant high morbidity and mortality. The adult form usually can be treated successfully if the left-to-right shunt is large enough to warrant repair.

Cavopulmonary Connection

Bradley and associates[40] from Ann Arbor, Michigan, report 85 consecutive patients (<7 months old) who underwent bidirectional superior cavopulmonary connection from December 1990 to February 1995. The average patient age was 5 ± 1 months (range, 5 weeks to 7 months). There were 5 hospital deaths, and PA thrombosis occurred in 3 patients. Younger age was significantly associated with PA thrombosis but not with operative death. Oxygenation improved significantly and spontaneously over the first 48 hours after operation, and younger age had a significantly adverse effect on oxygenation in the early postoperative period. Bidirectional superior caval connection can be performed successfully in infants younger than 6 months of age but is associated with PA thrombosis and postoperative hypoxemia. By waiting 4 to 6 months, if possible, the results of this operation are superior.

Reddy and associates[41] from San Francisco, California, analyzed data from 47 patients who underwent bidirectional cavopulmonary shunts and had preoperative and postoperative angiograms for review. Changes in the various measures of PA size after bidirectional shunt varied considerably, but the increase in the diameter was significant only for lower lobe arteries. Patients who underwent PA augmentation at the time of cavopulmonary shunt had significantly smaller indices before PA augmentation than those who did not undergo PA repair. Patients with PA augmentation also had significantly greater changes in the right and left PA index after bidirectional shunt. The more appropriate measure of PA growth is the indexed cross-sectional area of the lower lobe branch of the right and left PAs, which is less likely to be altered surgically with systemic pulmonary shunts, PA repair, and the bidirectional cavopulmonary anastomosis itself. The concern over growth after the bidirectional cavopulmonary shunt continues, and most people suggest the Fontan repair be completed within 6 to 12 months after the bidirectional cavopulmonary shunt.

Gardiner and associates[42] from London, United Kingdom, followed 119 patients undergoing total cavopulmonary connection between March 1987 and December 1993, to evaluate the incidence and determinants of arrhythmia by use of ambulatory electrocardiographic monitoring. Median age at surgery was 6 years (range, 0.5 to 20 years), and median follow-up was 5 years (range, 2 to 9 years). Ambulatory electrocardiograms were made before and after surgery and serially during follow-up. There were 17 early deaths, including 8 among 20 patients who had new arrhythmia documented in the operating room or intensive care unit. Of the 102 patients who survived more than 30 days after surgery, the proportion free of new arrhythmia or first arrhythmia symptoms was 93% at 2 years and 78% at 5 years. Most of the arrhythmia during follow-up was transient, so that the proportion of patients without arrhythmia was similar before and during follow-up. To date, there has been only 1 late arrhythmic death. The low prevalence of clinically important arrhythmia during medium-term follow-up supports the total cavopulmonary connection as a preferred procedure for Fontan repair.

Van Arsdell and associates[43] from Toronto, Ontario, Canada, report 38 patients who received a superior vena cava-PA anastomosis in association with biventricular repair. Patients were divided into 4 groups on the basis of indication for operation. Group A included 19 patients who had a small right ventricle defined by tricuspid annulus z values or predicted right ventricular volume. Group B included 11 patients who had a functionally compromised right ventricle. Group C included 4 patients who received an SVC-PA anastomosis as a facilitation to biventricular repair. Group D included 4 patients defined by acute postoperative right ventricular dysfunction. Ages ranged from 5 months to 51 years (median 4 years). There were 14 different underlying primary diagnoses in the cohort and multiple associated anomalies. Operative mortality was 11% in group A, 18% in group B, 0% in group 3, and 75% in group D. Follow-up was completed in 37 of 38 patients, ranging from 1 to 174 months (mean 46 ± 37). At follow-up, 22 patients are without symptoms, and 8 patients have mild symptoms. There is no clinical evidence of cyanosis or protein-losing enteropathy. With the use of this adjunctive approach, acceptable intermediate-term outcomes were obtained in patients having an anatomically or functionally compromised pulmonary ventricle. This anastomosis safely facilitates repair in a subset of patients, but results for this procedure when used as a salvage operation for right ventricular dysfunction have not been satisfactory.

Aortic and Pulmonic Valvular Stenosis

Shaddy and associates[44] from Salt Lake City, Utah, measured the frequency of panel-reactive human lymphocyte antigen (HLA) class I alloantibodies before, 1 month after, and 3 months after allograft implantation in 9 children who had cryopreserved valve allograft used in pediatric heart surgery. After allograft implantation, panel-reactive HLA class I alloantibodies increased from 3% before surgery to 63% at 25 days and 100% at 3 months. Control patients showed no increase in panel-reactive HLA class I alloantibodies over time. Cryopreserved valved allografts induce a marked HLA alloantibody response that increases to broad panel reactivity within 3 months after surgery. This HLA sensitization has potential not only for causing deleterious effects on allograft function but also for limiting the future opportunity of heart transplantation in these patients.

Early intervention is necessary in neonates with critical AS. The advent of alternative therapy, particularly balloon aortic valvuloplasty, requires a reappraisal of the traditional surgical approach, including the efficacy of initial transvalvular gradient reduction and freedom from recurrence of obstruction in the longer term. The report by Gildein and associates[45] from Melbourne, Australia, describes a series of 33 consecutive infants who underwent surgical aortic valvotomy in the first month of life. The hospital mortality was 18%, with a 5-year probability of survival of 66%. Fourteen reinterventions, 9 reoperations, and 5 balloon dilatations were required at a median age of 0.8 years (range 9 days to 6 years). Three patients died after reintervention (1 early and 2 late). The median follow-up time was 5.8 years (range 0.2 to 14 years). At last follow-up Doppler investigation, the average Doppler mean and peak gradients were 34 mm Hg and 18 mm Hg. Open valvotomy in neonatal AS allows the use of an appropriate surgical approach with low initial mortality and satisfactory 5-year freedom from reintervention.

van Son and associates[46] from San Francisco, California, assessed 22 patients with a mean age of 6 years with bicuspid in 11, tricuspid in 9, or quadricuspid in 2 aortic valves who underwent valvuloplasty for AS in 9, AR in 7, and a combination in 6. Previous procedures included balloon aortic valvuloplasty in 3 and open surgical valvotomy in 1. Median pressure gradient across the valve was 80 mm Hg. Surgical valvuloplasty techniques included thinning of the leaflets in 18, commissurotomy in 15, suspension of reconstructed leaflets to the aortic wall in 10, closure of leaflet fenestration in 5, shortening of free edge of prolapsed cusp in 4, repair of torn leaflets in 3, and augmentation of scarred leaflets with autologous pericardium in 3. Concomitant subvalvular and supravalvular stenosis was repaired in 9 and 4 patients, respectively. In 5 patients during the same hospital stay, a failed valvuloplasty was converted into a valve replacement with a pulmonary autograft because of residual or resultant stenosis in 3 or regurgitation in 2. There were no early or late deaths. At a median follow-up of 16 months, the median pressure gradient across the valve in 15 patients with preoperative stenosis or combined stenosis and regurgitation was 16 mm Hg. Of the 22 patients, the aortic valve functioned normally, defined as mild stenosis or regurgitation or both, in 14 patients including 5 with valve replacement. There were 4 patients who had residual stenosis with gradients of 40 to 60 mm Hg, 2 patients had regurgitation and 2 patients had combined stenosis with gradients of 40 to 50 mm Hg and regurgitation. Outcome after valvuloplasty was examined according to the valve structure: 6 of 9 tricuspid valves functioned normally, whereas only 3 of 13 nontricuspid valves functioned normally. Patients with a nontricuspid aortic valve and regurgitation had a high probability of requiring immediate valve replacement. The actuarial freedom from significant native stenosis or regurgitation at 24 months was 82% for tricuspid valves and 36% for nontricuspid valves. These authors suggest that surgically aortic valvuloplasty should be the preferred approach when the aortic valve is tricuspid, but in contrast, AVR with a pulmonary autograft should be considered in the presence of a nontricuspid aortic valve, especially when the valve is regurgitant or when surgical valvuloplasty has failed.

Starnes and associates[47] from Los Angeles, California, report 24 aortic root replacements with a pulmonary autograft in pediatric patients younger than 18 years of age. Of this group, 8 were infants and children with complex left ventricular outflow tract obstruction (aged 9 days to 22 months). The diagnoses were interrupted aortic arch/VSD/subaortic stenosis in 3, recurrent AS in 2, AS and subaortic stenosis in 1, and AS/subaortic stenosis, MS and MR in 2. All patients had undergone 1 to 3 previous operations. Preoperative echocardiographic peak left ventricular outflow gradients were 72 ± 25 mm Hg, and aortic annulus size was 7 ± 2 mm (range 4 to 11 mm). Surgical technique included replacement of the aortic root with the pulmonary autograft combined with incision of the conal septum to relieve subaortic stenosis or accommodate for size discrepancy between the aortic and pulmonary root, and a pulmonary homograft was placed in the right ventricular outflow tract. There were no perioperative or late deaths at follow-up from 2 to 25 months. Three children had complications with diaphragmatic paresis in 1, delayed pericardial effusion in 1, and AV block requiring a pacemaker in 1. Follow-up echocardiographic findings showed absent AR in 3, trivial AR in 5, and no significant LV outflow tract obstruction. Pulmonary homograft regurgitation was absent in 5, trivial in 2, and moderate in 1. Right ventricular outflow tract gradient by echocardiogram was trivial in 7, with a significant gradient of 55 mm Hg in 1 infant. It is hoped that these excellent results can be duplicated by other centers to deal with the perplexing problem of recurrent left ventricular outflow tract obstruction in young patients.

Baskett and associates[48] from Halifax, Nova Scotia, Canada, report the results of surgery for 48 homograft valves, which were cryopreserved onsite and implanted to reconstruct the right ventricular outflow tract in 44 children (aged 3 days to 20 years; mean 6 years). There was blinded serial echocardiographic follow-up in all 45 valves in the 41 survivors. Homograft valves were replaced because of pulmonary insufficiency in 3, or stenosis and insufficiency in 1. Freedom from reoperation was 90% at 50 months. During the follow-up period, 15 valves developed progressive pulmonary insufficiency of at least 2 grades and, in 3 valves, transvalvular gradients developed ($\geq$ 50 mm Hg). The freedom from echocardiographic failure defined as 2 or more grades of pulmonary regurgitation or of 50 mm Hg or higher was 44% at 50 months. Young age, low operative weight, small graft size, and homograft retrieval-to-cryopreservation time of less than 24 hours were significantly associated with failure. The type of donor valve (pulmonary vs aortic), donor age, and blood group mismatch were not associated with failure, although the blood group mismatch approached significance. Homografts function well as conduits between the pulmonary ventricle and PAs if long-term valve competency is not crucial. However, many homografts rapidly become insufficient, and this is an important implication for the choice of a valve if the indication for valve replacement is to protect a ventricle failing due to pulmonary insufficiency. Short periods between homograft retrieval and cryopreservation enhance viability and antigenicity, suggesting an immunological basis for graft failure.

Elkins and associates[49] from Oklahoma City, Oklahoma, reviewed results in 195 survivors of the Ross operation performed between 1986 and 1995. Freedom from reoperation was 89% $\pm$ 3% at 5 years and 92% $\pm$ 3% for the autograft alone. Early autograft valve failures after 6 months or less were due to technical error in 2 patients and persistent endocarditis in 1. Late autograft valve failure at 1 to 6 years was due to aortic annulus dilatation in 5 patients, bacterial endocarditis in 1, and valve degeneration in 2. Six autograft valves were replaced, and 5 were repaired. Reoperation for pulmonary homograft stenosis was required in 5 patients at 1 to 5 years involving obstruction of the conduit distal to the pulmonary valve. This study reveals a low incidence of reoperation for either autograft dysfunction or homograft obstruction. Autograft dysfunction can be corrected by autograft repair in patients with central insufficiency and aortic annular dilation.

Moore and associates[50] from Boston, Massachusetts, performed a retrospective review of 148 children (>1 month of age) who underwent balloon dilation for AS. Dilation was successful in 87% of patients, with a procedural mortality rate of 0.7%. The average immediate peak-to-peak gradient reduction was 56 ± 20%, and prior valvotomy was the only factor that significantly reduced the immediate gradient reduction after dilation (47 vs. 58%). Survival after dilation was 95% at 8 years; 75% of patients were free of repeat intervention 4 years after dilation, whereas 50% remain free of repeat intervention at 8 years. Asymmetrically thick valve leaflets and prior aortic valvotomy decreased the risk of repeat intervention. AR grade of 3 or more and residual gradient after dilation increased the risk of repeat intervention. The 8-year survival rate after dilation of 95%, with 50% of patients free of repeat intervention, indicates that, in appropriate skilled hands, balloon valvotomy is quite effective as a palliative management strategy prior to the need for valve replacement.

Hawkins and associates[51] from Salt Lake City, Utah, report the need for surgery after aortic valvuloplasty in 60 patients with congenital AS (age, 1 day to 27 years; mean, 7 years). Operation was required in 23 patients (38%) at a mean of 44 ± 37 months after valvuloplasty because of severe AR in 13 and recurrent or residual AS in 10. Severe AR was invariably due to avulsion of a cusp from the annulus, with resulting cusp prolapse and insufficiency (Figure 11-12). Operative intervention consisted of valve replacement in 14 patients and valve repair in 9. Actuarial freedom from surgical intervention after balloon valvuloplasty was 88% at 1 year, 70% at 5 years, and 51% at 9 years. All patients survived operation, and there was 1 late death. The average follow-up was 27 ± 20 months. Echocardiographic follow-up for the valve repair patients revealed a mean residual AS gradient of 32 mm Hg and mild AR or less in all patients. These authors found a 5% to 7% requirement for operation yearly after balloon valvuloplasty. These authors find a relatively high incidence of severe AR requiring operation after balloon valvuloplasty, a complication usually associated with a higher balloon/annulus ratio than 1.0. Other institutions have not reported this prevalence of AR requiring relatively early operation.

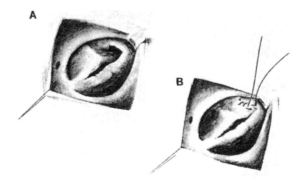

Figure 11-12. Pathological process and repair of aortic insufficiency after balloon aortic valvuloplasty in a patient with a bicuspid valve. In patients with severe aortic insufficiency, typically there is avulsion of one cusp from the annulus with resulting cusp prolapse **(A)**. Repair in this situation involves reattachment of the avulsed leaflet to the annulus using interrupted monofilament suture **(B)**. Reprinted with permission from Hawkins et al.[51]

Tricuspid Atresia

Ho and associates[52] from London, United Kingdom, examined 53 hearts with tricuspid atresia and 58 normal hearts matched for age. Using a microscopic-morphometric method, they analyzed the percentage field area occupied by interstitial fibrous tissue in 4 sites of the ventricular mass. A comparison of sample sites showed no significant variations between normal and malformed hearts, and results from a homogeneity of regression coefficients suggested that the 2 groups shared the same basic relation of proportion of fibrosis with age. There was, however, a clear separation between the extent of fibrous tissue in the 2 groups of hearts: tricuspid atresia hearts were consistently more fibrotic than normal hearts. These authors suggest that increased fibrosis in tricuspid atresia may be an inherent part of the malformation and not necessarily due to changes produced by cyanosis and volume or pressure overload.

Pulmonary Stenosis

Gildein and associates[53] from Melbourne, Australia, report the immediate and medium-term results of pulmonary valve dilation in 18 neonates in whom valvuloplasty was attempted. The procedure was accomplished in 14 patients, and the angiographically determined diameters of the pulmonary and tricuspid valves at the time of the procedure were 5.6 ± 1.5 and 14.0 ± 5.4 mm, respectively. The mean Doppler gradient decreased from 71 ± 27 to 27 ± 14 mm Hg. Perforation of the right ventricular outflow tract was a major complication in 3 patients, with 1 fatal event. Prostaglandin could be discontinued 1 to 5 days after the procedure. On follow-up, 3 children required a second balloon dilation with good results. There were 7 patients monitored for more than 9 months (mean follow-up, 34 ± 16 months), with a residual gradient of 12 ± 7 mm Hg. These authors showed good results with treatment of a difficult patient group. Interestingly, no patients had small tricuspid valves, but the majority had quite small pulmonary valve rings. Thus, the practice of recommending transannular patching of the hypoplastic pulmonary valve annulus in this lesion may need to be reviewed.

Redington and Somerville[54] from London, United Kingdom, undertook palliative stenting in 12 patients with complex pulmonary atresia and aortopulmonary collaterals. Each patient had at least 1 stenotic but balloon-dilatable collateral that supplied at least 3 lung segments. Twelve stents were deployed in 11 patients; in 1 patient it was not possible to traverse the stenotic area with a stent. There was no effect in 1 patient who had multiple stenoses distal to the stented area. There was excellent palliation in the remainder, with arterial oxygen saturation of 45% to 79% before stenting (mean 64% ± 12%), rising to 67% to 90% (mean 78% ± 10%) at discharge. One patient was referred for surgery to secure blood flow to a nearly totally occluded side branch to the right upper lobe traversed by the stent. There was excellent symptomatic response in the remainder, with an early increase in exercise duration. Late arterial

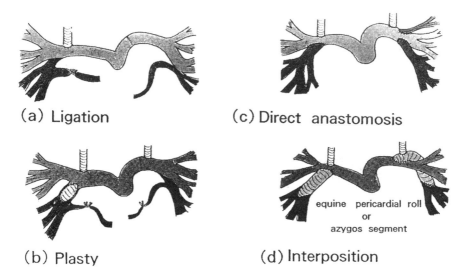

(a) Ligation

(c) Direct anastomosis

(b) Plasty

(d) Interposition

equine pericardial roll
or
azygos segment

FIGURE 11-13. Basic procedures to unifocalize intrapulmonary arteries in patients with central pulmonary arteries. **a,** Ligation of major anteroposterior collateral artery or coil embolization; **b,** repair of stenotic communication of intrapulmonary arteries with or without patch; **c,** direct anastomosis between intrapulmonary arteries; **d,** interposition between intrapulmonary arteries with azygos vein graft or pericardial tube graft (roll). Reprinted with permission from Yagihava et al.[55]

desaturation occurred in 2 patients. Stenting of stenotic collaterals can achieve palliation in a number of patients in this selected subgroup, and it appears to be an important new therapy for these complex patients.

Yagihara and associates[55] from Osaka, Japan, reported 50 patients with pulmonary atresia and VSD with major aortico-pulmonary collateral arteries who underwent unifocalization at ages ranging from 2 months to 26 years (mean 6 ± 7 years). A total of 84 staged procedures and 5 other palliative procedures were done in 49 patients. Basic procedures included ligation or coil embolization, repair of stenotic communications, direct patch and anastomosis between intrapulmonary arteries, and interposition between intrapulmonary arteries with xenograft or pericardial tube grafts (Figures 11-13 and 11-14). In addition, construction of a central PA with a xenograft pericardial tube was performed in 36 patients. There were 5 deaths after operation among those undergoing these 89 reparative operative procedures. Intracardiac repair after previous unifocalization has been performed in 26 patients. The right-to-left ventricle systolic pressure ratio immediately after intracardiac repair ranged from 0.24 to 0.91 (mean 0.54). One patient died shortly after intracardiac repair because of thrombosis within the PA. Postoperative catheterization showed that pulmonary resistance correlated significantly with the number of functioning pulmonary vascular segments rather than with the condition of central PAs. These authors show excellent results for this very difficult group of patients. It appears that surgical unifocalization leading to subsequent repair is feasible in a certain number of patients despite extremely hypoplastic or absent central PA.

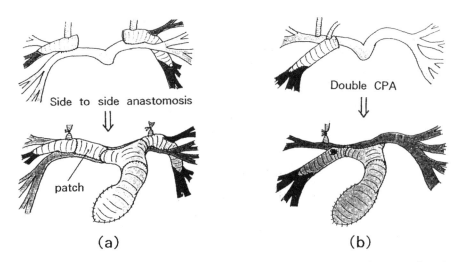

FIGURE 11-14. Construction of supplemental central pulmonary artery with xenograft pericardial tube in patients with slender central pulmonary arteries. In **upper left,** proximal side of tube is anastomosed to central pulmonary artery in side-to-side fashion. Upper right shows "double central pulmonary arteries" (CPA). **Lower illustrations** show how to reconstruct central pulmonary arteries at time of intracardiac repair. **a,** tube was connected to external conduit after enlargement of central pulmonary arteries with use of patch. **b,** tube was unified together with native central arteries. Reprinted with permission from Yagihara et al.[55]

Kreutzer and associates[56] from Boston, Massachusetts, reported presentation, evolution, and management of 12 adults with isolated pulmonary artery stenosis with a mean age of 36 years and a range from 17 to 51 years. Presenting symptoms were dyspnea and fatigue; perfusion scans revealed multiple segmental abnormalities of flow distribution in all patients. Right ventricular pressure was suprasystemic in 2, systemic in 1, and more than half-systemic in 7. All had multiple, bilateral, nonuniform stenoses in segmental and subsegmental arteries. Balloon pulmonary angioplasty to decrease right ventricular hypertension and improve pulmonary flow distribution was performed in 11 patients; vessel diameter increased by more than 50% in 10, distal PA pressure increased by more than 30% in 6, and right ventricular pressure decreased by more than 30% in 5. There was 1 death shortly after the procedure from pulmonary hemorrhage. Immediate procedural success was achieved in 9 of 11 patients; at a mean follow-up of 52 ± 32 months, 7 patients had sustained symptomatic improvement. There have been marked improvements in the treatment of pulmonary artery stenosis, both with dilatation and stents. Patients who have been considered previously as inoperable can now be treated successfully by this modality by those groups with considerable experience with this technique.

Patent Ductus Arteriosus

Dessy and colleagues[57] in Rotterdam, The Netherlands, evaluated 52 patients who had undergone successful transcatheter closure for patent ductus arteriosus during a 5-year period. Forty-nine were re-examined between March 1995 and June 1995. Clinical and echocardiographic examination and lung scintigraphy were performed. The Rashkind patent ductus arteriosus occluder device was used in the patients in this study presenting with a patent ductus arteriosus diagnosed by clinical, 2-dimensional echocardiographic and Doppler flow examinations. The initial procedure was successful in 52 patients (93%). Two patients underwent a second procedure without any problems because of significant residual shunting at 7 and at 26 months after the first procedure. All patients had isolated patent ductus arteriosus. Follow-up evaluation demonstrated protrusion into the left pulmonary artery of the occluder device in 5 of 49 patients (10%). In these patients, maximal flow velocity in the left pulmonary artery was significantly increased. Decreased lung perfusion defined as less than 40% of total pulmonary blood flow was found in 7 of 49 patients (14%). Although mean left pulmonary artery perfusion was decreased in patients with protrusion of the device, there was considerable overlap with patients without protrusion. Thus, these data demonstrate that protrusion of the occluder device after patent ductus arteriosus closure into the left pulmonary artery is an infrequent finding. It may be associated with increased maximal flow velocity in the left pulmonary artery and diminished left lung perfusion.

Hijazi and associates[58] from Boston, Massachusetts, and Ann Arbor, Michigan, reported their experience with transcatheter closure of PDA in infants 8 kg or smaller with single or multiple Gianturco coils and comparative results for PDA of 2.5 mm or less versus PDA greater than 2.5 mm. There were 24 infants with a median age of 0.7 years (range 2 weeks to 1.5 years) and a median weight of 6.5 kg (range 2.3 to 8 kg) who had 14 coils placed by transvenous route, 10 by transarterial route. The median PDA diameter was 2.7 mm (range 0.4–5.2 mm). PDA diameters of less than 2.5 mm were present in 10, and all had complete closure. PDA diameters of 2.5 mm or more were present in 14, and closure was complete in 10 patients, 9 of whom required multiple coils. There was immediate complete closure of the PDA with a diameter as large as 5.2 mm that has persisted at a median follow-up of 1.2 years. Closure was unsuccessful in 4 patients, each of whom required multiple coils. Complications included transient loss of femoral pulse in 2 infants, mild left PA obstruction in 2, and nonretrievable coil migration to the right lung in one. These authors conclude that transcatheter closure is effective therapy for small infants with a PDA diameter of less than 5.2 mm and that this procedure can be performed in neonates as small as 2.3 kg. Transcatheter closure of PDA as an outpatient is becoming more common in the older patient and has an excellent track record. The ability to apply this method to a small infant is worthwhile goal, but the procedure should be limited to centers with considerable expertise in pediatric interventional catheterization and with surgery available should it be required. Further studies will be necessary to determine the optimal use of this procedure.

In a study by Galal and associates[59] from Riyadh, Saudi Arabia, and Boston, Massachusetts, 35 patients (mean age 44 months, mean weight 13 kg) underwent anterograde PDA occlusion with Gianturco coils (coil group). These patients were compared with 35 age- and weight-matched patients who underwent PDA closure with the Rashkind umbrella device (device group). The mean

PDA diameter at its narrowest point was 2.8 mm in the coil group and 2.7 mm in the device group. There was immediate closure angiographically in 20 (57%) of 35 in the coil group compared with 9 (26%) of 35 for the device group. Color-flow mapping before discharge revealed complete closure in 30 (86%) of 35 in the coil group compared with 18 (51%) of 35 in the device group. Mean fluoroscopy time was 19 minutes (median 14 minutes) and 15 minutes (median 13 minutes) for the coil and device, respectively. Four coils and 1 device embolized down the PA; all were successfully retrieved in the catheterization lab. Coil closure of the small-to-moderate PDA is safe and effective. It is more effective than the Rashkind device for achieving immediate closure. More clinical trials with the coil technique are warranted to establish the long-term results.

Shim and associates[60] from Ann Arbor, Michigan, reviewed 75 patients who underwent coil occlusion of a PDA and who had residual shunting investigated by Doppler echocardiography. Residual shunts were found in 31 patients (41%) on the day of the procedure, and spontaneous closure was noted in 17 (55%) at 2 weeks to 20 months of follow-up. Of the 75 patients studied, 5 (7%) required a second coil procedure, and 10 (13%) remained with persistent residual shunts at most recent follow-up. Actuarial analysis estimated a 6% ± 5% prevalence of residual shunts 20 months after a single coil procedure and 3% ± 3% after all coil procedures. Minimal ductal diameter was associated with immediate complete ductal occlusion by a single coil. No association was identified between ductal angiographic type and outcome of coil occlusion. Small residual shunts are common after initial coil embolization, but most close spontaneously. A number of interventionalists now will place multiple coils until complete ductal closure is demonstrated.

Kimball and associates[61] from Cincinnati, Ohio, evaluated 14 premature infants with an average weight of 1 kg or less who underwent PDA ligation, with echocardiographic evaluation before, immediately after, and 24 hours after ligation. Data were compared with those of 14 preterm infants without PDA. Infants with PDA had higher values for ventricular performance, including mean fractional area change, and lower values for wall stress before ligation than did the control group. At 24 hours after ligation, ventricular performance was not significantly changed, but there were significant increases in blood pressure and systemic vascular resistance and no changes in wall stress or contractility. Ventricular performance is higher in premature infants with PDA because afterload is lower. Although ductal ligation increases blood pressure and systemic resistance, wall stress and ventricular performance are maintained. These results suggest that the premature newborn maintains ventricular performance during stress, at least in part, by manipulation of afterload.

Arrhythmias

Naheed and associates[62] from Chicago, Illinois, studied 30 consecutive patients with fetal SVT, with management prenatally in 17 and postnatally in 13. The fetal SVT mechanism was 1:1 AV conduction in 22 patients and SVT with AV block (atrial flutter) in 8. At the postnatal transesophageal procedure,

SVT was induced in 27 of 30; AV reentrant tachycardia in 25 (93%); and intraatrial reentrant tachycardia in only 2 of 27 (7%). Hydrops was present in 12 of 30 fetuses; sustained SVT (> 12 hours) and lower gestation at presentation correlated with hydrops, but mechanism of tachycardia and heart rate did not. Gestational age at delivery was significantly greater in those who received intrauterine management despite earlier presentation. AV reentrant tachycardia was the predominant mechanism of SVT in the fetus, and there was a high association of SVT with AV block in utero and accessory AV connections. Outcome at 1 to 7 years was excellent regardless of severity of illness at clinical presentation. These authors demonstrate very clearly the benefit of tertiary care management with the perinatologist, neonatologist, and cardiologist working together. With such management, there appeared to be a decrease in morbidity related to hydrops and a definite decrease in prematurity and cesarean section delivery.

Reciprocating SVT may have several clinical presentations, with symptoms often more severe during exercise or emotional stress. This study by Drago and associates[63] from Rome, Italy, shows, by using transesophageal atrial pacing, the factors related to syncope during exercise. Between May 1989 and June 1994, transesophageal atrial pacing was performed at rest and during exercise in 75 children (aged >6 years) with suspected or documented episodes of paroxysmal SVT. Reciprocating SVT could be induced both at rest and during exercise in 22 patients (8 girls, 14 boys; mean age 11 ± 2.7 years; range 7 to 15 years) with ventriculoatrial interval less than 70 msec in 11 patients and greater than 70 msec in 11. At rest, all patients had palpitations caused by the induction of tachycardia. After conversion to sinus rhythm, when tachycardia was induced during exercise, symptoms did not change in 14 patients (group A), whereas symptoms worsened (presyncope) in 8 (group B). The statistical analysis showed a significant difference of mean reciprocating SVT rate at rest between the 2 groups (group A, 211 ± 23 beats per minute; group B, 173 ± 33 beats per minute) and reciprocating SVT rate variation from rest to exercise (group A, 62 ± 18 beats per minute; group B, 105 ± 24 beats per minute). These data suggest that children with low tachycardia rate during normal activities may have syncope more frequently, independent of the tachycardia rate during exercise or emotional stress.

To assess the efficacy and safety of current pharmacologic therapy for SVT in infants, Weindling and associates[64] from Boston, Massachusetts, reviewed 112 infants treated between July 1985 and March 1993. The SVT mechanism was determined by esophageal electrophysiologic study and involved an accessory pathway in 86, AV nodal reentry in 10, atrial muscle reentry in 11, and an ectopic atrial tachycardia in 5 patients. Of 6 infants not treated, none had clinical recurrence of SVT. Of the 106 patients treated, 70% remained free of tachycardia while receiving digoxin, propranolol, or both. Class I antiarrhythmic agents were necessary for 13 patients, and class III agents were required for another 13 infants. Verapamil was used in 1 infant with AV nodal reentry tachycardia. Nine infants with complex clinical presentations were believed to have failed medical management and underwent radiofrequency ablation. Five patients died: 4 of complications related to structural heart disease, and 1 shortly after radiofrequency ablation was performed. No deaths appeared to be related to antiarrhythmic medications. No drug-related side effects requiring medication change occurred, and no proarrhythmia was observed. Thus medical therapy appears to be effective and safe in infants with SVT. Radiofrequency ablation should be reserved for rare infants who fail aggressive medical regimens or when the situation is complicated by ventricular dysfunction, severe symptoms, or complex congenital heart disease.

Mehta and associates[65] from Johnson City, Tennessee, report the use of atenolol in 22 children younger than 18 years of age with clinical SVT. Once-a-day oral atenolol was started as monotherapy, and tachycardia in 13 patients (59%) was well controlled long-term. The effective dosage ranged between 0.3 and 1.3 mg/kg/day, with a median effective dose of 0.7 mg/kg/day. There were adverse effects in 5, with colic and diarrhea in 1 infant, reactive airway disease in 1 patient, recurrent headache in 1, drowsiness and daydreaming in school in 1, and fatigue in 1 other patient. Atenolol appears useful as monotherapy for children with various types of SVT who benefit from β-blocker effect. Despite its relative cardioselective effect, some patients experienced adverse reactions.

Studies have suggested that interatrial septal aneurysms may be the initiating mechanisms of SVT in newborns and infants. A retrospective study was performed by Miga and associates[66] from Charleston, South Carolina, to determine the incidence of interatrial septal aneurysms in 30 infants with atrial arrhythmias (SVT, atrial flutter, or frequent premature atrial contractions) and their possible relation to the mechanism of atrial arrhythmias. An interatrial septal aneurysm was defined as dilatation of the septum greater than 5 mm beyond the plane of the atrial septum and associated with redundant tissue and abnormal mobility. The study patients were compared with age- and sex-matched control subjects. Four (13%) of the 30 study patients and 2 (7%) of 30 control individuals had an interatrial septal aneurysm. In contrast to previous reports, this study demonstrates that there is not a significant relation between the presence of interatrial septal aneurysms and the onset and recurrence of atrial arrhythmias.

Perry and associates[67] from San Diego, California; Houston, Texas; Atlanta, Georgia; and Boston, Massachusetts, studied the efficacy and safety of intravenous amiodarone in young patients with critical drug-resistant arrhythmias. Forty patients were enrolled, with 25 of 40 having early postoperative tachyarrhythmias and 21 of 25 having early successful treatment. Ventricular tachyarrhythmias were treated in 12: 7 had successful therapy and 6 died. No deaths were related to the drug. Atrial tachyarrhythmias were present in 11: 10 of 11 had immediate success, but 3 later died. Junctional ectopic tachycardia occurred in 14, which was treated with success in 13 of 14, with no deaths. There were 3 other patients with SVT, with successful treatment in 2 and no deaths. Mild hypotension during the amiodarone bolus occurred in 4 patients, and 1 patient experienced bradycardia requiring temporary pacing. None of the 9 of 40 deaths were attributed to amiodarone. This potent antiarrhythmic appears safe and effective for most young patients and can be lifesaving in certain situations when standard therapy is ineffective.

Schaffer and associates[68] from Denver, Colorado; Portland, Oregon; Norfolk, Virginia; and Omaha, Nebraska, report results of the Pediatric Radiofrequency Ablation Registry regarding the incidence, significance, and factors associated with inadvertent AV block during radiofrequency catheter ablation in childhood and adolescence. AV block occurred in 23 of 1964 ablations (1.2%), 14 as third-degree block (3 transient) and 9 as second-degree block (5 transient). Heart block occurred from 5 seconds to 2 months (mean 4 days; median 15 seconds) after the onset of the energy application. Transient cases lasted from 1 hour to 1 month, with a mean of 9 days and a median of 7 days. Inadvertent block was related to ablation site: 3 of 111 (3%) anteroseptal, 11 of 106 (10%) midseptal, and 2 of 197 (1%) right posteroseptal sites. Heart block occurred in 5 of 314 ablations (2%) for atrioventricular and nodal reentrant tachycardia. Compared with matched subgroups, radiofrequency ablation experience was the only significant risk factor for the occurrence of AV block. Inadvertent AV block may occur during, or late after, catheter ablation. It is associated with ablations for (1) anterior and midseptal accessory pathways and AV nodal reentry and (2) relative institutional inexperience.

Gonska and associates[69] from Göttingen, Germany, reported 16 patients in whom ventricular arrhythmias occurred 11 to 42 years after repair of congenital heart defects. There were 15 patients with a history of symptomatic sustained or nonsustained VT, and 1 had frequent nonsustained VT. Catheter ablation was carried out in the temperature-controlled mode, and follow-up was 6 to 33 months with a mean of 16 months. A right ventricular origin of the tachycardia in the surgically corrected area could be determined in all patients, and ablation was carried out without complications. Immediate noninducibility was achieved in 15 of the 16 patients, and 1 patient in whom VT was again inducible 1 week later was successfully treated with amiodarone. Antiarrhythmic drugs were discontinued in 11 patients. During follow-up, none had recurrence of the tachycardia that had been ablated. These authors present impressive results for radiofrequency ablation in patients with VT after successful repair of congenital defects. Since these conditions are potentially life threatening, it is hoped that this new approach can be generalized to larger groups of patients.

Sudden Cardiac Death

Steinberger and associates[70] from Minneapolis, Minnesota, studied the hearts of 70 patients 21 years of age or younger who died suddenly. Twenty patients were less than 1 year of age, and 50 were 1 to 21 years old. The cardiac findings were compared to those in 68 age-matched controls with known cardiac disease who did not die suddenly. Significant cardiac abnormalities were present in 13 (65%) of the 20 infants; 10 (50%) had anomalies of the aortic origin of the coronary arteries. Among the 50 older patients, cardiac abnormalities were found in 40 (80%), among whom coronary arterial anomalies existed in 12 (24%). Anomalies of aortic origin more frequently involved the left main coronary artery than the right coronary artery in both groups (Table 11-1).

Fontan Procedure

Fogel and associates[71] from Philadelphia, Pennsylvania, used MRI to evaluate cardiac function in 35 patients with a functional single ventricle at

TABLE 11-1
Sudden Death in Young Patients

Findings	Age<1 yr (n = 20)	Age 1–21 yr (n = 50)
Age		
Range	1 day to 1 yr	1–21 yr
Mean ± SEM	4.3 ± 1.1 mo	12.8 ± 1.5 yr
Males	14 (70%)	31 (62%)
Females	6 (30%)	19 (38%)
Cardiac abnormalities	13 (65%)	40 (80%)
Coronary arterial anomaly	10 (50%)	12 (24%)
Ectopic* aortic origin only	2 (R-1, B-1)	4 (R-2, L-2)
Acute angle aortic origin only	3 (L-3)	2 (L-2)
Both of the above	4 (L-4)	6 (L-4, R-2)
Ostial stenosis	1 (R-1)	0
Myocarditis	0	14 (28%)
Hypertrophic cardiomyopathy	1 (5%)	6 (12%)
Other cardiac abnormality	2 (10%)	8 (16%)
No cardiac abnormality	7 (35%)	10 (20%)

* Includes eccentric, wrong sinus, and high aortic origins (see text definitions).
B = both coronary arteries; L = left coronary artery; R = right coronary artery.
Reproduced with permission from Steinberger et al.[70]

various stages of Fontan reconstruction: 15 in the pre-hemi-Fontan stage, 11 after the hemi-Fontan operation, and 9 after the Fontan procedure. There was no difference from the pre-hemi-Fontan stage 6 to 9 months after the hemi-Fontan procedure in end-diastolic volume, mass, ventricular output, or centroid motion. Patients in the Fontan group demonstrated a marked decrease in all indices, indicating significant volume unloading and decrease in mass and ventricular performance. These authors did not show the volume unloading with the hemi-Fontan procedure that has been reported previously with studies within the first week or 2 after this procedure. One possible explanation for this difference is that the authors did not study the same patients sequentially, but used different patients for the 3 groups. In addition, aortopulmonary collateral flow after the hemi-Fontan operation, as well as change in blood flow distribution with increased flow to the head and neck after hemi-Fontan, may also have contributed to these results.

Jacobs and associates[72] from Philadelphia, Pennsylvania, report on 400 patients younger than 2 years of age who underwent hemi-Fontan operation, with mean age at operation of 9 months (range, 2 to 24 months). The operation included association of SVC with the branch PA, augmentation of the central PA, occlusion of the inflow of the SVC in the right atrium, and elimination of other sources of pulmonary blood flow. Operative mortality was 31 (8%) of 400 patients. In the last 200 patients, operative mortality was 4%. Younger age at operation was not an independent risk factor for mortality, but urgent operation in the presence of a hemodynamic burden requiring concomitant procedures was associated with increased mortality. It is hoped that these impressive results for use of the hemi-Fontan at an early age in patients with complex disease can be duplicated by other centers dealing with a large number of patients with complex single-ventricle anatomy.

Forbes and associates[73] from Houston, Texas, and Columbus, Ohio, evaluated 23 patients who initially received a systemic-to-PA shunt as an initial procedure before subsequent Fontan palliation. In 8 of these patients (group 1), bidirectional cavopulmonary anastomosis was performed before the age of 3 years, and in 4 (group 2), it was performed after the age of 10 years. The remaining 11 patients (group 3) were maintained with their initial shunt until they underwent Fontan palliation. Serial echocardiographic analysis was used to evaluate left ventricular volume, mass, and systolic pump function. Through 10 months of follow-up, group 1 patients showed significant decreases in indexed end-diastolic volumes after cavopulmonary anastomosis, whereas patients in groups 2 and 3 showed progressive increases in volume. Indexed ventricular mass decreased moderately after bidirectional cavopulmonary anastomosis in group 1 and was unchanged in groups 2 and 3. The ejection fraction decreased significantly in group 2 versus group 1 patients after cavopulmonary anastomosis. Oxygen saturation measurements before and after bidirectional shunt revealed a significant increase in group 1, from 73% to 86%, and a decrease in group 2, from 82% to 73%. Bidirectional cavopulmonary anastomosis facilitates ventricular volume unloading and promotes regression of LV mass in younger children (< 3 years of age) in preparation for a Fontan operation. In contrast, bidirectional cavopulmonary anastomosis is of questionable value in older children as a staging procedure for Fontan palliation. The older patients in this study had an increase in volume associated with a marked decrease in ejection fraction and systemic oxygen saturation after cavopulmonary anastomosis, indicating the marked deleterious effect of this procedure in this small subgroup.

Kreutzer and associates[74] from Boston, Massachusetts, reported 8 patients (8 to 25 years old) with tricuspid atresia in 4, double-inlet left ventricle in 3, and double-outlet right ventricle in 1, who underwent conversion to a lateral tunnel procedure. Before conversions, patients had decreased exercise tolerance in 8, arrhythmias in 6, effusions in 4, and protein-losing enteropathy in 8. At catheterization, all had a low cardiac index (average 1.9 ± 0.7), 5 had elevated pulmonary vascular resistance (> 3 Wood units), and 3 had right pulmonary venous return obstruction by compression of an enlarged right atrium. Fenestrated lateral tunnel reconstruction was undertaken 7.3 ± 3.6 years after atriopulmonary anastomosis, with 1 early death related to low output. After the lateral tunnel procedure, 2 patients had no clinical improvement, but 5 patients had either marked or partial improvement with the right pulmonary vein compression resolved in 3 patients after conversion. Conversion to a lateral tunnel procedure can be extremely helpful in patients, particularly those who have partial pulmonary vein compression by a large bulging right atrium.

McElhinney and associates[75] from San Francisco, California, report 7 patients (aged 8 to 20 years) after atriopulmonary connection with severe right atrial dilatation in 7, Fontan pathway obstruction in 4, progressive CHF in 4, atrial tachyarrhythmias in 4, right atrial thrombus in 1, obstruction of pulmonary veins by an enlarged right atrium in 1, and subaortic stenosis in 1. After evaluation of options, they performed revision of the atriopulmonary connection to extracardiac in 5 and intraatrial conduit cavopulmonary anastomosis in 2. One patient with severe cachexia died in the early postoperative period with massive effusions. Two patients eventually required permanent pacing for atrial dysrhythmia or complete heart block secondary to subaortic fibromuscular resection in 1, and 2 demonstrated marked improvement in unstable preoperative rhythm disturbances. At a median follow-up of 17 months, 4 of the 6 survivors were functioning at higher New York Heart Association levels than preoperatively, and 1 had recently undergone heart transplantation. In properly selected patients with atrial complications, revision of prior Fontan connection to extracardiac or intracardiac conduits can provide improved palliation.

Kaulitz and associates[76] from Hannover, Germany, analyzed 72 patients who underwent total cavopulmonary anatomy anastomosis at ages ranging from 7 to 219 months. There were 23 patients with mean PA pressures higher than 15 mm Hg, elevated pulmonary resistances greater than 3 $U \cdot m^2$, or elevated end-diastolic pressure greater than 12 mm Hg. Associated systemic or pulmonary venous anomalies were present in 22 patients (30%), and AV valve incompetence was present in 21 patients (29%). The overall operative mortality was 10%, and variables with significant effect on postoperative mortality were systemic or pulmonary venous anomalies, AV valve incompetence, mean PA pressure greater than 15 mm Hg, and prolonged cardiopulmonary bypass time. Postoperative morbidity resulted mainly from atrial arrhythmias, occurring in 20%. Clinical signs of protein-losing enteropathy or atrial thrombi were rare (3% and 6%, respectively). Postoperative hemodynamic data from 48 surviving patients revealed a mean transpulmonary gradient of 6.3 mm Hg, systemic venous pressure greater than 12 mm Hg in only 10 patients, and cardiac index less than 3 in 18 patients. These authors show reasonable results for Fontan operation in a group of rather complex univentricular hearts.

Goldman and associates[77] from London, United Kingdom, used inhaled nitric oxide in 10 consecutive children with oxygen saturations of 85% or less and compared them with 5 children with saturations greater than 85% after a Fontan operation. Exposure to nitric oxide resulted in a significant increase in saturation from 64% ± 5% to 82% ± 2% and reduction in transpulmonary gradient from 12 ± 1 to 10 ± 1 mm Hg in patients with baseline saturations of 85% or less. Baseline saturation was a predictor of response with a greater response in those with lower saturations. In contrast, no significant effects were noted in PaO_2 or transpulmonary gradient in patients with baseline saturations greater than 85%. A trial of inhaled nitric oxide should be considered in clinically unstable desaturated patients after the fenestrated Fontan operation.

Sommer and colleagues[78] in New York, New York, evaluated 5 children (4 to 8 years old at the time of cardiac catheterization) 0.5 to 24 months after operation for occlusion of a persistently patent Fontan fenestration. An 8 mm × 10 cm Gianturco coil was delivered to straddle the fenestration with established techniques for coil occlusion of patent ductus arteriosus. Complete occlusion occurred in 4 of 5 patients, in 2 of 4 before they left the catheterization laboratory. One patient had a residual angiographic shunt, but had complete closure within 24 hours as detected by echocardiography. In 1 patient who had a residual shunt at 24 hours, the fenestration was completely closed at 1 month after coil placement. One patient had residual shunting at 2 months, but saturations have increased 15% to 17% since coil placement. No embolization, clinical hemolysis, thromboembolic events, or hemodynamic deterioration occurred among patients during a 1- to 14-month follow-up. Thus, persistently patent fenestration after Fontan operation may be closed with a Gianturco coil. This universally available alternative to umbrella devices may make a fenestrated Fontan a more appealing option to centers that had not considered it previously.

Manning and associates[79] from Boston, Massachusetts, reviewed 324 patients undergoing a Fontan operation, with 227 having no prior cavopulmonary shunt (group 1) and 97 having cavopulmonary shunt before Fontan operation (group 2). Arrhythmias were classified as altered sinoatrial node function, SVT, or AV block. The prevalence of both transient and fixed altered sinoatrial node function was similar for the 2 groups after cavopulmonary shunt or primary Fontan and averaged 10% despite a heterogeneous patient population. Conversion from cavopulmonary shunt to Fontan in group 2 resulted in a higher prevalence of altered sinoatrial node function in the early postoperative period (transient 24%, fixed 24%) and on follow-up: group 1, 8%, and group 2, 17%. In group 2, 40 of 82 patients without arrhythmia after first intervention had an arrhythmia after the Fontan procedure; of 14 patients with arrhythmia after the first operation, 10 had 1 after the second intervention. In conclusion, a multistage operative pathway to Fontan reconstruction is associated with a higher early risk of altered sinoatrial node function. Whether this finding will carry over to clinically important conduction disturbances or arrhythmia is not clear at present.

Feldt and associates[80] from Rochester, Minnesota, observed 427 patients who survived 30 days after Fontan operation and analyzed these patients for protein-losing enteropathy. This problem occurred in 47 of 427 patients. The cumulative risk for development of this problem by 10 years was 13% among 30-day survivors. Five-year survival after the diagnosis of protein-losing enteropathy was 46%. Hemodynamic studies performed coincidently with the diagnosis of protein-losing enteropathy have shown increased systemic venous pressure, decreased cardiac index, increased pulmonary vascular resistance, and increased ventricular end-diastolic pressure. Medical management was only partially successful. Statistical analysis has shown that factors related to protein-losing enteropathy were ventricular anatomy, increased preoperative ventricular end-diastolic pressure, longer operative bypass time, increased length of hospital stay, and postoperative renal failure. This problem should be anticipated in any patient who has undergone a Fontan operation with suboptimal results. Maximizing hemodynamics and decreasing right atrial pressure, even if creation of an ASD is required, may help in some patients. An immunological component has been suggested because of the response to steroid therapy observed in some patients.

Laschinger and associates[81] from Baltimore, Maryland, used an extracardiac lateral tunnel in 14 patients undergoing Fontan procedures, or a conduit in combination with staged or simultaneous bidirectional Glenn shunts. Fenestrations were created in 4 patients: 2 each in extracardiac lateral tunnel and extracardiac lateral conduit patients. Aortic cross-clamping was completely avoided in 12 patients. There were no operative deaths and in follow-up from 6 to 54 months (mean 28 months), all patients are in New York Heart

Association class I or II and remain in normal sinus rhythm. Late protein-losing enteropathy was seen in 1 patient and was successfully treated by creation of a stented fenestration to the systemic atrium. Late catheterization revealed unobstructed extracardiac lateral tunnel function and low pulmonary pressures. Advantages of the extracardiac Fontan include avoidance of aortic cross-clamping in most patients, the hemodynamic benefits of total cavopulmonary connection, avoidance of atriotomy and intraatrial suture line, preservation of sinus rhythm, drainage of the coronary sinus to the low pressure atrium, allowance for early/late fenestrations, and prevention of baffle leaks and intraatrial obstruction. It is unclear whether the conduit will be large enough to allow for the necessary increase in unobstructed venous return as the child grows.

Canobbio and associates[82] from Los Angeles, California; Rochester, Minnesota; and Boston, Massachusetts, report 33 pregnancies after Fontan operation for various types of univentricular heart disease. There were 15 livebirths (45%) from 14 mothers, 13 spontaneous abortions, and 5 elective terminations. In the 14 women with livebirths, the median number of years between operation and pregnancy was 4, with a range of 2 to 14 years. Reported prepregnancy problems included atrial flutter in 1 and ventricular dysfunction, AR, and atrioventricular valve regurgitation in another. One patient developed SVT during pregnancy and had conversion to sinus rhythm. No maternal complications were reported during labor, delivery, or in the immediate puerperium. There were 6 female and 9 male infants, with mean gestational age of 37 weeks and a median weight of 2 kg. One infant had an ASD. At follow-up, all mothers and infants were alive and well. It is hoped that these encouraging results of relatively smooth pregnancies after Fontan operation can be repeated in other patients. Most of these patients probably had reasonably good ventricular function. Those patients who have clearly depressed ventricular function after Fontan operation should avoid pregnancy until more data are obtained.

Vitullo and associates[83] from Chicago, Illinois, report 9 patients who underwent Fontan revision at a mean age of 11 ± 5 years and a mean interval from initial Fontan operation to revision of 3 ± 2 years. The reasons for revision included marked impairment in exercise capacity and chronic fatigue in 6 patients, 3 of whom also had serious atrial arrhythmias. Classic Glenn shunt was present in 5 of 6 patients, and the mean right atrial pressure was greater than the pressure of the Glenn shunt. A significant gradient between right and left PA wedge and ventricular end-diastolic pressures was present in 3 of 6, indicating pulmonary vein obstruction from the bulging atrial septum or partitioning patch. The remaining 3 patients had revision because of malabsorption in 1, hepatomegaly and obstructed right pulmonary veins in 1, and TR in 1. Revision was accomplished with creation of a lateral tunnel and Glenn reconnection in 6 patients, Glenn reconnection in 2, and creation of a lateral atrial tunnel in 1. Four patients had additional procedures. There was 1 death from sepsis, and hospital discharge was accomplished in 8 patients in 8 ± 3 days. One patient died 8 months postoperatively after VF from attempted cardioversion for atrial flutter. The remaining patients had marked improvement in exercise capacity, improvement in duration and tolerance to arrhythmias on less medication, and resolution of malabsorption up to 37 months postoperatively. Patients who deteriorate following Fontan procedures should be carefully examined for potentially remedial surgical problems, as demonstrated in the study. A bulging atrial septum, which may be present in patients who underwent atrial to PA connections, can compress right pulmonary veins and cause significant symptoms.

Cetta and associates[84] from Rochester, Minnesota, compared 339 consecutive patients who had a Fontan operation at the Mayo Clinic between 1987 and 1992 with 500 patients who had operations performed between 1973 and 1986. Recent overall early mortality decreased from 16% to 9%, despite increased anatomic complexity of patients. One-year survival improved to 88% from 79%, and 5-year survival improved to 81% from 73%. Patients with common AV valve, those who took daily preoperative diuretic medications, or those with either postoperative renal failure or elevated postbypass right atrial pressure were at an increased risk for early mortality. Young age was not found to be a risk factor for early mortality. Early mortality for patients with heterotaxia decreased dramatically: recent 30-day mortality was 15%, compared with 41% previously. These authors show an excellent outcome without the use of atrial baffle fenestration. The length of hospital stay, with a mean of 14 days, appears high. In the recent cohort, 36% patients had chest drainage that was defined as prolonged (> 14 days), and 24% of patients were hospitalized longer than 21 days. These hospitals stays appear significaly prolonged compared with those of recent series wherein fenestration was more commonly applied; however, a direct comparison is not available. These data suggest that routine fenestration is not necessary in many patients who require Fontan operation.

Patent Foramen Ovale

The study by Stone and associates[85] from Baltimore, Maryland, investigated whether there is an association between the degree of interatrial shunting across a patent foramen ovale, as determined by saline contrast TEE, and the risk of subsequent systemic embolic events, including stroke. Thirty-four patients found to have patent foramen ovale during TEE were divided into 2 groups on the basis of the maximum number of microbubbles in the left heart in any single frame after intravenous saline contrast injection: group 1 (n = 16) with a "large" degree of shunt ($\geq$20 microbubbles), and group 2 (n = 18) with a "small" degree of shunt ($\geq$3 but <20 microbubbles). Patients were followed during a mean period of 21 months for subsequent systemic embolic events, including transient ischemic attack and stroke. Five (31%) of the patients with large shunts had subsequent ischemic neurologic events, whereas none of the patients with small shunts had embolic events. These events occurred despite antiplatelet or anticoagulant therapy. It was concluded that patients with a large degree of shunt across a patent foramen ovale, as determined by contrast TEE, are at a significantly higher risk for subsequent adverse neurologic events than are patients with a small degree of shunt.

Congenital Heart Disease

Harinck and associates[86] from Utrecht and Maastricht, The Netherlands, measured transcutaneous oxygen saturation in 12 cyanotic adults with congenital heart disease and 27 control subjects during simulated commercial flights of 1.5 and 7 hours in a hypobaric chamber. Ten of these patients and 6 control subjects were also evaluated during 2 actual flights of approximately 2.5 hours. Oxygen saturations averaged 86% ± 8% at sea level (range 69% to 98%) and showed a maximal decrease to 78% ± 5% (range 73% to 87%) and to 79% ± 8% during simulated flight (range 69% to 94%). During the actual flight, the maximal decrease in oxygen saturation was 6%. In-flight reduction of capillary PO_2 was considerable in the control subjects, but not in the patients. The flights had no influence on capillary blood pH, PCO_2, bicarbonate, or lactic acid levels in either patients or control subjects. These data are useful in advising patients concerning commercial air travel. It appears to be safe unless patients have control saturations that are quite low.

Buskens and associates[87] from Rotterdam, The Netherlands, performed a prospective follow-up study of 6922 scanned fetuses in pregnant women without known risk factors who were selected for routine fetal ultrasound examination between 16 and 24 weeks gestation. Follow-up until 6 months postpartum was available for 82%. By comparing prenatal diagnosis with postnatal diagnosis, a total of 80 cases of congenital malformations were diagnosed during the study: 44 cases of congenital heart disease, 40 cases of noncardiac malformations, and a combination of the 2 in 4 cases. The fetal 4-chamber view was considered abnormal in 7 women who were referred for extensive fetal ultrasound examination, and 2 proved to be carrying an affected fetus. Similarly, prenatal referral of 14 women because of suspected noncardiac malformations yielded 12 such cases. The fetal 4-chamber view had a sensitivity of 5%. These results indicate that the current mode of routine prenatal screening for congenital malformations is inefficient, particularly for cardiac anomalies. This study should alert physicians that a normal fetal ultrasound does not rule out congenital heart disease, even major abnormalities. Perhaps with more experienced ultrasonographers, this record will improve considerably.

Cardiomyopathy

Schwartz and associates[88] from Boston, Massachusetts, present a disciplinary diagnostic approach to pediatric cardiomyopathy of genetic etiology. Cardiomyopathy remains one of the leading cardiac causes of death in children although, in the majority of cases, the cause is unknown. The diagnostic evaluation of children with cardiomyopathy is complicated by the large number of rare genetic causes, broad range of clinical presentations, and the array of specialized diagnostic tests and biologic assays. These authors provide a differential diagnosis of genetic conditions associated with cardiomyopathy classified as inborn errors of metabolism, malformation syndromes, neuromuscular disorders, and familial isolated cardiomyopathy disorders. This type of approach should assist in identifying more specific etiologies and perhaps hasten the day when genetic testing and treatment will be possible for at least some of these rare conditions.

Theodoro and associates[89] from Rochester, Minnesota, report 25 pediatric patients who underwent extended left ventricular septal myectomy because of hypertrophic cardiomyopathy. Ages ranged from 2 months to 20 years with a mean of 11 years. Moderate-to-severe MR was present in 17. Medical therapy had failed in all patients, and 1 patient had undergone pacemaker treatment without improvement. Left ventricular outflow gradients ranged from 50 to 154 mm Hg (mean 100 ± 25). Concomitant cardiac procedures included mitral valve repair in 2, implantable defibrillator in 1, and closure of ASD in 1. Intraoperative premyectomy gradients ranged from 20 to 117 mm Hg (mean 60 ± 26), and postmyectomy gradients ranged from 0 to 20 mm Hg (mean 7 ± 6). Postmyectomy MR was reduced to regurgitant fractions of 0% to 12%, and no patient required MVR. A pacemaker was required in 1 patient because of complete heart block and, on subsequent follow-up, sinus rhythm had returned. There was no early mortality and no aortic or mitral valve injury or VSD. Follow-up ranged from 10 months to 20 years, with a mean of 6 years. There were no late deaths. LV outflow gradient by echocardiography was a mean of 14 mm Hg (median 5 mm Hg). All patients were in sinus rhythm, and reoperation because of recurrent left ventricular outflow obstruction was necessary in only 2 patients at 3 and 13 years. All patients except 1 had either no symptoms or minimal symptoms. These excellent results indicate the ability to relieve obstruction by myectomy. Most patients with this operation have a marked improvement in symptoms. Although it is hoped they will show improvement in terms of long-term outlook, this has not been the case for previous surgical series.

McCully and associates[90] from Rochester, Minnesota, analyzed data for 65 patients (aged 20 to 70 years old) with hypertrophic cardiomyopathy who had surgical treatment between 1986 and 1992. Of the patients, 95% were in New York Heart Association (NYHA) functional class III or IV before surgery: 95% had dyspnea, 62% had angina, 63% had near-syncope, and 23% had syncope. The overall early mortality rate was 4.6%; there was no mortality among the 45 patients who underwent isolated septal myectomy. At the 1-year postoperative evaluation, 89% of survivors were in NYHA functional class I or II, and 47% believed that they had 100% improvement. Significant improvement was seen in 67% of patients with dyspnea, 90% with angina, 86% with near-syncope, and 100% with syncope. The 5-year survival rate was 92%. This study affirms the efficacy of surgical treatment for hypertrophic cardiomyopathy for patients who are symptomatic despite optimal medical treatment.

Complications After Surgery

Taggart and associates[91] from London, United Kingdom, report serial measurements of myoglobin, the MB isoenzyme of creatine kinase, and the highly specific markers of myocardial damage cardiac troponin T and I at 1, 6, 24, 48, and 72 hours after operation in 40 patients undergoing pediatric cardiac surgery. Operative procedures included closure of ASD, VSD, and arterial switch for TGA. The control group included thoracotomy for extracardiac operations. Significant increases were seen in myoglobin and CK-MB, but not troponin in the control group. There were significant increases in all 4 biochemical markers in all the cardiac operations, particularly in the VSD and TGA group.

These increases were about 5 times greater than those previously reported in adult patients and suggest that the pediatric myocardium may be more vulnerable than adult myocardium to injury during cardiac surgery.

Shekerdemian and associates[92] from London, United Kingdom, investigated the effect of negative-pressure ventilation on cardiac output in 11 children in the early postoperative period after right heart surgery. Cardiac output was calculated by direct Fick method, and oxygen consumption was measured by respiratory mass spectrometry. Cardiac output was measured during intermittent positive-pressure ventilation and after 15 minutes of negative-pressure ventilation. Negative-pressure ventilation improved the cardiac output by a mean of 46% with mixed venous saturation increasing by 5%. The systemic and pulmonary vascular resistances were reduced significantly during negative-pressure ventilation. Negative-pressure ventilation improves cardiac output in children after total cavopulmonary connection and tetralogy of Fallot repair and may prove to be an important therapeutic option in children with low cardiac output state.

Interrupted Aortic Arch

Serraf and associates[93] from Le Plessis-Robinson, France, report 79 consecutive patients who underwent surgical repair of interrupted aortic arch. Median age at operation was 9 days (range 1 day to 6 years), and median weight was 3 kg (range 2 to 20 kg). All but 1 were in severe CHF, and 32% had oliguria or anuria. Type A interrupted arch was present in 37 cases, type B in 41 patients, and type C in 1 patient. There was an associated single VSD in 35 cases, 24 patients had associated complex defects, and 30 had significant subaortic stenosis. Aortopulmonary window was found in 4 patients, truncus arteriosus in 8, TGA in 5, double-outlet right ventricle in 1, single ventricle in 3, multiple VSDs in 2, and superior-inferior ventricles in 1. Single-stage repair was performed in 64 patients, and 15 underwent multistage repair. Arch repair consisted of direct anastomosis in 59 patients, patch augmentation in 8, and conduit interposition in 10. PA banding was performed in 10 patients, and 19 underwent concomitant repair of complex associated lesions. Subaortic stenosis was addressed by myotomy or myectomy in 5; creation of a double-outlet left ventricle, aortopulmonary anastomosis, and conduit insertion between the right ventricle and PA bifurcation in 4; left-sided VSD patch in 5; and no direct treatment in 6. Mean duration of hypothermic circulatory arrest, cross-clamp time, and cardiopulmonary bypass time were 39 ± 16 minutes, 61 ± 25 minutes, and 143 ± 40 minutes, respectively. Postoperative mortality rate was 19%, and overall mortality rate was 31%. The results improved with time, with an overall operative mortality of 12% since 1990. Univariate analysis revealed that early survival was influenced by preoperative renal function, cerebral bleeding, number of cardioplegic injections, and date of operation. Echocardiographic measurements of the left heart-aorta complex with preoperative z values as low as −4 demonstrated rapid growth after repair. In the presence of subaortic stenosis, improved survival was obtained with a left-sided patch for VSD closure. There were 26 reoperations in 23 patients with recoarctation in 7, left bronchial compression in 2, second-stage repair in 8, right ventricle-PA conduit replacement in 3, and miscellaneous in 4. Survival at 5 years for the entire series was 70% and, in the presence of subaortic stenosis, it was 60%. Interrupted aortic arch remains a surgical challenge with continually improving results. The associated subaortic stenosis and small annulus continue to provide further challenges. However, this study and others have shown remarkable growth in this area after successful arch repair.

Anomalous Coronary Artery

Lambert and associates[94] from Paris, France, report 39 consecutive patients with anomalous origin of the coronary from the PA who had restoration of a 2-coronary-artery system. Median age at surgery was 19 months (range 3 months to 38 years). LV function was normal in 13 patients, and direct aortic implantation was performed in 34 patients (87%), associated with mitral valvuloplasty in 3 patients. Hospital death occurred in 5 patients (13%), and 2 patients were lost to follow-up. Mean follow-up was 40 ± 42 months. There were no late deaths after 1 month, and the survival rate was 84%. At the last follow-up, LV shortening fraction was normal in 86%. Left ventricle dilation persisted in 73%, and 12 of the survivors (39%) had abnormal regional wall motion of the left ventricle. A perfusion defect with incomplete redistribution was observed in 8 patients on thallium-201 imaging, which was performed in 45% of survivors. Total mortality was related only to preoperative shortening fraction: 12% versus 25%; no factor was related to shortening fraction recovery. Despite no late deaths and shortening fraction recovery, left ventricle dilation and ischemic segments of the left ventricle persisted at the long-term follow-up.

1. Noto N, Ayusawa M, Karasawa K, Yamaguchi H, Sumitomo N, Okada T, Harada K: Dobutamine stress echocardiography for detection of coronary artery stenosis in children with Kawasaki disease. J Am Coll Cardiol 1996 (April);27:1251–1256.
2. Muzik O, Paridon SM, Singh TP, Morrow WR, Dayanikli F, DiCarli MF: Quantification of myocardial blood flow and flow reserve in children with a history of Kawasaki disease and normal coronary arteries using positron emission tomography. J Am Coll Cardiol 1996 (September);28:757–762.
3. Ino T, Akimoto K, Ohkubo M, Nishimoto K, Yabuta K, Takaya J, Yamaguchi H. Application of percutaneous transluminal coronary angioplasty to coronary arterial stenosis in Kawasaki disease. Circulation 1996 (May 1);93:1709–1715.
4. Kato H, Sugimura T, Akagi T, Sato N, Hashino K, Maeno Y, Kazue T, Eto G, Yamakawa R: Long-term consequences of Kawasaki Disease. Circulation 1996 (September 15);94:1379–1385.
5. Kaine SF, Smith EO, Mott AR, Mullins CE, Geva T: Quantitative echocardiographic analysis of the aortic arch predicts outcome of balloon angioplasty of native coarctation of the aorta. Circulation 1996 (September 1);94:1056–1062.
6. Rao PS, Galal O, Smith PA, Wilson AD: Five- to nine-year follow-up results of balloon angioplasty of native aortic coarctation in infants and children. J Am Coll Cardiol 1996 (February);27:462–470.
7. Mavroudis C, Backer C, Muster A, Rocchini A, Rees A, Gevitz M: Taussig-Bing anomaly: Arterial switch versus Kawashima intraventricular repair. Ann Thorac Surgery 1996 (May);61:1330–1338.
8. van Son JAM, Reddy VM, Silverman NH, Hanley FL: Regression of tricuspid regur-

gitation after two-stage arterial switch operation for failing systemic ventricle after atrial inversion operation. J Thorac Cardiovasc Surg 1996 (February);111:342–347.

9. Nakanishi T, Momoi N, Satoh M, Yamada M, Terada M, Nakazawa M, Momma K, Imai Y: Growth of the neopulmonary valve annulus after arterial switch operation in transposition of the great arteries. Circulation 1996 (November 1);94(suppl II): II–27–II–31.

10. Bonnet D, Bonhoeffer P, Piechaud JF, Aggoun Y, Sidi D, Planche C, Kachaner J: Long-term fate of the coronary arteries after the arterial switch operation in newborns with transposition of the great arteries. Heart 1996 (September);76:274–279.

11. Meijboom F, Szatmari A, Deckers JW, Utens EMWJ, Roelandt JRTC, Bos E, Hess J: Long-term follow-up (10 to 17 years) after Mustard repair for transposition of the great arteries. J Thorac Cardiovasc Surg 1996 (June);111:1158–1168.

12. Serraf A, Nakamura T, Lacour-Gayet F, Piot D, Bruniaux J, Touchot A, Sousa-Uva M, Houyel L, Planche C: Surgical approaches for double-outlet right ventricle or transposition of the great arteries associated with straddling atrioventricular valves. J Thorac Cardiovasc Surg 1996 (March);111:527–535.

13. Lacour-Gayet F, Serraf A, Komiya T, Sousa-Uva M, Bruniaux J, Touchot A, Roux D, Neuville P, Planche C: Truncus arteriosus repair: influence of techniques of right ventricular outflow tract reconstruction. J Thorac Cardiovasc Surg 1996 (April); 111:849–856.

14. Tweddell JS, Berger S, Frommelt PC, Pelech AN, Lewis DA, Fedderly RT, Frommelt MA, McManus TS, Mussatto KA, Kessel MW, Litwin SB: Aprotinin improves outcome of single-ventricle palliation. Ann Thorac Surg 1996 (November);62: 1329–1336.

15. Delius RE, Rademecker MA, de Leval MR, Elliott MJ, Stark J: Is a high-risk biventricular repair always preferable to conversion to a single ventricle repair? J Thorac Cardiovasc Surg 1996 (December);112:1561–1569.

16. Oski JA, Canter CE, Spray TL, Kan JS, Cameron DE, Murphy AM. Embolic stroke after ligation of the pulmonary artery in patients with functional single ventricle. Am Heart J 1996 (October);132:836–840.

17. Belli E, Serraf A, Lacour-Gayet F, Inamo J, Houyel L, Bruniaux J, Planche C: Surgical treatment of subaortic stenosis after biventricular repair of double-outlet right ventricle. J Thorac Cardiovasc Surg 1996 (December);112:1570–1580.

18. Cohen MS, Jacobs ML, Weinberg PM, Rychik J: Morphometric analysis of unbalanced common atrioventricular canal using two-dimensional echocardiography. J Am Coll Cardiol 1996 (October);28:1017–1023.

19. Ueda Y, Fukushige J, Ueda K: Congestive heart failure during early infancy in patients with ventricular septal defect relative to early closure. Pediatric Cardiology 1996 (November-December);17:382–386.

20. Du ZD, Roguin N, Barak M, Bihari SG, Ben-Elisha M: High prevalence of muscular ventricular septal defect in preterm neonates. M J Cardiol 1996 (November 15);78: 1183–1185.

21. Acherman RJ, Smallhorn JF, Freedom RM: Echocardiographic assessment of pulmonary blood supply in patients with pulmonary atresia and ventricular septal defect. J Am Coll Cardiol 1996 (November 1);28:1308–1313.

22. Moritz A, Marx M, Wollenek G, Domanig E, Wolner E: Complete repair of PA-VSD with diminutive or discontinuous pulmonary arteries by transverse thoracosternotomy. Ann Thorac Surg 1996 (February);61:646–650.

23. Baufreton C, Journois D, Leca F, Khoury W, Tamisier D, Vouhe P: Ten-year experience with surgical treatment of partial atrioventricular septal defect: risk factors in the early postoperative period. J Thorac Cardiovasc Surg 1996 (July);112:14–20.

24. Kreutzer J, Perry SB, Jonas RA, Mayer JE, Castaneda AR, Lock JE: Tetralogy of Fallot with diminutive pulmonary arteries: preoperative pulmonary valve dilation and transcatheter rehabilitation of pulmonary arteries. J Am Coll Cardiol 1996 (June);27:1741–1747.

25. Norgard G, Gatzoulis MA, Moraes F, Lincoln C, Shore DF, Shinebourne EA, Redington AN: Relationship between type of outflow tract repair and postoperative right ventricular diastolic physiology in tetralogy of Fallot. Circulation 1996 (December 15);94:3276–3280.

26. Bigras JL, Boutin C, McCrindle BW, Rebeyka IM: Short-term effect of monocuspid valves on pulmonary insufficiency and clinical outcome after surgical repair of tetralogy of Fallot. J Thorac Cardiovasc Surg 1996 (July);112:33–37.

27. Atallah-Yunes NH, Kavey REW, Bove EL, Smith FC, Kveselis DA, Byrum CJ, Gaum WE: Postoperative assessment of a modified surgical approach to repair of tetralogy of Fallot, long term follow-up. Circulation 1996 (November 1);94(suppl II):II-22–II-26.

28. Sideris EB, Leung M, Yoon JH, Chen C-R, Lochan R, Worms A-M, Rey C, Meier B. Occlusion of large atrial septal defects with a centering buttoned device: Early clinical experience. Am Heart J 1996 (February);131:356–359.

29. Ende DJ, Chopra PS, Syamasundar R: Transcatheter closure of atrial septal defect or patent foramen ovale with the buttoned device for prevention of recurrence of paradoxic embolism. Am J Cardiol 1996 (July 15);78:233–236.

30. Heller J, Hagege AA, Besse B, Desnos M, Marie FN, Guerot C: "Crochetage" (notch) on R wave in inferior limb leads: a new independent electrocardiographic sign of atrial septal defect. J Am Coll Cardiol 1996 (March);27:877–882.

31. Pascoe RD, Oh JK, Warnes CA, Danielson GK, Tajik AJ, Seward JB: Diagnosis of sinus venosus atrial septal defect with TEE. Circulation 1996 (September 1);94:1049–1055.

32. Mehta SK, Super DM, Anderson RL, Harcar-Sevcik RA, Babjak M, Liu X, Bahler RC. Parental hypertension and cardiac alterations in normotensive children and adolescents. Am Heart J 1996 (January);131:81–88.

33. Saji T, Ozawa Y, Ishikita T, Matsuura H, Matsuo N: Short-term hemodynamic effect of a new oral PGI_2 Analogue, Beraprost, in primary and secondary pulmonary hypertension. Am J Cardiol 1996 (July 15);78:244–247.

34. Luciani GB, Chang AC, Starnes VA: Surgical repair of transposition of the great arteries in neonates with persistent pulmonary hypertension. Ann Thorac Surg 1996 (March);61:800–805.

35. Bando K, Turrentine MW, Sharp TG, Sekine Y, Aufiero TX, Sun K, Sekine E, Brown JW: Pulmonary hypertension after operations for congenital heart disease: Analysis of risk factors and management. J Thorac Cardiovasc Surg 1996 (November);112:1600–1609.

36. Kubota H, Furuse A, Kotsuka Y, Yagyu K, Hirata K, Murakawa Y: Midterm results of the rotation-advancement flap method for correction of partial anomalous pulmonary venous drainage into the superior vena cava. J Thorac Cardiovasc Surg 1996 (July);112:1–7.

37. Delius RE, de Leval MR, Elliott MJ, Stark J: Mixed total pulmonary venous drainage: still a surgical challenge. J Thorac Cardiovasc Surg 1996 (December);112:1581–1588.

38. Bando K, Turrentine MW, Ensing GJ, Sun K, Sharp TG, Sekine Y, Girod DA, Brown JW: Surgical management of total anomalous pulmonary venous connection. Circulation 1996 (November 1);94(suppl 2):II-12–II-16.

39. Najm HK, Williams WG, Coles JG, Rebeyka IM, Freedom RM: Scimitar syndrome: Twenty years' experience and results of repair. J Thorac Cardiovasc Surg 1996 (November);112:1161–1169.

40. Bradley SM, Mosca RS, Hennein HA, Crowley DC, Kulik TJ, Bove EL: Bidirectional superior cavopulmonary connection in young infants. Circulation 1996 (November 1);94(suppl II):II-5–II-11.

41. Reddy VM, McElhinney DB, Moore P, Petrossian E, Hanley FL: Pulmonary artery growth after bidirectional cavopulmonary shunt: Is there a cause for concern? J Thorac Cardiovasc Surg 1996 (November);112:1180–1192.

42. Gardiner HM, Dhillon R, Bull C, de Leval MR, Deanfield JE: Prospective study of the incidence and determinants of arrhythmia after total cavopulmonary connection. Circulation 1996 (November 1);94(suppl II):II-17–II-21.

43. Van Arsdell GS, Williams WG, Maser CM, Streitenber KS, Rebeyka IM, Coles JG, Freedom RM: Superior vena cava to pulmonary artery anastomosis: an adjunct to biventricular repair. J Thorac Cardiovasc Surg 1996 (November);112:1143–1149.

44. Shaddy RE, Huner DD, Osborn KA, Lambert LM, Minich LL, Hawkins JA, McGough EC, Fuller TC: Prospective analysis of HLA immunogenicity of cryopre-

served valved allografts used in pediatric heart surgery. Circulation 1996 (September 1)94:1063–1067.

45. Gildein HP, Kleinert S, Weintraub RG, Wilkinson JL, Karl TR, Mee RBB. Surgical commissurotomy of the aortic valve: Outcome of open valvotomy in neonates with critical aortic stenosis. Am Heart J 1996 (April);131:754–759.

46. van Son JAM, Reddy VM, Black MD, Rajasinghe H, Haas GS, Hanley FL: Morphologic determinants favoring surgical aortic valvuloplasty versus pulmonary autograft aortic valve replacement in children. J Thorac Cardiovasc Surg 1996 (June); 111:1149–1157.

47. Starnes VA, Luciani GB, Wells WJ, Allen RB, Lewis AB: Aortic root replacement with the pulmonary autograft in children with complex left heart obstruction. Ann Thorac Surg 1996 (August);62:442–449.

48. Baskett RJ, Ross DB, Nanton MA, Murphy DA: Factors in the early failure of cryopreserved homograft pulmonary valves in children: preserved immunogenicity? J Thorac Cardiovasc Surg 1996 (November);112:1170–1179.

49. Elkins RC, Lane MM, McCue C: Pulmonary autograft reoperation: incidence and management. Ann Thorac Surg 1996 (August);62:450–455.

50. Moore P, Egito E, Mowrey H, Perry S, Lock JE, Keane JF: Midterm results of balloon dilation of congenital aortic stenosis: predictors of success. J Am Coll Cardiol 1996 (April);27:1257–1263.

51. Hawkins JA, Minich LL, Shaddy RE, Tani LY, Orsmond GS, Sturtevant JE, McGough EC: Aortic valve repair and replacement after balloon aortic valvuloplasty in children. Ann Thorac Surg 1996 (May);61:1355–1358.

52. Ho SY, Jackson M, Kilpatrick L, Smith A, Gerlis LM: Fibrous matrix of ventricular myocardium in tricuspid atresia compared with normal heart. Circulation 1996 (October 1);94:1642–1646.

53. Gildein HP, Kleinert S, Goh TH, Wilkinson JL: Treatment of critical pulmonary valve stenosis by balloon dilatation in the neonate. Am Heart J 1996 (May); 1007–1011.

54. Redington AN, Somerville J: Stenting of aortopulmonary collaterals in complex pulmonary atresia. Circulation 1996 (November 15);94:2479–2484.

55. Yagihara T, Yamamoto F, Nishigaki K, Matsuki O, Uemura H, Isizaka T, Takahashi O, Kamiya T, Kawashima Y: Unifocalization for pulmonary atresia with ventricular septal defect and major aortopulmonary collateral arteries. J Thorac Cardiovasc Surg 1996 (August);112:392–402.

56. Kreutzer J, Landzberg MJ, Preminger TJ, Mandell VS, Treves ST, Reid LM, Lock JE: Isolated peripheral pulmonary artery stenoses in the adult. Circulation 1996 (April);93:1417–1423.

57. Dessy H, Hermus JPS, van den Heuvel F, Oei HY, Krenning EP, Hess J. Echocardiographic and radionuclide pulmonary blood flow patterns after transcatheter closure of patent ductus arteriosus. Circulation 1996 (July 15);94:126–129.

58. Hijazi ZM, Lloyd TR, Beekman RH, Geggel RL: Transcatheter closure with single or multiple Gianturco coils of patent ductus arteriosus in infants weighing ≤ 8 kg: retrograde versus antegrade approach. Am Heart J 1996 (October);132:827–835.

59. Galal O, de Moor M, Al-Fadley F, Hijazi ZM. Transcatheter closure of the patent ductus arteriosus: Comparison between the Rashkind occluder device and the anterograde Gianturco coils technique. Am Heart J 1996 (February);131:368–373.

60. Shim D, Fedderly RT, Beekman RH, Ludomirski A, Young ML, Schork MA, Lloyd TR: Follow-up of coil occlusion of patent ductus arteriosus. J Am Coll Cardiol 1996 (July)28:207–211.

61. Kimball TR, Ralston MA, Khoury P, Crump RG, Cho FS, Reuter JH: Effect of ligation of patent ductus arteriosus on left ventricular performance and its determinants in premature neonates. J Am Coll Cardiol 1996 (January);27:193–197.

62. Naheed ZJ, Strasburger JF, Deal BJ, Benson DW, Gidding SS: Fetal tachycardia: mechanisms and predictors of hydrops fetalis. J Am Coll Cardiol 1996 (June);27: 1736–1740.

63. Drago F, Turchetta A, Calzolari A, Giordano U, Di Ciommo V, Santilli A, Pompei E, Ragonese P. Reciprocating supraventricular tachycardia in children: Low rate

at rest as a major factor related to propensity to syncope during exercise. Am Heart J 1996 (August);132:280–285.

64. Weindling SN, Saul JP, Walsh EP. Efficacy and risks of medical therapy for supraventricular tachycardia in neonates and infants. Am Heart J 1996 (January);131: 66–72.

65. Mehta AV, Subrahmanyam AB, Anand R: Long-term efficacy and safety of atenolol for supraventricular tachycardia in children. Pediatr Cardiol 1996 (July-August); 17:231–236.

66. Miga DE, Case CL, Gillette PC. Interatrial septal aneurysms and atrial arrhythmias in infants. Am Heart J 1996 (October);132:776–778.

67. Perry JC, Fenrich AL, Hulse JE, Friedman JK, Friedman RA, Lamberti JJ: Pediatric use of intravenous amiodarone: Efficacy and safety in critically ill patients from a multicenter protocol. J Am Coll Cardiol 1996 (April);27:1246–1250.

68. Schaffer MS, Silka MJ, Ross BA, Kugler JD: Inadvertent atrioventricular block during radiofrequency catheter ablation. Circulation 1996 (December 15);94: 3214–3220.

69. Gonska BD, Cao K, Raab J, Eigster G, Kreuzer H: Radiofrequency catheter ablation of right ventricular tachycardia late after repair of congenital heart defects. Circulation 1996 (October 15);94:1902–1908.

70. Steinberger J, Lucas RV Jr., Edwards JE, Titus JL: Causes of sudden unexpected cardiac death in the first two decades of life. Am J Cardiol 1996 (May 1);77:992–995.

71. Fogel MA, Weinberg PM, Chin AJ, Fellows KE, Hoffman EA: Late ventricular geometry and performance changes of functional single ventricle throughout staged Fontan reconstruction assessed by MRI. J Am Coll Cardiol 1996 (July);28:212–221.

72. Jacobs ML, Rychik J, Rome JJ, Apostolopoulou S, Pizarro C, Murphy J, Norwood WI: Early reduction of the volume work of the single ventricle: the hemi-Fontan operation. Ann Thorac Surg 1996 (August);62:456–462.

73. Forbes TJ, Gajarski R, Johnson GL, Reul GJ, Ott DA, Drescher K, Fisher DJ: Influence of age on the effect of bidirectional cavopulmonary anastomosis on left ventricular volume, mass and ejection fraction. J Am Coll Cardiol 1996 (November 1);28: 1301–1307.

74. Kreutzer J, Keane JF, Lock JE, Walsh EP, Jonas RA, Castaneda AR, Mayer JE: Conversion of modified Fontan procedure to lateral atrial tunnel cavopulmonary anastomosis. J Thorac Cardiovasc Surg 1996 (June);111:1169–1176.

75. McElhinney DB, Reddy VM, Moore P, Hanley FL: Revision of previous Fontan connections to extracardiac or intraatrial conduit cavopulmonary anastomosis. Ann Thorac Surg 1996 (November);62:1276–1283.

76. Kaulitz R, Ziemer G, Luhmer I, Kallfelz HC: Modified Fontan operation in functionally univentricular hearts: preoperative risk factors and intermediate results. J Thorac Cardiovasc Surg 1996 (September);112:658–664.

77. Goldman AP, Delius RE, Deanfield JE, Miller OI, de Leval MR, Sigston PE, Macrae DJ: Pharmacological control of pulmonary blood flow with inhaled nitric oxide after the fenestrated Fontan operation. Circulation 1996 (November 1);94(suppl II):II-44-II-48.

78. Sommer RJ, Recto M, Golinko RJ, Griepp RB. Transcatheter coil occlusion of surgical fenestration after Fontan operation. Circulation 1996 (August 1);94:249–252.

79. Manning PB, Mayer JE, Wernovsky G, Fishberger SB, Walsh EP: Staged operation to Fontan increases the incidence of sinoatrial node dysfunction. J Thorac Cardiovasc Surg 1996 (April);111:833–840.

80. Feldt RH, Driscoll DJ, Offord KP, Cha RH, Perrault J, Schaff HV, Puga FJ, Danielson GK: Protein-losing enteropathy after the Fontan operation. J Thorac Cardiovasc Surg 1996 (September);112:672–680.

81. Laschinger JC, Redmond JM, Cameron DE, Kan JS, Ringel RE: Intermediate results of the extracardiac Fontan procedure. Ann Thorac Surg 1996 (November);62: 1261–1267.

82. Canobbio MM, Mair DD, Van Der Velde M, Koos BJ: Pregnancy outcomes after the Fontan repair. J Am Coll Cardiol 1996 (September);28:763–767.

83. Vitullo DA, Deleon SY, Berry TE, Bonilla JJ, Chhangani SV, Cetta F, Quinones JA,

Bell TJ, Fisher EA: Clinical improvement after revision in Fontan patients. Ann Thorac Surg 1996 (June);61:1797–1804.

84. Cetta F, Feldt RH, O'Leary PW, Mair DD, Warnes CA, Driscoll DJ, Hagler DJ, Porter CJ, Offord KP, Schaff HV, Puga FJ, Danielson GK: Improved early morbidity and mortality after Fontan operation: the Mayo Clinic experience, 1987 to 1992. J Am Coll Cardiol 1996 (August);28:480–486.

85. Stone DA, Godard J, Corretti MC, Kittner SJ, Sample C, Price TR, Plotnick GD. Patent foramen ovale: Association between the degree of shunt by contrast TEE and the risk of future ischemic neurologic events. Am Heart J 1996 (January);131: 158–161.

86. Harinck E, Hutter PA, Hoorntje TM, Simons M, Benatar AA, Fischer JC, de Bruijn D, Meijboom EJ: Air travel and adults with cyanotic congenital heart disease. Circulation 1996 (January 15);93:272–276.

87. Buskens E, Grobbee DE, Frohn-Mulder IME, Stewart PA, Juttmann RE, Wladimiroff JW, Hess J: Efficacy of routine fetal ultrasound screening for congenital heart disease in normal pregnancy. (July 1) Circulation 1996;94:67–72.

88. Schwartz ML, Cox GF, Lin AE, Korson MS, Perez-Atayde A, Lacro RV, Lipshultz SE: Clinical approach to genetic cardiomyopathy in children. Circulation 1996 (October 15);94:2021–2038.

89. Theodoro DA, Danielson GK, Feldt RH, Anderson BJ: Hypertrophic obstructive cardiomyopathy in pediatric patients: results of surgical treatment. J Thorac Cardiovasc Surg 1996 (December);112:1589–1599.

90. McCully RB, Nishimura RA, Tajik AJ, Schaff HV, Danielson GK: Extent of clinical improvement after surgical treatment of hypertrophic obstructive cardiomyopathy. Circulation 1996 (August 1);94:467–471.

91. Taggart DP, Hadjinikolas L, Wong K, Yap J, Hooper J, Kemp M, Hue D, Yacoub M, Lincoln JC: Vulnerability of paediatric myocardium to cardiac surgery. Heart 1996 (September);76:214–217.

92. Shekerdemian LS, Shore DF, Lincoln C, Bush A, Redington AN: Negative-pressure ventilation improves cardiac output after right heart surgery. Circulation 1996 (November);94(suppl II):II-49-II-55.

93. Serraf A, Lacour-Gayet F, Robotin M, Bruniaux J, Sousa-Uva M, Roussin R, Planche C: Repair of interrupted aortic arch: A ten-year experience. J Thorac Cardiovasc Surg 1996 (November);112:1150–1160.

94. Lambert V, Touchot A, Losay J, Piot JD, Henglein D, Serraf A, Lacour-Gayet F, Planche C: Midterm results after surgical repair of the anomalous origin of the coronary artery. Circulation 1996 (November 1);94(suppl II):II-39-II-43.

12

Transplantation

General Topics

Cost Savings in De-Listing Patients on the Transplant Waiting List

Levine and associates[1] from Detroit, Michigan, retrospectively contrasted the medical outcome of patients removed from the heart transplant considera-tion list because of clinical improvement with the outcome of transplant recipi-ents. Of 60 patients awaiting transplantation, 18 were removed from the list (group A) and 42 received transplant or died (group B). Group A significantly improved regarding exercise oxygen uptake, ejection fraction (EF), and hemo-dynamics. For more than 2 years after transplantation or delisting, both groups had comparable symptoms (New York Heart Association class I to II) and cardiovascular mortality (1 of 18 for group A vs. 3 of 32 for group B) but lower hospitalizations for group A (0.5 ± 0.6 of 27 months per patient) versus group B (2.8 ± 2.1 of 23 months per patient). Despite 2 patients who had been re-moved from the list requiring transplantation, savings for delisting exceeded \$2.2 million. Thus medical therapy allows transplant recipient list removal with clinical improvements sustained for 1 to 3 years at significant cost savings.

HLA Matching in Transplantation Outcomes

Hosenpud and colleagues[2] determined the effects of human lymphocyte antigen (HLA) matching in cardiac and single-lung transplantation. Using the joint Thoracic Transplant Registry of the United Network for Organ Sharing and the International Society for Heart and Lung Transplantation, all adult primary heart and single-lung transplant procedures performed in the United States from October 1987 through December 1993 were analyzed to determine the effects of HLA matching on transplant mortality. Both total HLA matches and matches at individual HLA loci were considered. Including HLA matching, 16 potential risk factors for heart transplant outcome and 16 potential risk factors for lung transplant outcome were subjected to multivariate analysis. A total of 10,752 heart transplants and 1239 lung transplants were included in the independent analyses for each organ. For heart transplantation, there was a progressive reduction in risk for greater matching. The primary benefit of matching appeared to be at the A and DR loci. For lung transplantation, any matching had an independent positive effect on outcome, but the relationship between numbers of HLA matches and relative risk was not present and ranged from risk ratios of 0.7 to 0.9. Only matching of the A locus appeared to influence

579

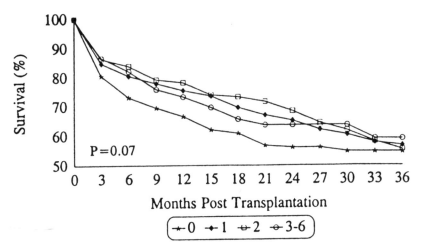

FIGURE 12-1. Univariate actuarial survival analysis over a period of 3 years after lung transplantation. There is a trend toward reduced survival in those patients with the poorest HLA compatibility with their donor organs (0 antigens matched). Reprinted with permission from Hosenpud et al.[2]

outcome. Thus, these data demonstrate that HLA matching independently affects survival in both heart and single-lung transplantation (Figure 12-1).

Myocardial Injury

Fyfe and colleagues[3] evaluated perioperative ischemic myocardial injury in the first 4 weekly endomyocardial biopsies and/or autopsy myocardium from 140 consecutive orthotopic heart transplantation recipients in the period 1984 to 1991 by grading the severity of coagulative myocyte necrosis as absent, 0; mild-focal, 1; moderate-multifocal, 2; or severe-confluent, 3, and determining the evolution of morphological features of its healing. Coagulative myocardial necrosis, often with contraction bands, was noted in 124 patients (89%). Twenty-four patients (17%) had grade 3 coagulative myocardial necrosis; of those patients, 4 died within 30 days of transplantation. At 1 year after transplantation, survival was similar in patients with and without severe injury. Increased cold ischemic time, but neither donor age nor intensity of inotropic support, correlated with more severe early ischemic injury. Perioperative ischemic myocardial injury inflammation was characterized by a predominantly polymorphonuclear/histiocytic infiltrate that contained lymphocytes and plasma cells expanding the interstitium, but not encroaching upon and separate from adjacent viable myocytes (Figure 12-2). Histological features of the perioperative ischemic myocardial injury developed and resolved more slowly than those of typical myocardial infarct necrosis in nonimmunosuppressed patients. At 4 weeks, coagulative myocardial necrosis persisted in 20% of patients and residual healing in nearly half of them. Diagnostic rejection was observed concurrently with perioperatively ischemic myocardial injury in 54

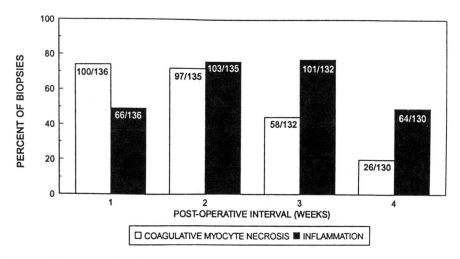

FIGURE 12-2. Temporal evolution of coagulative myocyte necrosis and inflammation in perioperative ischemic myocardial injury. Numbers in bars indicate numbers with feature/total biopsies examined. Necrosis was present most frequently in the earliest biopsies (76% and 72%
at weeks 1 and 2, respectively); inflammation was maximal at 2 and 3 weeks (76% and 77%,
respectively). Reprinted with permission from Fyfe et al.[3]

of 533 biopsies (10%). Thus, diagnosed by conventional histological criteria,
perioperative ischemic myocardial injury is common early after heart transplantation and has a protracted healing phase that can mimic or coexist with
histological evidence of rejection. Extensive perioperative ischemic myocardial
injury has a deleterious impact on short-term survival, but the long-term impact of this phenomenon remains to be shown.

Conduction Abnormalities After Transplantation

To study the long-term evolution, determinants, and clinical relevance of
the conduction abnormalities after orthotopic heart transplantation, Leonelli
and associates[4] from Lexington, Kentucky, and Houston, Texas, followed 87
patients for a mean of 105 ± 72 weeks. Patients were divided into 3 groups
according to the characteristics of their electrocardiograms compared with
their initial electrocardiogram recorded at study entry. The first group consisted of 24 patients whose initial electrocardiogram was normal, and subsequent electrocardiograms remained normal throughout the study. The second
group included 27 patients who developed electrocardiographic evidence of
progressive conduction system damage. The third group comprised 36 patients
whose initial electrocardiogram was abnormal and subsequent electrocardiograms remained unchanged during follow-up. Although the hemodynamic
and echocardiographic evaluations of right and left ventricular function were
initially similar among the 3 groups, groups 2 and 3 demonstrated a significant
deterioration of LV ejection fraction (62% ± 12% to 55% ± 16% and 62% ±
8% to 57% ± 14%, respectively) and cardiac index (2.7 ± 0.6 to 2.3 ± 0.5

and 3.0 ± 0.9 to 2.5 ± 0.9 L/min/m^2, respectively) while patients in group 1 maintained their normal baseline indices. Incidence and progression of coronary artery disease (CAD) as well as frequency of rejection episodes were comparable among the groups. Mortality was higher in the 2 groups with evidence of conduction defects. Sudden death associated with complete heart block (2 patients) or ventricular arrhythmias (3 patients) was exclusively confined to patients with evidence of progressive electrocardiogram abnormalities. We conclude that after orthotopic heart transplantation, stable or progressive conduction system damage on the electrocardiogram is associated with left ventricular dysfunction and increased mortality. Sudden death is not uncommon among patients demonstrating worsening cardiac conduction and, in some cases, is related to the development of potentially preventable complete heart block.

Myocardial Viability of Native Hearts: Assessment with ^{99m}Tc Sestamibi

Medrano and colleagues[5] in Houston, Texas, evaluated myocardial viability in 15 consecutive patients with ischemic cardiomyopathy who underwent orthotopic cardiac transplantation. An intravenous injection of ^{99m}Tc sestamibi was administered 1 to 6 hours before transplantation. Rotational tomography of the excised, intact, native hearts was performed to quantify the extent of myocardial hypoperfusion. The hearts were sliced and reimaged on a gamma camera followed by pathological quantification of the extent and severity of scarred and normal myocardium. Samples of normally and abnormally perfused myocardium had gamma well counting to determine tissue radioactivity and were examined under light microscopy for delineation of myocardial structure after trichrome staining. The mean extent of scintigraphic scar quantitated through the use of rotational tomography was 45% of the left ventricle and correlated closely with pathological scar (r = .89), despite a slight overestimation (Fig. 12-3). Scintigraphic scar size determined with planar imaging of the myocardial slices also correlated closely with pathological scar size (r = .88). A good correlation existed between tissue ^{99m}Tc sestamibi activity determined through well counting and histologic evidence of myocardial viability (r = .89). Most hypokinetic and 40% of akinetic/dyskinetic myocardial segments contained scintigraphically and histologically normal myocardium. ^{99m}Tc sestamibi scintigraphy may be used to quantify accurately the extent of myocardial scarring in similar patients. In addition, the relative sestamibi activity in perfusion defects, measured several hours after administration, is a good indicator of myocardial viability determined by microscopy.

Transplantation for Chagas' Disease

de Carvalho and colleagues[6] in São Paulo, Brazil, prospectively investigated the long-term follow-up of 10 patients with end-stage chronic Chagas'

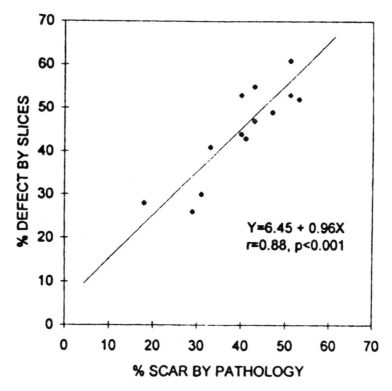

FIGURE 12-3. Linear regression analysis of defect size based on planar scintigraphy of myocardial slices on pathological scar size. Reprinted with permission from Medrano et al.[5]

heart disease who underwent heart transplantation. Immunosuppression was based on cyclosporine and azathioprine. *Trypanosoma cruzi* reactivation was prevented with benzonidazole. Besides allograft rejection surveillance, *T. cruzi* infection was monitored through blood tests, myocardial biopsies, and serological tests. During a mean follow-up period of 34 ± 38 months (range, 73 to 124 months), 7 patients remained alive and in New York Heart Association functional class I. Life expectancy was 78% for the second year and 65% for 10 years. Rejection was less frequent in the patients with Chagas' disease than in age- and sex-matched control patients (Figure 12-4). There was a decreased severity of rejection in the Chagas group as well. *T. cruzi* parasitemias detected on 3 occasions were successfully treated with benzonidazole. There were no signs of recurrence of the disease in the allograft. Thus, these results suggest an important role of heart transplantation in the treatment of chronic Chagas' heart disease. There was a low frequency of *T. cruzi* infection reactivation, as well as signs of recurrence of the disease in the allograft.

Cyclosporine Effects on Brain Function

Grimm and colleagues[7] in Klagenfurt, Austria, measured cognitive brain function and quality of life in out-of-hospital cardiac transplant candidates

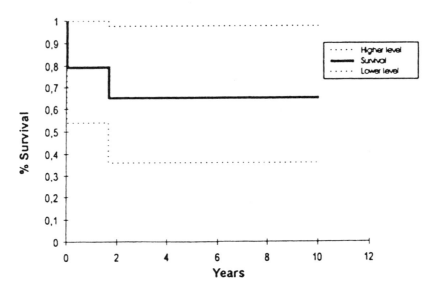

FIGURE 12-4. Life expectancy curve for patients with CCHD after heart transplantation. Kaplan-Meier method and respective 95% cardiac index (CI). Reprinted with permission from de Carvalho et al.[6]

(n = 55; left ventricular ejection fraction, 19.9%; mean age, 54 years). After transplantation, the patients were serially reevaluated at 4 months (n = 25) and at 12 months (n = 19). Brain function was measured objectively by cognitive P300 evoked potentials. Standard psychometric tests were performed. Cognitive P300 evoked potentials were impaired in cardiac transplant patients compared with 55 age- and sex-matched healthy subjects. After transplantation, P300 measures were normalized at 4 months but declined again at 12 months. Stepwise multiple regression analysis revealed that cumulative cyclosporine dosage was the only predictor of individual cognitive brain function at 4 and 12 months (Figure 12-5). Thus, objective cognitive P300 auditory evoked potential measurements indicate that cognitive brain function is significantly impaired in patients suffering from stable end-stage CHF. The decline in long-term cognitive brain function after successful cardiac transplantation may be related to cyclosporine neurotoxicity.

Nitric Oxide Synthase mRNA and Contractile Function

Lewis and colleagues[8] prospectively studied 16 patients in the first year after cardiac transplantation at the time of surveillance endomyocardial biopsy. Clinical data, the results of biopsy histology, and echocardiographic and Doppler evaluation of left ventricular systolic and diastolic function were recorded. Total RNA was extracted from biopsy specimens, and mRNA for β-actin detected by reverse transcription–polymerase chain reaction using human specific primers was used as a constitutive gene control. Inducible nitric oxide synthase mRNA was similarly detected by reverse transcription–poly-

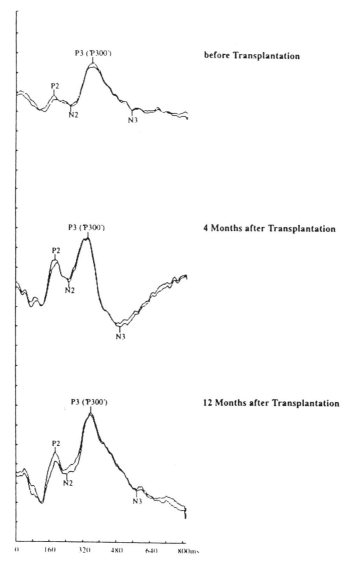

FIGURE 12-5. Cognitive P300 auditory evoked potential recordings (double tracing) of a 59-year-old woman before transplantation, 4 months after transplantation, and 12 months after transplantation. Graph shows recordings during rare tone delivery (20% at 2000 Hz). P2 indicates positive peak number 2; N2, negative peak number 2; P3 ('P300'), positive peak number 3 (P300 peak); and N3, negative peak number 3. Reprinted with permission from Grimm et al.[7]

merase chain reaction using human specific primers. The inducible nitric oxide synthase protein was detected in biopsy frozen sections by immunofluorescence. Myocardial cyclic GMP was measured by radioimmunoassay, and serum nitrogen oxide levels were measured by chemiluminescence. Inducible nitric oxide synthase mRNA was detected in allograft myocardium at some point in each patient and in 59 of 123 biopsies (48%) overall. In individual patients, inducible nitric oxide synthase mRNA expression was episodic and time depen-

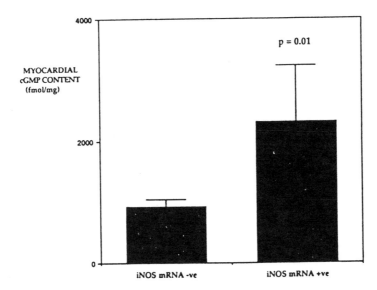

Figure 12-6. Bar graph showing myocardial cGMP content. Myocardial cGMP content was significantly increased ($p = .01$) in 5 biopsies with iNOS mRNA expression (iNOS mRNA +ve) compared with 5 biopsies without iNOS mRNA expression (iNOS mRNA −ve). Reprinted with permission from Lewis et al.[8]

dent, and the frequency of expression was highest during the first 180 days after transplantation. Inducible nitric oxide synthase protein associated with inducible nitric oxide synthase mRNA was detected by immunofluorescence in cardiac myocytes. Inducible nitric oxide synthase mRNA expression was not related to the histolic grade of rejection or to serum levels of nitric oxide, but was associated with increased levels of myocardial cGMP and with both systolic and diastolic LV contractile dysfunction as measured by echocardiography and Doppler (Figure 12-6). These data identify a relation between inducible nitric oxide synthase mRNA expression and contractile dysfunction in the human cardiac allograft.

Allograft Vascular Disease and Other Complications

Early Endothelial Dysfunction

Davis and colleagues[9] in Boston, Massachusetts, evaluated the relation between early endothelial dysfunction and the development of allograft atherosclerosis serially with intravascular ultrasound in 20 patients who had undergone heart transplantation. Endothelium-dependent vasomotion was assessed in these patients by serial intracoronary acetylcholine infusion, and the percent change in diameter was measured by quantitative angiography. The development of atherosclerosis was studied by use of intravascular ultrasound in the same 20 patients by quantifying the changes in intimal index and maximal

TABLE 12-1
Segment Analysis (n = 46): Early Endothelial Function and Development of Intimal Pathology

	Constrictors (n = 23)	Dilators (n = 23)	p
ACH response	−23.9 ± 2.6%	7.1 ± 1.5%	<.01
NTG response	10.2 ± 3.3%	13.4 ± 2.6%	NS
Intimal index			
Baseline	5 ± 3%	1 ± 1%	NS
Year 1	12 ± 4%	13 ± 1%	<.05
Change during initial year	7 ± 2%	2 ± 1%	<.05
Maximal intimal thickness			
Baseline	100 ± 50 μm	20 ± 20 μm	NS
Year 1	240 ± 60 μm	70 ± 30 μm	<.05
Change during initial year	140 ± 40 μm	50 ± 20 μm	<.05

ACH, acetylcholine; and NTG, nitroglycerin.

Values are mean ± SE.

Reproduced with permission from Davis et al.[9]

intimal thickness with 46 matched coronary segments between initial and 1-year follow-up studies. Coronary segments with endothelial dysfunction demonstrated constriction of 5% or more in 23 patients and a significantly greater increase in mean change in intimal index and change in maximal intimal thickness by 1 year after transplant compared with segments with normal endothelial function (Table 12-1). No other variables predicted the development of allograft arteriosclerosis in the initial year after transplant. Thus, paired studies that used intravascular ultrasound showed that early endothelial dysfunction predicts the development of allograft arteriosclerosis during the first year after transplantation.

Endothelin-1

Ravalli and colleagues[10] in New York, New York, used immunohistochemistry to investigate the role of endothelin-1 in transplant coronary heart disease. Endothelin-1 immunoreactivity and cellular localization were assessed in human coronary arteries with transplant coronary artery disease (n = 13) and in normal coronary arteries (n = 10) with single- and double-label immunohistochemistry. The intensity of immunostaining was determined by a semiquantitative method. Diffuse and intense endothelin-1 immunoreactivity was found in 11 of 13 patients with transplant coronary artery disease (85%), primarily in myointimal cells, and in lesser amounts in macrophages and endothelial cells. In contrast, normal coronary arteries had only faint immunostaining localized to the endothelial layer. Mean semiquantitative grade was higher in transplant coronary artery disease than in normal arteries (1.8 vs. 0.7). Endothelin-1 was more frequently present in lipid-rich, atheromatous lesions than in lipid-poor, proliferative ones. Intimal neovessels consistently immunostained for endothelin-1. Thus, these data suggest that immunoreactivity for endothelin-1 is significantly increased in transplant coronary heart disease, possibly as a result of stimulatory cytokines and growth factors that are upregulated in the posttransplant state. These results suggest a possible role for this mitogenic peptide in the pathogenesis of graft atherosclerosis.

Early Development

After heart transplantation, CAD of the graft is the major factor limiting long-term survival. Gao and colleagues[11] from Stanford, California, assessed the time of first appearance of angiographic CAD in relation to clinical variables and clinical events in heart transplant patients. One hundred thirty-nine consecutive patients who underwent heart transplantation and developed angiographic CAD were classified according to early (<2 years) versus late (>2 years) posttransplantation initial detection of CAD. The early-onset group (64 patients) had more rapid progression to ischemic events than did the late-onset group (75 patients), with 59% of the late group and only 35% of the early group free from ischemic events by 5 years after initial detection. There was no significant relationship between clinical or laboratory variables and ischemic events. The early group did have a significantly higher incidence of antecedent cytomegalovirus infection. These authors concluded that accelerated graft CAD develops at variable times after heart transplantation and that the early appearance of graft CAD may be a marker of intrinsically more aggressive disease. Cytomegalovirus infection was associated with the earlier onset of graft CAD. Patients with early development of graft CAD should potentially be given priority for interventional strategies.

Morphological Observations in Epicardial Coronary Arteries

Arbustini from Pavia, Italy, and Roberts from Dallas, Texas,[12] examined 39 cardiac allografts in place for more than 2 months and 37 grafts for 2 months and made a number of observations. (1) Allograft vascular disease affects all layers of the epicardial coronary arteries and, usually, the intramural coronary arteries in the outer one-half of the left ventricular wall. (2) The resulting intimal lesion is relatively uniform, consisting mainly of cellular and acellular fibrous tissue; it is diffuse, affecting all segments of the major and minor epicardial coronary arteries. (3) The degree of resulting luminal narrowing is similar in most 5-mm coronary segments, making coronary angiography hazardous in reliably predicting the degree of luminal narrowing. (4) The extensive adventitial fibrosis and the extensive fibrous tissue infiltration of the subepicardial tissue probably inhibit dilation and remodeling of the epicardial coronary arteries and, indeed, may constrict them. (5) Luminal narrowing of the epicardial coronary arteries after transplantation may be the consequence of both intraluminal lesions and exterior compression from the surrounding fibrous tissue. (6) Intraluminal and intralesion thrombus is commonly observed as are multiluminal channels in coronary plaques, suggesting that organization of thrombi plays some role in the progression of posttransplant epicardial CAD. (7) The coronary lesions developing after cardiac transplantation are morphologically quite different in composition from those occurring in natural (nontransplantation) atherosclerosis. (8) Inflammatory cellular infiltrates are often extensive in the subepicardial tissues, and the infiltrates in this area may be extensive even when intersitial myocardial inflammatory infiltrates are minimal or absent.

Dichotomous Pattern One to Nine Years After Transplantation

Transplant CAD is an important cause of death after cardiac transplantation. Tuzcu and colleagues[13] from Cleveland, Ohio, evaluated intravascular ultrasound as a tool for detection and quantitation of this disease. They performed intravascular ultrasound imaging in 132 patients, 1 to 9 years after transplantation. Of the 1188 coronary artery segments, 706 were imaged. At least 1 site with atherosclerosis was found in 83% of patients. Atherosclerosis was noted in 64% of proximal, 43% of mid, and 26% of distal segments. Disease was diffuse in 48% and focal in 52%. Focal atherosclerosis was more common in proximal than in mid and distal segments. Atherosclerosis was detected in more than 80% of patients, with proximal segments more frequently involved. These results suggest that transplant CAD has a dual etiology based on the dichotomous pattern of atherosclerosis seen by intravascular ultrasound.

Case-Matched Ultrasound Study

Lim and colleagues[14] in Stanford, California, determined whether the incidence and severity of transplant CAD as detected by intracoronary ultrasound in heart-lung transplant recipients are less than those encountered in heart transplant recipients. They studied the left anterior descending (LAD) coronary artery with the use of intracoronary ultrasound imaging in 22 heart-lung transplant recipients at the time of routine annual coronary angiogram. Twenty-two heart transplant recipients were case-matched for numbers of years after transplant at ultrasound study, recipient age, donor age, and diagnosis of nonischemic cardiomyopathy. Mean intimal area, intimal index, Stanford class, and incidence of at least moderate disease (Stanford class ≥3) were measured and calculated in each group and compared between the 2 groups. Mean intimal area, mean intimal index, mean Stanford class, and incidence of Stanford class of 3 or higher were significantly lower in the heart-lung transplant recipient group (Figure 12-7).

Bradycardia

Sinus node dysfunction, primarily sinus bradycardia, frequently occurs after orthotopic heart transplantation and may lead to permanent pacemaker implantation. Bertolet and colleagues[15] from Gainesville, Florida, evaluated the use of theophylline, an adenosine receptor antagonist, as a drug to reverse

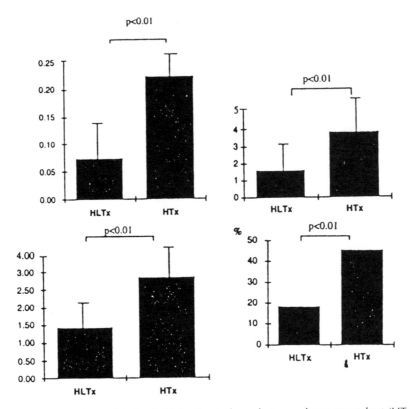

Figure 12-7. Comparison of intimal thickening indexes between heart transplant (HTx) and heart-lung transplant (HLTx) recipients. **A,** Intimal index; **B,** intimal area (in mm^2); **C,** Stanford class; and **D,** incidence (%) of at least moderate disease (Stanford class ≥ 3). Data are expressed as mean $\pm$ SD. Reprinted with permission from Lim et al.[14]

bradyarrhythmias after orthotopic heart transplantation. Twenty-nine transplant patients (group 1) were given theophylline when bradyarrhythmia developed after transplantation. Data in these patients were compared with those in a control group of 18 patients without bradyarrhythmia (group 2), who were not given theophylline. The mean heart rate in group 1 increased from 62 to 89 beats per minute after theophylline, while the mean heart rate in group 2 was 88. Patients in group 1 required more days of temporary atrial pacing (3.5 vs. 1.5) before the administration of theophylline than did patients in group 2. The length of hospital stay did not differ between the groups. These authors concluded that the use of theophylline for posttransplant bradyarrhythmias increased heart rate and facilitated the withdrawal of chronotropic support.

Hyperlipidemia

Hyperlipidemia occurs frequently after heart transplantation, and accelerated CAD remains the major cause of morbidity and mortality in patients who

TABLE 12-2
Recent Clinical Studies of Single-Agent Statin Therapy After Heart Transplantation

Study	Drug	Daily Dose (mg)	n	Follow-up (mo)	TC%	ΔLDL%	ΔTG%	ΔHDL%	Myositis/ Myalgias	Rhabdomyolysis: 10 × CK + Symptoms
Kuo et al, 1989[16]	L	20–60	11	15 [3–41]	−27	−34	+5	+5	0	0
Kobashigawa et al, 1990[17]	L	10–20	44	≥6	−26	−26	−22	−2	NR	1 (at 40 mg)
Ballantyne et al, 1992[18]	L	20	15	13 (6–30)	−21	−31	−8	+8	1	0
Peters et al, 1993[19]	L	20	35	NR	−24	NR	−5	NR	0	0
Anguita et al, 1994[20]	L	10–40	63	13	−15	−21	−17	+3	2	1 (believed 2° to colchicine)
Hidalgo et al, 1995[21]	L	10	18	2	−15	−21	−2	−2	1	0
Barbir et al, 1991[22]	S	10	12	8	−38	−42	−25	+9	0	0
Vanhaecke et al, 1994[23]	S	5–15	26	12	−27	−40	−21	−2	0	1 (at 15 mg)
Campana et al, 1994[24]	S	10	20	4	−12.5	−21.3	−4	+10	0	0
Pflugfelder et al, 1995[25]	S	10	13	12	−24	−39	−21	+2	0	0
Kobashigawa et al, 1995[26]	P	20–40	47	12	−22*	−27*	−32*	+21*	0	0

* Compared with control group (n = 50) rather than baseline value.

CK = creatine kinase; HDL = high-density lipoprotein cholesterol; L = lovastatin; LDL = low-density lipoprotein cholesterol; NR = not reported; P = pravastatin; S = simvastatin; TC = total cholesterol; TG = triglyceride; Δ = change.
Reproduced with permission from Ballantyne et al.[27]

survive more than 1 year after heart transplantation. The risk and benefits of lipid-lowering therapy after heart transplantation remain to be fully defined, and national guidelines for lipid-lowering drug therapy do not specifically address dyslipidemia in transplant recipients. Since the initial reports in the 1980s of rhabdomyolysis in heart transplant patients receiving high-dosage lovastatin, results of 11 posttransplantation studies that used lovastatin, simvastatin, or pravastatin at lower dosages as drug monotherapy have been published. These studies have shown an overall 1% incidence of rhabdomyolysis defined as creatine kinase more than 10 times the upper limit of normal plus muscle symptoms (Table 12-2). One randomized, controlled prospective trial has investigated the effects of lipid-lowering pharmacotherapy on patient outcome and cardiac transplant recipients. At 1-year follow-up in this nonblinded, single-center trial, patients treated with pravastatin (20 or 40 mg/day) initiated within 2 weeks of transplantation had a significant reduction in mortality rate and a significantly lower incidence of transplant arteriopathy. A number of important issues remain unanswered regarding treatment guidelines in patients with hyperlipidemia after heart transplantation. In January 1995, Ballantyne and associates[27] in Houston, Texas, began the Heart Transplant Lipid Registry with 12 participant centers to gather prospective data on the efficacy and safety of lipid-lowering drug therapies in the treatment of dyslipidemia after heart transplantation.

Coronary Thrombosis

Arbustini and associates[28] from Pavia, Italy, and Dallas, Texas, investigated at autopsy or at retransplantation the frequency and characteristics of coronary thrombosis in 76 cardiac allografts: 37 were in place 2 months or less (early) and 39 were in place for 2 to 99 months (late). The 76 allografts were inserted in 69 patients: 1 in 56 patients, and 2 allografts in 13 patients, 7 of whom subsequently died and had an autopsy. An average of 140 sections from 70 5-mm long segments of 8 epicardial coronary arteries were examined from each of the 76 allografts with both hematoxylin-eosin and Movat pentachrome stains. Thrombus was found in only 1 coronary artery (3%) (the right one) of the 37 early allografts, and in 24 of 39 late allografts (61%). Of the latter 39 grafts, 29 (79%) had allograft vascular disease (AVD), and 24 (83%) of them had coronary thrombosis. Of the 312 epicardial coronary arteries (4 major and 4 minor) examined in the 39 late cases, 66 arteries (21%) contained thrombus. Of the 24 late cases with thrombus in at least 1 artery, thrombus was present in 66 (34%) of the 192 epicardial coronary arteries examined: in 6 of the 8 arteries in 3 patients; in 5 arteries in 2 patients; in 4 arteries in 1 patient; in 3 arteries in 5 patients; in 2 arteries in 6 patients, and in a single artery in 7 patients. In all 66 arteries with thrombus (24 patients), the thrombus was larger than 5 mm. The thrombus in the late cases was entirely nonocclusive (mural) in 51 (77%) of the 55 epicardial coronary arteries containing thrombus and entirely occlusive in 10 arteries (15%). It consisted exclusively of multiluminal channels in 6 arteries (9%) and combinations in 1 artery (2%). Acute myocardial infarcts were present in 3 patients, all of whom had occlusive thrombi. In all 10 arteries with occlusive thrombi, the thrombus was larger than the underlying plaque, and no occlusive thrombi were located over ulcerated plaques. These observations demonstrate that thrombus is common in epicardial coronary arteries at least 2 months after cardiac transplantation.

Heart Transplantation in the Young

Surgical approaches to single-ventricle physiological abnormalities have included Fontan palliation or transplantation. No cost expenditures have been published. This study by Gajarski and associates[29] from Houston, Texas, compared expenditures between the Fontan procedure and heart transplantation. Between 1988 and 1992, records of 82 patients who underwent the Fontan procedure and 26 who underwent transplant were retrospectively reviewed. Charges for Fontan or transplant procedures were accrued from the date of surgical admission until discharge or patient death and included hospital, physician, and diagnostic laboratory charges. Additionally, the frequency and cost of postoperative hospital readmissions, outpatient evaluations, and diagnostic procedures were recorded for each patient. Estimated expenditures for each evaluated factor were based on 1992 to 1993 dollar charges. The total expenditure (surgery plus yearly follow-up) for transplantation exceeded that for the Fontan procedure ($96,475 vs $29,730). Although both groups had similar follow-up periods and mortality rates, numbers of hospital readmissions and postoperative diagnostic tests were higher among transplant recipients. Within 1 postoperative year, at least 4 high-risk patients who had undergone Fontan procedures required listing for transplantation; the total cost of their combined procedures (approximately $80,000 + $3,000 to $5,000 annual outpatient charges) was markedly greater than the cost of the Fontan procedure alone. Although the expenditure for heart transplantation far exceeds that for the Fontan procedure, Fontan palliation in high-risk patients is ultimately more costly and increases postoperative morbidity. In this subgroup, these investigators recommend heart transplantation as the initial, definitive procedure because it may increase long-term survival rates and minimize health care expenditures.

The pediatric myocardium has been shown to thicken markedly during steroid administration for the treatment of pulmonary or neurologic disease. Yet in the pediatric heart transplant patient, left ventricular thickening is sometimes used as a marker for rejection without accounting for steroid immunosuppression. Kimball and associates[30] from Cincinnati, Ohio, studied left ventricular thickness in 11 pediatric cardiac transplant patients. Left ventricular thickness (mass) was first measured during the entire posttransplant course. Second, thickness was measured before and during rejection. Last, to separate the independent effects of rejection and steroids on left ventricular mass, echocardiograms were reviewed in the immediate posttransplant period, when the protocol prescribed dramatic changes in steroid doses and rejection episodes were rare. Specifically, the donor heart underwent 5 evaluations: at donation, at peak steroid dose, 5 days after peak steroid dose, at moderate steroid dose, and at very low (maintenance) dose. Left ventricular mass changed most dramatically and consistently during the first 20 to 40 days after transplant. Thereafter, mass had little consistent change and did not change significantly during any of the 52 rejection episodes. Mass increased 5 days after peak steroid dose (54 ± 30 to 74 ± 38 g/ht$^{2.7}$) and decreased during low (maintenance) levels of steroids. Thickening was associated with cumulative steroid dose and age. Thus, in pediatric heart transplant patients, as in other pediatric diseases, left ventricular thickening is associated with steroid administration. Thickening may be an unreliable marker for acute cellular rejection.

Eke and associates[31] from Loma Linda, California, studied the neurodevelopmental outcome of 38 infants undergoing cardiac transplantation by use of deep hypothermic circulatory arrest before the age of 4 months. Outcome in the 22 boys and 16 girls was tested up to 2.5 years after transplantation by using the Bayley scales of infant development. Operation was performed using a bloodless prime that resulted in hematocrits of 5%; no surface precooling was used. Duration of arrest ranged from 42 to 70 minutes, with a mean duration of 56 minutes. The mean Bayley psychomotor development index was 91, with a range of 50 to 130; and mental developmental index was 88, with a range of 50 to 130. No relation was found between the rate of cooling and the duration of arrest on the Bayley scores. There continues to be controversy regarding the neurologic effect of circulatory arrest in infancy. An accompanying editorial by Jonas (Ann Thorac Surg 1996;61:779–780) suggests that until further data are forthcoming, surgeons undertaking transplantation for congenital defects would be wise to limit circulatory arrest to less than 45 minutes whenever possible and to avoid its use altogether in situations in which surgical outcomes are comparable with other techniques.

1. Levine TB, Levine AB, Goldberg AD, Tobes M, Narins B, Lesch M: Clinical status of patients removed from a transplant waiting list rivals that of transplant recipients at significant cost savings. Am Heart J 1996 (December);1323:1189–1194.
2. Hosenpud JD, Edwards EB, Lin H-M, Daily OP: Influence of HLA matching on thoracic transplant outcomes. An analysis from the UNOS/ISHLT* Thoracic Registry. Circulation 1996 (July 15);94:170–174.
3. Fyfe B, Loh E, Winters GL, Couper GS, Kartashov AI, Schoen FJ: Heart transplantation-associated perioperative ischemic myocardial injury. Morphological features and clinical significance. Circulation 1996 (March 15);93:1133–1140.
4. Leonelli FM, Dunn JK, Young JB, Pacifico A: Natural history, determinants, and clinical relevance of conduction abnormalities following orthotopic heart transplantation. Am J Cardiol 1996 (January 1);77:47–51.
5. Medrano R, Lowry RW, Young JB, Weilbaecher DG, Michael LH, Afridi I, He Z-X, Mahmarian JJ, Verani MS: Assessment of myocardial viability with ^{99m}Tc sestamibi in patients undergoing cardiac transplantation. A scintigraphic/pathological study. Circulation 1996 (September 1);94:1010–1017.
6. de Carvalho VB, Sousa EFL, Vila JHA, da Silva JP, Caiado MR, de R. Araujo SR, Macruz R, Zerbini EJ: Heart transplantation in Chagas' disease: 10 years after the initial experience. Circulation 1996 (October 15);94:1815–1817.
7. Grimm M, Yeganehfar W, Laufer G, Madl C, Kramer L, Eisenhuber E, Simon P, Kupilik N, Schreiner W, Pacher R, Bunzel B, Wolner E, Grimm G: Cyclosporine may affect improvement of cognitive brain function after successful cardiac transplantation. Circulation 1996 (September 15);94:1339–1345.
8. Lewis NP, Tsao PS, Rickenbacher PR, Xue C, Johns RA, Haywood GA, von der Leyen H, Trindade PT, Cooke JP, Hunt SA, Billingham ME, Valantine HA, Fowler MB: Induction of nitric oxide synthase in the human cardiac allograft is associated with contractile dysfunction of the left ventricle. Circulation 1996 (February);93:720–729.
9. Davis SF, Yeung AC, Meredith IT, Charbonneau F, Ganz P, Selwyn AP, Anderson TJ: Early endothelial dysfunction predicts the development of transplant coronary artery disease at 1 year posttransplant. Circulation 1996 (February);93:457–462.
10. Ravalli S, Szabolcs M, Albala A, Michler RE, Cannon PJ: Increased immunoreactive endothelin-1 in human transplant coronary artery disease. Circulation 1996 (November 1);94:2096–2102.
11. Gao SZ, Hunt SA, Schroeder JS, Alderman EL, Hill IR, Stinson EB: Early development of accelerated graft coronary artery disease: Risk factors and course. J Am Coll Cardiol 1996 (September);28:673–679.
12. Arbustini E, Roberts WC: Morphologic observations in the epicardial coronary arteries and their surroundings late after cardiac transplantation (allograft vascular disease). Am J Cardiol 1996 (October 1);78:814–820.
13. Tuzcu EM, DeFranco AC, Goormastic M, Hobbs RE, Rincon G, Bott-Silverman C, McCarthy P, Stewart R, Mayer E, Nissen SE: Dichotomous pattern of coronary atherosclerosis 1 to 9 years after transplantation: Insights from systematic intravascular ultrasound imaging. J Am Coll Cardiol 1996 (March 15);27:839–846.
14. Lim TT, Botas J, Ross H, Liang DH, Theodore J, Hunt SA, Oesterle SN, Yeung AC: Are heart-lung transplant recipients protected from developing transplant coronary artery disease? A case-matched intracoronary ultrasound study. Circulation 1996 (October 1);94:1573–1577.
15. Bertolet BD, Eagle DA, Conti JB, Mills RM Jr, Belardinelli I: Bradycardia after heart transplantation: Reversal with theophylline. J Am Coll Cardiol 1996 (August);28:396–399.
16. Kuo PC, Kirshenbaum JM, Gordon J, Laffel G, Young P, DiSesa VJ, Mudge GH, Vaughan DE: Lovastatin therapy for hypercholesterolemia in cardiac transplant recipients. Am J Cardiol 1989 (September 15);64:631–635.

17. Kobashigawa JA, Murphy FL, Stevenson LW, Moriguchi JD, Kawata N, Kamjoo P, Brownfield E, Wilmarth J, Leonard L, Chuck C, Drinkwater D, Laks H: Low-dose lovastatin safely lowers cholesterol after cardiac transplantation. Circulation 1990 (November);82:IV-281–283.
18. Ballantyne CM, Radovancevic B, Farmer JA, Frazier OH, Chandler L, Payton-Ross C, Cocanougher B, Jones PH, Young JB, Gotto AM: Hyperlipidemia after heart transplantation: report of a 6-year experience, with treatment recommendations. J Am Coll Cardiol 1992 (May);19:1315–1321.
19. Peters JR, Kubo SH, Olivari MT, Knutson KR, Hunninghake DB: Treatment of hyperlipidemia in heart transplant recipients with gemfibrozil ± lovastatin, Am J Cardiol 1993 (June 15);71:1485–1488.
20. Anguita M, Alonso-Pulpon L, Arizon JM, Cavero MA, Valles F, Segvia J, Perez-Jimenez F, Crespo M, Concha M: Comparison of the effectiveness of lovastatin therapy for hypercholesterolemia after heart transplantation between patients with and without pretransplant atherosclerotic coronary artery disease. Am J Cardiol 1994 (October 15);74:776–779.
21. Hidalgo L, Zambrana Jl, Blanco-Molina A, Lopez-Granados A, Concha M, Casares J, Perez-Jimenez F: Lovastatin versus bezafibrate for hyperlipemia treatment after heart transplantation. J Heart Lung Transplant 1995 (May–June);14:461–467.
22. Barbir M, Rose M, Kushwaha S, Akl S, Mitchell A, Yacoub M: Low-dose simvastatin for the treatment of hypercholesterolemia in recipients of cardiac transplantation. Int J Cardiol 1991 (November);33:241–246.
23. Vanhaecke J, Van Cleemput J, Van Lierde J, Daenen W, De Geest H: Safety and efficacy of low dose simvastatin in cardiac transplant recipients treated with cyclosporine. Transplantation 1994 (July 15);58:42–45.
24. Campana C, Iacona I, Regazzi MB, Gavazzi A, Perani G, Raddato V, Montemartini C, Vigano M: Efficacy and pharmacokinetics of simvastation in heart transplant recipients. Ann Pharmacother 1995 (March);29:235–239.
25. Pflugfelder PW, Huff M, Oskalns R, Rudas L, Kostuk WJ: Cholesterol-lowering therapy after heart transplantation: A 12-month randomized trial. J Heart Lung Transplant 1995 (July–August);14:613–622.
26. Kobashigawa JA, Katznelson S, Laks H, Johnson JA, Yeatman L, Wang XM, Chia D, Terasaki PI, Sabad A, Cogert GA, Trosian K, Hamilton MA, Moriguchi JD, Kawata N, Hage A, Drinkwater DC, Stevenson LW: Effect of pravastatin on outcomes after cardiac transplantation. N Engl J Med 1995 (September 7);333:621–627.
27. Ballantyne CM, Bourge RC, Domalik LJ, Eisen HJ, Fishbein DP, Kubo SH, Lake KD, Radovancevic B, Taylor DO, Ventura HO, Yancy CW Jr, Young JB: Treatment of hyperlipidemia after heart transplantation and rationale for the heart transplant lipid registry. Am J Cardiol 1996 (September 1);78:532–535.
28. Arbustini E, Dal Bello B, Morbini P, Grasso M, Diegoli M, Fasani R, Pilotto A, Bellini O, Pellegrini C, Martinelli L, Campana C, Gavazzi A, Specchia G, Viganò M, Roberts WC: Frequency and characteristics of coronary thrombosis in the epicardial coronary arteries after cardiac transplantation. Am J Cardiol 1996 (October 1);78:795–800.
29. Gajarski RJ, Towbin JA, Garson A Jr: Fontan palliation versus heart transplantation: A comparison of charges. Am Heart J 1996 (June);131:1169–1174.
30. Kimball TR, Witt SA, Daniels SR, Khoury PR, Meyer RA: Frequency and significance of left ventricular thickening in transplanted hearts in children. Am J Cardiol 1996 (January 1);77:77–80.
31. Eke CC, Gundry SR, Baum MF, Chinnock RE, Razzouk AJ, Bailey LL: Neurologic sequelae of deep hypothermic circulatory arrest in cardiac transplant infants. Ann Thorac Surg 1996 (March);61:783–788.

Author Index

Subject Index

Myocarditis, idiopathic, 398–99
  left ventricular endocardial surface,
     histological changes and,
     398

Natriuretic peptide, increased levels of,
     unstable angina, 174–75
Natural disasters, as risk factor for
     myocardial infarction,
     190–91
Neutrophil platelet adhesion, unstable
     angina, 177–78
Nifedipine, metoprolol and, *vs.*
     monotherapy, stable angina,
     158–59
Nitrate tolerance, coronary artery
     disease, 130
Nitric oxide
  continuing platelet activation,
     inhibition, unstable angina,
     183–85
  deficiency, angina, 169–70
  production, hypercholesterolemia,
     24–25
Nitric oxide synthase
  congestive heart failure, 364
  in endothelial cells, downregulation,
     22–23
No-reflow phenomenon
  myocardial infarction, 205
  reperfusion outcomes/injury, 317–18
Non-Q wave infarction, prognosis in,
     236–37
Noncardiac procedures, cardiac risk in,
     341–44

Obesity, effect on blood presure, 406–7
Oral anticoagulants
  mechanical heart valve replacement,
     425
  myocardial infarction, 224
Outflow obstruction, left ventricular,
     echocardiographic features,
     hypertrophic
     cardiomyopathy, 388–89
Oxidative stress
  congestive heart failure, 373–74
  coronary endothelial dysfunction,
     26–27

Pacemaker
  insertion of, clinical outcome, 259
  United States survey, 453–54
Pain, during percutaneous transluminal
     angioplasty, 267–69
Papillary muscle rupture, coronary
     artery disease, 128–29
Patent ductus arteriosus, in young,
     558–60

Patent foramen ovale, in young, 569
Pediatric cardiovascular disease,
     527–78
  arrhythmias, 560–63
  atrial septar defect, 545–47
  atrioventricular canal, 540–42
  cardiomyopathy, 570–71
  cavopulmonary connection, 551–52
  coarctation of aorta, 528–32
  complications after surgery, 571–72
  congenital heart disease, 569–70
  coronary artery, anomalous, 573
  double-outlet right ventricle, 540
  Fontan procedure, 563–69
  interrupted aortic arch, 572–73
  Kawasaki disease, 527–28
  partial atrioventricular septar defect,
     544
  patent ductus arteriosus, 558–60
  patent foramen ovale, 569
  pulmonary atresia, 543
  pulmonary hypertension, 547–48
  pulmonary stenosis, 556–58
  pulmonary venous drainage,
     anomalous, 548–50
  scimitar syndrome, 550–51
  single ventricle, 538–40
  sudden cardiac death, 563
  systemic arterial hypertension, 547
  Taussig-Bing anomaly, 532–33
  tetralogy of Fallot, 544–45
  total anomalous pulmonary venous
     connection, 550
  transplantation, 592–94
  transposition of great arteries,
     533–36
  tricuspid atresia, 556
  truncus arteriosus, 536–38
  valvular stenosis, aortic, pulmonic,
     552–55
  ventricular septal defect, 542
Percutaneous transluminal angioplasty,
     259–71
  angioscopic predictors, early adverse
     outcome, 263–65
  body mass index, as risk factor,
     259–61
  CK-MB fraction, release of, 266–67
  complications, 271–73
    abrupt closure, 271
    AMI, 273
    elastic recoil, 271–73
  coronary thrombi, as risk factor,
     261–62
  delayed, after AMI, 270–71
  diabetic patients, 265–66
  follow-up, 274
    arterial remodeling after, 274–76
    creatine kinase levels after, 280–81

TERMS COMMONLY ABBREVIATED

AF	=	atrial fibrillation
AMI	=	acute myocardial infarction
AR	=	aortic regurgitation
AS	=	aortic valve stenosis
ASD	=	atrial septal defect
AV	=	atrioventricular
AVR	=	aortic valve replacement
BBB	=	bundle branch block
BP	=	blood pressure
CABG	=	coronary artery bypass grafting
CAD	=	coronary artery disease

Coronary arteries:

LAD	=	left anterior descending
LC	=	left circumflex
LM	=	left main
CHF	=	congestive heart failure

Cholesterol:

HDL	=	high density lipoprotein
IDL	=	intermediate density lipoprotein
LDL	=	low density lipoprotein
VLDL	=	very low density lipoprotein
EF	=	ejection fraction
HC	=	hypertrophic cardiomyopathy
LA	=	left atrial
LV	=	left ventricular
MR	=	mitral regurgitation
MS	=	mitral stenosis
MVP	=	mitral valve prolapse
MVR	=	mitral valve replacement
PA	=	pulmonary artery
PS	=	pulmonic valve stenosis
PDA	=	patent ductus arteriosus
PTCA	=	percutaneous transluminal coronary angioplasty
RA	=	right atrial
RV	=	right ventricular
SVT	=	supraventricular tachycardia
TF	=	tetralogy of Fallot
TGA	=	complete transposition of the great arteries
TR	=	tricuspid regurgitation
VF	=	ventricular fibrillation
VPC	=	ventricular premature complex
VSD	=	ventricular septal defect
VT	=	ventricular tachycardia
WPW	=	Wolff-Parkinson-White

TERMS COMMONLY ABBREVIATED

AF = atrial fibrillation
AMI = acute myocardial infarction
AR = aortic regurgitation
AS = aortic valve stenosis
ASD = atrial septal defect
AV = atrioventricular
AVR = aortic valve replacement
BBB = bundle branch block
BP = blood pressure
CABG = coronary artery bypass grafting
CAD = coronary artery disease
Coronary arteries:
  LAD = left anterior descending
  LC = left circumflex
  LM = left main
CHF = congestive heart failure
Cholesterol:
  HDL = high density lipoprotein
  IDL = intermediate density lipoprotein
  LDL = low density lipoprotein
  VLDL = very low density lipoprotein
EF = ejection fraction
HC = hypertrophic cardiomyopathy
LA = left atrial
LV = left ventricular
MR = mitral regurgitation
MS = mitral stenosis
MVP = mitral valve prolapse
MVR = mitral valve replacement
PA = pulmonary artery
PS = pulmonic valve stenosis
PDA = patent ductus arteriosus
PTCA = percutaneous transluminal coronary angioplasty
RA = right atrial
RV = right ventricular
SVT = supraventricular tachycardia
TF = tetralogy of Fallot
TGA = complete transposition of the great arteries
TR = tricuspid regurgitation
VF = ventricular fibrillation
VPC = ventricular premature complex
VSD = ventricular septal defect
VT = ventricular tachycardia
WPW = Wolff-Parkinson-White